Bill and Sue Alto
1905 33rd Avenue South
Seattle, WA 98144

YO-CAW-652

Oxford Handbook of
Tropical
Medicine

Second Edition

Michael Eddleston
Centre for Tropical Medicine,
Oxford

Stephen Pierini
Locum GP and volunteer doctor to the
indigenous tribes of the Xingu reserves, Brazil

Robert Wilkinson
Wellcome Trust Career Fellow in Clinical Tropical
Medicine, Imperial College London and Institute of
Infectious Diseases and Molecular Medicine, University of
Cape Town

Robert Davidson
Consultant Physician and Honorary Senior Lecturer,
Department of Infectious Diseases,
Northwick Park Hospital, London

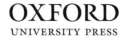

OXFORD
UNIVERSITY PRESS

OXFORD
UNIVERSITY PRESS

Great Clarendon Street, Oxford OX2 6DP

Oxford University Press is a department of the University of Oxford.
It furthers the University's objective of excellence in research, scholarship,
and education by publishing worldwide in

Oxford New York

Auckland Bangkok Buenos Aires Cape Town Chennai
Dar es Salaam Delhi Hong Kong Istanbul Karachi Kolkata
Kuala Lumpur Madrid Melbourne Mexico City Mumbai Nairobi
São Paulo Shanghai Taipei Tokyo Toronto

Oxford is a registered trade mark of Oxford University Press
in the UK and in certain other countries

Published in the United States
by Oxford University Press Inc., New York

A catalogue record for this title is available from the British Library

ISBN 0 19 852509 5

10 9 8 7 6 5 4 3 2 1

Typeset by Cepha Imaging Pvt Ltd

Printed in Italy

on acid-free paper by Legoprint S.p.A

Foreword

David A. Warrell
Head, Nuffield Department of Clinical Medicine,
University of Oxford

Some 10 years ago, two 'fresh-faced' Oxford clinical students approached me with a crazy notion; to write a handbook of clinical tropical medicine. I sent them away, less than sympathetically, with the admonition: 'Why not try learning some tropical medicine before you start writing about it!' Fortunately, my reproach did not break their young hearts. Quite the opposite in fact; the book was written, admittedly with some outside help and encouragement which Michael Eddleston and Stephen Pierini fully acknowledged, and with some reliance on sources such at the *Oxford Textbook of Medicine* and the *Oxford Handbook of Clinical Medicine*.

Michael Eddleston had conceived the idea for the book while doing research on poisoning and envenoming in Anuradhapura, Sri Lanka. He was struck by the lack of access to information among health professionals, particularly junior doctors working in isolation. This was partly due to poor distribution of published materials, even WHO publications. Recognizing the usefulness of pocket references such as the *Oxford Handbook of Clinical Medicine*, he resolved to produce a similar publication on medicine in the developing world.

OHTM was first published in 1999 to general critical acclaim. It was compact, reasonably comprehensive, and consistently practical in its emphasis. Its format was particularly attractive and original, making the contents easy to navigate and inviting search for further information and the addition of locally-relevant information on strategically-placed blank pages. My initial misgivings have been replaced by admiration. I have been delighted to discover *OHTM* in use all over the world, revealed protruding from the pockets of doctors and medical students from Peru (Gorgas Course) to Bangladesh (Chittagong Medical College) and from Sri Lanka (University of Colombo) to Nigeria (Kaltungo General Hospital). Of course, the book was not perfect. Perversely, my copy always seems to fall open at page 321 where an egg of *Schistosoma mansoni*, with characteristic side-spike, is mislabelled as *S. haematobium*. There were a few unfortunate typos (e.g. hyper-aesthetic rather than hypo-aesthetic skin patch in leprosy). Snake bite, which kills or maims hundreds of thousands of children and agricultural workers each year, surely deserves more than one page, compared to, for example, non-venereal treponematoses. Generally, however, it was hard to fault the editors' allocation of space among so many important and competing entities.

OHTM has been marvellously well reviewed and very widely noticed. Google yielded >15,000 hits in a fifth of a second! The most amusing and perceptive comments were provided by Rani Beharry and Jay S. Keystone in *Emerging Infectious Diseases* 2000;6(2). They correctly inferred that the editors were medical students but concluded: 'We should judge an excellent book such as this one by its contents and not by the prestige of its authors. As Butch Cassidy said to the Sundance Kid, 'Who are those guys?' In this case it doesn't matter.' Even more convincing were the opinions of doctors who had put *OHTM* to the test and found it useful 'in the field', in the rural tropics, for example in Togo, Malaŵi, Cambodia and Guyana (Amazon 5* reviews). The *British Medical Journal*'s reviewer carped at the inappropriateness of some of *OHTM*'s diagnostic and treatment recommendations but kindly concluded: 'It's not the fault of the book that so much of its advice can't be followed in the developing world; it's more a reflection of the socio-economic conditions in which tropical and other diseases flourish.' Conversely, other reviewers complemented the authors on omitting unrealistic procedures and recommending drugs which, while not always being ideal, were likely to be available locally.

Now, 5 years on, we have a second edition. Has a medical student's brain child matured, and, in the process, lost its charm and focus? Has the expanded list of contributors enhanced its quality and authority or jeopardized its uniformity of style? Have criticisms of the first edition been addressed or ignored? In short, is it a better and more useful book?

Recruitment of a large body of recognized experts, active in their fields of interest, is the most notable departure in this new edition. The original editorial duo has metamorphosed into a successful physician and a successful medical practitioner, both now clinical investigators in their own right with impeccable credentials for writing on tropical medicine. They have 'been there', they have 'seen it', they have 'done it' and they have been prolific in publishing results of original research in this field. The editorial team has been strengthened by the addition of two physicians experienced in tropical medicine, Robert Wilkinson and Robert Davidson. Both are now based in London but remain active in research in Africa, respectively in tuberculosis and leishmaniasis. A cadre of distinguished section editors has presided over each subject area. Most have substantial experience of living and working in tropical developing countries. Punctuality and a high standard of writing and accuracy have been rigorously enforced, as I learned to my cost when I was summarily dismissed from the authorship for failing to fulfil a deadline! And yet, the refreshing style and welcoming, accessible format of *OHTM-1* has not been compromised.

I have thoroughly enjoyed reading the proofs of *OHTM-2* and I look forward to seeing the book in print, resplendent with 32 new coloured plates of attractively-stained parasites and pathogens. The order of sections follows some sense of priority but I was glad to pass quickly from the somewhat prosaic 'WHO/UNICEF approach to the Integrated Management of Childhood Illness' to the more compelling subject of malaria, surely one of the world's most fascinating and important diseases. Coverage is comprehensive, including almost all the familiar tropical diseases together with a proper inclusion of malnutrition and other non-infectious conditions such as diabetes mellitus and cardiovascular disease which are now of overwhelming importance in the developing world. The editors have certainly not followed too slavishly any traditional definitions of tropical medicine. Control and prevention are not always sufficiently emphasized. The opportunity to educate patient, family, friends, and neighbours should never be missed in home visit, clinic, dispensary, or hospital. Therapeutic doctors and other medical staff should never be allowed to forget their responsibility of encouraging disease prevention, even at the bed side.

OHTM-2 is replete with up-to-date, useful, and relevant information for those medical personnel challenged by a perplexing diversity of unfamiliar diseases in a developing country, where limited resources force the clinician back on nearly-forgotten clinical skills, a minimum of investigations and an algorithmic approach to diagnosis and treatment. Where hard copy still beats electronic tinsel, whether for convenience or resilience, or where there is simply no alternative, this new edition of *OHTM* (400g) will win over many of the most stick-in-the-mud tropical medicine specialists from their conventional 'bibles', such as *Manson's Tropical Diseases* (21st ed 5kg).

.......but still only one page on snake bite!

Oxford
May 2004

Preface

Introduction

The 1st edition of the *Oxford Handbook of Tropical Medicine* was published in 1999. It had been written by Michael Eddleston and Stephen Pierini to fill a gap between handbooks of clinical medicine, which were unsuitable for use in resource-poor settings, and WHO guidelines, which were appropriate but not available in a collected format.

The 1st edition was very popular, not least because of its tough plastic binding which meant it really could be carried around in one's pocket and used as a ready reference.

For the 2nd edition, Eddleston and Pierini decided on a completely new approach: Robert Davidson and Robert Wilkinson were brought in as co-editors; 29 international experts contributed sections to the book. Some experts wrote everything from scratch, others just read through and commented on what we had written. Many others were involved in advising, correcting, and improving the text. Every sentence has been checked, and scarcely a paragraph remains un-altered. New sections have been added, reflecting the fact that medicine in the tropics is not just 'tropical medicine' in the old-fashioned sense of parasitic and infectious diseases. Guidelines from the WHO and other sources have been incorporated where possible.

We have tried to make this edition wiser than the first edition, as well as more comprehensive. We have tried to restrict the length so it might be affordable in most countries, and remain pocket-sized.

Making this book specific to your local areas – a request

Clinical medicine differs in different environments, and it is impossible to write a handbook which will be ideal for all continents and both urban and rural settings. However, we feel that there is enough in common across the tropics for a book like this to be useful to junior doctors, medical assistants, and nurses, supplying them with advice and guidance, often drawn up by the WHO. Readers will have to be critical and selective, deciding what is relevant for their own circumstances and facilities. The blank pages and lines have been left like this to allow each reader to make notes, adapting the book to his or her circumstances. We expect the reader to attack the algorithms with pencils, changing them to reflect their experience of local practice. We wish to stimulate, not prescribe.

We ask that readers send us back comments and criticisms so that we may improve the book in future editions. You can send your comments to us via the OUP website: http://www.oup.co.uk/isbn/0-19-852509-5.

Royalties

All royalties from the sale of this book are donated to Tropical Health Technology (PO Box 50, Fakenham, Norfolk, NR21 8XB, UK. Tel: +44 (0)1328 855 805. Fax: +44 (0)1328 853 799. http://www.tht.ndirect.co.uk Email: thtbooks@tht.ndirect.co.uk). THT's mission is to provide essential books, microscopes, and diagnostic bench aids for health workers in the poorest settings.

Contents

Colour plates

Contributors

The editors would like to thank the contributors for all their work revising and updating the Handbook, in particular Milly Davis and Tony Moody who reviewed the whole book for drug doses and diagnostics, respectively.

Saad Abdalla
Imperial College Faculty of
Medicine
St. Mary's Campus
Praed Street
London W2 1NY
Chapter 14

Theresa Alain
Elgar House
Southmead Hospital
North Bristol NHS Trust
Bristol
Chapter 13

Suzanne Anderson
Department of Paediatrics
Imperial College University of
London Faculty of Medicine
St. Mary's Campus
Norfolk Place
London W2 1PG
Chapter 1

Tania Araujo-Jorge
Lab. of Cell Biology
Oswaldo Cruz Institute
Oswaldo Cruz Foundation - Fiocruz
Av. Brasil 4365
Pav. Carlos Chagas
Rio de Janeiro RJ 21045-900
Brazil
Chapter 3

Tony Berendt
Bone Infection Unit
Nuffield Orthopaedic Centre
Oxford
Chapter 12

Anneli Björersdorff
Research Centre for Zoonotic
Ecology and Epidemiology
Kalmar
Sweden
Chapter 3

Francois Chappuis
Médecins Sans Frontières - Swiss
section &
Travel and Migration Medicine Unit
Department of Community
Medicine
Geneva University Hospital
rue Micheli-du-Crest 24
1211 Geneva 14
Switzerland
Chapter 3

David Dance
Consultant Microbiologist
Health Protection Agency
Derriford Hospital
Plymouth
Devon PL6 8DH
Chapter 3

Robert Davidson
(editor)

Mildred Davis
Chesterfield
Derbyshire
all (doses)

Michael Eddleston
(editor)

Jeremy Farrar
University of Oxford Clinical
Research Unit
The Hospital for Tropical Diseases
190 Ben Ham Tu
Quan 5
Ho Chi Minh City
Viet Nam
Chapter 8

Allen Foster
International Centre for Eye Health
London School of Hygiene and
Tropical Medicine
Keppel St
London
Chapter 10

David Goldblatt
Institute of Child Health
University College London and
Great Ormond Street Hospital for
Children
30 Guilford Street
London WC1N 1EH
Chapters 3, 17

James Hakim
Department of Medicine
University of Zimbabwe
PO Box A 178
Avondale Harare
Zimbabwe
Chapter 4

Stan Houston
Departments of Medicine and
Public Health Science
2E4.12 WC Mackenzie Ctr.
University of Alberta
Edmonton AB
Canada T6G 2B7
Chapter 2C

Oliver Howes
Division of Psychological Medicine
Institute of Psychiatry
London SE5 8AF
Chapter 9

Michael Jacobs
Centre for Hepatology
Royal Free & University College
Medical School
Rowland Hill Street
London NW3 2PF
Chapter 3

Saskia van der Kam
Medecins Sans Frontieres –
Holland
Plantage Middenlaan 14, 1018 DD
Amsterdam
Holland
Chapter 15

Beate Kampmann
Academic Department of
Paediatrics
Imperial College London
St. Mary's Campus
London
Chapter 2

Clement Kiire
Southport & Ormskirk Hospital
Wigan Road
Ormskirk L30 2AZ
Chapter 7

Diana Lockwood
Hospital for Tropical Diseases
Mortimer Market
London WC1E 6JB
Chapters 8, 11

Monir Madkour
Department of Internal Medicine
Military Hospital
Riyadh
Kingdom of Saudi Arabia
Chapter 3

Ben Marshall
Southampton University
Hospitals
Southampton SO16 6YD
Chapter 5

Tony Moody
Dept of Clinical Parasitology
Hospital for Tropical Diseases
London WC1E 3BG
all (Laboratory)

Sita Nanayakkara
Chapter 6

Chris Parry
Department of Medical
Microbiology and Genitourinary
Medicine
Duncan Building
University of Liverpool
Liverpool L69 3GA
Chapter 3

Geoffrey Pasvol
Dept of Infection & Tropical
Medicine
Imperial College University of
London Faculty of Medicine
Lister Unit
Northwick Park Hospital
Harrow
Middlesex HA1 3UJ
Chapter 2A

Mary Penny
Instituto de Investigación
Nutricional

Av La Molina 1885
La Molina
Lima 33
Peru
Chapter 2

Stephen Pierini
(editor)

Graham Taylor
Department of Genitourinary
Medicine
Imperial College University of
London Faculty of Medicine
St. Mary's Campus
Norfolk Place
London W2 1PG
Chapter 2B

Ian Ternouth
Taranaki Base Hospital
New Zealand (Prev Parirenyatwa
Hospital, Zimbabwe)
Chapter 4

Robert Wilkinson
(editor)

Abbreviations

>	more than
<	less than
$\uparrow$	raised
$\downarrow$	lowered
$\rightarrow$	leading to
%	per cent
~	approximately
+ve	positive
−ve	negative
1°	primary
2°	secondary
A_2	aortic component of second heart sound
ABG	arterial blood gases
ACE	angiotensin-converting enzyme
ACS	acute confusional state
ACTH	adrenocorticotrophic hormone
AD	autosomal dominant (genetic inheritance)
AF	atrial fibrillation
AFB	acid-fast bacilli
AFP	acute flaccid paralysis
AHA	autoimmune haemolytic anaemia
AHF	Argentinian haemorrhagic fever
AIDS	acquired immunodeficiency syndrome
ALL	acute lymphoblastic leukaemia
ALS	advanced life support
ALT	alanine transferase
AML	acute myeloblastic leukaemia
ANS	autonomic nervous system
APBA	allergic bronchopulmonary aspergillosis
AR	autosomal recessive (genetic inheritance)
ARF	acute renal failure
ARDS	acute respiratory distress syndrome
ARI	acute respiratory infection
ASO	antistreptolysin O
AST	aspartate transaminase
ATLS	advanced trauma life support

ATN	acute tubular necrosis
AV	atrioventricular
AXR	abdominal X-ray (plain)
Ba	barium
BAL	bronchoalveolar lavage
BCG	Bacille Calmette Guerin
bd	bis die (twice a day)
BHF	Bolivian haemorrhagic fever
BL	Burkitt's lymphoma
BLS	basic life support
BMI	body mass index
BNF	British National Formulary
BOOP	bronchiolitis obliterans organizing pneumonia
BP	blood pressure
BPM	beats per minute
CA	carcinoma
Ca^{2+}	calcium ions
CABG	coronary artery bypass graft
CAH	chronic active hepatitis
Cal	calorie
CAP	community-acquired pneumonia
CBD	common bile duct
CCF	congestive cardiac failure
CCHF	Crimean-Congo haemorrhagic fever
CDC	Centers for Disease Control and Prevention, Atlanta, USA
CF	cystic fibrosis
CID	*Clinical Infectious Diseases*
CK	creatinine kinase
CK-MB	creatinine kinase cardiac isoenzyme
Cl^-	chloride ions
CLL	chronic lymphocytic leukaemia
cm	centimetre
CMI	cell-mediated immunity
CML	chronic myeloid leukaemia
CMV	cytomegalovirus
CNS	central nervous system
COPD	chronic obstructive pulmonary disease
CPR	cardiopulmonary resuscitation
Cr	creatinine
CRF	chronic renal failure

CSF	cerebrospinal fluid
CT	computerized tomography
CVA	cerebrovascular accident (stroke)
CVI	Children's Vaccine Initiative
CVS	cardiovascular system
CXR	chest X-ray
D&V	diarrhoea and vomiting
DCL	disseminated cutaneous leishmaniasis
DCT	direct Coomb's test
DEC	diethylcarbamazine
DHF	dengue haemorrhagic fever
DIC	disseminated intravascular coagulation
dl	decilitre
DM	diabetes mellitus
DNA	deoxyribonucleic acid
DOTS	directly observed treatment strategy
DT	diphtheria toxoid
DTP	diphtheria toxoid, pertussis, and tetanus toxoid
DVT	deep vein thrombi
dxm	dexamethasone
EBV	Epstein-Barr virus
ECF	extracellular fluid
ECG	electrocardiogram
EEV	equine encephalitis virus
eg	for example
EHEC	enterohaemorrhagic *E. coli*
ELISA	enzyme linked immunosorbant assay
EPI	Expanded Programme on Immunization
ERCP	endoscopic retrograde cholangiopancreatography
ESR	erythrocyte sedimentation rate
ETEC	enterotoxigenic *E. coli*
ETT	exercise treadmill test
EUA	examination under anaesthesia
F	female
FBC	full blood count
FCPD	fibrocalculous pancreatic diabetes
FDP	fibrinogen degradation product
Fe	iron
FEV_1	forced expiratory volume in first second
FFP	fresh frozen plasma

FHx	family history
FOB	faecal occult blood
ft	feet (measurement)
g	gram
G$^+$	Gram-stain positive
GBS	Guillain-Barre syndrome
GCS	Glasgow coma scale
GFR	glomerular filtration rate
GH	growth hormone
GI	gastrointestinal
GN	glomerulonephritis
G6PD	glucose-6-phosphate dehydrogenase
GTN	glyceryl trinitrate
GTT	glucose tolerance test
GU	genitourinary
HA	haemaglutanin
HAV	hepatitis A virus
Hb	haemoglobin
HBeAg	hepatitis B virus e antigen
HBsAg	hepatitis B virus surface antigen
HBV	hepatitis B virus
HCC	hepatocellular carcinoma
HCV	hepatitis C virus
HDV	hepatitis D virus
HELLP	haemolysis, elevated liver enzymes and low platelet counts
HF	haemorrhagic fever
HHV-8	human herpes virus-8 (KSAV)
Hib	*Haemophilus influenzae* type b
HIV	human immunodeficiency virus
HL	Hodgkin's lymphoma
HLA	human lymphocyte antigen
HMMA	4-hydroxy-3-methoxymandelic acid
HMS	hyperreactive malarial splenomegaly
hrs	hours
HSV	herpes simplex virus
HT	hypertension
HTLV	human T-cell lymphotrophic virus
HUS	haemolytic-uraemic syndrome
Hx	history
IBD	inflammatory bowel disease

ICP	intracranial pressure
ID	intradermal
IDD	iodine deficiency
IDDM	insulin-dependent diabetes mellitus
IHD	ischaemic heart disease
IMCI	WHO's Integrated Management of Childhood Illness
IM	intramuscular
INR	international normalized ratio
IPV	injected polio vaccine
ITP	idiopathic thrombocytopenic purpura
ITU	intensive therapy unit
IU	international unit
IUD	intrauterine contraceptive device
IV	intravenous
IVU	intravenous urography
J	joule
JE	Japanese encephalitis
JVP	jugular venous pressure
K^+	potassium ions
KCCT	kaolin cephalin clotting time
kg	kilogram
kJ	kilojoule
KOH	potassium hydroxide
kPa	kiloPascal
KS	Kaposi sarcoma
KSAV	Kaposi sarcoma associated virus
l	litre
LBBB	left bundle branch block
LBRF	louse borne relapsing fever
LD	lymphocyte depleted
LDH	lactate dehydrogenase
LFT	liver function test
Li^+	lithium ions
LIF	left iliac fossa
LN	lymph node
LOC	level of consciousness
LP	lymphocyte predominant
LP	lumbar puncture
LPS	lipopolysaccharide
LV	left ventricle

LVF	left ventricular failure
m	metre
M	male
MALT	mucosa-associated lymphoid tissue
max	maximum
MC	mixed cellularity
MC	mucosal leishmaniasis
MCH	mean cell haemoglobin
MCV	mean cell volume
mg	milligram
Mg^{2+}	magnesium ions
MI	myocardial infarction
mins	minutes
MI	myocardial infarction
mm	millimetre
mmHg	millimetres of mercury
mmol	millimol
MMR	measles, mumps, and rubella vaccine
MND	motor neurone disease
MoH	Ministry of Health
mosmol	milliosmol
MR	measles and rubella vaccine
MRDM	malnutrition-related diabetes mellitus
MST	morphine sulphate
mths	months
MUAC	mid-upper arm circumference
N	north
NA	neuraminidase
Na^+	sodium ions
ND	notifiable disease (WHO)
NE	north east
NG	nasogastric
NGO	Non-governmental Organization
NGT	nasogastric tube
NHL	non-Hodgkin's lymphoma
NIDDM	non-insulin-dependent diabetes mellitus
NS	nodular sclerosing
NSAID	non-steroidal anti-inflammatory drug
N&V	nausea and/or vomiting
O_2	oxygen

OCP	oral contraceptive pill
od	omni die (once daily)
OGS	oxygenic steroid
O/p	outpatient
OPV	oral polio vaccine
ORS	oral rehydration solution
OTM	Oxford Textbook of Medicine
$PaCO_2$	partial pressure of carbon dioxide in arterial blood
PAM	primary amoebic meningoencephalitis
PAN	polyarteritis nodosa
PCP	Pneumocystis carinii pneumonia
PCV	packed cell volume
PDPD	protein deficient pancreatic diabetes
PE	pulmonary embolism
PEFR	peak expiratory flow rate
pg	picogram
PGL	persistent generalized lymphadenopathy
PHT	portal hypertension
PID	pelvic inflammatory disease
PIM	post-infective malabsorption
PKDL	post kalar dermal leishmania
PML	progressive multifocal leukoencephalopathy
PMN	polymorphonuclear neutrophils
PNG	Papua New Guinea
PNS	peripheral nervous system
PO	per os (by mouth)
PO_4	phosphate
PR	per rectum (by the rectum)
PRV	polycythaemia rubra vera
PT	prothrombin time
PTB	pulmonary tuberculosis
PTH	parathyroid hormone
PTT	partial thromboplastin time
PV	per vaginam (by the vagina)
qds	quater die sumendus (to be taken 4 times a day)
q2h	every 2 hours
q4h	every 4 hours, etc
RA	rheumatoid arthritis
RBBB	right bundle branch block
RBC	red blood cell

RDA	recommended daily allowances
RF	rheumatic fever
RHF	right heart failure
RIF	right iliac fossa
RIG	anti-rabies immunoglobulin
RMSF	Rocky Mountain spotted fever
RNA	ribonucleic acid
RR	respiratory rate
RSV	respiratory syncytial virus
RUQ	right upper quadrant
RV	right ventricular
RVF	Rift Valley fever
RVF	right ventricular failure
SAH	subarachnoid haemorrhage
SBE	subacute bacterial endocarditis
SC	subcutaneous
SCC	short course chemotherapy
SE	south east
SG	specific gravity
SIADH	syndrome of inappropriate ADH secretion
SLE	systemic lupus erythematosus
SOL	space-occupying lesion
SSPE	subacute sclerosing panencephalitis
STI	sexually transmitted disease
SVC	superior vena cava
TB	tuberculosis
TBRF	tick borne relapsing fever
Td	tetanus toxoid and low-dose diphtheria toxoid vaccine
tds	ter die sumendus (to be taken 3 times a day)
TFC	therapeutic feeding centre
TFT	thyroid function test
TIA	transient ischaemic attack
TIBC	total iron binding capacity
TMP/SMX	trimethoprim/sulfamethoxazole (co-trimoxazole)
TMR	Tropical Medicine Resource (The Wellcome Trust)
TSH	thyroid-stimulating hormone
TSS	tropical splenomegaly syndrome
TT	tetanus toxoid vaccine
TURP	transurethral resection of the prostate
UC	ulcerative colitis

U&E	urea and electrolytes – and creatinine
UK	United Kingdom
URT	upper respiratory tract
URTI	upper respiratory tract infection
USS	ultrasound scan
UTI	urinary tract infection
UV	ultraviolet
VEEV	Venezuelan equine encephalitis virus
VF	ventricular fibrillation
VHF	viral haemorrhagic fever
VMA	vanillyl mandelic acid
VSD	ventriculo-septal defect
VT	ventricular tachycardia
VZV	varicella-zoster virus
WCC	white cell count
WHO	World Health Organization
wks	weeks
yrs	Years
ZN	Ziehl-Neelson

WHO/UNICEF approach to the Integrated Management of Childhood Illness

Section editor   **Suzanne Anderson**

Diarrhoea, pneumonia, measles, malaria, and malnutrition — and often a combination of these conditions — account for more than 70% of deaths and health facility visits among children under five years of age in developing countries (see below). Most of these deaths are preventable and easily treated, but the goal of effectively applying cost-effective interventions is still not achieved in many parts of the world.

Major causes of death globally in children under five

• Pneumonia (together with malnutrition)	20%
• Diarrhoea (" " ")	12%
• Malaria (" " ")	8%
• Measles (" " ")	5%
• HIV/AIDS (" " ")	4%
• Perinatal (" " ")	22%
• Other (" " ")	29%
• One or more of these conditions (together with malnutrition)	60%

Children differ from adults in two important respects: they are growing and developing, and they are dependent on others for sustenance and protection. To achieve sufficient growth and to develop and thrive, children require adequate nutrition, essential health care, protection from the environment, and an emotionally nurturing family.

The loss of food security and disruption to health services through political unrest, famine, and debt and the growing impact of HIV/AIDS on family structure all contribute to the erosion of child health. Child health programmes therefore need to address the child's whole well-being and not just individual conditions.

Surveys reveal that many sick children are not adequately assessed and treated by health care providers when parents seek help and that parents are poorly advised. Additionally, first-level health facilities in low-income countries often have minimal or non-existent diagnostic facilities such as radiology and laboratory services, and drug supplies may be scarce or irregular. Doctors working in such an environment therefore have to rely on history and symptoms and signs of disease in order to determine a diagnosis and a subsequent course of management that makes best use of available resources. Because there is considerable overlap in the signs and symptoms of the major childhood illnesses, a single diagnosis for a sick child is often inappropriate. To address this challenge, the WHO and UNICEF have developed a strategy called the *Integrated Management of Childhood Illness* (IMCI).

What is the IMCI and how is it achieved?

IMCI is an integrated approach to childhood illness in the under-fives that includes both preventive and curative elements implemented by families and communities, as well as by health care providers in resource-poor settings. Its main aims are:

- Improving the skills of health providers
- Speeding up the referral of sick children
- Promoting appropriate health-seeking behaviours as well as emphasizing disease prevention through immunization and improved nutrition

An algorithmic approach has been used to produce a series of guidelines for the diagnosis and management of the sick child. These algorithms have been, and continue to be, refined and adapted to country-specific disease epidemiology and to local guidelines and policies. The full IMCI guidelines are beyond the scope of this handbook. However, copies of the IMCI guidelines can be obtained directly from the WHO[1] or UNICEF.

Summary of case management

The training course developed by the WHO and UNICEF teaches the following case management process:
1. First assess the child, asking questions of the mother, examining the child, and checking immunization status.
2. Classify the child's illness and decide whether to (i) refer urgently, (ii) give specific medical treatment and advice, or (iii) give simple advice on home management.
3. Identify specific treaments — give urgent treatments only to children who are being referred.
4. Give practical treatment instructions. Teach the mother how to give oral drugs, how to increase fluids during diarrhoea, and how to treat simple infections at home. Advise the mother on the signs that indicate the child should immediately be brought back to the clinic, and when to return for follow-up.
5. Assess feeding in children <2 yrs and those with low weight for age. Record any feeding problems and provide counselling on feeding problems.
6. Organize follow-up.

Summary of patient assessment

1. Check for the following general danger signs that indicate the child is severely ill:
- Cough or difficulty in breathing which might indicate pneumonia.
- Diarrhoea (whether acute watery diarrhoea, dysentery, or persistent diarrhoea) and dehydration.
- Fever and presence of stiff neck. Management then depends on whether the locality is a high malaria risk area or not.
- Evidence of measles.
- Ear problems or mastoiditis.
- Severe pallor suggestive of significant anaemia.
2. Assess nutritional status in all children, identifying severely malnourished children who need referral to hospital.
3. Check the child's immunization status and give vaccines as required.

---

1 WHO website *http:/www.who.int/child-adolescent-health/integr.htm*

HIV/AIDS

An estimated 1800 children become infected with HIV worldwide each day, with 90% of infections acquired perinatally (vertically). Of these, 95% come from developing countries: 90% from sub-Saharan Africa, but with an increasing number in India, South-East Asia, and countries of the former Soviet Union.

Identification and management of HIV/AIDS was not included in the original IMCI guidelines. However, in many sub-Saharan African countries it is now the leading cause of childhood death, reducing all the gains made in reducing infant mortality in urban populations over the past 20 years. A number of algorithms are now being developed, and Fig. 1.1 shows the algorithm recently developed in Kwa–Zulu Natal, South Africa — a high prevalence environment in which access to diagnostic facilities is limited.[2]

Despite the lack of availability of antiretroviral drugs in resource-poor settings, effective interventions, including treatment of intercurrent infection, co-trimoxazole prophylaxis of *Pneumocistis jiroveci* pneumonia, and family support can be implemented if health care workers effectively identify infected children. In addition, the provision of antiretroviral therapy, for both children and their mothers, is likely to be an achievable goal in many disadvantaged countries in the near future.

Tuberculosis

TB is increasing in prevalence across the world, with the rising number of HIV cases contributing to the rise in prevalence. Children present a particular diagnostic dilemma since the disease may present insidiously, is difficult to diagnose, and is likely to cause high morbidity and mortality with dissemination to the brain and other vital organs. In an attempt to improve the rate and accuracy of diagnosis in resource-poor settings, a number of workers have attempted to produce TB scoring systems to aid the health care provider.[3,4] These are not included in the IMCI and need to be evaluated according to local HIV co-infection rates. However, the particular problems associated with TB diagnosis in children and the increasing impact of HIV/TB co-infection warrant their inclusion in this handbook.

2 Horwood C et al. (2003) Diagnosis of paediatric HIV infection in a primary health care setting with a clinical algorithm. Bull World Health Organ, **81**:858–66.

3 Fourie B et al. (1998) Use of a TB score chart in an HIV endemic area. Int J Tubercle Lung Dis, **2**:116–23.

4 Hesseling AC et al. (2002) Review. A critical review of diagnostic approaches used in the diagnosis of childhood tuberculosis. Int J Tuberc Lung Dis, **6**:1038–45.

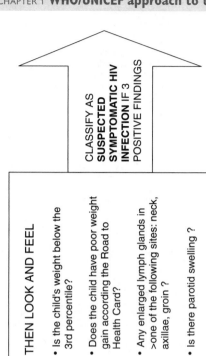

ASK	THEN LOOK AND FEEL
• Does the child have pneumonia today ?	• Is the child's weight below the 3rd percentile?
• Has the child had any diarrhoea in the past 3 months ?	• Does the child have poor weight gain according the Road to Health Card?
• Has the child any episode of persistent diarrhoea (≥ 14 days) in the past 3 months ?	• Any enlarged lymph glands in >one of the following sites: neck, axillae, groin ?
• Has the child an ear discharge or had one in the past ?	• Is there parotid swelling ?

CLASSIFY AS **SUSPECTED SYMPTOMATIC HIV INFECTION** IF 3 POSITIVE FINDINGS

Fig. 1.1 Classification of suspected symptomatic HIV infection.

Malaria[1]

Section editor **Geoffrey Pasvol**

WHO revised guidelines

New, extensively revised WHO guidelines for the management of severe falciparum malaria have been published: WHO (2000) Severe falciparum malaria. *Trans Roy Soc Trop Med Hyg*, **94**: Suppl. 1. They are also available on the website of the Royal Society of Tropical Medicine and Hygiene *www.rstmh.org* or the WHO's website *mosquito.who.int/docs/hbsm_toc.htm*.

Combination chemotherapy

The rapid spread of drug resistance has meant that chloroquine, as a single agent, is no longer effective in much of the world for the treatment of *P. falciparum* malaria. Limited cases of chloroquine-resistant vivax malaria have also been reported. The use of combination therapies to reduce the development of drug resistance is advocated. However, therapy with the combination of two antifolate drugs, sulfadoxine and pyrimethamine (SP) is also proving less effective. Drugs such as mefloquine and Malarone® (a combination of atovaquone and proguanil) are very expensive and unaffordable for mass administration in Africa. The addition of an artemesinin derivative (e.g. artesunate) to these combination therapies provides another strategy to overcome the problem of drug resistance (discussed in White NJ *et al.* (1999) *Lancet*, **353**, 1965).

---

1 Sources: (detailed account) White NJ (2002) *Manson's tropical diseases*, 21st Edn, pp 1205–95, Saunders; (less detailed account) Pasvol G (2004) *Infectious diseases* (ed. Cohen and Powderly), Chapter 166, pp. 1579–91, Mosby.

Introduction

Malaria is a disease caused by four species of protozoan parasites of the genus *Plasmodium* — namely *P. falciparum*, *P. vivax*, *P. ovale*, and *P. malariae*.

Almost two billion people in endemic areas are at risk of malaria, and each year it is estimated that up to 250 million clinical cases occur and over one million die, largely among African infants and young children. The manifestations of malaria may be extremely variable, not only from geographical region to region and village to village, but also from person to person. These differences are due to many factors and include mosquito biting and breeding habits, the infecting parasite species (*P. falciparum* resulting in the most severe forms of disease), genetic and acquired resistance of the host, and compliance with drug treatment.

Life cycle and transmission

The life cycle of the malarial parasite alternates between the sexual cycle in the invertebrate host (the female *Anopheles* mosquito) and the asexual cycle in the vertebrate host (in this case human). Transmission occurs when the mosquito, requiring blood for the development of her eggs, bites the human host and injects sporozoites (see Fig. 2A.1) into the bloodstream which then invade hepatocytes, where they develop into liver schizonts. When each schizont ruptures, thousands of merozoites are released which invade red blood cells and initiate that part of the cycle responsible for all the clinical manifestations of the disease.

Incubation periods

P. falciparum usually 7–14 days but may be longer (up to six weeks) in those with partial immunity or those on inadequate prophylaxis. *P. vivax* 12–17 days and *P. ovale* 15–18 days but a small percentage of these two species, perhaps 5–10%, may produce symptoms many months or even years later as a result of the reactivation of a dormant form in the liver called the hypnozoite. *P. malariae* without a hypnozoite form has an average incubation period of 18–40 days.

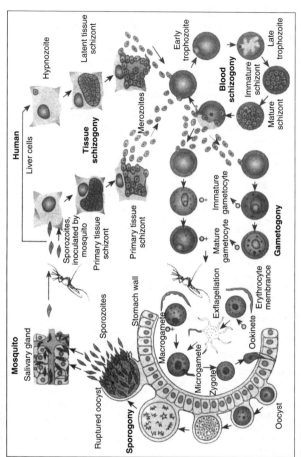

Fig. 2A.1

Epidemiology

Malarial transmission depends upon a number of factors including:

- Mosquito longevity (lifespan)
- Ambient temperature (shortens the cycle in the mosquito)
- Population density of both mosquito and humans
- Mosquito's human-biting habit
- Host immune response
- Whether the drugs used in treatment have any activity against the gametocytes.

In endemic areas, transmission may be measured using either the parasite rate (% of the population who are positive for malarial parasites on blood film) or the spleen rate (% of population with splenomegaly), although the latter is less reliable since an enlarged spleen may be a result of other diseases. Neither method, however, reflects the clinical impact of mortality or morbidity of the disease on a given population.

Two distinct patterns of malarial transmission emerge which represent extremes:

- *Stable* malaria where there is intense all year round transmission. The disease predominantly affects young children and pregnant women. Adults might be positive on blood film but are rarely ill with malaria.
- *Unstable* malaria, which affects all ages and occurs in areas of seasonal or low transmission.

Malaria control in stable areas is problematic, since interventions that reduce transmission, but do not eradicate the disease, may impair the development of naturally acquired immunity in the population, resulting in a pattern of unstable disease.

Protection against malaria

Many innate factors of resistance against infection were first identified in falciparum malaria. Acquired resistance to malaria is slow to develop and the immune mechanisms involved are still unclear.

Innate immunity: Falciparum malaria remains the best example of a selective agent that results in genetic polymorphisms in the host that might provide partial protection against severe disease. Certain genetic variants of the red cell, notably sickle cell trait, glucose 6-phosphate dehydrogenase (G6PD) deficiency, thalassaemia trait, and ovalocytosis, may partially protect against severe disease. The lack of Duffy antigen (the receptor for merozoites of *P. vivax*) on red cells in most West Africans may account for their, as yet undisputed, protection against this infection.

Acquired immunity: Acquired immunity is believed to require repeated exposure to malarial infection, possibly with differing genetic variants of the parasite. In areas of stable transmission, neonates are usually protected by maternal antibodies for the first 6 months or so of life, followed by a period of increased susceptibility during which it is thought that immunity to severe disease is slowly acquired (*antidisease immunity*). Depending upon the level of transmission, *antiparasite immunity* appears later, at around 10 yrs of age, when the parasite rate may be as high as 50%. Adults tend to get less severe bouts of disease but when they do, parasite densities are generally lower than in children.

Without reinfection, immunity wanes after about 5 yrs. Pregnancy, severe illness, and surgery also lead to reduced immunity. Malnutrition does not appear to increase susceptibility to disease, although if present it will increase mortality and morbidity. Surprisingly, HIV infection has not been found to have a major effect on the severity of malarial disease.

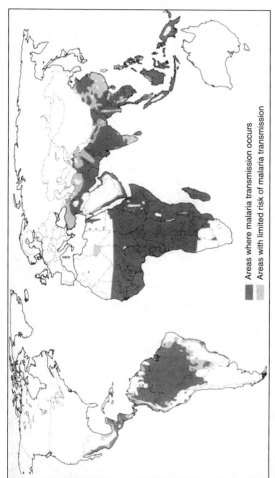

Areas where malaria transmission occurs
Areas with limited risk of malaria transmission

Fig. 2A.2

Clinical features

- *P. falciparum* infection generally follows a relatively mild or uncomplicated course. However, in some patients, particularly young children and non-immune adults, falciparum malaria may become a severe life-threatening disease.
- *P. ovale*, *P. malariae*, and *P. vivax* infection, on the other hand, rarely result in severe disease or death except in cases of splenic rupture. Chronic infection or infection of pregnant women with these 'benign' species however may lead to marked morbidity (e.g. anaemia).
- Two major features distinguish falciparum infection from the benign malarias and may account for differences in severity. First, only falciparum results in high parasite densities in the blood and, second, only falciparum demonstrates the feature of 'sequestration' in which mature parasites specifically adhere to endothelial cells in the post capillary venules of critical organs such as the brain.

Falciparum malaria

The clinical presentation of mild malaria in adults with rigors is well known. There is usually a history of travel to or residence within an endemic area. Even the best compliance with the most effective antimalarial chemoprophylaxis cannot exclude the diagnosis of malaria. There may be a prodromal period of tiredness and aching. The features of a classical paroxysm are:

- An abrupt onset of an initial 'cold stage' associated with a dramatic rigor (paroxysm) in which the patient visibly shakes
- An ensuing 'hot stage' during which the patient may have a temperature of well over 104°F (40°C), may be restless and excitable, and may vomit or convulse
- Finally, the 'sweating stage' during which the patient's temperature returns to normal (defervesces) and sleep may ensue.

Such a paroxysm can last 6–10 hours; a prolonged asymptomatic period may follow lasting 38–42 hours in the case of vivax and ovale malaria and 62–66 hours in *P. malariae* infections. In falciparum malaria the periodicity of fever tends to be less predictable and the fever may be continuous. There may be accompanying headache, cough, myalgia (flu-like symptoms), diarrhoea, and mild jaundice.

Malaria is rarely, if ever, the cause of lymphadenopathy, pharyngitis, or a rash, and alternative explanations need to be considered for these specific symptoms. In children, the illness may often be non-specific and misleading with fever, early cough, vomiting, diarrhoea, anaemia, and hypoglycaemia. Jaundice, pulmonary oedema, and renal failure are rarer in children than adults, although progression to other severe complications is usually faster (1–2 days) in children.

Pregnant women: Malaria during pregnancy increases the risk of miscarriage, stillbirth, prematurity, low birth weight, and neonatal death, as well as maternal morbidity and mortality. High fever is thought to contribute to foetal distress.

- The risk is greatest is in primigravidae in areas of unstable malaria.
- Cerebral malaria is more common — in Thailand 50% of mortality due to cerebral malaria occurs in pregnant women.
- Parasitaemia is usually higher, anaemia more profound, hypoglycaemia and pulmonary oedema more common than in non-pregnant women.

- Congenital transmission is rare, usually occurring in non-immune individuals infected with *P. vivax* or *P. malariae*. Neonatal illness presents with fever, haemolytic anaemia, and failure to thrive in the first days/weeks of life.

Complications

Falciparum malaria may progress to severe disease and death (malignant tertian malaria; see p. 16). In patients living in endemic areas in whom parasites persist after treatment or who are soon reinfected, anaemia is common and further attacks, due to recrudescence of blood forms, may occur. In Thailand, 30% of patients with falciparum malaria develop symptomatic *P. vivax* infection within 2 months without re-exposure to parasites, implying an initial mixed infection.

The benign malarias

- *P. vivax* and *P. ovale*: may relapse up to 5 yrs after initial infection despite treatment which eliminates all blood forms. This is due to latent liver hypnozoites undergoing schizogony and re-entering the blood stream — a true relapse (as opposed to recrudescence).
- *P. malariae*: persistent parasites may cause recurrent fevers when the infection recrudesces even decades following 1° infection. The fevers decrease in frequency and severity over time. Anaemia and splenomegaly may occur.
- *P. malariae*: may lead to glomerulonephritis and nephrotic syndrome.
- *P. vivax*: a rare complication of *P. vivax* infection is splenic rupture (mortality 80%). It results from acute enlargement with or without trauma and presents with sudden and persistent abdominal pain, guarding, fever, shock, and a lowered haemocrit. *P. vivax* causes a post-malaria cerebellar syndrome.

Chronic malaria

The persistence of low-level parasitaemia in the blood may lead to 'chronic' malaria. Symptoms include recurrent acute attacks of malaria, anaemia, hepatosplenomegaly, diarrhoea, weight loss, and increased incidence of other infections (especially bacterial gastroenteritis). Chronic malaria may resolve, with the onset of partial immunity, or progress, with 2° complications: falciparum malaria is associated with an increased incidence of Burkitt's lymphoma due to impaired T-cell immunity.

Hyperreactive malarial splenomegaly: (formerly called tropical splenomegaly syndrome) may develop with recurrent infections. It is characterized by massive splenomegaly, profound anaemia, 2° infection, fever, and jaundice. There is hypersplenism with pancytopenia, hypergammaglobulinaemia, and a lymphocytic infiltrate in the liver. There is a marked elevation of serum IgM. Although malarial parasites are seldom found in the blood, the condition responds to prolonged courses of antimalarial prophylaxis.

Quartan malarial nephropathy: *P. malariae* infection appears to be a cause of nephrotic syndrome, particularly in West and East Africa. Malarial antigens are found in the renal glomerular basement membrane. The condition unfortunately does not respond to antimalarial prophylaxis.

Severe malaria

Severe malaria is the result of extensive multi-system involvement in falciparum malaria. The onset of severe disease can be rapid, with death (particularly in children) occurring in a matter of hours. In travellers from endemic regions, it is most frequently observed when the diagnosis is made late.

Cerebral malaria (CM) is the most important complication of falciparum malaria and has ~20% mortality. It most often occurs in non-immune adults and in children. CM is 'unrousable coma in the presence of peripheral parasitaemia where other causes of encephalopathy have been excluded'. However, any alteration in conscious status in the context of falciparum malaria should be taken seriously. Neck rigidity and photophobia are not usually seen and Kernig's sign is −ve. There may be one or more of: diffuse cerebral dysfunction with coma, convulsions (~50% generalized), focal neurological signs, brainstem signs such as abnormal doll's eye or oculovestibular reflexes, etc. Retinal haemorrhages occur in about 15% of cases. Neurological sequelae are found in at least 5% of survivors (10% in children) and include hemiparesis, cerebellar ataxia, cortical blindness, hypotonia, and mental retardation. In children, CM carries a 10–40% mortality, most deaths occurring within the first 24 hrs. Reduced consciousness may follow a febrile convulsion in a child. Malarial convulsions can occur at any temperature and post-ictal coma may last a few hours. In deep coma, abnormalities of posture and muscle tone are frequently seen. For young children use the Blantyre Coma Scale (see box) to grade the coma.

Respiratory distress (RD) is manifest by rapid laboured breathing, sometimes with abnormal rhythms of respiration. In children there may be intercostal recession, use of the accessory muscles of respiration, and nasal flaring — sometimes difficult to differentiate from an acute respiratory infection. RD in patients with malaria may be the result of a number of pathologies:

- In the majority of cases, particularly in children, it represents respiratory compensation for a profound metabolic acidosis. Severe metabolic acidosis (BE >12) is associated with an 8-fold increased risk of death in children. Rapid intervention is required.
- Effect of parasites on the respiratory centre in the brainstem.
- Lung infection because of the immunosuppression caused by malaria.
- Air hunger as a result of severe anaemia.
- Acute respiratory distress syndrome (ARDS) caused by direct alveolar capillary damage by parasites and neutrophils worsened by hypoalbuminaemia and iatrogenic fluid overload.

Each of these causes of RD requires a different form of treatment.

WHO criteria for severe malaria

One or more of:
- cerebral malaria (CM)
- respiratory distress (RD)
- severe normocytic anaemia
- renal failure
- hyperparasitaemia
- pulmonary oedema
- hypoglycaemia
- circulatory collapse
- spontaneous bleeding/DIC
- repeated generalized convulsions
- acidosis
- malarial haemoglobinuria

Other manifestations include:
- impaired consciousness, but rousable
- prostration, severe weakness
- jaundice
- hyperpyrexia

Blantyre Coma Scale

	Score
Best motor response	
• Localizes painful stimulus *	2
• Withdraws limb from painful stimulus **	1
• No response or inappropriate response	0
Best verbal response	
• Cries appropriately with painful stimulus, or if verbal, speaks	2
• Moan or abnormal cry with painful stimulus	1
• No vocal response to painful stimulus	0
Eye movements	
• Watches or follows (e.g. mother's face)	1
• Fails to watch or follow	0

To obtain 'coma score' add the scores from each section.

* Pressure with blunt end of pencil on sternum/supraorbital ridge
** Pressure with horizontal pencil on nail bed of finger or toe

Anaemia All patients with malaria sustain some fall in haemoglobin level. The anaemia is normocytic. Severe anaemia with a haematocrit of less than 15% (or Hb <5 g/dl) in the presence of parasitaemia greater than 10,000/mcl is a common presentation in African children. Pallor, breathlessness, gallop rhythm, RD, pulmonary oedema, and neurological signs are common features of severe anaemia. Anaemia is exacerbated by secondary bacterial infections, haemorrhage, and pregnancy. Hyperparasitaemia and/or G6PD deficiency can result in massive intravascular haemolysis. In children, repeated episodes of otherwise uncomplicated malaria may lead to chronic normochromic anaemia with dyserythropoietic changes in the bone marrow.

Children are prone to developing rapid, severe anaemia following *P. falciparum* infection, which may contribute to neurological and cardiopulmonary signs.

Jaundice is common in adult patients and is the result of a number of mechanisms including haemolysis, hepatocellular damage, and cholestasis. Both unconjugated and conjugated bilirubin may be raised to greater than 50 mcmol/l (3.0 mg/dl). Clinical signs of liver failure are unusual unless there is concomitant viral hepatitis.

Renal impairment may be pre-renal or renal in origin, usually occurs in adults, and is characterized by a raised serum Cr (>265 mcmol/l, 30 mg/dl) and urea, with oliguria or anuria (<400 ml urine/24 hrs in an adult) due to acute tubular necrosis. Renal impairment may occur at the time of maximal parasitaemia or even when the parasites have been cleared. In some cases, there is polyuria. Renal failure in malaria has a poor prognosis (~45% die).

Blackwater fever is massive haemoglobinuria (the urine becomes very dark) in the context of severe malaria. The cause is incompletely characterized but in some cases it follows treatment or prophylaxis with an oxidant drug such as primaquine. It is more common in patients with G6PD deficiency or other red cell enzyme deficiencies (e.g. pyruvate kinase).

Hypoglycaemia (whole blood glucose <2.2 mmol/l, 40 mg/dl) may be due to impaired liver function or quinine/quinidine-induced hyperinsulinaemia (pregnant women are particularly prone). It presents with anxiety, sweating, breathlessness, dilated pupils, oliguria, hypothermia, tachycardia, and light-headedness, eventually leading to decreased consciousness, convulsions, and coma. However, it can easily be missed in patients with disturbed conscious level. In a fasting adult, hepatic glycogen stores last approximately 2 days; in a child, maybe as little as 12 hrs. Hence, hypoglycaemia is common in 1–3 yr olds (especially those with CM, hyperparasitaemia, or convulsions). Hypoglycaemia indicates a poor prognosis and is a risk factor for neurological sequelae. It is not associated with signs of malnutrition.

Indicators of a poor prognosis

- Hyperlactataemia (>6 mmol/l or arterial pH <7.3)
- Hyperventilation
- Bleeding
- Convulsions
- Hyperparasitaemia (>10^6 ring stage forms/ml)
- ≥5% of polymorphs contain malarial pigment (haenozoin)
- Decerebrate posturing
- Hypothermia (<36.5°C)
- Sustained hyperthermia (>39°C)
- Severe anaemia (PCV <15% or Hb <5 g/dl)
- Deep coma (3–5 on GCS)
- Age <3 yrs
- Jaundice
- Uraemia (>21.4 mmol/l)
- Shock
- Hypoglycaemia (plasma glucose <2.2 mmol/l)
- Peripheral leucocytosis (>12,000/ml)
- ALT and AST raised three-fold above normal limits

Lactic acidosis: pH <7.3, or raised plasma and CSF lactate levels (plasma >15 mmol/l) and a low plasma HCO_3^- carry a poor prognosis, especially in children with CM. Lactate levels >5 mmol/l frequently exceed the buffering capacity of the body and result in metabolic acidosis. In these patients, particularly children, RD is not infrequent.

Fluid and electrolyte disturbances such as hypovolaemia and dehydration are common. Low Na^+, Cl^-, PO_4^-, Ca^{2+}, Mg^{2+}, and endocrine dysfunction are common, but seldom have major clinical implications except in the severely ill.

Acute respiratory distress syndrome carries a 50% mortality and may occur at a time when the patient is otherwise improving. Excessive fluid replacement exacerbates this complication and is suggested by an increase in respiratory rate (excluding aspiration or acidosis). Predisposing causes include hyperparasitaemia, renal failure, and pregnancy (may occur suddenly after delivery). Hypoxia may cause convulsions and death within a few hours.

Shock (algid malaria): cold, clammy, cyanotic skin (core skin temperature difference >10°C); weak rapid pulses; supine systolic BP <70mmHg (50 in children) suggests circulatory collapse. Shock in malaria is commonly due to 2° bacterial infection, metabolic acidosis, pulmonary oedema, dehydration, or a gastrointestinal bleed.

Disseminated intravascular coagulation (DIC) is due to pathological activation of the coagulation cascade. DIC may manifest with bleeding gums, epistaxis, petechiae, haematemesis, and/or melaena with significant blood loss. DIC occurs in less than 10% of patients, but is more common in non-immune people (especially travellers). Blood film shows thrombocytopenia and schistocytes (damaged red cells). There is a prolonged prothrombin time (PT) and an increase in fibrin degradation products (FDP).

Hyperpyrexia (rectal temperature >40°C) is more common in children. Associated with convulsions, delirium, and coma, and may result in permanent neurological sequelae or death.

Hyperparasitaemia in endemic areas is a parasite density >10^6 parasites/ml (about 20% cells infected), although in highly endemic areas patients may tolerate greater densities without accompanying clinical features.

Gastrointestinal symptoms are common in children. Nausea, vomiting, abdominal pain, and diarrhoea without blood or pus are frequently seen. There may also be ulceration of the stomach and duodenum, malabsorption, and an increase in bacterial infections (e.g. salmonella). Persistent vomiting requires urgent parenteral drug administration.

2° infection with septicaemia, pneumonia (e.g. following aspiration), urinary tract infection (following catheterization), and post-partum sepsis are common. Gram negative septicaemia may occur without any focus of infection.

Differential diagnosis

Malaria is a great mimic and must enter the differential diagnosis of several clinical presentations.

- The presentation fever needs to be differentiated from other endemic diseases such as typhoid, viral illnesses such as dengue fever and influenza, brucellosis, and respiratory and urinary tract infections. Less common causes of tropical fevers include leishmaniasis, trypanosomiasis, rickettsial infections, and relapsing fevers.
- The coma of CM needs to be differentiated from meningitis (including tuberculous meningitis), encephalitis, enteric fevers, trypanosomiasis, brain abscess, and other causes of coma.
- The anaemia of malaria can be confused with other common causes of haemolytic anaemia in the tropics such as that due to the haemoglobinopathies. The anaemia of malaria must be differentiated from that of iron, folate, or vitamin B12 deficiency.
- The renal failure of malaria must be distinguished from massive intravascular haemolysis, sickle cell disease, leptospirosis, snake envenoming, use of traditional herbal medicines, and chronic renal disease resulting from glomerulonephritis and hypertension.
- The jaundice and hepatomegaly of malaria must be distinguished from that of viral hepatitis (A, B, and E, cytomegalovirus, and Epstein–Barr virus infections), leptospirosis, yellow fever, biliary disease, and drug-induced disease including alcohol.

Clinical diagnosis on its own is notoriously inaccurate in the diagnosis of malaria and a blood film is desirable.

Laboratory diagnosis

Blood films

Specific diagnosis of malaria requires identification of parasites in smears of blood. See Fig. 2A.3 and thick/thin film methodology in box.

Maintain a high index of suspicion and carry out multiple blood films (at least three). Infection may exceptionally occur via transfusion, needlestick injury, during brief airport stopovers in endemic areas, and when infected mosquitoes 'alight' from airplane flights from endemic areas and bite individuals ('airport' malaria). In falciparum malaria, the presence of schizonts in peripheral blood samples may indicate severe infection, as these forms would normally sequester.

Pitfalls

- A single negative film does not exclude malaria. Repeat on three occasions. The patient may have been partially treated, suppressing patent infection. Malaria prophylaxis should be stopped whilst investigating for active infection.
- In endemic areas, a positive film does not prove that malaria is responsible for the current symptoms.
- Cross-contamination of slides is possible in bulk staining.
- Correlation between parasite density and disease severity may be poor — patients with a low parasitaemia may be very ill, whilst semi-immunes may harbour high parasitaemias with relatively few symptoms.
- Platelets, cell fragments, and impurities in the stain can be mistaken for malarial parasites.

Other methods of diagnosis

Currently available methods include serodiagnosis (only to be used exceptionally and in retrospect), monocytic malarial pigment, quantitative buffy coat (QBC) method, dipstick antigen capture tests (e.g. ParaSight F®, Malaria PF test®, and OptiMAL test®), and PCR.

Rapid dipstick methods

- The ParaSight F® and the Malaria PF Test® antigen capture tests use a monoclonal antibody to detect the histidine-rich protein II of *P. falciparum*. These are useful in those who have not had malaria before and require minimal expertise. However, they are expensive, not quantitative, and detect only the presence of *P. falciparum*.
- The OptiMAL® test detects parasite rather than human lactate dehydrogenase — hence pLDH. This test can distinguish falciparum from vivax infections.
- PCR is very useful in epidemiological studies.

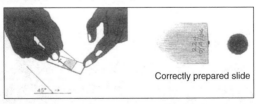

Correctly prepared slide

Fig. 2A.3

How to prepare a thick and thin film on the same slide

1. Clean the tip of the patient's left index finger.
2. Pierce the pulp of the fingertip with a sterile lancet or needle.
3. Squeeze the finger until a droplet of blood forms and place it onto the middle of a clean slide (holding the slide by the edges). This is for the thin film.
4. Place a further three droplets of blood onto the slide at a point to one side of the first droplet. These are for the thick film.
5. Using a second clean slide as a spreader, touch the first, small drop with the edge and allow the blood to run along its edge. With the spreading slide at 45°, push the spreader forwards slowly, ensuring even contact, so that the blood is spread as a thin film over the surface of the slide. See Fig. 2A.3.
6. Using the corner of the spreading slide, amalgamate the three drops of blood on the other half of the slide into a single small, denser film about 1 cm in diameter.
7. Label the slide with a pencil and allow to dry horizontally.

Problems: Badly positioned blood droplets, too much or too little blood, using a greasy slide, a chipped edge of the spreader slide.

Staining: (consult a laboratory manual for more details)

Giemsa stain may be used for both films but is costly and more difficult to do. Thin films must first be fixed in methanol then dipped in 10% Giemsa for 20–30 mins; thick films in 5% solution for 30 mins.

Field's stain uses two solutions, A and B, that are cheaper and more suited to rapid bulk staining. For thick films, dip dried slides into solution A for 5 secs, avoiding agitation. Wash in tap water (preferably neutral pH) for 5 secs, then dip into solution B for 3 secs. Wash again in water for 5 secs, then allow to dry vertically. The centre of the film may not be stained, but optimal parasite staining occurs at the edges of the film. For thin films use solution B (diluted 1:4 with a buffer) before solution A.

Leishman's stain may be used for thin films. 0.5 ml stain is added to each horizontal film and left for 30 secs; then 1.5 ml of buffered water is added and left for 8 mins. The slide is then washed in tap water.

Blood film identification of malarial parasites[2]

1. Are there one or more red-stained chromatin dots and blue cytoplasm?
   YES — go to 2. NO — what you see is not a parasite.
2. Are the size and shape correct for a malarial parasite?
   YES — go to 3. NO — what you see is not a malarial parasite.
3. Is there malarial pigment in the cell?
   YES — go to 7. NO — go to 4.
4. Does the parasite have one chromatin dot attached to blue cytoplasm in the form of a regular ring in the cytoplasm?
   YES —— this is a trophozoite. NO — go to 5.
5. Does the parasite have one chromatin dot attached to blue cytoplasm in the form of a small solid or regular ring or with a vacuole?
   YES — this is a trophozoite. NO — go to 6.
6. Is the parasite with one chromatin dot irregular or fragmented?
   YES — this is a trophozoite. NO — go to 8.
7. Does the parasite with malarial pigment have one chromatin dot?
   YES — go to 8. NO — go to 9.
8. Does the parasite have a vacuole or is it fragmented in some way?
   YES — this is probably a late trophozoite stage. NO — go to 11.
9. Does the parasite have 2 chromatin dots attached to a ring and have a vacuole?
   YES — this is a trophozoite. NO — go to 10.
10. Does the parasite have between 2 and 32 chromatin dots and pigment?
    YES — this is a schizont.
11. Is the parasite rounded or 'banana-shaped'?
    Rounded — go to 12. Banana-shaped — go to 14.
12. Does the rounded parasite have clearly stained chromatin and a deep blue cytoplasm?
    YES — this is a female gametocyte. NO — go to 13.
13. Does the rounded parasite have a reddish overall colour, so that the chromatin is indistinct?
    YES — this is a male gametocyte.
14. Does the 'banana-shaped' parasite have densely stained blue cytoplasm and bright red chromatin?
    YES — this is a female gametocyte. NO — go to 15.
15. Does the 'banana-shaped' parasite have a reddish overall colour, so that the chromatin is indistinct?
    YES — this is a male gametocyte.

2 WHO (1991) Basic malaria microscopy — learner's guide, WHO, Geneva.

	Early trophozoite (ring form)	Mature trophozoite
Plasmodium vivax	Thick rings, $1/3 – 1/2$ the diameter of the red cell 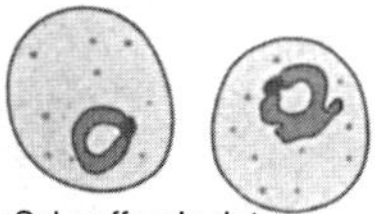 A few Schuffner's dots Accolé (Shoulder) forms and double dots less common than with *P. falciparum*	Ameboid rings, $1/2 – 2/3$ the diameter of the red cell Pale blue or lilac parasite with prominent central valuole 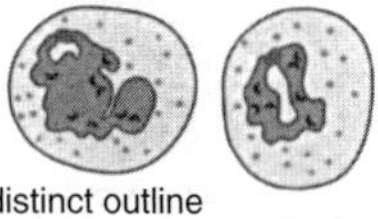 Indistinct outline Scattered fine yellowish-brown pigment granules or rods
Plasmodium ovale	Thick, compact rings, $1/3 – 1/2$ the diameter of the red cell 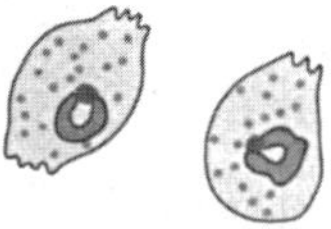 Numerous Schuffner's dots but paler than with *P. vivax*	Thick rings, less irregular than those of *P. vivax*, $1/3 – 1/2$ the diameter of the red cell 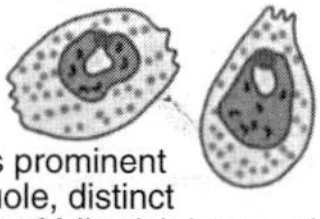 Less prominent vacuole, distinct outline Yellowish brown pigment which is coarser and darker than that of *P. vivax* Schuffner's dots prominent
Plasmodium falciparum	Delicate rings, $1/6 – 1/4$ the diameter of the red cell 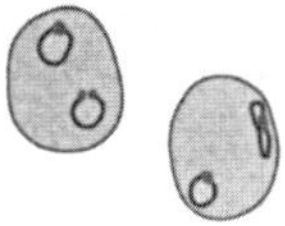 Double dots and Accolé forms common	Fairly delicate rings, $1/3 – 1/2$ the diameter of the red cell 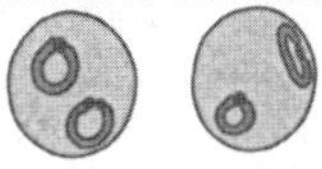 Red-mauve stippling (Maurer's dots or clefts) may be present Mature trophozoites are less often present in peripheral blood than ring forms
Plasmodium malariae	Small, thick, compact rings Small chromatin dot which may be inside the ring 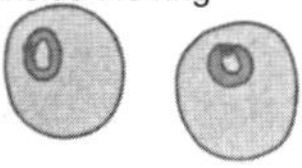 Double dots and Accolé forms rare	Ameboid form more compact than *P. vivax* Sometimes angular or band forms 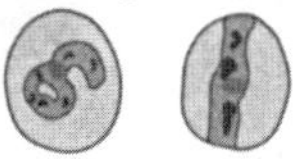 Heavy, dark-yellow-brown pigment No stippling unless ovestained

Fig. 2A.4 Diagrams of malarial blood cells. From Bain BJ (1995) *Blood cells. A practical guide.* Blackwell Science, Oxford (with permission).

	Early schizont	Late schizont
Plasmodium vivax	Rounded or irregular Ameboid Loose central mass of fine yellowish-brown pigment 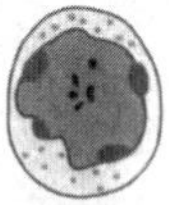 Schizont almost fills cell Schuffner's dots	12–24 (usually 16–24) medium-sized merozoites 1–2 clumps of peripheral pigment 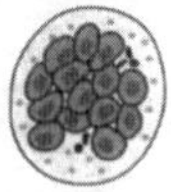 Schizont almost fills cell Schuffner's dots
Plasmodium ovale	Round, compact Darkish brown pigment, heavier and coarser than that of P. vivax 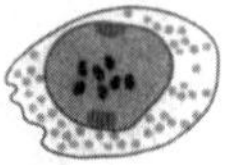 Schuffner's dots	6–12 (usually 8) large merozoites arranged irregularly like a bunch of grapes 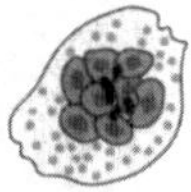 Central pigment Schuffner's dots
Plasmodium falciparum	Not usually seen in blood Very small, ameboid Scattered light-brown to black pigment	Not usually seen in blood 8–32 (usually few) very small merozoites; grouped irregularly Peripheral clump of coarse dark brown pigment
Plasmodium malariae	Compact, round, fills red cell 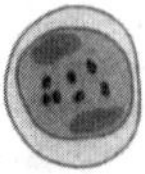 Coarse dark yellow-brown pigment	6–12 (usually 8–10) large merozoites, arranged symmetrically, often in a rosette or daisy head formation 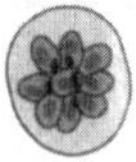 Central coarse dark yellowish-brown pigment

Fig. 2A.4 *Continued* Diagrams of malarial blood cells. From Bain BJ (1995) *Blood cells. A practical guide.* Blackwell Science, Oxford (with permission).

		Gametocyte	
		Macrogametocyte	Microgametocyte
Plasmodium vivax		Round or ovoid, almost fills enlarged cell Blue cytoplasm 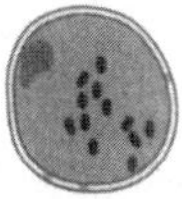 Eccentric compact red nucleus Scattered pigment	Round or ovoid, as large as a normal red cell but does not fill the enlarged red cell 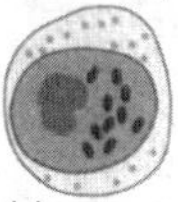 Faintly staining Larger, lighter red central or eccentric nucleus Fine, scattered pigment
Plasmodium ovale		Similar to *P. vivax* but somewhat smaller 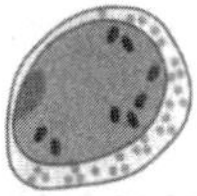 Pigment coarser and blacker, scattered but mainly near the periphery	Similar to *P. vivax* but smaller 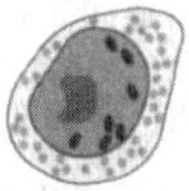
Plasmodium falciparum		Sickle or crescent shaped Deforms cell which often appears empty of haemoglobin 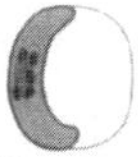 Blue cytoplasm Compact central nucleus with pigment aggregated around it	Oval or crescentic with blunted ends Pale blue or pink 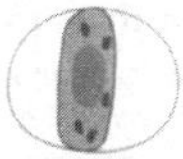 Large pale nucleus with pigment more scattered than in macrogametocyte
Plasmodium malariae		Similar to *P. vivax* but smaller, pink or oval, almost fills cell, blue with a dark nucleus 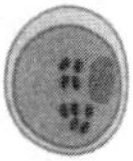 Prominent pigment concentrated at centre and periphery	Similar to *P. vivax* but smaller, pink or paler blue than macrogametocyte with a larger, paler nucleus 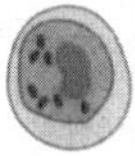 Prominent pigment

Fig. 2A.4 *Continued* Diagrams of malarial blood cells. From Bain BJ (1995) *Blood cells. A practical guide.* Blackwell Science, Oxford (with permission).

General management

Decide whether the patient has falciparum malaria or one of the 'benign' malarias. If there are signs of severe falciparum infection, do not wait for laboratory confirmation: weigh the patient and start treatment immediately.

Basic rules

- In many instances, especially in endemic areas, uncomplicated malaria can be treated on an outpatient basis.
- Await blood film results for uncomplicated malaria.
- Advise patients to return promptly if symptoms worsen or do not improve within 48 hrs.
- Beware of sending home children who have mild symptoms but high levels of parasitaemia, since they may deteriorate rapidly.

All patients will usually require antimalarial chemotherapy

Antimalarial treatment with an appropriate agent should be started immediately. Choose the drug bearing in mind likely compliance and side effects, local resistance, and costs (see p. 30). Take into account the locally recommended chemotherapy.

Most patients will need antipyretics and analgesics

If fever causes distress or the child is prone to febrile convulsions, give paracetamol. Avoid aspirin in children — both because of Reye's syndrome and because aspirin can exacerbate acidosis.

For hyperpyrexia, begin tepid sponging and fanning quickly to reduce the likelihood of febrile convulsions. Consider giving intramuscular antipyretics.

Adjunctive therapy for patients with severe disease

Consider the following:

1. **50% dextrose 50 ml** (children: 1.0 ml/kg) given by IV bolus if hypoglycaemic (blood glucose <2.2 mmol). Follow this with 10% dextrose IV with electrolytes (beware of hyponatraemia and hypokalaemia). Monitor blood glucose levels regularly, especially during infusion of quinine.

2. **Rehydration** is required in particular if diarrhoea and vomiting are present. Adults with severe falciparum malaria usually require 1–3l of isotonic saline over the first 24 hrs. However, avoid overhydration; the JVP and CVP are unreliable guides. Monitor renal output, BP hourly. Be careful to take into account volumes of fluids given with any IV drugs. If the patient remains oliguric, peritoneal dialysis (but preferably haemofiltration or haemodialysis) may be indicated.

3. **Blood** (and exchange) transfusion with pathogen-free, compatible fresh blood or packed cells.
   Blood transfusion may be urgent, particularly in children, if the haematocrit falls below 15% (Hb <5 g/dl) and is accompanied by acidosis or RD. Give blood 10 mg/kg over 30 mins, then a further 10 mg/kg over 2–3 hrs without diuretics in children with RD and severe anaemia. In DIC, fresh blood, clotting factors (fresh frozen plasma), and/or platelets should be given as required.

The overall clinical condition of the patient must be weighed against the risks incurred by transfusion. In some situations, especially with parasitaemias over 30%, consider exchange transfusion — although this has not been subject to a RCT.

4. **Oxygen and mechanical ventilation** may be required for patients with RD or significant raised intracranial pressure. Ensure that the airway is clear and the head of the bed is raised if distress is due to pulmonary oedema. If due to overhydration, reduce IV fluids and give IV furosemide. Haemofiltration may be used, if available.

5. **Diuretics** such as furosemide 20–80 mg IV. Should be given in pulmonary oedema — if there is no response, the dose can be increased up to 200 mg.

6. **Broad spectrum antibiotics** should be started immediately (after taking blood, urine stool cultures, etc.) if 2° bacterial infection is suspected. Suggestive features include a significantly raised neutrophil count and hypotension. Continue until specific sensitivities are known. Bacteraemia occurs in ~8% of children with severe anaemia, rising to ~12% in those under 30 months.

7. **Dopamine** may be given in shock through a central line if the BP or JVP are not maintained following the use of plasma expanders. Adrenalin should be avoided as it can exacerbate acidosis.

8. **Vitamin K** 10 mg IV by slow injection may help normalize the PT and PTT. Heparin should be avoided even in the face of DIC.

9. There is no role in cerebral malaria for systemic corticosteroids.

Cerebral malaria

Treat as above with the following additional specific measures:

- Nurse the patient on his/her side to avoid aspiration of vomit. Turn every 2 hrs.
- Unless anuric, the patient should be catheterized and have temperature, heart and respiratory rates, BP, and fluid balance measured regularly.
- Consciousness must be assessed regularly with the Glasgow or Blantyre Coma Scores.
- If convulsions arise — be alert since they may be subtle — treat with diazepam 0.15 mg/kg (up to a maximum of 10 mg in adults) by slow IV injection. (An alternative is diazepam 0.5 mg/kg rectally.)
- Avoid corticosteroids or other ancillary agents for cerebral oedema since they are of no proven benefit.

Antimalarial chemotherapy

- Aim to reduce the parasitaemia as quickly as possible, using oral agents if tolerated.
- Beware local patterns of resistance.
- If the species is unknown or there is mixed infection, treat as falciparum malaria.
- Parasite count may paradoxically rise during the first 24 hrs and does not necessarily indicate drug failure. If the parasite count has not fallen by at least 75% 48 hrs after starting therapy, the count should be rechecked and, if confirmed, a different antimalarial drug should be considered.
- During pregnancy, quinine is still the treatment of choice for severe falciparum malaria despite the remote possibility of induced abortion since preservation of the mother's life is paramount. Avoid mefloquine in the first trimester of pregnancy.

Antimalarial preparations and their recommended doses

1. *Quinine:* used in the treatment of falciparum malaria and emergency IV treatment of benign malaria where oral drugs are not tolerated.
   For uncomplicated disease give 10 mg/kg quinine salt PO tds. Once the parasites have been eradicated, give tetracycline 4 mg/kg PO qds, doxycycline 3 mg/kg PO od, or clindamycin 10 mg/kg PO bd, each for one week.
   For severe disease give a loading dose of 20 mg/kg of quinine IV over 4 hrs, followed by 10 mg/kg infused over 4 hrs every 8 hrs until oral therapy is tolerated.
- Oral doses which are vomited out within 1 hr of administration should be repeated immediately.
- Doses should be reduced by one-third in patients with liver dysfunction and/or in renal failure.
- Compliance with 7 days of oral quinine is poor because of the bitter taste; shorter regimens are acceptable as long as they are accompanied by a second drug (e.g. doxycycline).
- IV doses of quinine should be given in 500 ml of 5% dextrose solution into a large vein, over 4 hrs.
- Check if the patient has already received chloroquine, quinine, or mefloquine — if yes, omit the loading dose. Check that cardiac monitoring is available.
- Watch for hypoglycaemia (particularly in pregnant women), hyponatraemia, hypokalaemia. Reduce the rate of infusion if cardiac arrhythmias occur. Switch to oral drugs as soon as possible.
- Where IV access is unavailable, quinine may be given IM (20 mg/kg loading dose followed by 10 mg/kg tds) but beware of tissue damage and risk of heart block. (Tetanus has also been recorded where IM quinine injections have been given — check immunization status.) Dilute the preparation 5-fold and give in divided doses by deep IM injection into the anterior thigh.
2. *Artemisinins* are highly effective in clearing multidrug-resistant *P. falciparum* parasites. IM artemether is as effective as IM quinine (although recrudescence rates may be higher). Artesunate suppositories are quick, easy, and free of the risks associated with IV injections.

For uncomplicated disease give artesunate or artemether
10–12 mg/kg PO in divided doses over 3–7 days, plus a total of 25 mg/kg
mefloquine. If used alone, the total dose is given over 7 days (usually
4 mg/kg on day 1, 2 mg/kg on days 2 and 3, and 1 mg/kg on days 4–7).
For severe disease, give artesunate 2.4 mg/kg IV or IM initially, followed by 1.2 mg/kg at 12 and 24 hrs, then 1.2 mg/kg od. (60 mg of arte-
sunic acid is dissolved in 0.6 ml of 5% $NaHCO_3$, diluted to 3–5 ml with
5% dextrose and given IV or IM. 1 ampoule = 80 mg.)
Or give artemether, 3.2 mg/kg IM initially, followed by 1.6 mg/kg od.
Do not give IV.

3. **Mefloquine** is related to quinine and may be used for multidrug-resistant
   forms of *P. falciparum* but can only be taken orally. Adverse neuropsychiatric side-effects have been reported in using this drug both for prophylaxis (severe in 1:1500 cases) and in treatment (in 1:300 cases). The
   benefit of treating potentially life-threatening multidrug-resistant malaria
   outweighs this risk. Adverse effects may respond to chlorpromazine.
   Give 15 mg/kg base PO stat (+/− 2nd dose of 10 mg/kg 8–24 hrs later).
   (In the USA, 1 tablet = 228 mg base; elsewhere 1 tablet = 250 mg base.)
   • Do not administer mefloquine within 12 hrs of the last quinine dose.
   • Do not use in early pregnancy. Warn women to avoid conception
     within 3 months of taking mefloquine.
   • Avoid in severe disease because of the risk of neurological
     syndromes.
   • Do not use for treatment if taken as prophylaxis.

4. **Chloroquine:** the use of chloroquine for falciparum malaria is no
   longer recommended due to widespread resistance. However, it is still
   used in many parts of the world because it is cheap, easy to use, safe
   (e.g. in pregnancy), and works to some degree. It should not be used if
   it has been taken as prophylaxis. In these situations, treat with quinine,
   unless certain of sensitivity. Falciparum malaria in Central America
   (North of the Panama Canal) and the Middle East is still said to be
   chloroquine sensitive.
   Chloroquine is still the drug of choice for benign malaria in most parts
   of the world, although resistant strains are emerging (see below).
   For uncomplicated disease, give a total of 25 mg/kg base as 10 mg/kg
   base PO followed by either 10 mg/kg base at 24 hrs and 5 mg/kg base at
   48 hrs, or 5 mg/kg base at 12, 24, and 36 hrs.
   For P. vivax or P. ovale, add **primaquine** 0.25 mg base/kg od for
   14 days to obtain a radical cure (see below).
   For patients with G6PD deficiency, use an increased dose and longer
   intervals for primaquine (usually 45 mg once a week for 6 weeks) to
   avoid severe haemolysis. Watch out for black urine; reduce the dose if
   this occurs.
   IV route administration of chloroquine should be considered if a
   patient cannot swallow, has D&V, or if IV quinine/quinidine is not available. Rapid IV administration of chloroquine is dangerous and may result
   in fatal cardiovascular collapse and blindness.
   Give 10 mg/kg base at a constant rate by IV infusion over 8 hrs, followed by 15 mg/kg base over 24 hrs. If IV route is not available, give
   3.5 mg/kg base IM or subcutaneously q6h (up to total of 25 mg/kg base).

5. **Tetracycline/doxycycline:** used in conjunction with quinine in the treatment of *P. falciparum* infections and in patients hypersensitive to sulfadoxine-pyrimethamine. See quinine text for doses. Do not give in pregnancy and in young children under the age of 12, and decrease the dose in renal failure.

6. **Sulfadoxine–pyrimethamine (Fansidar®):** there is now widespread resistance to this drug combination. It is used after initial treatment with quinine, but is no longer routinely recommended.
   Give 20 mg/kg sulfadoxine plus 1 mg/kg pyrimethamine as a single dose. (3 tablets of Fansidar® is usual adult dose.)

7. **Quinidine:** if quinine is unavailable, quinidine (a related compound) may be given. It is important to have cardiac monitoring available during IV infusion of this drug as it is more cardiotoxic (largely because less is bound to plasma proteins).
   Give 7.5 mg/kg base IV at a constant rate over 1 hr, followed by 0.02 mg base/kg/min.

8. **Halofantrine:** used in the treatment of uncomplicated chloroquine-resistant *P. falciparum* infections usually when other drugs are unavailable or have failed to work.
   Give 8 mg/kg PO repeated at 6 and 12 hrs on an empty stomach. Repeat 1 week later in those without immunity.
   - Needs ECG monitoring due to cardiotoxicity.
   - Side-effects include QT interval prolongation and ventricular arrhythmias, particularly in patients with coronary heart disease, cardiomyopathy, and congenital heart disease. Do not take in combination with arrhythmogenic drugs or drugs that cause electrolyte disturbances.
   - Do not use to treat recrudescent infections within 28 days of primary mefloquine therapy.

9. **Atovaquone/proguanil (Malarone®):** a new drug that is now licensed in some countries for the treatment of uncomplicated falciparum malaria where resistance to other drugs is suspected. It is however expensive. Each tablet contains proguanil hydrochloride 100 mg and atovaquone 250 mg.
   Give adult and child >40 kgs, 4 tablets od for 3 days; child 11–20 kg, 1 tablet; 21–30 kg, 2 tablets; 31–40 kg, 3 tablets, all od for 3 days.

10. **Amodiaquine:** can be effective against R1, R2, and R3 chloroquine-resistant *P. falciparum* (see section on drug resistance). IV preparations are not available, although the related amopyroquin is administered IM.

Radical cures and primaquine in benign malaria

- Treatment with a blood schizontocidal drug, such as quinine, will not eliminate parasites from the liver. Therefore, patients infected with *P. vivax* or *P. ovale* are also given primaquine to kill the liver hypnozoites and prevent recrudescence later. *P. malariae* does not produce persistent liver forms.
- Since primaquine is also gametocidal, it is sometimes given to patients infected with *P. falciparum* in non-endemic regions. This prevents the blood gametocytes being taken up by local mosquitoes and possibly initiating local foci of infections.
- A major drawback is primaquine's ability to cause severe intravascular haemolysis in patients with G6PD deficiency. Weekly doses of 45 mg are better tolerated in such patients than daily doses of 15 mg for 14–21 days.
- Relatively primaquine-resistant strains of *P. vivax* have been reported in the Pacific region that require at least 6 mg/kg total dose (~2× normal dose).

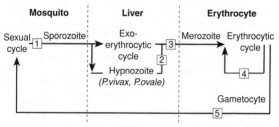

Fig. 2A.5 Stage specificity of antimalarial drugs.

Chemoprophylaxis

Chemoprophylaxis against malaria rarely provides full protection and measures should be taken at all times to reduce mosquito bites. Insecticide-treated bednets should be used: they reduce morbidity and mortality from malaria in children. Individuals should be aware of malarial symptoms, which may be non-specific, and report early for a blood film if malaria is suspected.

Travellers to malarial areas should preferably begin prophylaxis 1 week (2–3 weeks in the case of mefloquine) before arrival, and must continue for 4 weeks after departure, except in the case of Malarone, where prophylaxis may be commenced the day before entry into a malarious area and ended 7 days after return.

Any febrile illness occurring within 1 year of travel could be malaria. For long-term non-immune residents consideration should be given to the balance between the risks of infection and the side-effects of chemoprophylaxis. It may be possible to target prophylaxis during the transmission season alone.

Drugs used in prophylaxis

1. **Proguanil:** used for prophylaxis in pregnant women and non-immune individuals in areas of low risk only. It is more commonly used in combination with chloroquine (see below).
   Dose 200 mg PO od in adults, including pregnant women. Children <1 yr 25 mg/day; 1–4 yrs 50 mg/day; 5–8 yrs 100 mg/day; and 9–14 yrs 150 mg/day. A folic acid supplement should be taken during pregnancy.

2. **Chloroquine** is used in combination with proguanil in low-risk areas, in pregnant women, and other individuals who cannot tolerate other antimalarials.
   Dose: 300 mg (as base) PO weekly in adults, including pregnant women. Children require 5 mg/kg weekly.
   - Chloroquine binds to melanin in the retina, causing concern that long-term prophylaxis may lead to visual impairment/blindness. Total lifetime exposure therefore should not exceed 100g (~6 yrs of continuous usage). Twice-yearly retinal screenings should be performed in anyone who has taken 300 mg of chloroquine weekly for >6 yrs.

3. **Mefloquine** is now a favoured drug for the prophylaxis of malaria in many areas where chloroquine resistance is present.
   Dose: 250 mg PO weekly in adults; in children >45 kg 62.5 mg weekly in children 3 months–5 yrs, 125 mg for 6–8 yrs, 187.5 mg for 9–14 yrs). Mefloquine is not recommended in neonates.

4. **Doxycycline:** useful as an alternate to mefloquine for short term prophylaxis of up to 8 weeks.
   Dose: 1.5 mg/kg PO od, up to a max of 100 mg. Do not use in children <12 yrs and in pregnant and lactating women. Conception should be avoided for >1 week after its use.

5. **Pyrimethamine-dapsone (Maloprim®):** used in areas of chloroquine resistance (with chloroquine to cover P. vivax) when mefloquine or doxycycline are contraindicated. However, availability has become a limiting factor.
   Dose: 12.5 mg pyrimethamine plus 100 mg dapsone (1 tablet of Maloprim) PO weekly for adults. Children: 1–5 yrs ¼ dose, 6–11 yrs ½ dose, >11 yrs full adult dose.
   Pyrimethamine-sulfadoxine (Fansidar®) is no longer used for prophylaxis due to the risk of Stevens–Johnson syndrome and bone marrow toxicity.

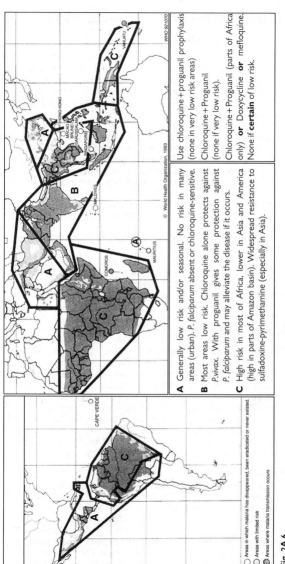

A Generally low risk and/or seasonal. No risk in many areas (urban). *P. falciparum* absent or chloroquine-sensitive.

B Most areas low risk. Chloroquine alone protects against *P. vivax*. With proguanil gives some protection against *P. falciparum* and may alleviate the disease if it occurs.

C High risk in most of Africa, lower in Asia and America (high in parts of Amazon basin). Widespread resistance to sulfadoxine-pyrimethamine (especially in Asia).

Use chloroquine + proguanil prophylaxis (none in very low risk areas)

Chloroquine + Proguanil (none if very low risk).

Chloroquine + Proguanil (parts of Africa only) **or** Doxycycline **or** mefloquine. None if **certain** of low risk.

© World Health Organization, 1993

WHO 92/070

○ Areas in which malaria has disappeared, been eradicated or never existed.
○ Areas with limited risk
● Areas where malaria transmission occurs

Fig. 2A.6

Multidrug-resistant malaria and treatment failure

Resistance of malarial parasites to conventional drugs is a growing problem across the world (see Fig. 2A.7), particularly with *P. falciparum*. In certain areas, notably in South-East Asia, prophylaxis with chloroquine or pyrimethamine-sulfadoxine, and treatment with mefloquine or pyrimethamine-sulfadoxine are no longer recommended. *P. vivax* resistance has been reported in areas of South-East Asia.

Chloroquine resistance is classified as follows:

- **R1:** recrudescence occurs <4 wks after apparently successful treatment.
- **R2:** despite improvement with treatment, parasitaemia persists and increases soon afterwards, heralding a clinical deterioration in the patient.
- **R3:** complete resistance in which the patient continues to deteriorate (and the parasitaemia increases) despite treatment, until chloroquine is replaced by an effective drug.

Treatment failure is defined as a failure of either symptoms to begin to improve or the parasite count to have fallen by 75% within 48 hrs. It is possible with any drug and may result from:

- Inadequate treatment (patient non-compliance or oral drug vomited)
- Parasite resistance to drug
- Poor drug quality
- Non-malarial cause for the symptoms.

Reassess the patient and if malaria is still thought to be the cause, change to a different treatment and ensure that the patient is compliant with therapy.

Future perspectives

There was once the belief that a combined strategy of treatment, prophylaxis, control measures, and a successful vaccine would eradicate malaria. The aim of eradication has been dismissed, largely because the assumptions that were made at the time of planning were not practical. The current aims are to reduce morbidity, prevent mortality, and reduce socio-economic loss. Efforts continue around the world to produce an effective vaccine — an elusive goal, although several are currently being tested. The sequencing of the malarial parasite's genome will hopefully lead to the development of new drugs to obviate the problem of resistance. Until that time, however, education must remain one of our strongest tools.

Role of education

- To promote prompt and effective diagnosis and treatment, educating the population as to when to seek treatment, when prophylaxis is required, and the importance of compliance with treatment.
- To reduce contact between mosquito and humans, particularly the development and implementation of insecticide-treated bednets.
- To control mosquito breeding by draining stagnant water, removing litter and debris that retain water and provide a mosquito breeding ground, and using larvicides and larvivorous fish in mosquito breeding pools. DDT spraying is still widely used but may eventually be replaced by new methods.

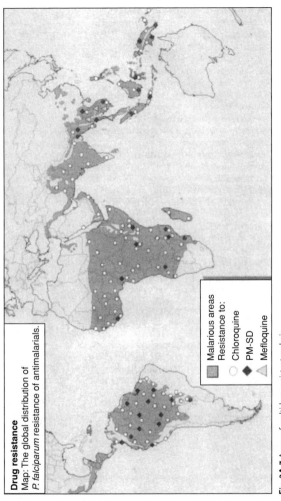

Drug resistance
Map: The global distribution of
P. falciparum resistance of antimalarials.

Malarious areas
Resistance to:
○ Chloroquine
◆ PM-SD
◁ Mefloquine

Fig. 2A.7 Areas of multidrug-resistant malaria.

HIV/sexually transmitted infections

Section editors   **G.P. Taylor**

Sexually transmitted infections (STIs)

The demonstration that treatment of STIs may reduce the transmission of HIV re-emphasizes the importance of these infections. STIs are also responsible for sterility, stillbirth, miscarriage, blindness, brain disease, disfigurement, cancer, and death throughout the world. The burden on the medical services is immense — several hundred million new cases are treated each year. Only two means of decreasing HIV transmission have thus far been shown to work:

- Syndromic treatment of STIs
- Government promotion of condom use

Control requires a multidisciplinary approach

- Correct diagnosis
- Effective early treatment
- Education on avoidance of contact and prevention of transmission
- Promotion and provision of condoms
- Tracing, treating, and counselling of sexual partners
- Appropriate clinical follow-up.

It is essential that persons are treated when first seen and counselled to modify their sexual behaviour.

Syndromic approach to diagnosis and treatment

Where diagnostic facilities and effective therapies are available, all persons attending a STI clinic should be screened using laboratory tests for HIV, syphilis, chlamydia, and gonorrhoea infection. However, many cases will be treated in primary health centres where these laboratory facilities are unavailable. As a result, the WHO has developed a syndromic approach to empirical treatment that is based on the commonly seen clinical signs and symptoms. This approach is presented in the second half of this section.

These charts have been designed to provide a framework for evaluation and treatment, but they should not replace clinical judgement based on local knowledge. They need to be trialled in, and adapted for, local circumstances.

- Single-dose antibiotics should be used whenever possible.
- Where repeated oral doses are prescribed for ambulatory patients, drug administration should be supervised if at all possible.
- Particular attention must be made to local patterns of antibiotic resistance when these are known, particularly for gonococcus and, to a lesser extent, chancroid.

Causes of STIs and reproductive tract infections

Microbe	*Condition*
• ***Bacteria***	
Neisseria gonorrhoeae	Gonorrhoea
Gardnerella vaginalis plus anaerobic bacteria	Bacterial vaginosis
Haemophilus ducreyi	Chancroid
Calymmatobacterium granulomatis	Donovanosis
Treponema pallidum	Syphilis
Chlamydia trachomatis	Urethritis/cervicitis
	Lymphogranuloma venereum
• ***Fungi***	
Candida albicans	Candidiasis
• ***Protozoa***	
Trichomonas vaginalis	Trichomoniasis
• ***Viruses***	
HIV	AIDS
Herpes simplex virus	Genital herpes
Human papillomavirus	Genital warts
• ***Arthropods***	
Phthirus pubis	Pubic lice
Sarcoptes scabiei	Scabies

Other microbes can be passed sexually (e.g. hepatitis B and CMV) but are not considered STIs.

HIV infection/AIDS

The human immunodeficiency viruses are the cause of the acquired immunodeficiency syndrome (AIDS) pandemic that is currently sweeping through the world. Most disease is caused by HIV-1 — it is more virulent and widespread than HIV-2 which mostly occurs in west Africa.

The viruses attach to and enter immune cells that bear the CD4 protein on their surface. CD4-positive lymphocytes co-ordinate the body's immune response and as their numbers fall during the late stages of AIDS, profound immunosuppression occurs. This lays the patient open to a variety of infections that would not normally cause disease in an immunocompetent person — so-called 'opportunistic' infections. The specific opportunistic infections that occur will depend on both the area of the world and the patient's degree of immunosuppression. Certain tumours, caused by viruses, are more common in AIDS patients: lymphomas (due to EBV) and Kaposi sarcoma (herpesvirus KSAV or HHV-8).

There is currently no vaccine and no cure for the viral infection itself. Good therapies have been developed, however, for many of the opportunistic infections. Combination antiretroviral treatment (ART) can control viral replication and allow a considerable restoration of immune function that can last for many years.

The three stages of the disease

1. An acute retroviral illness, similar to mononucleosis, that occurs in ~50% of patients 2–5 weeks post-infection.
2. An asymptomatic stage during which the body's immune system attempts to control the virus. (Note that the virus is not latent at this stage but in balance with the immune system. Billions of virus particles are produced and destroyed each day.)
3. A symptomatic stage as the immune system's function becomes compromised. The patient suffers from opportunistic infections as well as the direct effects of HIV itself.

Transmission routes

- Unprotected intercourse (both heterosexual and homosexual)
- The mother to fetus or infant before, during, or after birth (virus is passed from an infected mother to her child in milk)
- Receipt of infected blood products
- Injections or treatments with unsterile needles, syringes, or skin-piercing instruments.

STIs — particularly those that cause genital ulceration — increase the risk of sexual transmission. In the developing world, heterosexual intercourse appears to be the major mode of transmission for adults, followed by blood transfusion and contaminated needles. Children are at risk of infection perinatally and from blood transfusion.

Clinical features

Acute retroviral illness

This occurs in some patients 10–30 days post-exposure and lasts 3–21 days. It is similar to infectious mononucleosis with a variety of signs and symptoms — malaise, fever, sore throat, myalgia, anorexia, anthralgia, headache, diarrhoea, nausea, generalized lymphadenopathy, macular eruption involving trunk and arms, thrombocytopenia. Rare complications include aseptic meningoencephalitis and mono/polyneuritis. Atypical lymphocytes may be seen in the blood film. There may be significant temporary immunosuppression during the acute infection.

Asymptomatic HIV infection

Lasts for a variable period of time before immune system dysfunction produces symptoms. In the USA ~50% of HIV +ve individuals develop symptoms by 10 yrs. The length of the asymptomatic period in the developing world is unclear — it may be shorter, reflecting the generally lower level of health compared to the USA. The only sign of infection during this period may be generalized lymphadenopathy, probably due to HIV.

Symptomatic HIV infection

Weight loss and weakness are common manifestations. Opportunistic infections attack multiple systems (see following pages). Certain opportunistic infections become more common as the CD4 count falls — reflected in the WHO's proposals for staging HIV infection and disease by clinical signs and symptoms.

WHO clinical staging system for HIV infection and disease

The following staging system has been developed for epidemiological purposes. It may prove useful for estimating a patient's prognosis and following the development of AIDS. The system can be adapted for each locality. The presence of any of these manifestations in a previously healthy adult should suggest HIV infection. Any suspicion of HIV infection should be confirmed by laboratory tests after discussion with and consent of the patient.

HIV encephalopathy: clinical findings of disabling cognitive and/or motor dysfunction interfering with activities of daily living, progressing over weeks to months, in the absence of a concurrent illness or condition other than HIV infection that could explain the findings.

HIV wasting syndrome: weight loss >10% of body weight, plus either unexplained chronic diarrhoea (>1 month) or chronic weakness and unexplained prolonged fever (>1 month).

Performance scale Developed by the WHO for the staging of HIV infection and AIDS and compatible with the clinical staging system shown in the opposite box.

Performance level

1. Asymptomatic, normal activity
2. Symptomatic, normal activity
3. Bedridden <50% of the day during the last month
4. Bedridden >50% of the day during the last month

Clinical stage 1

- Asymptomatic
- Persistent generalized lymphadenopathy (PGL)

Clinical stage 2

- Weight loss <10% of body weight
- Minor mucocutaneous lesions (seborrhoeic dermatitis, prurigo, fungal nail infections, recurrent oral ulcerations, angular cheilitis)
- Zoster within the last 5 yrs
- Recurrent upper respiratory tract infections (including bacterial sinusitis)

Clinical stage 3

- Weight loss >10% of body weight
- Unexplained chronic diarrhoea for >1 month
- Unexplained prolonged fever (intermittent/constant) for >1 month
- Oral candidiasis (thrush)
- Oral hairy leukoplakia
- Pulmonary tuberculosis within the past year
- Severe bacterial infections (pneumonia, pyomyositis)

Clinical stage 4

- HIV wasting syndrome
- Pneumocystis carinii pneumonia (PCP)
- Toxoplasmosis of the brain
- Cryptosporidiosis with diarrhoea, for >1 month
- Cryptococcosis, extrapulmonary
- Cytomegalovirus (CMV) disease of an organ other than liver, spleen, or lymph nodes
- Herpesvirus infection, mucocutaneous for > 1 month, or visceral of any duration
- Progressive multifocal leukoencephalopathy (PML)
- Any disseminated endemic mycosis
- Candidiasis of the oesophagus, trachea, bronchi, or lungs
- Atypical mycobacteriosis, disseminated
- Non-typhoid salmonella septicaemia
- Extrapulmonary tuberculosis
- Lymphoma
- Kaposi sarcoma
- HIV encephalopathy
- Invasive cervical cancer

Laboratory diagnosis of HIV infection

There are three main purposes for which HIV antibody testing is performed:

1. Transfusion/transplant safety: screening of donated blood and organs to prevent HIV transmission.
2. Surveillance: unlinked and anonymous testing for monitoring the prevalence of, and trends in, HIV infection over time in a given population.
3. Diagnosis of HIV infection: voluntary testing of serum from asymptomatic persons or from persons with clinical signs and symptoms suggestive of HIV infection or AIDS.

The first objective requires extremely sensitive tests that will pick up all contaminated blood/organs and thus prevent them from entering the blood/organ supply. The third objective requires very specific tests so that there are few false positives (i.e. HIV −ve people are not told that they are infected). The second objective requires tests that are sensitive and specific but not to the same degree as the other two objectives.

Diagnostic tests for HIV infection should never be considered as positive, and the patient informed, until they have been confirmed by a second assay.

Counselling

If you decide to offer an HIV test, counselling is essential. Studies indicate that a patient who knows him or herself to be infected will practise safer sexual practices if the HIV testing is accompanied by counselling and if future psychological support is provided.

- **Pre-test counselling:** ensures that the patient understands the purpose of the test and the consequences of a positive result.
- **Post-test counselling:** helps the patient come to terms with a positive result or to encourage HIV-negative individuals to practise low-risk behaviour.

A physician should be able to discuss the diagnosis of HIV infection, the transmission of the virus and its prevention, and the best ways of staying healthy with HIV and of taking care of common HIV/AIDS-related problems.

Clinical presentation and management

A list of the main causes for each manifestation of AIDS, in order of significance, should be established for each country, in light of the available information.

- While opportunistic infections are important causes of disease in patients with AIDS, the infections that are common in HIV-negative patients also tend to be common in HIV-infected patients in the same area. They are often simply more severe and life-threatening in the latter.
- The infections and conditions that are characteristic of patients with AIDS in a certain locality will also occur in other immunosuppressed patients (e.g. those with haematological malignancies).

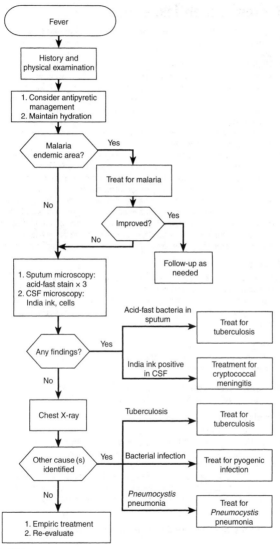

Fig. 2B.1

Systemic manifestations

Always consider TB as a cause of systemic illness in HIV-infected persons. The manifestations of TB in such a person are extremely diverse (see Chapter 2C).

1. **Weight loss** may be the first sign of HIV infection. After treatment for an intercurrent infection, some patients gain weight again but often only for a short time. Accelerated weight loss is a sign of disease progression (some lose up to 40% of their weight and die in extreme cachexia). No specific cause is identified in most patients; however, post-mortem studies have identified TB in many patients.

2. **Weakness and anorexia** are frequently present, but may be absent even at times of great weight loss.

3. **Fever** Hx and Ex first to look for localizing signs (Chapter 3). If these are absent, the fever may be an 'HIV-associated fever'. This is defined as a fever with a duration of >2 weeks as the only clinical presentation in a patient with a prior history of symptomatic HIV infection, or in a known HIV-positive patient with an asymptomatic prior history. The fever is often intermittent and accompanied by night sweats and chills.

However, when resources are limited, the identification of non-HIV aetiologies for fever may sometimes be impossible. Fever due to HIV itself should only be considered after other treatable causes — a diagnosis of last resort.

Aetiology

- **Infections:** bacteria (*Salmonella* spp, *S. pneumoniae*, *H. influenzae*), mycobacteria (TB, atypical mycobacteria), fungus (cryptococcosis, histoplasmosis, *Pneumocystis jiroveci*—previously called *P. carinii*), virus (disseminated CMV, EBV), protozoa (*P. carinii*, *T. gondii*, *Leishmania* spp).
- **HIV** infection itself.
- **Malignancy:** lymphoma.
- **Drugs:** many possibilities.

When no alternative cause for the fever can be found, try discontinuing the patient's drugs one at a time.

4(i) **Lymphadenopathy:** defined as lymph node enlargement in a patient with symptomatic HIV infection.

Aetiology

- HIV infection itself
- Infections — bacterial (TB, syphilis), fungal (histoplasmosis), or viral (CMV)
- Malignancies — lymphadenopathic KS (not necessarily associated with cutaneous KS), lymphoma
- Dermatological conditions — seborrhoeic dermatitis, chronic pyoderma

A careful physical examination should identify any local or contiguous infection that might explain the lymphadenopathy. Infections prevalent in the region concerned should also be considered.

4(ii) **Persistent generalized lymphadenopathy (PGL)** is common in HIV +ve patients and is often due to HIV alone. It is defined as follows:

- More than 3 separate lymph node groups affected
- At least 2 nodes >1.5 cm in diameter at each site

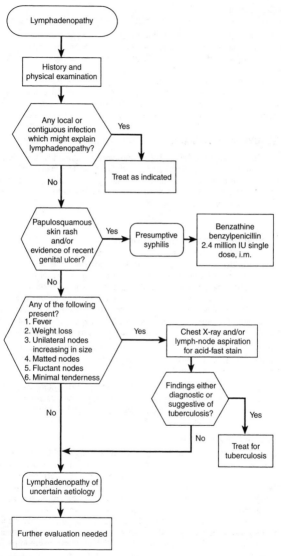

Fig. 2B.2

- Duration of >1 month
- No local or contiguous infection that might explain the lymphadenopathy

It is important to exclude the following treatable causes:
- Syphilis: (papulosquamous rash +/− evidence of recent genital ulcer)
- TB: (suggestive clinical signs → CXR and/or node aspiration for AFB)

If excluded, asymptomatic patients do not need further investigation. However, if nodes are rapidly enlarging, or there is nodal asymmetry or systemic symptoms, a lymph node must be biopsied to exclude lymphoma, lymphadenopathic KS, and infiltrative fungal or mycobacterial disease.

GPA/WHO flowcharts

The flowcharts presented in this section were developed by the Global Programme on AIDS (GPA) of the WHO to aid the management of HIV-infected persons in resource-poor settings with a high incidence of both malaria and TB. Similar flowcharts may be useful for the management of these patients in other settings.

Atypical mycobacterial infection

Non-tuberculous mycobacteria cause disseminated infection or pneumonia in patients with underlying illnesses. However, the prevalence of these diseases has increased markedly since the emergence of AIDS. They are environmental pathogens worldwide, but appear to occur less commonly in Africa compared to other parts of the world. Any of the known pathogenic mycobacteria can cause a febrile illness with weight loss, malaise, and night sweats. Other signs: anaemia, hepatosplenomegaly, lymphadenopathy, and widespread organ involvement particularly the GI tract.

Diagnosis: Ziehl–Neelsen staining of intracellular AFB in biopsies (also sputum, but not necessarily indicative of disease); specialized blood culture — allows differentiation from TB.

Management: clarithromycin 250–500 mg PO bd plus rifabutin 450–600 mg PO od plus ethambutol 15 mg/kg PO od. Therapy improves symptoms; it is not clear if it improves survival. Note that in many regions, the great majority of AFB will be TB.

Cytomegalovirus (CMV)

Most people have been infected by this herpesvirus by the age of 40. In nearly all cases, infection is asymptomatic; <10% have a self-limiting mononucleosis-like illness. In the immunocompromised host, however, it may cause a severe febrile illness with protean manifestations involving multiple organs. Chorioretinitis is the most common manifestation. GI involvement may include colon, oesophagus, and liver; CNS infection is rare. Other organs that may be involved include lungs and adrenal glands. Both lung and bowel involvement can be fatal — the former presents similarly to pneumocystosis; intense inflammation in the latter can result in perforation and peritonitis or haemorrhage. Untreated infection of the retina rapidly produces blindness.

CMV can be isolated from urine and blood from both symptomatic and asymptomatic persons. However, the diagnosis of CMV disease is often based on identification of typical inclusion bodies on histopathological examination, presence of IgM antibody, or seroconversion. The disease in most AIDS patients is a reactivation of a chronic/latent infection. Treatment with antiviral agents, such as ganciclovir or foscarnet, is able to treat disease and prevent reactivation but it is expensive.

Penicilliosis marneffei

A disseminated and progressive fungal infection that is well recognized in immunosuppressed patients in South-East Asia and South China. It may be misdiagnosed as TB or other disseminated fungal infection (histoplasmosis, cryptococcosis) due to its common mode of presentation: fever, anaemia, weight loss, skin lesions, sepsis, and/or lymphadenopathy. Other sites include lungs (painful, non-productive cough; CXR may show abscesses, cavities), liver, spleen; rarely bones, joints.

Diagnosis is via Giemsa stain of bone marrow, lymph node, or skin scraping for yeast-like organisms; serology.

Treatment: amphotericin B IV for 2 weeks followed by itraconazole for 6 weeks. Relapses are common — retreat with amphotericin B or fluconazole.

Side-effects of antiretroviral therapy (ART)

Side-effects may be early or late and can be life-threatening. Drug interactions are common especially with the protease inhibitors. Dose and/or drug modification is required with TB therapy except with nucleoside analogues. Details of drug interactions can be found at *http://www.hiv-druginteractions.org/*

Severe ART toxicities	Most likely candidates
Anaemia/neutropenia	Zidovudine (especially with co-trimoxazole)
Neuropathy	Stavudine, zalcitabine, didanosine (avoid stavudine plus INH)
Pancreatitis	Zalcitabine, didanosine
Hepatic steatosis	Stavudine, didanosine — avoid these together
Lactic acidosis	Stavudine, didanosine — in pregnancy
Hypersensitivity	Abacavir: life-threatening, don't rechallenge
Stevens–Johnson syndrome	Nevirapine
Hepatitis	Nevirapine
Psychiatric	Efavirenz
Nephrolithiasis	Indinavir
Diarrhoea	Protease inhibitors
Hyperlipidaemia	Protease inhibitors — excluding saquinavir
Lipoatrophy	Nucleoside analogues, stavudine >zidovudine
Lipodystrophy/insulin resistance	Protease inhibitors

Antiretroviral therapy (ART)

Treatment aims to allow immune (CD4 lymphocyte) reconstitution by limiting HIV-1 replication to very low levels. Inadequate ART results in the emergence of viral strains with reduced drug sensitivity. Three or four compounds are usually required. Strict adherence to therapy is essential. Treatment is lifelong and expensive.

- Monotherapy with zidovudine or nevirapine reduces mother-to-child transmission of HIV-1 infection. Zidovudine can be useful in HIV-associated thrombocytopenia.
- Dual therapy has been shown to reduce morbidity and mortality but is less effective than triple therapy and results in the emergence of resistant viral strains.
- Triple therapy results in suppression of viral replication to below detectable levels in >80% of adult patients. The duration of response to the first regime can be longer than 5 years.

Second- and third-line therapy will successfully re-suppress viral replication in the majority of patients. Viral sequences determined on or shortly after discontinuing therapy can help select the best options but are very expensive and not widely available.

Currently licensed therapies inhibit two HIV enzymes: reverse transcriptase (RT) and protease. Two nucleoside analogues with either a non-nucleoside RT inhibitor or a protease inhibitor (PI), or three nucleoside analogues are most commonly prescribed. Optimal first-line therapy has not been determined. ART combinations which include either an NNRTI or a PI triple are generally superior to nucleoside/tide combinations. Choice will be determined by availability including cost and acceptability (including adherence issues and toxicity). The use of a small dose of ritonavir to 'boost' other PI concentrations has significantly improved the pharmacokinetic profile of PIs.

Starting therapy. The optimum time to start therapy is patient dependent. AIDS-defining illness (except TB) is uncommon with CD4 lymphocytes count above 200/ul whole blood.

Prior to starting ART, the CD4 lymphocyte count is the best monitor. An initial viral load (HIV-1 RNA copies/ml plasma) is useful to predict CD4 decline. Viral load is the best assay to monitor therapy. If the viral load is undetectable, CD4 lymphocyte counts rarely alter management except to discontinue prophylaxis for opportunistic infections.

Treatment failure. Can be virological (virus detected in plasma repeatedly), immunological (CD4 decline), or clinical (morbidity). Virological failure by itself is not an indication to change or discontinue therapy. Patients on ART have lower morbidity and mortality than matched untreated patients. Clinical failure may not reflect virological failure.

Adult dose recommendations for ART

Reverse transcriptase inhibitors	Food restrictions
1. Nucleoside analogues	
• Zidovudine 250–300 mg bd	
• Lamivudine 150 mg bd	
• Stavudine 40 mg bd (>60 kg), 30 mg bd (<60 kg)	
• Didanosine EC 400 mg od (>60 kg), 250 mg od (<60 kg)	Empty stomach
• Abacavir 300 mg bd	
• Zalcitibine 0.75 mg tds (toxic, now rarely prescribed)	
2. Nucleotide analogue	
• Tenofovir 245 mg od	With food
3. Non-nucleoside analogues	
• Nevirapine 200 mg bd (od for first 2 weeks)	
• Efavirenz 600 mg od	
4. Protease inhibitors	
• Ritonavir 600 mg bd	With/after food
• Indinavir 800 mg tds	Water ± low-fat meal
• Saquinavir 1200 mg tds	With food
• Nelfinavir 1250 mg bd	With food
• Amprenavir capsules 1200 mg bd	
5. Boosted protease inhibitor regimen	
• Saquinavir 1000 mg + ritonavir 100 mg bd	
• Lopinavir 400 mg + ritonavir 100 mg bd	With food
• Indinavir 800 mg + ritonavir 100 mg bd	
• Amprenavir 600 mg + ritonavir 100–200 mg bd	
6. Fixed-dose combinations	
• Combivir® (zidovudine 300 mg + lamivudine 150 mg) 1 bd	
• Trizivir® (zidovudine 300 mg + lamivudine 150 mg + abacavir 300 mg) 1 bd	
• Kaletra® (lopinavir 133.3 mg + ritonavir 33.3 mg) 3 bd	

Cutaneous manifestations

Many people with HIV have cutaneous manifestations (see box), some of which are fairly specific for AIDS. Others are non-specific and may be signs of systemic disease — biopsy and scraping are required for a diagnosis. The skin of AIDS patients often becomes dry and atrophic, and the hair becomes thinner, losing its colour.

A generalized papular pruritic reaction occurs in many African HIV +ve patients, often as a first sign of infection. In certain high-risk groups, it is quite specific for HIV infection. The cause is not known. Papules, scratch marks, and hyperpigmented macules are symmetrically distributed over the body, particularly the extensor arm surfaces, back of the hands, ankles, and dorsum of the feet. They last throughout the patient's illness.

Kaposi sarcoma (KS)

A tumour of endothelial cells, caused by the Kaposi sarcoma-associated virus (KSAV or HHV-8; a sexually-transmitted herpesvirus), that presents with lesions of the skin and in many cases the viscera. Two other forms are recognized: classic KS (in equatorial Africa) that is slowly progressive in adults (aggressive in children/adolescents) and limited to one anatomical region, particularly the feet; and an indolent skin tumour of elderly men in the USA and elsewhere.

Clinical features: the multiple lesions are nodular and pigmented, appearing black on black skin and purple on pale skin. Early lesions, being small, macular, and erythematous, are often difficult to recognize. While mostly asymptomatic, especially at first, the lesions may become infiltrated or ulcerate. They occur on all parts of the body, not just the skin, and are rarely limited to one anatomical region. Lesions on the face, soles, and in the oral cavity are common. Visceral disease may occur without skin involvement — the only visible lesion may be in the oral cavity. Oral lesions (a) are often not raised and (b) may result in bleeding, pain, and dysphagia. KS commonly involves lymph nodes (producing lymphoedema), GI tract (mostly stomach, duodenum, rectum; rarely resulting in intestinal obstruction, bleeding) and lungs (dyspnoea, cough, chest tightness, bronchoconstriction; rarely fever). However, any organ may be involved.

Diagnosis: can be made clinically in most cases; a punch biopsy otherwise shows characteristic histology (biopsy very rarely leads to haemorrhage).

Management: the clinical course of KS is often indolent, patients normally dying from intercurrent infections. However, pulmonary KS can be rapidly fatal. The lesions may respond to chemotherapy; relapse is common. Local treatment such as surgical excision, radiation, or topical liquid nitrogen can be used for individual lesions on the face or in the mouth. Combination ART is, where affordable, the first line of therapy particularly for cutaneous KS.

Cutaneous manifestations of AIDS

Neoplasia	Kaposi sarcoma	Non-Hodgkin's lymphoma
	Squamous cell CA	Basal cell CA
Infections	Herpes zoster	Herpesvirus infections
	Superficial fungal infections	Angular cheilitis
	Chancroid	Cryptococcosis
	Histoplasmosis	Human papillomavirus
	Impetigo	Lymphogranuloma venereum
	Molluscum contagiosum	Mycobacterial infection
	Syphilis	Furunculosis
	Folliculitis	Pyomyositis
Others	Pruritic papular dermatitis	Seborrhoeic dermatitis
	Drug eruptions	Vasculitis
	Xeroderma	Psoriasis
	Granuloma annulare	Thrombocytic purpura
	Telangiectasia	Hyperpigmentation
	Dry atrophic skin	Hair changes

Gastrointestinal (GI) manifestations

Studies of AIDS patients in different parts of the world have begun to identify the most common causes of GI disease. It is becoming clear that these differ between regions (e.g. *Cryptosporidium* spp and CMV are the most common gut pathogens in parts of Africa and in India, respectively). Further studies should help define the most common causes of the GI signs and symptoms in each region, with clear advantages for treatment when diagnostic work-up is limited.

1. **Chronic diarrhoea:** defined as 'liquid stools 3 or more times per day, continuously or episodically for >1 month, in a patient with symptomatic HIV infection'.

Aetiology: although the cause is often not identified, possibilities include:
- Infections — cryptosporidiosis, *Isospora belli*, *Giardia lamblia*, *Salmonella* spp, *Shigella flexneri*, *Campylobacter* spp., *Entamoeba histolytica*, CMV, *Strongyloides stercoralis*, atypical mycobacteria.
- Malignancies — KS, lymphoma.
- Idiopathic (possibly HIV infection).

2. **Colitis:** may present with severe abdominal cramps and distension, rebound tenderness, and megacolon. Watery diarrhoea (+/− blood) is common. The cause is often not identified; possibilities include CMV and ulcerative KS.

3. **Dysphagia:** commonest cause is treatable oesophageal candidiasis; other causes include CMV and herpes virus.

Oesophageal candidiasis: anyone with weight loss and dysphagia due to oral candidiasis requires treatment with fluconazole (50–100 mg PO od for 14–30 days or, if required, 400 mg IV on day 1, then 200 mg IV until clinical response). Recurrence is common after stopping antifungals. Diagnosis is presumed if patient with oral candida complains of dysphagia. Imaging or endoscopy of the oesophagus is only required if treatment with fluconazole is ineffective.

4. **Perianal discomfort:** anogenital ulcerations are caused by herpes viruses, *T. pallidum* and *H. ducreyi*; perianal warts by human papillomavirus.

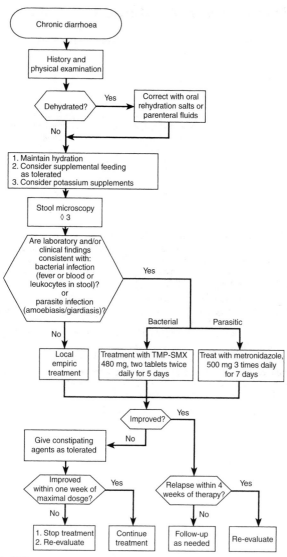

Fig. 2B.3

Respiratory manifestations

Persistent or worsening cough, chest pain, dyspnoea, cyanosis, or tachypnoea

Aetiology:
- **Infections**   TB — see Chapter **2C**
  PCP
  Bacterial pneumonia (*S. pneumoniae*) — see Chapter **2E**
  Also fungal infections (cryptococcus, histoplasmosis, coccidioido-mycosis), atypical mycobacteria, CMV, toxoplasmosis, *Nocardia asteroides*, *Candida albicans*, *Legionella pneumophila*
- Malignancies — KS, lymphoma
- Others — lymphoid interstitial pneumonitis (rare in adults)

These may be exacerbated by
- Pleural effusion/empyema (TB, bacterial infection, or cancer)
- Pneumothorax (TB, PCP, or cancer)
- Pericardial effusion (TB)

Histoplasmosis and coccidioidomycosis

Although these fungi are normally local infections of the lung (see p. 304), they can cause disseminated disease in AIDS patients. Early signs are non-specific or pulmonary, including: cough, fever, malaise, weight loss, and interstitial infiltrates on CXR. D&V may occur.

Management: haematogenous spread may result in rapid deterioration, so therapy should be started in severe cases on clinical suspicion (+/– the presence of serum antibody). Give:
1. Amphotericin B 0.5–1 mg/kg IV od for 6 weeks (to a maximum total of 3 g), then
2. Amphotericin B 0.5 mg/kg IV at weekly intervals to prevent relapse.

Mild cases, or those unable to tolerate amphotericin, can be treated with:
- Itraconazole 200 mg PO tds for 3–4 days, then 200 mg for 6 weeks *or*
- Fluconazole 400 mg PO/IV od for 6 weeks

Maintenance: itraconazole 200 mg PO bd for life.

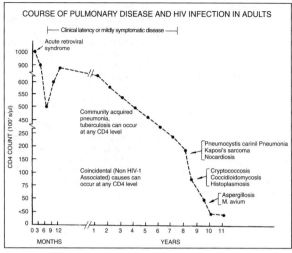

Fig. 2B.4

Pneumocystosis

The causative organism, *Pneumocystis jiroveci,* formerly *P. carinii*, is a ubiquitous microbe and does not cause disease in the immunocompetent. It is a common cause of pneumonia (*Pneumocystis* pneumonia — PCP) in adult AIDS patients, except in Africa where it occurs in HIV +ve infants. In contrast, in Brazilian and Thai AIDS patients, *Pneumocystis carinii* is common. Respiratory failure results from a fibrotic reaction caused by fungal multiplication in the alveolar septal walls throughout the lungs.

Clinical features: are initially insidious and easily missed (a few have a fulminant infection). Include dyspnoea and non-productive cough; rarely, mild pleuritic chest pain. Auscultation reveals rales and wheeze only at an advanced stage. Similarly, early CXR may be normal; later they show bilateral interstitial and alveolar infiltrates in middle and lower zones, usually with peripheral sparing. Cavities may form. Severe clinical symptoms in the absence of findings on examination or CXR is highly suggestive of PCP. Extrapulmonary infection has been reported. Pneumothorax can be a life-threatening complication.

Diagnosis: pneumocystosis is strongly suspected in a patient who does not have TB but has bilateral pulmonary infiltrates resistant to antimicrobials. Examination of Silver stained lavage from bronchoscopy is the ideal investigation. When bronchoscopy is not available, non-invasive induced sputum method has proved sensitive — stain sputum after inhalation of 3% nebulized saline.

Management:

1. Co-trimoxazole 100–120 mg/kg/day IV/P0 in 2–4 divided doses, *or* pentamidine isethionate 4 mg/kg IV od. Both regimens for 21 days.
2. If the patient is **cyanosed**, the simultaneous administration of corticosteroids decreases risk of death. Give:
   - Prednisolone 40 mg bd for 5 days, *followed by*
   - 40 mg od for 5 days, *then*
   - 20 mg od for 10 days.
   Alternatively, give methylprednisolone IV.
3. 2° chemoprophylaxis:
   - Co-trimoxazole 960 mg PO od, *or*
   - Dapsone 100 mg PO od, *or*
   - Pentamidine isethionate 300 mg by aerosol every 4wks.
   All regimens for life unless CD4 persistently >200 cells/ul on combination ART.
4. Primary chemoprophylaxis: in regions where PCP is a significant clinical problem, prophylactic treatment (Co-trimoxazole 480 mg PO OD) should be started for all patients with symptomatic HIV infection or CD4 counts <200/ul.

Neurological manifestations

1. **Headache:** defined as a headache in a patient with symptomatic HIV infection, often persistent or severe, and rapidly increasing or not responding to common drugs used for pain relief. It can be with or without fever.

Aetiology
- Infections — chronic meningitis due to tuberculosis, cryptococcus, or chronic HIV infection; rarely meningoencephalitis due to *Toxoplasma* or viruses (e.g. CMV)
- Malignancies — lymphoma
- Drug side-effects — zidovudine

Causes of headache (see p. 398) not related to HIV infection, particularly malaria, and bacterial meningitis, should be identified and treated.

2. Progressive behaviour changes and dementia (subacute AIDS encephalopathy)

Cognitive dysfunction may be common in AIDS patients. It has an insidious onset; signs/symptoms include:
- Loss of concentration and recent memory
- Mental slowing
- Motor signs such as tremor and slowness
- Apathy
- Social withdrawal
- Unco-ordination

In time, it progresses to: severe dementia, mutism, incontinence, paraplegia.

This condition appears to be due to direct HIV infection of the CNS — no association has been found between this condition and opportunistic infections. However, progressive multifocal leukoencephalopathy (see p. 66) can cause similar signs.

3. **Meningism:** acute HIV infection may cause signs of meningism. If chronic, it is likely to be due to cryptococcus or tuberculosis.

4. **Visual impairment:** commonly due to CMV infection or toxoplasmosis.

5. **Focal neurological signs including seizures:** most commonly due to *T. gondii* or B-cell lymphoma. Candida, cryptococcus, and mycobacteria also cause space-occupying lesions in the CNS.

6. **Peripheral neuropathy (see p. 440):** due to HIV, other viruses, vasculitis, compression by a lymphoma, alcohol, and increasingly by drug therapy (isoniazid, antiretrovirals).

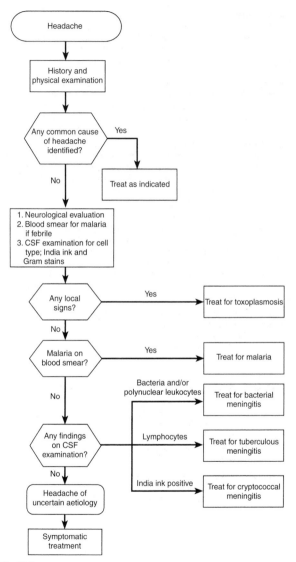

Fig. 2B.5

Toxoplasmosis

Infection by *Toxoplasma gondii*, an obligate intracellular parasite, is a common infection of normal adults that is normally asymptomatic but may rarely result in a mononucleosis-like syndrome. Primary infection of women in the early stages of pregnancy results in fetal infection and serious congenital malformations.

Following acute infection, a latent infection ensues that may become reactivated in immunocompromised patients. In this situation, toxoplasmosis is a serious disease, primarily of the brain but also involving lungs, heart, and chorioretina. Focal *Toxoplasma* encephalitis with brain abscesses is a common manifestation in AIDS; a rarer diffuse form is rapidly fatal.

Transmission: via licking fingers or eating food (incl. vegetables) contaminated with oocytes from cat faeces or ingesting tissue cysts in undercooked meat from domesticated animals. Infection occurs in multiple animal species but the cat appears to be the definitive host. Mother to fetus transmission occurs in humans but there is little evidence of other human-to-human transmission.

Clinical features: if symptomatic, a primary infection presents as a mononucleosis with discrete, non-tender lymphadenopathy without suppuration. After reactivation in an immunosuppressed patient, subacute CNS disease can occur, presenting with focal brain signs: commonly hemiparesis, speech abnormalities, cranial nerve lesions, altered higher function, coma. Diffuse cerebral involvement presents with generalized CNS dysfunction without focal signs. Pneumonitis manifests as fever with cough and dyspnoea; chorioretinitis is uncommon.

Diagnosis: isolation of toxoplasma from blood/body fluids during acute infection; demonstration of tissue cysts in Giemsa-stained tissue sections or centrifuged body fluids; characteristic lymph node histology (reactive follicular hyperplasia, epithelioid histocytes blurring germinal centre margins, focal cellular distension of sinuses); serology.

Management:
- Pyrimethamine 200 mg PO in divided doses on day 1, then 75–100 mg PO od, *plus*
- Sulfadiazine 1–1.5g PO qds, *plus*
- Calcium folinate 3–5 mg PO every 3rd day
All for at least 6 weeks.

Maintenance therapy: pyrimethamine 25–50 mg PO daily and sulfadiazine 0.5–1 g qds daily for life.

Prevention: pregnant women and immunocompromised people should be warned not to eat undercooked meat and to take care of personal hygiene when in contact with domestic cats. Chemical prophylaxis with co-trimoxazole may be of value.

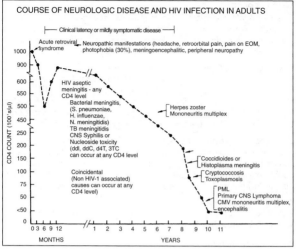

Fig. 2B.6

Cryptococcosis

This fungal infection often presents in AIDS patients as a subtle chronic meningitis. Rarely, it may manifest as fulminant disease with extraneural involvement. It is ubiquitous in the environment and therefore exposure is presumed to be common; overt infection is rare in the immunocompetent.

Early clinical features: include low-grade fever, headache, weight loss; neck stiffness occurs later with N&V +/– photophobia. If untreated, confusion and coma ensure. Focal signs are rare. CSF is clear; WBC may be absent or there may be a few PMN. Other sites: lungs (pneumonia gives high mortality), skin (non-specific lesions often painless on face/scalp; may be first sign), bone, GI tract. Blood WCC is generally unchanged.

Diagnosis: add 1 drop of sediment from >3 ml CSF to 1 drop India ink, mix and smear onto a slide under a coverslip (if correctly made, newsprint should be readable through it). Search the whole slide for cryptococci: double refractile cell wall, distinctly outlined capsule, refractile intracytoplasmic inclusions. Others: antigen in serum/CSF; fungal culture.

Management: suggested regimens:
- Amphotericin B 0.25 mg/kg IV, increasing to 1 mg/kg od, for 6 weeks, *plus*
- Flucytosine 50 mg/kg IV qds for 2 weeks

Maintenance therapy:
- Fluconazole 200 mg PO od for life.

Progressive multifocal leukoencephalopathy (PML)

This is caused by the JC polyomavirus and presents with altered mental status and/or limb weakness. Autopsy shows patchy areas of demyelination and necrosis, which show up as pale areas on a CT scan.

Diagnosis: Detection of JC virus in CSF by PCR.

Clinical course: is often indolent; patients normally die of other infections.

Management of the HIV +ve asymptomatic person

This involves both counselling and medical care.

Counselling

The general purpose is to promote and maintain the maximum possible level of psychological and physical health among infected people, their partners and relatives, their caregivers, and others who see themselves at risk of HIV infection. It has two particular aims:

- To support the ability of infected persons and those who care for them to cope with the stresses of HIV/AIDS
- To prevent the transmission of HIV to others

Medical management of asymptomatic persons with HIV has the following aims:

- Early detection of HIV-associated disease and treatment
- Primary prophylaxis when indicated
- Determination of the appropriate time to start antiretroviral therapy

Knowledge of the degree of immune deficiency by CD4 count assists in (i) interpretation of symptoms and determining when to initiate (ii) primary prophylaxis and (iii) antiretroviral therapy. Frequency of visits should increase as CD4 count falls. Where this is not practical, priority should be given to regular follow-up in clinic (e.g. q6m) with only minimal laboratory investigations (e.g. Hb, total WCC). Total lymphocyte count fluctuates greatly due to concurrent infections — it is only a crude guide to CD4 status and degree of immune deficiency. CD4 count is the best indicator of the immediate prognosis. Rate of CD4 decline indicates longer term prognosis. Viral RNA measurements prior to therapy add very little to management. Viral RNA load on treatment indicates a successful or failing ART regimen, and hence whether the CD4 count will rise or fall.

History: check for

- Fever
- Anorexia
- Cough
- Pruritus
- Night sweats
- Dysphagia
- Odynophagia
- Seizures
- Diffuse lymphadenopathy
- Weight loss
- Diarrhoea
- Worsening headache
- Visual symptoms
- Skin rash

Ask specifically about current medication.

Physical examination: should cover the following:
- **General:** weight loss, fever
- **Neurological system:** peripheral neuropathy, cognitive disorders
- **Skin changes:** herpes zoster, herpes simplex, folliculitis, tinea, KS, pruritus, seborrhoeic dermatitis, severe psoriasis
- **Oral cavity:** thrush, hairy leukoplakia, gingivitis, KS, lymphoma
- **Eyes:** perform a fundoscopy
- **Lymph nodes:** look for focal or diffuse enlargement
- **Lungs:** check for consolidation and crepitations
- **Abdominal examination:** hepatosplenomegaly
- **Genitalia:** chancre, ulcers
- **Anus:** ulcers, warts

Laboratory investigations and X-ray: in areas with limited resources, lab tests can be limited to Hb and total WCC. However, these investigations may be considered:
1. Tests to assess degree of immunodeficiency
- Total lymphocyte count (poor marker)
- CD4 lymphocyte count and percentage
- Plasma viral RNA (if on ART)
2. Tests to assess potential infection
- Serology: toxoplasmosis, CMV, syphilis, hepatitis B
- Tuberculin skin test (reduces with increasing immunosuppression)
- Complete blood count
- Liver function tests
- Chest X-ray

Drug therapy: primary prophylaxis and administration of vaccines is valuable. Local prevalence of the following infections will determine whether primary prophylaxis or vaccination should be offered:
- TB
- PCP
- Toxoplasmosis
- Pneumococcal pneumonia

Prevention and control

In the absence of either widely available antiretroviral drugs or vaccine, primary prevention is the only method of controlling the AIDS pandemic. Strategies to control HIV infection should be aimed at the main methods of transmission: sexual, parenteral, and vertical.

Sexual

Changing high-risk sexual behaviour through health education could have a major effect on sexual HIV transmission. It would also have a marked effect on STI transmission. Creative educational approaches, respecting cultural traditions, are necessary to make the population aware of the dangers of HIV infection and AIDS and to encourage protective measures. Several governments have now initiated such health education programmes. However, these programmes will have to be accompanied by approaches that influence the social and environmental determinants of risk to enable those vulnerable to infection to protect themselves.

Blood transfusion

Screening of blood donations for HIV antibody may result in high benefit-to-cost ratio for the prevention of AIDS in populations with a high infection rate. Drawbacks are cost, logistics, and the lack of detectable HIV antibodies for 3–6 weeks (with 3rd generation ELISAs) after infection in some persons. Efforts to identify and exclude high-risk donors have proven to be difficult, but they may be important in decreasing the risk of HIV +ve, sero-negative persons donating blood.

Injections

Prevention of infection through contaminated needles is feasible with the use of universal precautions. However, the use of disposable needles and syringes may be prohibitively expensive for some countries and health workers should be trained to give as few injections as possible and to sterilize reusable equipment. The risk from infected needlestick injuries to health workers appears to be very low — about 0.5% of persons receiving needlestick injuries with body fluids from an HIV-infected person become infected.

Vertical

Most importantly this involves the prevention of HIV infection in women of childbearing age, and advice on contraception to HIV +ve women. The WHO recommends that breastfeeding should remain the standard advice to pregnant women, including those known to be HIV +ve, where the 1° causes of infant deaths are infectious disease and malnutrition. Where this is not the case, HIV +ve women are advised not to breastfeed but to use a safe feeding alternative for their babies. Nevirapine, 200 mg orally given to the mother at delivery and 2 mg/kg given to the neonate within 72 hours, is safe and effective in reducing perinatal mother-to-child transmission of HIV. Single dose nevirapine often causes nevirapine resistance virus mutations. This impairs the future response to nevirapine-containing ART. Thus if combination ART is intended for mothers or children post-partum, combination ART should be used ante-partum to reduce mother-to-child transmission. If ART is stopped post delivery, continue the nRTIs for 5–10 days after stopping nevirapine, because of the long half-life of nevirapine.

Symptomatic management of STIs

Urethral discharge

Male patients complaining of urethral discharge and/or dysuria should be examined for evidence of discharge. If none is seen, gently massage the urethra from the ventral part of the penis towards the meatus. If microscopy is available, a urethral specimen should be collected — a Gram-stained urethral smear showing more than 5 PMNs per field (×1000) in areas of maximal cellular concentration is indicative of urethritis.

The major pathogens causing urethral discharge are:
- *Neisseria gonorrhoeae*
- *Chlamydia trachomatis*

Unless a diagnosis of gonorrhoea can be definitively excluded by laboratory tests, the treatment of the patient with urethral discharge should provide adequate coverage of these two organisms.

Recommended treatment regimens
- Therapy for uncomplicated gonorrhoea (see p. 91) *plus*
- Therapy for uncomplicated chlamydia (see p. 93)

Alternative regimen when tetracyclines are contraindicated or not tolerated
- Therapy for uncomplicated gonorrhoea (see p. 91) *plus*
- Erythromycin 500 mg PO qds

Alternative regimen where single-dose therapy for gonorrhoea is not available
- Co-trimoxazole 480 mg 10 tablets PO od for 3 days *plus*
- Doxycycline 100 mg PO bd *or* tetracycline 500 mg PO qds both for 7 days

This can only be used in areas where co-trimoxazole has been shown to be effective against uncomplicated gonorrhoea.

Follow-up
Patients should be advised to return if symptoms persist 7 days after start of therapy. Persistent or recurrent symptoms may be due to poor compliance, reinfection, infection with a resistant strain of *N. gonorrhoeae*, or infection with *T. vaginalis*. Where symptoms persist or recur after adequate treatment of the index patient and partner(s), both (or all) should be referred for laboratory investigation. The investigation should include a Gram stain to confirm the presence of urethritis and to look for *N. gonorrhoeae*. *T vaginalis* may be identified by microscopic investigation of a first voided urine sample, although this test has a fairly low sensitivity as compared to culture. If the presence of *T vaginalis* is confirmed, treat as per p. 96.

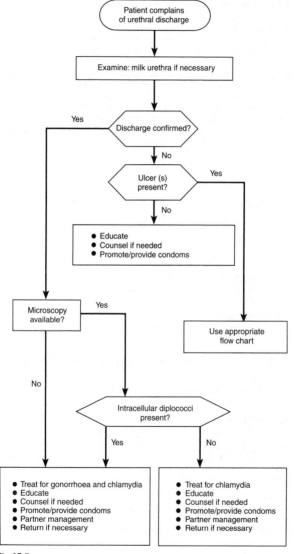

Fig. 2B.7

Genital ulcers

The frequency with which genital ulcers are caused by specific organisms varies dramatically in different parts of the world. Clinical differential diagnosis of genital ulcers is inaccurate, particularly in settings where several aetiologies are common. Clinical manifestations may be further altered in the presence of HIV infection.

After examination to confirm the presence of genital ulceration, treatment appropriate to local aetiologies and antibiotic sensitivity patterns should be given. For example, in areas where both syphilis and chancroid are prevalent, treat patients with genital ulcers for both conditions at the time of initial presentation to ensure adequate treatment in case of loss to follow-up. In areas where granuloma inguinale or LGV are prevalent, treatment for these conditions should be included.

Laboratory-assisted differential diagnosis is rarely helpful at the initial visit, and mixed infections are common. For instance, in areas of high syphilis incidence, a reactive serological test may reflect a previous infection and give a misleading picture of the patient's present condition.

Causes of genital ulcers: syphilis, chancroid, granuloma inguinale, LGV, HSV, scabies, drug reactions, Behcet's disease, carcinoma.

Note that a finding of vesicles or small ulcers, with a history of recurrent vesicles, suggests herpes simplex infection (see p. 97)

Recommended regimen
- Therapy for syphilis (see p. 87) *plus*
- Therapy for chancroid (see p. 95) *or*
- Therapy for granuloma inguinale (see p. 95) *or*
- Therapy for LGV (see p. 93)

Genital ulcer and HIV infection
In HIV-infected patients, prolonged courses of treatment may be necessary for chancroid. Moreover, where HIV is prevalent, an increasing proportion of cases of genital ulcer are likely to harbour herpes simplex virus. Herpetic ulcers may be atypical and persist for long periods in HIV-infected patients.

Follow-up
Patients with genital ulcers should be followed up weekly until the ulceration shows signs of healing.

Inguinal bubo

Inguinal bubo — an enlargement of the lymph nodes in the groin area — is rarely the sole manifestation of an STI and is usually found together with other genital ulcer diseases. Non-sexually transmitted local and systemic infections (e.g. lower limb infections) can cause swelling of the inguinal lymph nodes.

Recommended regimen
- Ciprofloxacin 500 mg PO bd for 3 days *plus either*
- Doxycycline 100 mg PO bd for 14 days *or*
- Erythromycin 500 mg PO qds for 14 days.

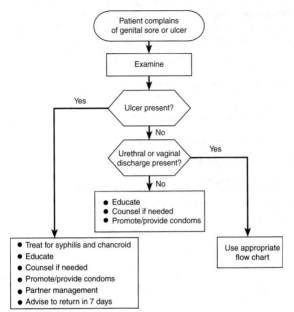

Fig. 2B.8

Scrotal swelling

Scrotal swelling can be caused by trauma, tumour, torsion of the testis, or epididymitis. Inflammation of the epididymis is usually accompanied by pain, oedema, and erythema, and sometimes by urethral discharge, dysuria, and/or frequency. The adjacent testis is often inflamed (orchitis), producing epididymoorchitis.

Sudden onset of unilateral swollen scrotum may be due to trauma or testicular torsion and requires immediate referral. The testis will be irreversibly damaged within 6 hrs — see below.

When not treated effectively, STI-related epididymitis may lead to infertility.

The most important causative agents are:

- Neisseria gonorrhoeae
- Chlamydia trachomatis

Recommended regimen

- Therapy for uncomplicated gonorrhoea (see p. 91) *plus*
- Therapy for chlamydia (see p. 93)

Adjuvants to therapy

Bed rest and scrotal elevation until local inflammation and fever subside.

Torsion of the testicle

The aim is to recognize this condition before the cardinal signs and symptoms are fully manifest, as a torted testis will survive for only about 6 hrs. If in any doubt, surgical exploration is required. It is more common in 15–30 year-olds, but may occur at any age.

Clinical features: sudden onset of pain in one testis, making walking very uncomfortable. Abdominal pain and N&V are common. Lifting or supporting the testis does not ease the pain (as it classically does in epididymitis). The testis is hot, swollen, and tender.

Differential diagnosis: includes epididymitis (tends to occur in older patients, with slower onset and symptoms of UTI), tumour, trauma, acute hydrocele.

Treatment: ask for consent for a possible orchidectomy (removal of the testis) and bilateral fixation (orchidopexy) before surgery to untwist the testis.

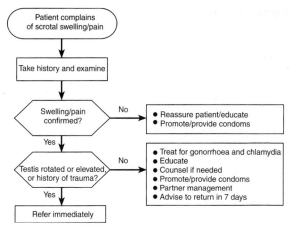

Fig. 2B.9

Vaginal discharge

Vaginal discharge is most commonly caused by vaginitis, but may also be the result of cervicitis.

Cervicitis is caused by
- Neisseria gonorrhoeae
- Chlamydia trachomatis

Vaginitis is caused by
- *Trichomonas vaginalis*
- *Candida albicans*
- *Gardnerella* spp *plus* anaerobic bacterial infection

Non-infectious causes of vaginal discharge (e.g. neoplasia, oestrogen deficiency, foreign body) often have a slower onset. Any form of immunosuppression, such as diabetes or AIDS, will predispose to *C. albicans* infection.

Effective management of cervicitis is more important from a public health point of view. However, it is often difficult to clinically distinguish between vaginitis and cervicitis. The symptom of vaginal discharge is neither sensitive nor specific for either condition. Recent studies suggest that an assessment of the woman's risk status helps greatly in making a diagnosis of cervicitis, but further evaluation of the following three flowcharts (see Figs. 2B.10–2B.12) is needed, particularly with regard to risk factors, which will vary from country to country. The risk factors listed below need to be adapted to the local situation.

Where it is not possible to differentiate between cervicitis and vaginitis, and risk assessment is positive, patients should be treated for both.

Recommended regimens

Cervicitis
- Therapy for uncomplicated gonorrhoea (see p. 91) *plus*
- Therapy for chlamydia (see p. 93).

Vaginitis
- Therapy for bacterial vaginosis (see p. 96) *and*
- Therapy for *Trichomonas vaginalis* (see p. 96) *and, where indicated*
- Therapy for *Candida albicans* (see p. 97).

WHO suggested risk factors

Either partner is symptomatic
Or two of: 1. age <21
　　　　　　　　2. single
　　　　　　　　3. >1 partner
　　　　　　　　4. new partner in last 3 months

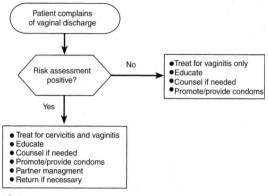

Fig. 2B.10

Locally derived risk factors

Either partner is symptomatic
Or two of: 1.
                2.
                3.
                4.

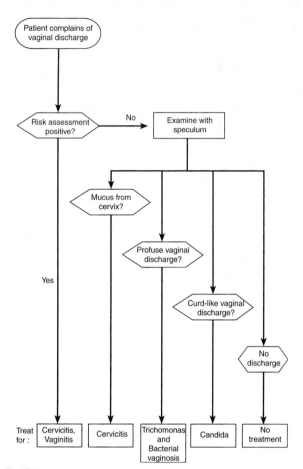

Fig. 2B.11

For all patients:	**For all infected patients:**
• Educate	• Manage partners
• Promote/provide condoms	• Organize follow-up
• Counsel	

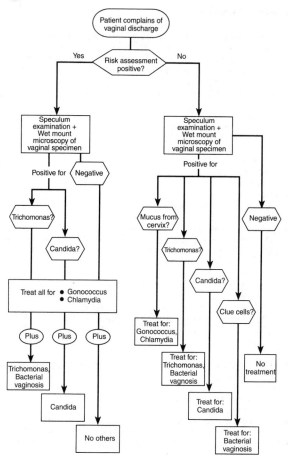

Fig. 2B.12

For all patients:
- Educate
- Promote/provide condoms
- Counsel

For all infected patients:
- Manage partners
- Organize follow-up

Lower abdominal pain

All sexually active women presenting with lower abdominal pain should be carefully evaluated for the presence of salpingitis (pelvic inflammatory disease — PID) and/or endometriosis. In addition, routine bimanual and abdominal examinations should be carried out on all women with a presumptive STI since some women with PID or endometriosis will not complain of lower abdominal pain.

Women with endometriosis may present with complaints of.:
- Vaginal discharge
- Bleeding
- Uterine tenderness on pelvic examination.
  Symptoms suggestive of PID include:
- Abdominal pain
- Dyspareunia
- Vaginal discharge
- Menorrhagia
- Dysuria
- Pain associated with menses
- Fever
- Nausea and vomiting

PID is difficult to diagnose because clinical manifestations are varied. PID becomes highly probable when one or more of the above symptoms are manifested in a woman with adnexal tenderness, evidence of lower genital tract infection, and cervical motion tenderness. Enlargement or induration of one or both fallopian tubes, tender pelvic mass, and direct or rebound tenderness may also be present. The patient's temperature may be elevated but is normal in most cases. In general, clinicians should err on the side of over-diagnosing and treating milder cases.

Hospitalization of patients with acute PID should be seriously considered when:
- The diagnosis is uncertain
- Surgical emergencies such as appendicitis and ectopic pregnancies have to be excluded
- A pelvic abscess is suspected
- Severe illness precludes management on an outpatient basis
- The patient is pregnant
- The patient is unable to follow or tolerate an outpatient regimen
- The patient has failed to respond to an outpatient regimen
- Clinical follow-up 72 hrs after the start of antibiotic therapy cannot be guaranteed.

Many experts recommend that all patients with PID should be admitted to hospital for treatment.

PID is caused by:
- N. gonorrhoeae
- C. trachomatis
- Anaerobic bacteria (Bacteriodes spp, G +ve cocci)
- (Gram-negative rods)
- (Mycoplasma hominis)

Since it is difficult to clinically differentiate between these organisms, therapy should be effective against all.

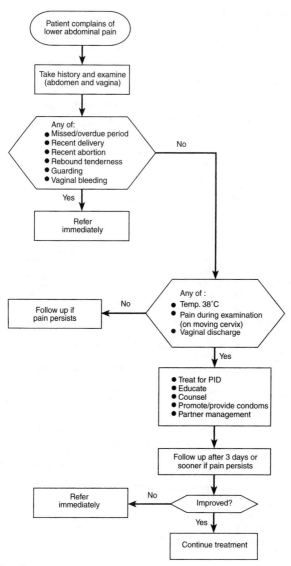

Fig. 2B.13

Inpatient therapy
Recommended regimens — use one of.
1. Ceftriaxone 250 mg IM od *plus*
   Doxycycline 100 mg PO/IV bd *or* tetracycline 500 mg PO qds *plus*
   Metronidazole 400–500 mg PO/IV bd *or* chloramphenicol 500 mg
   PO/IV qds
2. Clindamycin 900 mg IV q8h *plus*
   Gentamicin 1.5 mg/kg IV q8h
3. Ciprofloxacin 500 mg PO bd *or* spectinomycin 1 g IM qds *plus*
   Doxycycline 100 mg PO/IV bd *or* tetracycline 500 mg PO qds *plus*
   Metronidazole 400–500 mg PO/IV bd *or* chloramphenicol 500 mg
   PO/IV qds

For all three regimens, therapy should be continued until at least 2 days after the patient has improved and should then be followed with either:
- Doxycycline 100 mg PO bd *or*
- Tetracycline 500 mg PO qds

Both for 14 days.
Tetracyclines are contraindicated in pregnancy.

Outpatient therapy
Recommended regimen
- Single-dose therapy for uncomplicated gonorrhoea (see p. 91 — only ceftriaxone has been shown to be effective for PID; other single-dose regimens have not been formally evaluated) *plus*
- Doxycycline 100 mg PO bd *or* tetracycline 500 mg PO qds, for 14 days, *plus*
- Metronidazole 400–500 mg PO bd for 14 days

Alternative regimen where single-dose therapy for gonorrhoea is not available:
- Co-trimoxazole 480 mg 10 tablets PO od for 3 days, then 2 tablets PO bd for 10 days *plus*
- Doxycycline 100 mg PO bd *or* tetracycline 500 mg PO qds, both for 14 days, *plus*
- Metronidazole 400–500 mg PO bd for 14 days

This can only be used in areas where co-trimoxazole has been shown to be effective against uncomplicated gonorrhoea.

Adjuncts to therapy: removal of intrauterine contraceptive device (IUD)
The IUD is a risk factor for development of PID. Although the exact effect of removing an IUD on the response of acute salpingitis to antimicrobial therapy and the risk of recurrent salpingitis is unknown, removal of an IUD is suggested soon after microbial therapy has been initiated.
   When an IUD is removed, contraceptive counselling is essential.

Follow-up
Outpatients with PID should be followed up at 72 hours and admitted if their condition has not improved.

Syphilis

A worldwide disease caused by the spirochaete *Treponema pallidum*. The disease can be divided into four stages:

1. Local primary infection.
2. Dissemination associated with 2° syphilis.
3. A latent period during which infectivity is low. However, relapses into 2° syphilis may occur during the 1st 4 years after contact — the early latent period.
4. Late syphilis, which occurs after many years with widespread production of gummas (granulomatous lesions with a necrotic centre and surrounding obliterative endarteritis). Other manifestations result from long-term damage to the cardiovascular and central nervous systems.

Transmission: is almost exclusively through abraded skin at sites of sexual contact with infected persons. Other modes include congenital transmission (which produces severe disease in the infant) and infection by blood transfusion.

Clinical features

1° syphilis: 9–90 days after infection, a primary ulcer or chancre forms on the genitalia. It is typically solitary, 'punched out', indurated, and painless, with a clear exudate. It resolves over a few weeks. Atypical lesions occur and there may be multiple ulcers in HIV +ve patients. There is painless regional lymphadenopathy. The lesions are highly infective.

2° syphilis: coincides with the greatest number of treponemes in the body and blood, 1–6 months after contact. Specific features include:

- A transient, variable (not vesicular) rash particularly on trunk, soles, and palms
- In warm, moist areas where two skin surfaces are in contact, the papules enlarge and coalesce to form highly infectious plaques called *condylamata lata*
- Silver-grey lesions with red periphery on mucosal surfaces called mucous patches (e.g. snail track ulcers in the mouth)

There is also:

- Low-grade fever
- Malaise
- Generalized lymphadenopathy
- Arthralgias
- Occasionally, focal involvement of eyes, meninges, parotid glands, or viscera (kidney, liver, GI tract).

Late syphilis

The most common manifestations are areas of local tissue destruction in skin, bones, liver, and spleen due to **gumma** formation. Others include damage to the:

1. *Cardiovascular system* — ascending aorta aneurysm +/− aortic regurgitation and coronary artery stenosis.
2. CNS
   - Chronic meningitis — cranial nerve defects, hemiparesis, seizures
   - Parenchymal disease (general paralysis of the insane) — psychoses, dementia, hyperactive reflexes, tremor, speech, and pupillary (Argyll–Robertson) disturbances
   - Tabes dorsalis — shooting pains in limbs, peripheral neuropathy, ataxia, Charcot's joints, a positive Romberg's sign.

Diagnosis

During stages 1 and 2, repeated dark field microscopy for motile spirochaetes in lesion exudates; serology, either treponeme-specific (FTA, TPHA) for exposure or non-specific (VDPL, RPR) for active disease.

All patients with syphilis should be encouraged to have an HIV test since dual infection is common and has implications for assessment and management.

Management

Early syphilis (stages 1 and 2 or latent syphilis of <2 years' duration)

1. Benzathine penicillin G 2.4 million IU, IM stat as two injections into separate sites, **or**
   Procaine penicillin G 1.2 million IU, IM od for 10 days
2. For penicillin-allergic patients, alternatives include:
   Tetracycline 500 mg PO qds **or**
   Doxycycline 100 mg PO bd
   Both for 15 days

Late syphilis (not neurosyphilis) (includes latent syphilis of >2 years' or indeterminate duration)

1. Benzathine penicillin G 2.4 million IU, IM as two injections into separate sites, once weekly for 3 weeks, **or**
   Procaine penicillin G 1.2 million IU, IM od for 20 days
2. Alternatives for penicillin-allergic patients include:
   Tetracycline 500 mg PO qds (probably better) **or**
   Doxycycline 100 mg PO bd, both for 30 days.

However, penicillin is the preferred therapy and should be given whenever possible.

3. Some experts recommend examination of CSF in these patients for asymptomatic neurosyphilis.

Neurosyphilis

1. Aqueous benzylpenicillin G 12–24 million IU, administered IV od, in 4 hourly doses of 2–4 million IU, for 14 days, **or**
   Procaine penicillin G 1.2 million IU, IM od, **plus** probenecid 500 mg PO qds, for 10–14 days — ensure patient's outpatient compliance for this regimen.
2. Alternative regimen for penicillin-allergic patients:
   Tetracycline 500 mg PO qds **or**
   Doxycycline 200 mg PO bd
   Both for 30 days.
3. Consult a neurologist if possible and follow up carefully.

Follow-up early syphilis at 3, 6, and 12 months to assess treatment and possible reinfection.

Note that tetracyclines are contraindicated in pregnant women.

Management of pregnant women

Pregnant women should be treated with penicillin whenever possible. Alternatives include erythromycin 500 mg PO qds for 15 days (early syphilis) or 30 days (other forms of syphilis). Note that the effectiveness of erythromycin is highly questionable, particularly for neurosyphilis, and many failures have been reported. The baby should be evaluated and treated soon after birth. An extended course of a 3rd generation cephalosporin should probably be given to pregnant women whose allergy is not manifested by anaphylaxis.

Gonorrhoea

Gonorrhoea results from infection with the Gram-negative coccus, *Neisseria gonorrhoeae*. 1° infection through sexual contact usually involves the mucosal surfaces of the urethra, cervix, rectum, and oropharynx.

Without early effective treatment, both local and disseminated complications occur. Although sensitive to penicillin for many years, recent decades have seen the rise in strains resistant to penicillin, tetracycline, doxycycline, and other antibiotics. Conjunctival infection of neonates during vaginal delivery is a serious condition that may cause blindness if not treated early.

Clinical features: in **men**, urethral discharge and dysuria occur 2–5 days after infection. The discharge is initially mucoid, but becomes profuse and purulent (in contrast to non-gonococcal urethritis). Local complications include acute epididymitis, prostatis, periurethral abscess, and urethral stricture. In **women**, after 10-day incubation period, infection produces signs of cervicitis (+/– urethritis) — vaginal discharge, dysuria, and intermenstrual bleeding. Unlike men, many women are asymptomatic or have insufficient symptoms for medical presentation. Local complications include PID and perihepatitis. Frequency and urgency are uncommon in both men and women.

Haematogenous dissemination is a rare complication in untreated patients. It may result in meningitis, endocarditis, osteomyelitis, sepsis, or acute destructive monoarthritis with synovial effusion. Reactive polyarthropathy and papular/pustular dermatitis are recognized complications.

Diagnosis: gram-negative intracellular diplococci in smears — urethra in men (>90%), endocervix in women (less reliable); culture.

Management: all patients with gonococcal infection should also be treated for chlamydia since they often coexist, unless facilities are available to exclude specifically chlamydial infection. Sexual partners should be treated at the same time.

See box opposite for recommended regimens

Locally recommended regimens:
1. Uncomplicated infection:
2. Pharyngeal infection:
3. Disseminated infection:
4. Gonococcal conjunctivitis:

Pregnant patients:

Recommended regimes

1. *In uncomplicated genital and anal infection*
   - Ciprofloxacin 500 mg PO stat (*not during pregnancy*) or
   - Azithromycin 2g PO stat or
   - Ceftriaxone 125 mg IM stat or
   - Cefixime 400 mg PO stat or
   - Spectinomycin 2g, IM stat or
   - Kanamycin 2g IM stat or
   - Co-trimoxazole 480 mg 10 tablets od for 3 days
   Always use the locally recommended regimen.

2. *In disseminated infection*
   - Ceftriaxone 1g IV/IM od for 7 days or
   - Spectinomycin 2g IM bd for 7 days
   Extend the course to 14 days in meningitis, and 28 days in endocarditis.

3. *Gonococcal conjunctivitis in adults* is highly contagious. Treat with barrier nursing, in addition to frequent saline irrigation and antibiotics:
   - Ceftriaxone 125 mg IM stat or
   - Spectinomycin 2 g IM stat or
   - Ciprofloxacin 500 mg PO stat
   - (If above not available, alternative is kanamycin 2g IM stat)

4. *Neonatal gonococcal conjunctivitis*
   - Ceftriaxone 50 mg/kg IM stat, to a max. of 125 mg
   - (Alternative: Kanamycin 25 mg/kg IM stat, to a max. of 75 mg)
   - (Alternative: Spectinomycin 25 mg/kg IM stat, to a max. of 75 mg)

Neonatal patients should be reviewed at 48 hrs.

Neonatal gonococcal conjunctivitis can be prevented by careful cleaning of the infant's eyes immediately after birth and either 1% silver nitrate solution or 1% tetracycline ointment applied.

Chlamydial infections

Chlamydia trachomatis is an obligate intracellular bacterium that causes two STIs in adults, depending on the strain:
• An infection of urethra, endocervix, or rectum
• Lymphogranuloma venereum
It is also the cause of ocular trachoma, which is a major cause of blindness worldwide.

1. Urethritis/endocervicitis/proctitis

The D-K serotypes of chlamydiae have become the most common STI in the developed world. They are prevalent throughout the world, frequently coexisting with gonococcal infections, and are the most common cause of non-gonococcal urethritis (NGU) in men. Complications in men include epididymitis and, in homosexual men, chronic proctitis. Infection in women is often subclinical or non-specific. However, it is associated with cervicitis, salpingitis, and endometriosis and is a major cause of female subfertility worldwide.

Screening women through culture or serology and treating them for asymptomatic chlamydial infection should reduce complications.

2. Lymphogranuloma venereum (LGV)

A chronic STI caused by the L1, 2, and 3 strains. The 1° lesion is a painless genital ulcer (rarely visible in women) that heals in a few days. After a latent period of days or months, an acute, fluctuant inguinal lymphadenopathy (buboes) develops. With time, the buboes may spread locally and ulcerate → sinuses/fistulae. Subsequent chronic blockage of lymphatic drainage results in genital lymphoedema which is often quite severe in women.

Diagnosis: by microscopy, although this is difficult — intracellular inclusions may be seen on smears of material from lesions or bubo aspirate (immunofluorescence is helpful if available — ? refer); otherwise culture.

Management (see box for antibiotic regimens)
Uncomplicated anogenital infection: the addition of trimethoprim to a sulfonamide does not increase its activity against *C. trachomatis*. Treatment >7 days does not appear to improve the cure rate in uncomplicated infection. However, **compliance** for 7 days is critical. Because resistance to these regimens has not been observed, it is unnecessary to undertake a cure evaluation on completion of treatment. Patients should be asked to return if symptoms persist. **Partners** must be treated at the same time.

LGV: fluctuant lymph nodes should be aspirated through healthy skin. Incision and drainage, or excision, of nodes will delay healing and is contraindicated. (Late sequelae such as stricture/fistula, however, may require surgical intervention.)

Antibiotics regimens for chlamydial infection*

Uncomplicated anogenital infection:
- Doxycycline 100 mg PO bd for 7 days **or**
- Azithromycin 1g PO stat
- (Alternative: amoxicillin 500 mg PO tds for 7 days **or**)
- (Alternative: erythromycin 500 mg PO qds for 7 days **or**)
- (Alternative: ofloxacin 300 mg PO bd for 7 days **or**)
- (Alternative: tetracycline 500 mg PO qds for 7 days)

Uncomplicated anogenital infection during pregnancy:
- Erythromycin (base/ethylsuccinate) 500 mg PO qds for 7 days **or**
- Amoxicillin 500 mg PO tds for 7 days

LGV:
Doxycycline 100 mg PO bd for 14 days **or**
Erythromycin 500 mg PO qds for 14 days
(Alternative: tetracycline 500 mg PO qds for 14 days)

Neonatal chlamydial conjunctivitis
- Erythromycin syrup 12.5 mg/kg PO qds for 14 days
- (Alternative: co-trimoxazole 240 mg PO bd for 14 days)

*Recommended regimens are those **not** in brackets

Chancroid

An acute STI caused by the bacterium *Haemophilus ducreyi* that is characterized by painful ulceration and frequent bubo formation. It is highly infectious and a common cause of genital ulcers in Africa and South-East Asia. Chancroid is much more common in males, suggesting a female carrier state.

Clinical features: 3–7 days post-infection, painful papules form which rapidly develop into soft ulcers with undermined, ragged edges. Ulcers are haemorrhagic and sticky (often secondarily infected); if multiple, they may become confluent; they occur at sites of trauma during intercourse (extragenital is rare). Commonly 7–14 days later, inguinal nodes become involved: painful, matted, tethered to erythematous skin = bubo. A discharging sinus may develop, in time becoming a spreading ulcer. The lesions heal slowly and commonly relapse.

Diagnosis: clean the ulcer with saline, then remove material from the undermined edge; or aspirate pus from bubo. Gram stain the smear. *H. ducreyi* are Gram −ve rods (fine, short, round-ended) sometimes seen in 'shoal-of-fish' or 'railroad track' formation. Beware contaminating organisms. Culture is difficult.

Granuloma inguinale (donovanosis)

The bacterium *Calymmatobacterium granulomatis* causes chronic ulceration of genitals and surrounding tissues. Males are more frequently infected than females; patients' sexual partners are often uninfected.

Clinical features: 1–6 weeks following infection, an indurated painless papule forms which slowly develops into a 'beefy' granulomatous ulcer with characteristic rolled edges. The lesion is elevated, well defined, and bleeds easily with trauma. The usual sites are in the anogenital region, thighs, and perineum; rarely, intravaginal (or rectal) lesions may present with PV (or PR) bleeding. Healing is uncommon without treatment — 2° infection can follow → painful, destructive lesions, as can squamous cell carcinoma. Inguinal nodes are not involved unless there is 2° infection. Subcutaneous granulomas form which may be mistaken for enlarged lymph nodes (hence the name 'pseudobubo') — they may also become an abscess, discharging via a sinus, or an infected ulcer. Elephantoid enlargement of genitalia may occur during healing.

Diagnosis: crush a piece of granulation tissue from the active edge of the lesion between 2 slides, air dry, and stain with Giemsa or Gram stains. Large mononuclear cells are filled with the cytoplasmic Gram −ve rods (Donovan bodies — they look like closed safety pins due to bipolar staining).

Management of chancroid

- Ciprofloxacin 500 mg PO bd for 3 days *or*
- Erythromycin 500 mg PO qds for 7 days *or*
- Azithromycin 1 g PO stat *or*
- Ceftriaxone 250 mg IM stat.

Erythromycin should be used wherever possible — there is evidence that single-dose regimens are associated with an unacceptably high failure rate in some parts of the world and in HIV +ve patients, and that co-trimoxazole is less effective in parts of Africa and Asia.

Treatment outcome and the development of antibiotic resistance should be carefully monitored when the alternative regimens are used.

Management of donovanosis

No controlled trials have been published.
- Azithromycin 1g PO stat *or*
- Doxycycline 100 mg PO bd
- (Alternative: erythromycin 500 mg PO qds *or*)
- (Alternative: tetracycline 500 mg PO qds *or*)
- (Alternative: co-trimoxazole 960 mg PO bd)

No controlled trials have been published. Treatment should be continued for 7 days or until all lesions have completely epithelized, whichever is later.
- Azithromycin 1 g PO on first day, then 500 mg PO daily.

Trichomoniasis

Vaginal infection with *Trichomonas vaginalis* produces an irritating, pruritic (rarely bad smelling) discharge, 5–28 days post-infection. Dyspareunia, dysuria, and urethral infection occur in some patients; lower abdominal pain is rare. The discharge is copious, sometimes yellow or green, and pools in the posterior fornix. The vagina and exocervix become inflamed; colposcopy reveals cervical haemorrhages in 50% of symptomatic cases. However, the infection is frequently asymptomatic in women (? up to 50%) and in most men. It occasionally causes urethritis.

Diagnosis is by light microscopy. The parasite can readily be seen in a wet film of a posterior fornix smear as a motile, pear-shaped flagellate, particularly when the lighting is reduced.

Management

1. Metronidazole 2g PO stat or 400–500 mg PO bd for 7 days for both symptomatic and asymptomatic women, or tinidazole 2 g PO stat.
2. Notify and treat all sexual partners. Infection is most often asymptomatic in men, sometimes producing an NGU. The 7-day metronidazole regimen works well; efficacy of the single dose is less clear.
3. Patients should return after 7 days if symptoms persist. Failure can be due to resistance or reinfection. Patients often respond well to retreatment with the 7-day regimen.
4. Refractory infections should be treated with metronidazole 2 g PO od plus 500 mg applied intravaginally each night for 3–7 days.
5. During pregnancy, metronidazole may only be used at the minimum effective dose during the 2nd and 3rd trimesters (2 g PO stat).

Bacterial vaginosis

Bacterial vaginosis is a common form of vulvovaginitis that is often milder than either candidiasis or trichomoniasis. It is caused by coinfection with *Gardnerella vaginalis* and anaerobic bacteria such as *Bacteroides* and *Prevotella* spp. *G. vaginalis* alone appears to be insufficient to cause bacterial vaginosis.

Clinical features: most women have a grey/white, homogenous discharge with bubbles and a pungent odour, that adheres to the vaginal wall; it is usually not present in large quantities. Dysuria, dysparaeunia, and abdominal pain are uncommon — marked abdominal pain should raise the suspicion of concurrent conditions. Erythema and oedema are uncommon. The cervix is not involved; a cervical discharge suggests concurrent infection.

Diagnosis is by microscopic examination of a wet smear for 'clue cells' — vaginal epithelial cells that are covered with tiny coccobacilli — and the presence of large clumps of coccobacilli in Gram-stained smears. The discharge has few neutrophils. Loss of natural acidity is a useful clue to bacterial vaginosis and trichomoniasis. Litmus paper testing of the discharge shows the pH is >4.5.

Management

- Metronidazole 400–500 mg PO bd, for 7 days. In single dose of metronidazole 2 g is an alternative if adherence is likely to be poor.
- Partners are not routinely treated (although this may result in female re-colonization; if infection recurs in female, treat partner). However, he should be assessed for other STIs.

Genital herpes

A condition that is caused by herpes simplex viruses, predominantly HSV-2 (70–95%). Recurrent infection occurs frequently with reactivation of the latent virus from the dorsal root ganglia. Asymptomatic shedding is common and an important cause of reinfection. Infections are often prolonged and severe in the immunocompromised.

Transmission occurs by direct contact with infected genital secretions. After an incubation period of 2–7 days, local infection and inflammation result in multiple vesicular lesions that rapidly ulcerate. The ulcers are greyish and extremely painful; they occur on the penis in men and the vagina, cervix, vulva, and perineum in women, often accompanied by a vaginal discharge (also found in anus). 1° infection is accompanied by fever, malaise, and inguinal lymphadenopathy; extragenital involvement occurs in lip to 20% of cases. Encephalitis is a recognized complication of genital herpes.

Diagnosis: culture, serology; rarely, multinucleated giant cells in scrapings from suspected lesions (also found in VZV infection).

Management

- **First clinical episode** (take a careful history): aciclovir 200 mg PO 5× daily for 7 days to reduce formation of new lesions, duration of pain, time required for healing, and viral shedding, but probably not the rate of recurrence.
- **Recurrences:** aciclovir 200 mg PO 5× daily for 5 days or, if recurs >6 times/year, aciclovir 400 mg PO bd continuously. Recurrences become less common with increasing duration, so some experts recommend stopping aciclovir after 1 year so that recurrence rates can be reassessed. The minimum continuous dose that will suppress recurrence should be determined empirically. However, aciclovir does not stop viral shedding. Recommend the use of condoms.
- **HIV +ve patients:** HSV infection may be destructive in immunocompromised persons. Treat with aciclovir 400 mg PO 3–5× daily. Persistence and recurrences are common.

Candida vaginitis

Not normally a STI, it results from overgrowth of a commensal vaginal fungus, *Candida albicans*. Antibiotic therapy, pregnancy, and immunosuppression all predispose. Discharge is thick, curd-like, white (rarely, a scanty discharge) with Gram +ve fungal hyphae but no PMN. Visualization of hyphae is made easier by the addition of 10% KOH to clear the epithelial cells. Intense vulval pruritus and erythema are characteristic. The perineum may be involved; endometritis is rare but it can be followed by 2° bacterial infection. Occasionally, a woman can infect her partner → balanitis.

Management

- Miconazole or clotrimazole 200 mg intravaginally od for 3 days
- Clotrimazole 500 mg intravaginally stat **or** fluconazole 150 mg PO stat
- (Alternative: nystatin 100,000 IU intravaginally od for 14 days)

Tuberculosis[1]

Section editor **Stan Houston**

[1] This chapter is intended for use in conjunction with the relevant national TB programme manual.

Current global situation and trends

Tuberculosis (TB) has been curable for more than 50 years, yet it continues to cause an immense burden of morbidity and mortality. Approximately one-third of the world's population is infected with *Mycobacterium tuberculosis*, with 8–10 million developing active TB and ~3 million dying of TB each year (almost half of whom are co-infected with HIV). About 95% of cases occur in low-income countries and 75% are in the 15–50 age group. Both globally and within countries, there is a striking link between poverty and TB.

Two important developments have occurred in the past two decades:
- TB incidence has increased dramatically in communities highly endemic for HIV.
- The emergence of drug resistance jeopardizes both individual treatment and control of the disease in communities. In 1993, WHO declared TB a global emergency.

Modern TB treatment regimens of 6–8 months are highly effective in curing patients and preventing transmission. TB treatment is among the most cost effective of all health interventions. In recent years TB has been recognized as a health and development priority with substantial expansion of TB control programmes.

Many years of experience, including both disastrous failures and gratifying successes, have led to the recognition of several basic principles of TB treatment and control:
- TB treatment and control is first and foremost a public health activity since identifying and curing infectious patients is the most important element in reducing transmission in the community.
- In every setting, TB patients are more likely to be poor and disadvantaged, with more difficulties accessing health care.
- Thus it is vital that the public sector take responsibility for ensuring the proper functioning of the programme, usually through the establishment of a National Tuberculosis Programme, and that treatment be provided free of charge to patients.
- Many of the functions of successful TB treatment and control (see box) can only be provided effectively through a well-organized programme structure, usually operating nationwide.
- Finally, the TB programme must be integrated with the general health services of the community since that is where TB cases present.

Elements of the WHO TB control strategy

- *Sustained political commitment*
- *Microscopy:* case detection among symptomatic patients attending health services using sputum smear microscopy
- *SCC/DOT:* standardized short-course chemotherapy (SCC) using regimens of 6–8 months for at least all confirmed smear-positive cases. Good case management includes directly observed therapy (DOT) during the intensive phase for all new sputum-positive cases, during the continuation phase of regimens containing rifampicin, and throughout a re-treatment regimen.
- *Drug supply:* establishment and maintenance of a system to supply all essential anti-TB drugs, and to ensure no interruption in their availability.
- *Recording and reporting:* establishment and maintenance of a standardized recording and reporting system, allowing assessment of treatment results.

Microbiology

Mycobacteria are slender, curved, aerobic bacilli whose cell wall components make them acid-fast on Ziehl–Neelsen (ZN) staining. Members of the genus *Mycobacterium* are listed in the box.

M. tuberculosis multiplies slowly so that up to 6 weeks are required for culture. Correspondingly, disease due to *M. tuberculosis* tends to progress slowly, and responds slowly to treatment in comparison with infections due to common pyogenic bacteria.

Transmission

M. tuberculosis is acquired by the inhalation of microscopic droplets produced by individuals with active pulmonary TB, during coughing, sneezing, or speaking. Overcrowded, poorly ventilated conditions increase the risk of transmission as does duration of exposure. Other sources of *M. tuberculosis* infection, except for handling TB cultures in the laboratory, are extremely rare.

M. bovis is a pathogen in cattle and can infect a wide range of domestic and wild animals. As with *M. tuberculosis*, it is primarily transmitted by droplet inhalation, but human infection can occur through ingestion of unpasteurized milk from infected cows.

Disease and pathogenesis

TB infection

Aerosolized droplets containing *M. tuberculosis* enter alveoli and initiate a non-specific response. The bacilli are ingested by macrophages and transported to regional lymph nodes. They may either be contained there or spread via the lymphatics or bloodstream to other organs. With the development of cell-mediated immunity, cytokines secreted by lymphocytes recruit and activate macrophages, which organize into the granulomas characteristic of TB, surrounded by lymphocytes, effectively walling in the organisms.

In an immunocompetent host, most granulomas heal. They can sometimes be seen on CXR; more commonly the lesion is not detectable radiographically and a positive tuberculin skin test (TST) is the only evidence of infection. Although the lesions become fibrotic, bacilli can persist intracellularly in macrophages in a quiescent state capable of reactivation at a later time. This is known as 'latent tuberculous infection'.

Active TB disease

On average ~10% of adults infected with *M. tuberculosis* ultimately develop active TB, with about half of this risk occurring in the first 1–2 years after infection and the other half distributed over the remainder of the individual's lifetime. A number of factors can substantially increase the risk of disease reactivation (see box).

In a minority of cases, particularly infants or those with depressed cell-mediated immunity, 1° infection is not contained and symptomatic or disseminated disease (progressive 1° TB) develops directly from 1° infection.

Post-primary TB

Occurs as a reactivation of latent infection, often years or even decades after the 1° infection.

The genus *Mycobacterium* includes:

- **M. tuberculosis** complex (*M. tuberculosis, M. bovis, M. bovis BCG, M. africanum*): very closely related organisms of which *M. tuberculosis* is the most important human pathogen.
- **M. leprae**, the cause of leprosy, is an important mycobacterial pathogen of humans.
- *Mycobacteria other than TB:* mainly environmental organisms which cause a spectrum of relatively uncommon human diseases (e.g. *M. avium* complex, *M. kansasii, M. fortuitum, M. marinum.*) *M. ulcerans* is the cause of Buruli ulcer, a destructive cutaneous mycobacteriosis seen with increasing frequency in West Africa. Person to person transmission has not been observed with these organisms. This group will not be considered further in this chapter.

Risk factors for development of active TB disease in individuals infected with *M. tuberculosis*

- HIV — the most powerful known factor
- Recent infection — the risk/year of developing active disease is much greater in the first 1–2 years after infection
- Age — weakened immunity at the extremes of age
- Malnutrition, including vitamin D deficiency
- Diabetes mellitus
- Silicosis
- Intercurrent infections (eg. measles, visceral leishmaniasis)
- Toxic factors (eg. alcohol and smoking)
- Poverty — probably many biologic mechanisms involved
- Immune suppression (e.g. corticosteroid therapy, malignancy)
- 'Herd immunity' — members of populations with little historical exposure to TB appear to be more susceptible to disease.

Clinical features

Many settings where TB care is provided will not have access to some of the high technology diagnostic equipment mentioned below, which may be required for the diagnosis of less common forms of TB. However, most cases of TB can be diagnosed with very basic resources, in particular smear microscopy.

Primary TB: symptomatic primary TB is mainly a disease of children. It may be suspected clinically in the presence of fever, malaise, and cough, particularly in the setting of recent TB exposure. The diagnosis may be assisted by documenting TST conversion or supported by a positive TST in a patient likely to have been negative previously. A positive smear or even culture is uncommon. A CXR may show enlarged hilar or paratracheal lymph nodes with or without lung consolidation. A diagnosis of symptomatic primary TB is an indication for anti-TB therapy.

Post-primary or reactivation TB: one or more non-specific systemic symptoms are usually present including weight loss, anorexia, fever, night sweats, or malaise.

In adults, pulmonary TB (PTB) is the most common presentation. It is also the most important type of TB epidemiologically since it accounts for most transmission. However, TB may affect any organ in the body resulting in organ-specific symptoms and signs. Extrapulmonary TB is more common in children and in HIV-infected patients.

Pulmonary TB (PTB): involves the lung parenchyma. A history of cough is present in most cases. A cough of long duration is unlikely to be due to common respiratory infections, hence cough lasting >2–3 weeks is an indication for sputum smear microscopy. The cough may be productive but often is not. Haemoptysis, chest pain, breathlessness may also be present in some patients.

Examination is often normal or the findings non-specific. Some patients may look ill and wasted with a fever and tachycardia, but some patients, even with infectious TB, appear surprisingly well. Chest examination may reveal localized crackles or a pleural effusion. Finger clubbing indicates that a diagnosis other than TB is likely, but prolonged PTB or lung damage from past PTB can cause bronchiectasis and clubbing.

Approximately 65% of PTB cases are sputum smear positive. Sputum smear positivity is more likely in patients who are (a) most infectious (smear-positive patients are several times more likely to transmit TB than are those who are smear-negative, even if culture positive) and (b) sickest. A positive smear for acid-fast bacilli in a high TB prevalence area almost always indicates TB.

Smear-negative pulmonary TB: smear-negative PTB is common but difficult to diagnose accurately. Underdiagnosis is clearly undesirable since an opportunity for effective treatment is missed. Overdiagnosis also creates problems, using scarce resources from a very important health programme, overlooking other treatable diagnoses, and undermining the TB programme's credibility in the community. Monitoring the proportion of smear-negative vs. smear-positive pulmonary patients in a programme is a useful indicator of any tendency to overdiagnosis of TB. Roughly, the 'expected' proportion of smear-positive:smear-negative is 2:1.

Pleural TB: An effusion can often be detected on physical examination and confirmed by X-ray or by diagnostic aspiration with a small gauge needle. In high TB endemic areas, and in the absence of obvious alternative explanations such as heart failure, acute pneumonia, or disseminated KS, TB will be the most common cause of a 'straw-coloured' effusion. TB effusions are exudates (fluid protein > half that in serum) and the stained smear contains increased lymphocytes but is seldom positive for acid-fast bacilli. Culture of pleural biopsy tissue is very sensitive and histology of the biopsy usually shows granulomas.

Complications of pulmonary TB: haemoptysis can be life-threatening. Pneumothorax can occur. Dissemination to other organs can occur before treatment is started. Chronic complications include post-TB bronchiectasis, extensive lung fibrosis, and aspergillomas (fungus balls) in persistent cavities.

TB lymphadenitis: can involve any site, most frequently cervical lymph nodes. Nodes may initially be rubbery and non-tender, becoming matted or fluctuant (cold abscess), sometimes progressing to the development of chronic draining sinuses. They may have been present for weeks or months, and are seldom acutely inflamed. Sometimes TB lymph nodes enlarge or discharge during anti-TB therapy. These characteristics, and the asymmetrical involvement, help to distinguish TB adenitis from persistent generalized lymphadenopathy of HIV.

Often a needle aspiration will find a pocket of pus in the node, and this may be smear-positive in some cases (especially if HIV infected). Definitive diagnosis is by surgical biopsy with histologic examination and/or culture where available.

Bone TB: most commonly affects the spine (Pott's disease). Vertebral collapse may ultimately produce a characteristic angular deformity. Some patients develop features of spinal cord compression. Paravertebral cold abscesses or psoas abscesses may accompany Pott's disease and may be relieved by needle drainage — they do not generally require open surgical drainage.

The presence of a characteristic 'step' kyphosis in a TB-endemic area is virtually diagnostic of spinal TB. X-ray changes with intervertebral disc and adjacent bony involvement +/− paravertebral soft tissue densities are characteristic but do not distinguish between TB and other infections such as brucellosis. A cold abscess when present can be aspirated for culture. Imaging-guided biopsy requires sophisticated resources. Spinal TB responds well to drug treatment. Patients with severe deformities or with progressive neurologic compromise might benefit from neurosurgical stabilization if available, but neurologic improvement often occurs with medical therapy alone. TB of other joints such as hip and knee generally require biopsy for diagnosis and respond well to chemotherapy.

Miliary TB: most commonly affects infants and the immunosuppressed. There is a history of gradual onset fever, malaise, and weight loss in the absence of other apparent causes. Clinical suspicion is raised in a child with known or likely recent contact with an infectious TB patient. Physical findings are commonly non-specific, but include hepatomegaly, slight splenomegaly, tachypnoea, and neck stiffness (meningitis may complicate miliary TB). Progression to death occurs in the absence of therapy.

Chest X-ray characteristically shows diffuse, tiny, nodular opacities. Sputum smear examination and TST are often negative; where available, biopsy of liver, bone marrow, lymph nodes, or lung parenchyma may yield acid-fast bacilli or granulomata.

TB meningitis: is most commonly seen in children and the immunosuppressed. Clinical presentation includes headache, irritability, vomiting, decreased consciousness, or any unexplained progressive central neurologic syndrome. The history is usually less acute than in bacterial meningitis. Neck stiffness may be mild at first, later opisthotonus; coma may occur. Cranial nerve palsies (III, IV, VI, and VIII particularly) occur, reflecting basilar distribution of the disease. Seizures and focal neurologic deficits may also occur.

Diagnosis rests on CSF examination. There is typically a lymphocytosis with raised protein and decreased glucose — in early disease, mild changes may be present. CSF should also be examined for cryptococcus if there is a possibility of HIV infection. Unless concentrated the CSF is rarely positive for acid-fast bacilli; cultures may become positive in most cases.

Once a diagnosis has been made on the basis of clinical features, suggestive CSF abnormalities, and the absence of a likely alternative diagnosis, TB treatment should be started immediately. The available evidence and most expert opinion supports adjunctive therapy with corticosteroids.

Abdominal TB: gastrointestinal TB may present as partial bowel obstruction with a history of fever. It can occur at any site in the GI tract, most commonly the terminal ileum. The diagnosis is likely to be made at surgery or endoscopy. Granulomatous hepatitis is characterized by a systemic illness with laboratory evidence of cholestasis and diagnosed on liver biopsy. Peritoneal TB may be suspected on the basis of ascites without another obvious cause such as liver disease and portal hypertension — the ascites has the same characteristics as TB pleural fluid (see above). The peritoneum has a characteristic appearance on direct inspection; peritoneal biopsy, ideally taken at laparoscopy, with culture and histology provides a definitive diagnosis.

Pericardial TB: is often first suspected on the basis of globular enlargement of the cardiac silhouette on CXR in patients being investigated for a variety of systemic and cardiorespiratory symptoms. It is seen more frequently in HIV-infected patients. A pericardial rub or clinical features of tamponade (elevated jugular venous pressure, pulsus paradoxus, hypotension) may be present. Ultrasound readily confirms the presence of an effusion. Pericardial fluid has the same characteristics as pleural fluid (see above). The risk of tamponade acutely, and constriction later on, may be reduced by adding corticosteroids for the first 6–12 weeks of TB treatment.

Genitourinary TB: can involve any part of the male or female genitourinary tract. Presentation is subacute and diagnosis usually requires TB culture or histology of biopsies. Renal TB presents with dysuria, hematuria, flank pain, or mass. The urine contains pus cells on microscopy, but is negative on culture for common bacteria. Genital tract TB in women presents as infertility, pelvic pain, mass, or abnormal bleeding. Epididymal swelling is the most common presentation of genital TB in males.

TB in children

The risk of progression to disease following *M. tuberculosis* exposure is greater in infants and young children and the death rate may be very high among those infants who develop TB. By contrast, children between around 7 and 12 years of age have the lowest risk of any age group of developing active TB. Even where culture and other facilities are available, diagnosis of childhood TB is difficult. Sputum smears are usually negative in children with PTB. A history of close contact with a smear-positive pulmonary TB case is essential information. A positive TST is also strongly suggestive of TB in a child with unexplained illness, particularly in younger children in whom the 'background' rate of TST positivity is low. Scoring systems have been developed to rationalize the diagnosis of childhood TB — none has been well validated, but they may provide useful guidance.

Example of a scheme to aid diagnosis of TB in children[2]

1. Score chart for child with suspected TB

Score	0	1	3
Length of illness	<2 weeks	2–4 weeks	>4 weeks
Weight for age	>80%	60–80%	<60%
Family TB (past or present)	None	Reported by family	Proved sputum +ve

2. Score for other features if present:

• Positive tuberculin skin test (TST)	3
• Large painless lymph nodes: firm, soft, and/or sinus in neck, axilla, and groin	3
• Unexplained fever, night sweats, no response to malaria treatment	2
• Malnutrition, not improving after 4 weeks	3
• Angle deformity of the spine	4
• Joint swelling, bone swelling, or sinuses	3
• Unexplained abdominal mass or ascites	3
• CNS: change in temperament, convulsions, or coma	3

3. If the TOTAL score is 7 or more — treat for TB

Treat children with a score less than 7 if:
• CXR is characteristic of TB infection, or
• The child does not respond to two 7-day courses of two different antibiotics

2 Dr Keith Edwards, University of Papua New Guinea, published in Crofton *et al.* (1997) *Clinical tuberculosis*, MacMillan.

Diagnosis

Sputum smears

Three sputa should be examined whenever a cough has been present for >2–3 weeks. In patients who travel some distance to the clinic, the 1st specimen is collected at first presentation, the 2nd is an early morning sputum collected at home on the day the patient returns for follow up, and the 3rd is collected in clinic that day. In patients who cannot produce sputum, or in suspected PTB with repeated negative sputum smears, induction with 3% hypertonic saline significantly improves the sensitivity of smear and culture. Gastric lavage is useful in children, where culture facilities are available.

Chest X-ray

CXR is not routinely necessary for the diagnosis and management of TB. A normal CXR makes PTB unlikely, but CXRs cannot distinguish reliably between TB and other diseases or between changes of current and past TB. The interpretation of CXR varies according to the skill of the reader and between readers. They do not predict infectiousness (as the sputum smear does), nor supply the definitive identification provided by culture. CXR is useful in patients with undiagnosed chest symptoms who are repeatedly smear negative.

Tuberculin skin testing (TST)

Relies on the fact that cell-mediated hypersensitivity typically develops within 8 weeks of infection with *M. tuberculosis*. The test involves intra-dermal injection of PPD (purified protein derivative). The diameter of skin induration (swelling; not redness) is measured at 48–72 hours. Training and experience in interpreting skin test responses is critical to achieving accurate results. In most situations, 10mm of induration to a standard tuberculin dose is the cut-off point between positive and negative; 5mm is considered to be positive in an HIV-infected individual. Both false negative and false positive TST results occur commonly. The stronger the TST response, the less likely it is to be a false positive.

Uses of the TST

- Epidemiologic — determining prevalence or incidence in populations or specific groups such as health care workers.
- Diagnostic — to aid in assessing the likelihood of TB as the cause of a clinical illness. In high-prevalence countries, this use is largely limited to children because of the high 'background' prevalence of TST positivity in the adult population.
- Determination of candidates for 'chemoprophylaxis' (e.g. paediatric contacts of pulmonary TB patients, HIV-infected individuals).

Diagnosis of sputum-negative PTB

Reassessment and repeat sputum examination after 2–3 weeks, following a therapeutic trial of a broad-spectrum antibiotic, may clarify the diagnosis. CXR, interpreted with the cautions mentioned below, may help to estimate the likelihood of TB in suspects who remain smear-negative. Before diagnosing smear-negative PTB, consider alternative diagnoses such as:

- Pneumonia
- Asthma
- Chronic bronchitis
- Bronchiectasis
- Lung abscess
- Lung cancer
- Non-TB respiratory complications of HIV infection

In some TB programmes, a decision to start treatment for smear-negative PTB can only be made by a doctor or individual with particular expertise in TB.

A 'therapeutic trial' of treatment

A therapeutic trial is widely used by some practitioners to diagnose TB. Therapeutic trials have not been validated, and this approach risks creating confusion among health care workers. If 'therapeutic trials' are to be used, then:

1. All efforts to make a diagnosis should have been exhausted.
2. The endpoint used to determine success or failure should be established before starting treatment and should be objective (eg. fever, weight gain).
3. The duration of the trial should be established at the beginning: fever can be expected to settle within 14 days of starting treatment in most cases, and weight gain should be evident by 4 weeks.
4. The drugs used for the trial should have antimycobacterial activity (isoniazid, ethambutol, and pyrazinamide) but not be effective against other infections (rifampicin and streptomycin).
5. The patient's status as a 'trial patient' should be clearly established in the local TB programme.

A false positive TST can be caused by:

- BCG: TST response following BCG is variable; BCG in infancy is unlikely to account for a strongly positive TST in adulthood
- Exposure to environmental mycobacteria
- Incorrect interpretation

A false negative TST can be caused by:

- Normal variation
- Long interval since infection
- Reduced cell-mediated immune response (HIV, old age, corticosteroid therapy, measles, malnutrition)
- Severe illness, including overwhelming TB
- Incorrect TST technique or interpretation

Treatment

Aims of treatment
- To cure the patient.
- To prevent transmission in the patient's family and community.
- To prevent development of resistant bacilli.

Principles of anti-TB therapy
- Use at least 2 drugs to which the organism is presumed to be sensitive.
- Administer treatment for an adequate duration (6–8 months with the regimens used in most national TB programmes).
- Ensure that each patient completes the full course of therapy with a high level of adherence.

First- and second-line anti-TB drugs (see box opposite)
Treatment is the same regardless of disease site, although some advise a prolonged consolidation phase for TB meningitis and bone disease (12 months total). Anti-TB drugs should be provided in the form of fixed-dose combination (FDC) tablets which make monotherapy impossible and provide a further defence against the development of drug resistance.

Anti-TB drug dosage and standard regimens
Most national TB programmes have a standard regimen and a re-treatment regimen — the latter for patients who have defaulted, failed treatment, or relapsed.

Anti-TB drug (abbreviation)	Recommended dose (mg/kg) od	3×/week
Isoniazid (H)	5	10
Rifampicin (R)	10	10
Pyrazinamide (Z)	25	35
Streptomycin (S)	15	15
Ethambutol (E)	15	30
Thiacetazone (T)	2.5	N/A

First-line regimen (WHO) 2HRZE 4HR **or** 2HRZE 4H3R3
- Isoniazid, rifampicin, pyrazinamide, and ethambutol od for 2 months
- Followed by isoniazid and rifampicin either od or 3×/week for 4 months

First-line regimen (International Union Against Tuberculosis and Lung Disease) 2HRZE 6HE
- Isoniazid, rifampicin, pyrazinamide, and ethambutol od for 2 months
- Followed by isoniazid and ethambutol od for 6 months

'Re-treatment regimen' (defaulters, treatment failure, relapse). 2HRZES 1HRZE 5H3R3E3
- Isoniazid, rifampicin, pyrazinamide, ethambutol, and streptomycin od for 2 months
- Followed by isoniazid, rifampicin, pyrazinamide, ethambutol od for 1 month
- Followed by isoniazid, rifampicin, ethambutol 3×/week for 5 months

Anti-TB drugs

- **Isoniazid** (INH; 'H'): potent anti-TB activity. Main serious adverse effect is liver toxicity.
- **Rifampicin** (rifampin in North America; 'R'): essential to the success of modern short course TB therapy (<12 months). Rifampicin is characterized by a high rate of drug interactions (induces liver enzymes and lowers serum levels of warfarin, anticonvulsants, oral contraceptives, some antiretrovirals, etc). It can cause hepatitis.
- **Pyrazinamide** ('Z'): 'sterilizing' activity allows treatment courses of 6 months. May cause vomiting, arthralgias, less commonly hepatitis. Contribution to first-line regimens limited largely to the first 2 months of therapy.
- **Ethambutol** ('E'): main role is prevention of resistance to other drugs, particularly when 1° resistance to one or more first-line agents is possible. Main serious adverse effect is ocular toxicity, which is uncommon at recommended doses.
- **Thiacetazone** ('T'): formerly used in conjunction with isoniazid in the continuation phase. Largely abandoned in high HIV-prevalence countries because of high rates of Stevens–Johnson syndrome in HIV-co-infected patients.
- **Streptomycin** ('S'): now limited to second-line or re-treatment regimens because of the cost of needles and syringes and the desire to avoid unnecessary injections in the HIV era. Ototoxicity (vertigo >hearing loss) and renal toxicity are the main adverse effects. The drug should be avoided or dosage adjusted carefully in renal dysfunction. Contraindicated in pregnancy.

Special groups

- Isoniazid causes peripheral neuropathy more commonly in diabetic, malnourished, alcoholic, and pregnant patients; and in those with pre-existing neuropathy. Give pyridoxine 10–15 mg/d to prevent peripheral neuropathy.
- Women on oral contraceptives must use another form of contraception (e.g. an IUD) during rifampicin therapy and for 4–8 weeks after stopping rifampicin.
- Pregnancy: TB drugs, except for streptomycin, may be used in pregnancy. Any theoretical risks to the fetus are much less than the risks from untreated TB.

Third-line anti-TB drugs

Recently, some programmes have acquired 'third- line' anti-TB drugs for the treatment of multidrug-resistant (MDR) TB. Treatment of MDR TB is much longer (>18 months), much more toxic, much more costly, and considerably less effective than treatment of drug-sensitive TB. Therefore it must only be introduced in settings where a DOTS (directly observed therapy, short course) programme is established and demonstrating good outcomes. MDR TB treatment requires supervision of every treatment dose, a well-structured programme with guidelines, appropriate laboratory resources, assured drug supply, and access to expert advice, as recommended by the WHO 'Green Light Committee'.

Monitoring treatment: sputum-positive patients should be monitored by sputum smear examination after 2 months of treatment and prior to treatment completion. All other patients should be monitored clinically.

Monitoring for adverse drug reactions is essential.

Concordance: patients usually feel better soon after starting treatment, so may lose the motivation to continue therapy for many months. Treatment completion is essential for cure and prevents the development of drug resistance. The treating health care worker and the TB programme must ensure that patients complete TB therapy. This is most likely to succeed if the patient and community are active and informed participants and aware of the risks of drug resistance. The relationship between the patient and program or clinic staff is a major factor promoting concordance.

Resistance: small numbers of M. tuberculosis are mutants naturally resistant to single TB drugs. Combination chemotherapy ensures that these resistant organisms will be killed by other drugs. Poor choice of treatment or poor concordance with therapy results in selection for these resistant organisms.

Treatment failure: follow guidelines in the national TB manual or the re-treatment regimen on p. 110.

TB control

Smear-positive PTB patients transmit infection. Curing smear-positive cases is the 1° means of reducing TB transmission in the community.

Once availability and quality of treatment have been established, the next priority is case finding. This activity must be integrated with the primary health care service since it depends upon recognition and appropriate investigation (most importantly by sputum smear examination) of TB suspects by primary health care workers.

Bacille Calmette Guerin (BCG): is a live attenuated vaccine derived from *M bovis*. Protective efficacy ranges from 0 to 80% for reasons which remain controversial. BCG provides some protection against miliary TB and TB meningitis, and should be given at birth to all children in high TB-prevalence countries (except those with symptomatic HIV disease). BCG has little or no impact on the rate of infectious TB in a community.

Household and close contacts of TB cases: Symptomatic contacts should be investigated for active TB. Chemoprophylaxis should be offered to asymptomatic household contacts aged <5 years, of smear-positive PTB patients.

In high-prevalence countries, HIV prevention is an important form of TB control.

Cross-infection control

Health care workers are exposed to a significant occupational risk of TB, and HIV-infected subjects are at very high risk. The important infection control principles are:

- Early diagnosis and treatment of patients to minimize the period of infectiousness.
- Encourage patients to cover their mouths when coughing or sneezing.
- Early identification and respiratory isolation of TB suspects pending diagnosis.
- Increased natural ventilation and sunlight in TB wards and clinics.
- Encourage health care workers to be tested for HIV and employ those with HIV where there is lower risk of TB exposure (e.g. non-clinical jobs, paediatrics).

Wearing of common surgical masks by staff provides very limited protection against TB. The infectious droplets are too small to be blocked by these masks and the masks do not seal around the mouth.

In the laboratory, most TB risk occurs in handling of TB cultures. The risk in handling specimens and preparing sputum smears is much lower. Patients should cough sputum specimens in a separate, well-ventilated area. Wearing of masks by lab staff is not needed.

TB and HIV

TB incidence has increased up to 6-fold in some communities affected by the HIV pandemic. HIV prevalence is up to 80% among TB patients in these places. TB is the most common cause of death in patients with HIV. The main mechanism involved is suppression of cell-mediated immunity (CD4 helper T-cells and macrophages) by HIV which impairs the immune response to TB.

Differences in management of TB in HIV +ve patients

Presentation: most patients with HIV-related TB do not know their HIV status. Some have clinical features of HIV infection: oral candidiasis, chronic diarrhoea, skin and hair changes, peripheral neuropathy, herpes zoster scars, etc. However, since TB can occur early during the course of immune suppression, other clinical features of HIV are often absent. Extrapulmonary TB is common in HIV +ve patients, particularly lymphadenopathy, pleural and pericardial effusions, miliary TB, and meningitis. However, PTB continues to be the most common form of TB.

The radiographic appearance of PTB in HIV +ve patients sometimes differs from the classical appearances, roughly according to the individual's degree of immune suppression. HIV +ve patients less commonly have upper lobe disease and cavities and more commonly have hilar adenopathy, effusions, and miliary and nodular shadowing.

Diagnosis: sputum smear microscopy is slightly less sensitive in HIV +ve patients. Differential diagnosis of lung disease in the HIV +ve includes:

- Bacterial (most often pneumococcal) pneumonia: a short history and a response to antibiotic therapy is suggestive.
- *Pneumocystis jiroveci* pneumonia: it is less common in some tropical settings but characteristic features are a history of cough and fever for weeks, severe dyspnoea and hypoxia, diffuse changes on X-ray, and a response to high-dose co-trimoxazole therapy.
- Pulmonary Kaposi's Sarcoma: most patients have cutaneous or mucosal lesions (e.g. on the hard palate).

Treatment regimens: the same drug regimens are used in HIV +ve and uninfected patients, so knowledge of HIV status is not required to provide anti-TB treatment. Sputum conversion rates and initial cure rates are similar in HIV +ve patients and those without HIV provided modern rifampicin-containing regimens are used. Recurrence rates and re-infection rates are higher. Mortality during and after treatment is markedly increased among patients with HIV, with most deaths being due to HIV-related causes other than TB.

Increasing numbers of patients have access to ART. Treatment with anti-TB and antiretroviral drugs can lead to complex and clinically important drug interactions:

- Rifampicin reduces serum levels of most protease inhibitors and some non-nucleoside reverse transcriptase inhibitors such as nevirapine.
- Immune reconstitution reactions can result in temporary clinical deterioration when ART is started early in the course of TB treatment.

One strategy is to delay ART until completion of the intensive phase of TB treatment and use of a non-rifampicin-containing continuation phase such as 6 months of isoniazid and ethambutol. Seek expert advice if ART and TB therapy are to be given together.

There are potential benefits to patients with HIV and TB from giving prophylaxis with co-trimoxazole. Consult national guidelines on this issue.

Compared to HIV uninfected people, persons with HIV have:
• A much higher risk of progressive primary disease following infection.
• A much higher risk of reactivation of latent TB infection — about 10% per year (compared to 10% in a lifetime in HIV uninfected people).
• After successful treatment of TB, an increased risk of re-infection with a new strain of M. tuberculosis.
TB increases HIV replication and may enhance progression to AIDS.

Treatment of latent TB infection in HIV-infected patients: HIV +ve individuals, who are also TST-positive and who have no evidence of active TB disease, have significantly less risk of developing active TB if given 'chemoprophylaxis' — though the benefit declines with time, especially if the patient continues to live in a community where the risk of TB transmission is high. Isoniazid for 6–9 months is standard, and seems not to cause increased isoniazid resistance. Large-scale 'chemoprophylaxis' programmes for people with HIV are uncommon in practice. Care must be taken that anti-TB drugs, especially rifampicin, are not used or distributed in ways that could promote development of resistance.

HIV testing of TB patients: TB patients are a 'sentinel' group, often selected for epidemiologic surveillance of the HIV epidemic. When treating individual patients, there is an ethical obligation to inform patients when strong clinical evidence of HIV infection is found and to provide them with the option of serologic testing to confirm or exclude HIV. Whether all TB patients should be offered HIV testing should be determined at local or national level based on availability of testing and 'counselling' resources and care for HIV infection, policies regarding voluntary testing and counselling, anticipated local reaction in relation to stigmatization of TB patients, and other local factors.

Diarrhoeal diseases

Introduction

Diarrhoea is defined as the passage of abnormally loose or fluid stools more frequently than normal. Normal bowel habit varies greatly from person to person, but recent onset of 3 or more liquid or loose stools per day is considered abnormal.

Infective diarrhoea is the second highest cause of death due to infection in the world, with ~3–4 million fatalities each year. 80% of deaths are in children under 2 yrs, specifically during and shortly after the introduction of complementary foods between 6–12 months. Breastfeeding, especially exclusive breastfeeding, confers significant protection against intestinal infections. Repeated attacks of diarrhoea initiate a vicious cycle of malnutrition, reduced immunity, and more intestinal infections.

An accurate history is vital for all cases of diarrhoea, since it will give clues to the aetiology and severity of disease. Include in the past medical history any similar episodes and any current medication.

The treatment of most diarrhoeal episodes depends on treating and preventing dehydration regardless of the aetiology of the infection. Antimicrobials are only recommended for dysentery and cholera, and for severe episodes with laboratory diagnosis in certain vulnerable groups (see below). Symptomatic antidiarrhoeal agents should be avoided in young children.

Some key questions to be asked
- How long has the diarrhoea been present?
- Is (or was) there fever or other systemic symptoms?
- What is the stool like — specifically is there blood (bright red or dark) and/or mucus?
- How frequent are the motions?
- Is there any abdominal pain — where?
- Is there a sense of tenesmus (incomplete emptying following defecation)?
- Has the patient vomited — how much, when, what?
- Has the patient been in contact with anyone with similar symptoms?
- Have they eaten or drunk anything unusual prior to the onset of symptoms?
- Is anyone else in the family ill?
- Is there a history of recent travel? Where?
- Has the patient been exposed to malaria?

In examining the patient, one should look for signs of dehydration and malnutrition, as well as for clues to determine the disease aetiology.

Classification of diarrhoea

It is useful to subdivide diarrhoeal diseases according to presence or not of blood in the stool, since the causative agents are largely different, but be aware that both shigellosis and Campylobacter infections may present as acute watery diarrhoea. Here we shall divide the diseases into acute diarrhoea with blood (dysentery) and acute diarrhoea without blood. Diarrhoea that continues more than 14 days is considered persistent or chronic and additional pathological conditions need to be considered and this condition is accorded a separate section.

Antimicrobial drugs

In the majority of cases, symptoms of diarrhoea improve with treatment of dehydration alone, without the need for antibiotics. In certain circumstances, however, antimicrobial drugs may be beneficial. These include:

- **Bloody diarrhoea (dysentery) that does not improve after 3 days of rehydration treatment**. If a specific cause is found it should be treated appropriately (see relevant section below). If no cause can be found, an antimicrobial effective against *Shigella* should be used in the first instance.
- **Cholera with severe dehydration**: any suspected case of cholera should be treated with an effective antimicrobial and control agencies notified.
- **Laboratory-proven symptomatic cases of G. intestinalis infection** that do not improve after 3 days of ORS therapy should be treated with an antimicrobial.
- **Laboratory-proven enteropathogenic E. Coli infections** respond to antibiotics and should be used in vulnerable hosts such as young babies.
- **Traveller's diarrhoea in adults**: duration is reduced when treated with an antibiotic such as ciprofloxacin.

Investigations

For general assessment in a hospital setting or if diarrhoea continues beyond 2–3 days include Hb, FBC, U&E, and glucose. However, most uncomplicated cases of diarrhoea can be managed without any laboratory tests. Stool culture and microscopy are often requested but few centres can offer diagnostic tests for all enteropathogens; mixed infections are common; single-stool cultures are insufficient for some pathogens; and results will often come back too late to influence management. Apart from investigation of outbreaks, surveillance, and research purposes, stool culture in uncomplicated cases should be limited to the exclusion of those pathogens for which antibiotic treatment is indicated (e.g. parasites, *Shigella* species, and *Vibrio cholerae*). If appropriate, do a blood film for malaria.

How to make a direct faecal smear

1. Write the patient's name on a clean slide.
2. Place a drop of sterile saline in the centre of the left-hand side of the slide and place a drop of iodine in the centre of the right-hand side of the slide. Fig. 2D.1
3. With a match or applicator, pick up a small portion of faeces (~2 mg — or about the size of a match head) and add it to the drop of saline. Repeat and add to the iodine. Mix the faeces with the drops to form suspensions. Fig. 2D.2

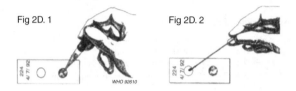

Fig 2D. 1

Fig 2D. 2

WHO 92610

4. Cover each drop with a coverslip. Fig. 2D.3
5. Examine each drop with the ×10 objective or, for identification, with the higher power objectives, searching in a systematic manner. When organisms are seen, switch to higher power for more detail. Fig. 2D.4

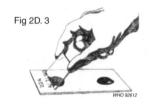

Fig 2D. 3

WHO 92612

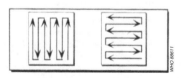

Fig 2D. 4

WHO 88611

Table 2D.1

Formed stool	Unformed/semi-solid/blood & mucus/liquid		
Faecal concentration for ova/cysts	With blood/mucus	Saline suspension for exudate, *Schistosoma mansoni* ova, and amoebic trophozoites	Bacteriological culture for *Shigellosis*, *Campylobacter*
Direct saline suspension for exudate/ova/cysts	Without blood/mucus	• Saline suspension for exudate, Protozoal trophozoites (*Giardia*, *Trichomonas hominis*, *Chilomastix*), • Faecal concentration for ova/cysts/oocysts/larvae • Faecal stain (modified Zn) for *Cryptosporidia*, *Cyclospora cayetanensis*	• Bacteriological culture • Enteric viral screen (latex agglutination for rotavirus)
	Liquid	As for 'without blood/mucus' with additional 'hanging drop' observation for Vibrio Cholera	Bacteriological culture including *V. Cholera.*
	From HIV and immune-compromised patient	As for 'without blood/mucus' with the addition of trichrome stain for *Microsporidia* sp.	

Acute diarrhoea with blood

The presence of blood in diarrhoea (dysentery) usually signifies ulceration of the large bowel. The most common bacterial agents causing dysentery in the tropics are *Shigella* (bacillary dysentery) and *Campylobacter*. Shigellosis can be a serious infection that progresses to complications and death. Dysentery should be treated on clinical diagnosis with antibiotics that cover *Shigella*. If the patient does not improve after 48 hours, the antibiotic should be changed taking into account stool culture findings if available. If culture results are negative or not available, change the antibiotic (e.g. from co-trimoxazole to nalidixic acid or ciprofloxacin).

Bacillary dysentery (shigellosis)

Shigella dysenteriae, Sh. flexneri, Sh. Boydii, and *Sh. sonneii* cause the disease known as bacillary dysentery, with the former two species responsible for most morbidity and mortality (which may reach 20% in untreated cases). The disease may occur both endemically and epidemically, with children most frequently affected. The incubation period in humans (the only natural host) is 1–5 days following direct person to person contact (from cases of asymptomatic excreters) or ingestion of contaminated water and food.

Clinical features: range from mild disease in which there is intermittent watery diarrhoea alone, to severe systemic complications. In severe cases, onset is usually rapid, with tenesmus, fever, and passage of frequent (up to 100/day) bloody mucoid stools. Intestinal complications include: toxic megacolon, perforation, and protein-losing enteropathy. Systemic complications include: dehydration, hypoglycaemia, and electrolyte imbalance (particularly hyponatraemia), haemolytic-uraemic syndrome, convulsions (particularly in children, often before the onset of diarrhoea), Reiter's syndrome, thrombotic thrombocytopenic purpura, pneumonia. Invasive disease may give 'rose spots' — crops of 2–4 mm papules which fade on pressure, usually appearing on the upper abdomen and lower chest.

Diagnosis: the clinical distinction between bacillary and amoebic dysentery is usually impossible. Stool microscopy may show leukocytes and haematophagus trophozoites of amoeba.

Management
1. Oral rehydration is sufficient for mild disease.
2. In severe disease, ampicillin or trimethoprim (or co-trimoxazole) should be given, although resistance is common in many places; quinolones such as ciprofloxacin are an alternative. Antimicrobial sensitivities should be sought from individual cultures wherever possible.

Prevention: no vaccine is currently available.

Causes of acute diarrhoea with blood

- Bacillary dysentery (shigellosis)
- Enterohaemorrhagic *E. coli*
- *Campylobacter* enterocolitis
- *Salmonella* enterocolitis
- *Yersinia* enterocolitis
- Amoebic dysentery
- *Balantidium coli* enterocolitis
- Massive *Trichuris* infection
- Antibiotic-associated colitis (pseudomembranous colitis)
- *S. mansoni* or *S. japonicum* infection

Enterohaemorrhagic *E. coli* (EHEC)

These bacteria produce vero cell cytotoxins similar to the toxin produced by *Shigella dysenteriae*. The most common EHEC is *E. coli* 0157. These bacteria have been associated with a number of outbreaks of inflammatory, haemorrhagic colitis and are implicated in the haemolytic-uraemic syndrome (HUS). Infections occur most frequently in the summer months. Contaminated food, particularly ground beef in hamburgers or milk, is the most common cause; cider, fruit, and vegetables may be contaminated by animal faeces. Cross-contamination of meat products has been responsible for outbreaks.

Clinical features: the illness may start with watery diarrhoea, blood appearing after 2–3 days. Vomiting and abdominal tenderness are common and the infection may be confused with appendicitis, intussusception, or inflammatory bowel disease. HUS is a serious life-threatening complication that occurs in 8–10% of children with known *E. coli* 0157 infection usually about a week after onset of diarrhoea. It is characterized by thrombocytopaenia, renal failure, and CNS involvement.

Diagnosis: stool culture is necessary to make the definitive diagnosis but is not generally available. The presence of an outbreak and exposure risk should be sought in the history.

Management

1. Oral rehydration and supportive care.
2. Antibiotic treatment is not indicated and has been associated with increased duration. Some, but not all, studies suggest that antibiotic use may increase the risk of the HUS. Antimotility drugs should be avoided.

Prevention: improve animal management practices, food preparation, and food storage.

Campylobacter enterocolitis

C. jejuni, *C. coli*, or *C. laridis* cause frequent epidemics in nurseries or paediatric wards and are common in the community in developing countries. Infective bacteria may continue to be excreted in the faeces up to 3 weeks after the cessation of diarrhoea. *Campylobacter* infect most mammals and birds and transmission may be by contact with animal or poultry excreta or contaminated food or water.

Clinical features: the disease is normally self-limiting in 5–7 days. Severe, disseminated infection can occur with concurrent malnutrition, hepatic dysfunction, malignancy, diabetes mellitus, renal failure, and immunosuppression. *Complications* include bacteraemia, meningitis, deep abscesses, cholecystitis, and reactive arthritis.

Diagnosis: clinically, the enterocolitis often starts with fever, abdominal pain, and watery diarrhoea, followed by bloody diarrhoea in some cases when it becomes indistinguishable from *Shigella* and *Salmonella* infections. Abdominal pain may be prominent and continue after diarrhoea settles. Diagnosis depends on Gram stain or dark field microscopy of faecal smears +/− culture. In severe disease, colonoscopic biopsy may be needed.

Prevention: Campylobacter infection is an almost ubiquitous zoonosis. Prevention depends on breaking the chain of food and water contamination. No vaccine is currently available.

Yersinia enterocolitis

Yersinia enterocolitica is a rare cause of diarrhoea in the tropics. There may be low-grade fever, bloody diarrhoea, and abdominal pain affecting mainly children <5 yrs, plus nausea, vomiting, headache, or pharyngitis. Infection may spread to cause: septicaemia; peritonitis; hepatic, renal and splenic abscesses; pyomyositis; and osteomyelitis, although such complications are more common in immunocompromised adults or in patients who are iron overloaded (e.g. haemochromatosis).

Diagnosis: culture from stool or other focal sites of infection.

Balantidium enterocolitis

Balantidium coli is a rare protozoal pathogen of humans. It exists in cyst and trophozoite forms, the former being responsible for transmission. Trophozoites invade the intestinal mucosa producing inflammation and ulceration.

Clinical features: infection closely resembles amoebic colitis and may take one of three forms:
- Asymptomatic carrier state (80%).
- Acute dysentery that may be associated with nausea, abdominal pain, and weight loss. This is potentially fatal.
- Chronic diarrhoea, frequently without blood.

Diagnosis: rests upon identification of the trophozoite in the faeces.

Management

Careful rehydration and symptomatic relief is usually sufficient for all three infections. Severe disease may require antibiotics:

• *Campylobacter* enterocolitis

In severe dysenteric type disease, use erythromycin. Resistant strains (especially *C. coli*) may need trimethoprim (or co-trimoxazole) or ciprofloxacin.

• *Yersinia* enterocolitis

In complicated disease, use combinations of gentamicin, cefotaxime, ciprofloxacin, or doxycycline.

• *Balantidium* enterocolitis

If necessary, tetracycline 500 mg PO qds for 10 days in severe disease. The parasite is also sensitive to ampicillin and metronidazole.

Salmonella enterocolitis

Salmonella typhimurium and *S. enteritidis* enterocolitis is an important public health problem in the developing world. Transmission is faeco-oral, usually by ingestion of contaminated food (they survive freezing at 20°C). The organisms are widely distributed among wild and domestic animals. The incubation period is 24–48 hrs (up to 72 hrs); bacteria are then excreted in the faeces for up to 8 weeks following infection. There are associations with both malaria and HIV infection.

Clinical features: range in severity according to the serotype involved. Two (often overlapping) clinical syndromes are seen.

- Acute enterocolitis: nausea and vomiting, headache, fever, and malaise, rapidly progressing to diarrhoea with cramping abdominal pains. Initially voluminous and watery, the stool changes to 'colitic stool' with blood and mucus as the disease progresses. There may be LIF pain and rebound tenderness. Infrequently, ileal involvement is dominant with symptoms mimicking appendicitis. Severe colitis may be complicated by toxic megacolon.
- Invasive salmonellosis: bacteraemia rates of 8% have been recorded, with higher rates for certain serotypes. Predisposing factors are: extremes of age, immunosuppression, malignancy, gastric hypoacidity (e.g. antacid use), concurrent severe disease, bartonellosis, and sickle cell disease. Systemic illness is characterized by swinging fevers, rigors, and general toxicity accompanying the diarrhoea, or a typhoid-like illness characterized by sustained fever, splenomegaly, rose spots, and minimal diarrhoea. There may be metastatic spread to meninges (almost exclusively in children < 2 yrs old), bones and joints, lungs, endocardium and arteries, liver, spleen, ovaries, or kidneys. A reactive arthritis is infrequently seen. Patients with chronic schistosomiasis are prone to 2° *Salmonella* bacteraemia since the bacteria live within the helminth and are protected from antibiotics.

Diagnosis: requires isolation of the bacteria from faecal samples or blood cultures. Sigmoidoscopy may be used in severely ill patients. *Salmonella typhi* does not usually present with diarrhoea and should not be confused with *Salmonella* enterocolitis.

Management

1. Careful rehydration and supportive care is usually sufficient.
2. Most antibiotics do not influence the clinical course and may prolong bacterial carriage.
3. To patients with severe colitis and/or invasive disease, plus those in whom the risk of developing severe disease is high (eg. neonates, immunosuppressed, and elderly), give ciprofloxacin 500 mg PO bd for 5 days.
4. Chloramphenicol, amoxicillin, or trimethoprim (or co-trimoxazole) may be effective in systemic disease, but local resistance is increasing. Cefotaxime is highly effective, where available.

Amoebic dysentery

Around 480 million people worldwide are infected by the protozoan *Entamoeba histolytica* and, although only about 10% are symptomatic, it is the third leading parasitic cause of death after malaria and schistosomiasis, with an annual mortality of ~100,000. Severe infection occurs in pregnant women, very young children, the malnourished, and people on steroids.

Transmission: occurs via the faeco-oral route, usually through food and drink becoming contaminated with human faeces. Prevalence is highest in areas where human faeces are used as fertilizer. Sexual transmission also occurs. Cysts are ingested and pass into the small and large intestine, dividing to form metacysts and trophozoites which produce further cysts. These are evacuated in the stool and remain viable and infective for several days (up to 2 months in cool, damp conditions). *E. histolytica* has the capacity to destroy almost any tissue in the body, with amoebic liver abscess being the most common extra-intestinal manifestation.

Clinical features: range from the asymptomatic carrier state to fulminant colitis with perforation and multi-organ involvement. Intestinal amoebiasis usually has an insidious onset with abdominal discomfort and diarrhoea becoming increasingly bloody and mucoid as severity increases. Tenesmus occurs in half the patients and is always associated with rectosigmoid involvement. On palpation, there is frequently tenderness over the caecum, transverse, and sigmoid colon and the liver may be enlarged and tender. Colonoscopy may reveal hyperaemic, necrotic ulcers covered with a yellowish exudate, particularly in the region of the flexures. Following repeated amoebic infection, an amoebal granuloma (amoeboma) may develop (most frequently at the caecum) where it may be palpable and mistaken for a malignant mass.

Extra-intestinal amoebiasis: the most common form is a liver abscess which may in turn give rise to pericardial, pleuropulmonary, cerebral, genitourinary, or cutaneous disease. It may occur without dysentery.

Diagnosis: is often difficult. Examine at least 3 stool samples using concentration and permanent stain techniques, preferably before administration of medications or contrast media since these interfere with amoebae recovery. The presence of *E. histolytica* trophozoites containing ingested erythrocytes is diagnostic of amoebiasis. However, the demonstration of cysts in a patient with GI symptoms does not necessarily indicate that amoebiasis is causing these symptoms. The cysts of the lumen-dwelling amoeba *E. dispar* is identical to invasive *E. histolytica* and cannot be distinguished microscopically. Techlab Entamoeba 11® is a faecal ELISA based on lectin detection that will differentiate invasive *E. histolytica* cysts or trophozoites from those of *E. dispar*.

Prevention: improved hygiene; no vaccine is yet available.

Management

1. Metronidazole 800 mg PO tds for 5 days followed by
2. Diloxanide furoate 500 mg tds for 10 days.
3. If there are signs of peritonism, add a broad spectrum antibiotic.

(Metronidazole is effective against the trophozoite, but because it has little effect on the cysts treatment should be followed by a luminal amoebicide such as diloxanide).

Trichuriasis (whipworm)

Thought to infect up to 25% of the world's population, *Trichuris trichuria* are 3–4 cm long and colonize the colon and rectum after ingestion of faecally contaminated soil.

Life cycle: ingested eggs hatch in the small intestine releasing larvae which mature in the villi for ~1 week before colonizing the caecum and colorectum. Released eggs pass out in the stool and can resist low temperatures, but not desiccation. The time from ingestion to appearance of eggs in the faeces is ~60 days. The perianal area is covered with eggs and autoinfection occurs by the eggs being carried from the anal margin directly to the mouth.

Clinical features: are often absent in mild infections. However, co-infection with *Ascaris lumbricoides* or hookworms (which is common) may result in RIF pain, vomiting, distension, flatulence, and weight loss. Heavy worm burden can result in lower GI haemorrhage, mucopurulent stool, and dysentery, with rectal prolapse. 2° infection with *E. histolytica* or *B. coli* can aggravate mucosal ulceration and exacerbate dysentery. In such cases there may be finger clubbing and growth retardation in children.

Diagnosis: is by detection of eggs in the stool. An egg count may be done and indicates the degree of infection (>30,000/g stool is heavy infection, implying the presence of several hundred adult worms). There may be anaemia and hypoalbuminaemia, though eosinophilia usually indicates concomitant *Toxocara* infection. Proctoscopy may reveal worms attached to a reddened, ulcerated rectal mucosa. AXR can show changes similar to those seen in Crohn's disease.

Management: mebendazole 500 mg or albendazole 400 mg, both PO once, are equally effective, although there may be regional differences in albendazole sensitivity. 3 day courses may be used for heavy infections.

Prevention: control is as for other soil-transmitted helminths.

Antibiotic-associated colitis

This condition was previously called pseudomembranous colitis or *Clostridium difficile* colitis. It is caused by infection with *C. difficile* following disruption of the normal bowel flora by broad-spectrum oral or IV antibiotic therapy. It is apparently rare in the tropics but is one of the most common causes of hospital acquired diarrhoeal infection in developed countries.

Clinical features: vary from the asymptomatic to toxic megacolon and are due to the production of toxins. Sigmoidoscopy shows characteristic yellow plaques (pseudomembranes) on the mucosa.

Management: metronidazole 800 mg PO stat, then 400 mg PO tds for 10 days. Oral vancomycin (0.5–2 g PO daily in 3–4 divided doses for 7–10 days) is an expensive alternative.

Prevention: careful use of broad-spectrum antibiotics.

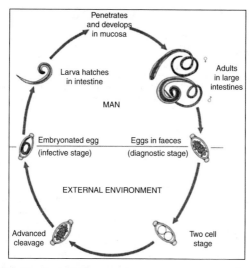

Fig. 2D.5 Life cycle of *T. trichiura*

Clindamycin

Because it is associated with potentially fatal antibiotic-associated colitis, clindamycin has few primary indications (staphylococcal joint and bone infections; intra-abdominal sepsis). However, the WHO considers clindamycin to be a valuable drug that should be used when other antibiotics are known to be ineffective or inappropriate for a given individual. It should be stopped immediately that diarrhoea occurs. It should also be borne in mind that in western countries the most common antibiotics associated with the development of antibiotic-associated colitis are the broad-spectrum β-lactams.

Acute diarrhoea without blood

See box opposite for causes.

Rotavirus

In developed countries, viral infections account for up to 60% of all gastro-enteritis in children < 5 yrs. In contrast, rotavirus cause < 5% of all episodes of diarrhoea in developing countries, but of episodes requiring hospitalization, 40–50% are due to rotavirus. Nearly all children in the tropics have been infected with rotavirus at least once before the age of 2 yrs.

Clinical features: vomiting is an early feature; fever is common; the diarrhoea is usually watery and large volume. Colicky abdominal pains, ill-defined tenderness, and exaggerated bowel sounds are common. The stool may have a characteristic smell.

Management: is supportive, aiming to prevent dehydration. Since rotavirus infection is common in infants, dietary management is especially important to avoid growth faltering and malnutrition. Continue breast-feeding. Lactose malabsorption is common but intolerance is usually only a clinical problem in severe cases. Children with mild diarrhoea should be encouraged to continue eating a normal diet in order to limit weight loss. If diarrhoea continues or is severe, lactose can be reduced by mixing milk with cereals or changing to a lactose free diet but calorie intake should be maintained. As with all diarrhoeal episodes, once the child improves or is hungry extra food should be given in order to make up for weight loss. Beware confusion with surgical causes of diarrhoea in the neonate such as Hirschsprung's disease, intussusception, and bowel atresia.

Prevention: highly contagious, rotavirus infection is difficult to prevent and is a frequent nosocomial infection. A rotavirus vaccine effective in reducing severe disease was developed and marketed but later withdrawn because of reports that risk of intussusception was increased. Alternative vaccines are being tested.

Other viral causes of diarrhoea

Astrovirus: are single-stranded RNA viruses that cause diarrhoea mainly in children and the elderly, with a worldwide distribution. Infection is indistinguishable from rotavirus but generally milder. Diagnosis is by electron microscopy only. Management is oral rehydration as necessary

Norwalk virus: is a human enteric calicivirus and the most important viral cause of food-borne diarrhoeal outbreaks in both developing and developed countries. It is also called 'winter vomiting' disease.

Clinical features: vomiting is usual at onset and may be severe; watery diarrhoea is rarely severe and usually lasts 12–24 hrs. Diagnosis is by PCR or ELISA.

Management: supportive.

Enteric adenovirus: two serotypes, 40 and 41, cause diarrhoea but seem more common in developed countries. Clinical features and management are similar to other viral diarrhoeas. Diagnosis is by electron microscopy or ELISA

Causes of acute diarrhoea without blood

1. *Malaria,* especially *P. falciparum* (see Chapter 2A)

2. *Viruses*
- Rotavirus
- Astrovirus
- Norwalk virus
- Enteric adenovirus

3. *Bacteria*
- Early stage or mild shigellosis, *Salmonella*, or campylobacter infections
- Enterotoxigenic *E. coli* (ETEC) (commonly causing traveller's diarrhoea)
- Enteropathogenic *E. coli* (EPEC)
- Enteroaggregative *E. coli* (EAEC)
- Enterotoxin-producing strains of *Staphylococcus aureus*
- Cholera
- *Clostridia* spp

4. *Protozoa*
- Giardiasis
- Cryptosporidiosis
- *Cyclospora cayetenesis*

5. *Strongyloidiasis*

6. *Food toxins*

Enterotoxigenic *E. coli* (ETEC)

ETEC accounts for 20% of diarrhoeal cases, second only to rotavirus as a cause of inpatient gastroenteritis in developing countries. Transmission is by the faeco-oral route either directly or via contaminated food or water. It may account for up to 80% of 'traveller's diarrhoea' which is said to affect between 20–50% of the estimated 12 million travellers from industrialized countries to the tropics/subtropics annually.

Clinical features: toxins stimulate Cl^-, Na^+, and water efflux into the intestinal lumen, resulting in voluminous, watery diarrhoea after an incubation period of 1–2 days. Vomiting and abdominal cramps are frequently a feature and up to 10 motions per day may be passed.

Diagnosis: depends upon culture of *E. coli* from the faeces and identification of the toxin which is usually only possible in specialist laboratories. By the time this is done, symptoms have usually subsided.

Management: rehydration. Trimethoprim or ciprofloxacin are most likely to be effective in severe disease.

Enteropathogenic *E. coli* (EPEC)

EPEC refer to strains of *E. coli* that include the classic pathogens O111 and O55 and other serotypes which display distinct localized adhesion to Hep-2 cells in culture and human intestinal mucosal cells. In severe infections, the mucosal brush border is lost by a process of vesiculation resulting in malabsorption and osmotic diarrhoea. EPEC are a major cause of infantile diarrhoea that can be devastating. Transmission is by the faeco-oral route. Epidemics of hospital-acquired infection occur and recent hospitalization is a risk factor for infection. It is also associated with traveller's diarrhoea.

Diagnosis: diagnosis rests upon culture of EPEC from the stool or duodenal aspirate. Serology is not reliable but may be the only tool available; DNA probes are available in specialist centres.

Clinical features: range from acute watery diarrhoea to relapsing severe and prolonged diarrhoea, usually with mucus but no blood. Initially there may be vomiting and fever. Epidemics can occur affecting mainly babies, and fatality in untreated epidemics can reach 50%.

Management: rehydration. If the diarrhoea is prolonged, special diets and, rarely, parenteral feeding and antibiotics may be necessary. Co-trimoxazole is recommended since ampicillin is unlikely to be effective, resistance being a problem. Bovine milk immunoglobulin concentrate from immunized cows is a promising new advance.

Prevention: no vaccine is yet available

Causes of traveller's diarrhoea

Enterotoxigenic *E. coli*	30–80%
Campylobacter jejuni	~20%
Shigella spp.	5–15%
Salmonella spp.	3–15%
Giardia intestinalis	0–3%
Unknown	15–20%

Enteroaggregative *E. coli* (EAEC)

These bacteria are recognized by their characteristic adherence pattern to Hep-2 cells. Recently identified, they are now known to be important pathogens in developing countries and seem to be particularly prone to cause persistent diarrhoea. Children of all ages are affected.

Clinical features: vary from asymptomatic to watery diarrhoea, often persistent. EAEC cause travellers' diarrhoea.

Diagnosis: definitive diagnosis is by Hep-2 cell assay

Management: supportive; ciprofloxacin is the most effective antibiotic.

Enterotoxin-producing *S. aureus*

Commonly spread from the milk of cows with staphylococcal mastitis, but may also grow in prepared foods. The incubation time is short; 2–6 hrs (since the enterotoxin is preformed).

Clinical features: vomiting rapidly followed by diarrhoea which may be very severe, though usually short-lived.

Management: supportive; antibiotics are useless.

Cholera

The enterotoxic *Vibrio cholerae* is the main cause of dehydrating diarrhoea in adults. Infections range from asymptomatic to acute fulminant watery diarrhoea, often described as a rice-water stool, which if untreated may be fatal.

Vibrios are Gram-negative, aerobic, comma-shaped rods that are oxidase positive and ferment both sucrose and glucose but not lactose. They can be divided into several serovars with *V. cholerae* 01 causing cholera. *V. cholerae* is killed by heating at 55°C for 15 mins and by most disinfectants, yet it can survive in saline conditions for up to two weeks at ambient temperatures. In most cases, the bacteria survive for only limited periods on foodstuffs, with the notable exception of chitinous shellfish upon which they may survive for 14 days if refrigerated.

Transmission: humans are the only known natural host. Infection usually requires a large infective dose and occurs via contaminated food or water. The incubation period ranges from a few hours to 5 days. Only a minority of infected people develop symptoms — studies suggest that there are ~40 asymptomatic carriers of El Tor to every symptomatic case (~5:1 for classical biotype). This is true both in endemic areas and during outbreaks; hence the need for meticulous hygiene.

Clinical features: symptomatic infection varies between mild self-limiting diarrhoea and severe watery diarrhoea of up to 30 litres per day. Even severe diarrhoea is painless; it leads to electrolyte imbalances, metabolic acidosis, prostration, and can cause death from dehydration within hours. Vomiting starts shortly after the onset of diarrhoea in 80% of cases. Shock typically follows ~12 hrs later, with impaired consciousness due to hypovolaemia and hypoglycaemia. This is particularly serious in children who, unlike adults, may have a mild fever. Renal failure, ileus, and cardiac arrhythmias accelerate death; the elderly or those with low gastric acid, such as alcoholics, are especially vulnerable. Muscular and abdominal cramps are common owing to loss of Ca^{2+} and Cl^- ions.

Diagnosis: in epidemics, the diagnosis may be made on clinical grounds alone. In non-epidemic periods or places, acute watery diarrhoea resulting in severe dehydration or the death of a patient over 5 yrs should suggest cholera. Dark field microscopy of faecal material shows comma-shaped bacteria darting about; this is quickly halted upon addition of diluted 01 antisera. Transportation of samples should be in alkaline peptone water and kept cool. Culture requires selective media such as TCBS agar. If possible, specimens should be sent to a reference laboratory for bio- and serotyping.

Management

1. In all but a few cases, treatment consists solely of meticulous attention to rehydration, usually with oral preparations. This will reduce mortality to less than 1%. See below for rehydration management. The most common error is underestimation of the volume of ORS or intravenous fluid required. In some emergency cases, where ORS was not available, sucrose and rice-water-based solutions have been given with success.

Epidemiology of *V. cholerae*

V. cholerae serovar 01 is the causative agent of cholera. There are two biotypes of the 01 serovar: *classical* and *El Tor*. Each of these biotypes is further divided into three serotypes: Ogawa, Inaba, and Hikojima.

The classical biotype caused the first six cholera pandemics in south Asia during the 19th and early 20th centuries. The El Tor biotype was first recognized in 1906 but until 1963 was restricted to Sulawesi. During the 1960s, the seventh pandemic started with spread of the El Tor biotype, Inaba serotype, out of Indonesia into South Asia, Africa, and, since 1991, Latin America. This biotype has now replaced the classical biotype throughout much of the world, except Bangladesh.

Other *V. cholerae* serovars cause a cholera-like illness. The 0139 serotype first appeared in southern India in 1992. Unlike other non-01 strains, it causes cholera with similar epidemiological and clinical pictures to 01 cholera. The major difference noted in Bangladesh is that it tends to affect adults. Previous exposure to the 01 serovar does not confer protection.

2. Antibiotics should be given to severe cases, where they have been shown to reduce both the volume and duration of diarrhoea.
- Doxycycline is the drug of choice for adults (except pregnant women) in whom a single dose of 300 mg is sufficient.
- Tetracycline 500 mg PO qds for 3 days can be given to adults, although resistance has been reported in central Asia and Africa.
- Follow local guidelines based on susceptibilities.
- Give children or pregnant women co-trimoxazole 30 mg/kg PO od. This may also be used for adults: 960 mg PO bd for 3 days.

Prevention: public health measures aimed at improving food and water hygiene and sanitation are the most important factors. Currently, oral killed whole-cell vaccines and a live attenuated vaccine are available. Their use in outbreaks has not been fully evaluated and should not deflect resources from treatment facilities and prevention of spread.

Health education: plays a major role in both preventing outbreaks and limiting the spread of infection once one occurs. This should not only concentrate upon ensuring food and water hygiene, but also measures such as disinfecting patients' clothing by boiling for 5 mins, drying out bedding in the sun, burying stools, etc. In larger health centres, patient excreta may be mixed with disinfectant (e.g. cresol) or acid before disposal in pit latrines. Semi-solid waste should be incinerated. Funerals have been a source of spread and preventive measures should be instigated to minimize the risk of mourners arriving from uninfected areas, and potential contamination from ritual washing of the dead and funeral feasts.

The cholera outbreak

It is obligatory to notify the WHO of all cholera cases. Suspected cases should be reported immediately by health authorities and laboratory confirmation sent as soon as it is obtained. This should be followed by weekly reports containing the number of new cases and deaths since the last report, the cumulative totals for the year, and if possible the age distribution and number of patients admitted to hospital, recorded by region or other geographical division. This data should be sent to WHO headquarters as well as to the appropriate regional office.

Usually there is a national co-ordinating committee to implement and regulate control and prevention measures, though often it is up to the front-line doctors to initiate the process and frequently they remain in close collaboration with national and international bodies. Mobile control teams may be needed in inaccessible areas or in countries with no national co-ordination and these are responsible for establishing and operating temporary treatment centres, training local staff, educating the public, carrying out epidemiological studies, collecting stool, food, and water samples for laboratory analysis, and providing emergency logistical support to health posts and laboratories. Emergency treatment centres may be needed if appropriate facilities do not exist or are swamped with patients. Strict isolation or quarantine measures are not needed. The most crucial factor affecting survival is access to treatment centres with trained staff and intravenous and oral rehydration capability.

Estimated minimum supplies needed to treat 100 patients during a cholera outbreak[1]

- 650 packets of ORS solution (1 litre)
- 120 bags of 1 litre Ringer's lactate solution[2], with giving sets
- 10 scalp vein sets
- 3 NG tubes, 5.3 mm outside diameter (16 French), 50cm long for adults
- 3 NG tubes; 2.7 mm outside diameter (8 French), 38 cm long for children.

For adults:
- 60 capsules of doxycycline 100 mg (3 caps per severely dehydrated adult patient) *or*
- *480 capsules of tetracycline 250 mg (24 capsules per severely dehydrated patient).*

For children or pregnant women:
- 300 tablets of co-trimoxazole 120 mg

If selective chemoprophylaxis is planned:
The additional requirements for 4 close contacts per severely dehydrated patient (~80 people) are:
- 240 capsules of doxycycline 100 mg (3 capsules per person) *or*
- 1920 capsules of tetracycline 250 mg (24 capsules per person).

Other necessary supplies:
- 2 large water dispensers with tap for bulk ORS manufacture
- 20 1-litre bottles, 20 half-litre bottles for ORS dispensing
- 40 200 ml cups
- 20 teaspoons
- 5 kg cotton wool
- 3 reels of adhesive tape.

1. The supplies listed are sufficient for IV fluid followed by oral rehydration salts for 20 severely dehydrated patients and for ORS alone for 80 patients.
2. If Ringer's lactate solution or similar solution is unavailable, physiological saline may be substituted.

Clostridium perfringens

Clostridium perfringens produces two forms of gastrointestinal disease: simple food poisoning (caused by type A) and necrotic enterocolitis (type C).

1. *Food poisoning* — see Table 2D.2
2. *Necrotic enterocolitis (pigbel)*

This is common in Uganda, South-East Asia, China, and the highlands of Papua New Guinea. It occurs when *C. perfringens* type C is eaten, normally in meat, by people who are malnourished, heavily infected with *Ascaris lumbricoides*, or have a diet rich in sweet potatoes. The latter two are associated with high levels of heat-stable trypsin inhibitors that inhibit the luminal proteases, preventing them inactivating the toxin.

Clinical features: symptoms usually begin 48 hrs following ingestion but may start up to one week later. It is classified into 4 types:

- Type I (*acute toxic*) presents with fulminant toxaemia and shock. It usually occurs in young children and carries an 85% mortality rate.
- Type II (*acute surgical*) presents as mechanical or paralytic ileus, acute strangulation, perforation, or peritonitis. It has 40% mortality.
- Type III (*subacute surgical*) presents later, with features similar to type II. Mortality is also ~40%.
- Type IV is of *mild diarrhoea* only, though it may progress to type III.

In types II and III a thickened segment of bowel is sometimes palpable. Blood and pus are passed with the stool in severe disease.

Diagnosis: isolation of *C. perfringens* from stool or peritoneal fluid culture. Serological diagnosis is also possible.

Management: type I and II disease require urgent surgery after appropriate resuscitation. Give IV chloramphenicol or benzylpenicillin and *C. perfringens* type C antiserum, where available. Milder cases may require glucose and electrolyte infusions, with IV broad-spectrum antibiotics if there are signs of extraintestinal spread. Give an antihelminthic effective against *Ascaris*. Oral food intake should begin after 24 hrs.

Prevention: immunization with type C toxoid has greatly reduced the incidence and severity of the disease in Papua New Guinea.

Table 2D.2 Food poisoning from bacteria or their toxins

Organism/toxin	Principal foods	Time after food	Clinical features
Staph. aureus	Meat, poultry, dairy produce	1–6 hrs	D, V, AP
B. cereus	Fried rice, sauces, vegetables	1–5 hrs 6–16 hrs	V D, AP
Red bean toxin		1–6 hrs	D, V
Scombrotoxin	Fish	1–6 hrs	D, flushing, sweating, mouth pain
Mushroom toxin		1–6 hrs	D, V, AP
Ciguatera	Fish	1–6 hrs	Fits, coma, renal/liver failure
Salmonella spp.	Meat, poultry, dairy produce	8–72 hrs (mean 12–36 hrs)	D, V, AP, fever
Campylobacter spp	Poultry, raw milk, eggs	1–10 days (mean 2–5 days)	D, AP
C. perfringens A	Cooked meat	8–24 hrs (mean 8–15 hrs)	D, AP, V
Vibrio parahaemolyticus	Seafood	4–96 hrs (mean 12 hrs)	D, V, AP, cramp, headache
Shigella spp.	Faecal contamination	1–7 days (mean 1–3 days)	D(bloody), V, fever
C. botulinum	Poorly canned food, smoked meats	2 hrs–8 days (mean 12–36 hrs)	Diplopia, paralysis
L. monocytogenes	Dairy produce, meat, vegetables, seafood	1–7 weeks	Septicaemia, septic abortion
E. coli	Dirty water	8–44 hrs	D, V, cramps
Y. enterocolitica	Pork and beef	24–36 hrs	Fever, AP, D

V = vomiting, D = diarrhoea, AP = abdominal pain

Giardiasis

Giardia intestinalis (also known as *G. lamblia*, *G. duodenalis*) is the most common human protozoan GI pathogen, having a worldwide distribution. Its prevalence rates can reach ~30% in the tropics, with infection being highest in infants and children. It causes 3% of traveller's diarrhoea.

Transmission: the cysts can survive for long periods outside the host in suitable environments (e.g. surface water). They are notably NOT killed by chlorination. Infection follows ingestion of cysts in faecally contaminated water (rarely food) or through direct person to person contact. Partial immunity may be acquired through repeated infections.

Clinical features: in endemic areas, the asymptomatic carrier state is common. Symptoms of acute disease usually begin within 3–20 days of infection; most patients recover within 2–4 weeks, although in 25% of travellers symptoms persist for up to 7 weeks. Diarrhoea is the major symptom; it is watery initially, becoming steatorrhoeic and often associated with nausea, abdominal discomfort, bloating, weight loss, and sometimes sulfurous, offensive burps.

Some patients develop a chronic diarrhoea associated with weight loss of up to 20% of ideal body weight, fat malabsorption, deficiencies (particularly of vitamins A and B12), and in some cases 2° hypolactasia.

Complications: in hyperendemic settings, infections are universal and usually asymptomatic but some studies have documented retardation of growth and development in severely affected infants and children, in whom malabsorption exacerbates malnutrition. Chronic giardiasis is associated with allergic and inflammatory conditions such as lymphoid nodular hyperplasia. Protein-losing enteropathy, lactose intolerance, and irritable bowel syndrome can also occur.

Diagnosis: detection of cysts (and occasionally trophozoites) in faecal samples by light microscopy. Examine 3 separate samples, since cysts are excreted only intermittently, and diagnostic sensitivity is low. Trophozoites may be detected in biopsies of small intestine mucosa. ELISA tests now exist for faecal *Giardia* antigens. Since mixed enteric infections and asymptomatic carriage of *Giardia* is so common, identification of the parasite does not guarantee that it is the causative agent of the diarrhoea. Serology is not useful because of cross-reactivity in non-infected individuals in endemic areas.

Management

1. Rehydration and symptomatic relief are usually sufficient.
2. If symptoms persist, an anti-giardial drug will decrease the severity and duration of symptoms. Drug failure due to resistance is increasing. Recommended drugs include metronidazole and tinidazole.

Prevention: attention to personal hygiene, appropriate treatment of water supplies, encouraging breastfeeding (shown to partially protect against infection).

Paromycin:
Oral aminoglycoside
approved for use giardia (in preg. women too)
modest effic. for crypto.

Handwritten annotations (top): c HIV <100 CD4 = chronic, <50 = cholera-like. can also get sclerosing cholangitis (infect. of biliary tract)

Cryptosporidiosis

The protozoan *Cryptosporidium parvum* is a common opportunistic infection in HIV +ve patients. It is also a common cause of childhood diarrhoea in the immunocompetent. Transmission is mainly through contaminated water. It accounts for up to 17% of childhood diarrhoea in the developing world, and infections contribute to growth faltering during the first year of life. Although usually mild, severe or persistent diarrhoea may occur.

Handwritten (right margin): C. hominus more common now. get a succ to other forms of diarr.

Clinical features: acute [watery] diarrhoea is indistinguishable from other aetiologies. *Cryptosporidium* should be sought in persistent (chronic) diarrhoea; in AIDS patients it may be severe, mimicking cholera, and/or very prolonged.

Handwritten: reg. O+P will miss this

Diagnosis: faecal detection of the oocysts (4–6 µm in diameter red spheres on modified ZN stain). Oocysts can also be seen in sputum on occasions.

Handwritten: ↳ acid fast, IFA, flourescent (50% schs.) A g defect assays (BEST) or PCR

Management: rehydration with symptomatic relief; as yet, no drug has been shown to be effective against this organism. Ø lactose

Handwritten: * 10% travelers diarrhea caused by Crypto. can use anti-motility drugs. Nitazoxanide may help speed recov. treat children. ⊗ PI helps resolve Crypto.

Cyclospora

Cyclospora cayetanensis is a protozoan coccidian parasite now recognized to be a frequent cause of diarrhoea in developing and developed countries. Transmission is via contaminated water or food; the largest outbreaks in USA were caused by contaminated imported raspberries.

Handwritten: watery diarrhea > 3 wks. duration (up to months)

Diagnosis: is by finding typical oocysts in faeces which are 7–10 µm diameter and contain a 'morula' of 8 spherical bodies. The oocysts are also irregularly acid-fast when stained with modified Zn stain.

Clinical features: watery diarrhoea which is most severe in non-immune travellers. Mild fever, fatigue, anorexia, and weight loss may occur. The illness can last for weeks.

Management: co-trimoxazole 960 mg bd for 7–10 days.

Handwritten: children 5mg/kg. main site of infect is jejunum. ALTS: Cipro?

Trophozoites of Giardia spp in stool isolates

Handwritten (right): Antimot. Loperomede Perogolde

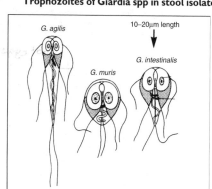

G. agilis

10–20µm length

G. muris

G. intestinalis

Strongyloidiasis

The nematode *Strongyloides stercoralis* commonly infects humans world-wide, particularly in parts of S. America and S.E. Asia. It is a serious condition in the immunosuppressed and may cause acute, relapsing, or persistent diarrhoea. There are two adult forms of the worm and two larval forms, one of which is infective.

Life cycle: Complex, since reproduction can take place in either of two cycles: an external cycle involving free-living worms or an internal cycle involving parasitic worms. Contamination of skin or buccal mucosa with larvae-containing soil permits initial penetration of larvae and infection. The larvae travel to the lungs and enter the bronchi, eventually passing into the small intestine, where they mature into adults. Eggs produced by the female pass out in the faeces and continue the external cycle.

Autoinfection occurs by either bronchial larvae producing progeny or filariform larvae not passing out in the stool but reinvading bowel or perianal skin. This can produce indefinite (up to 30 yrs) multiplication within the host, not requiring further infection. The pre-patent period from infection to the appearance of larvae in the stools is ~1 month.

Clinical features: Infection is asymptomatic in most instances, except for autoinfection through perianal skin. The immune response limits the infection to the small bowel and also the number of adult worms.

Larval penetration causes petechial haemorrhages and pruritus at the site of entry, frequently with a linear, red eruption (larva currens) as the larvae migrate under the skin. This is normally transient, but may be followed by congestion and oedema. A creeping urticarial rash may occur in pre-sensitized individuals following reinfection. Symptoms similar to bronchopneumonia with consolidation may result from larval invasion of the lungs which, together with eosinophilia, may resemble TPE. Watery diarrhoea with mucus is a frequent symptom; its intensity is dependent upon the worm burden. It often alternates with constipation. In severe cases, chronic diarrhoea with malabsorption may ensue.

In the immunosuppressed, malnourished, or debilitated, massive tissue invasion may occur. Complications include severe diarrhoea, ileus, hepatomegaly, and multi-system disease due to blood/lymphatic spread. Granulomas and/or abscesses occur in the liver, kidneys, and lungs; CNS involvement produces pyogenic meningitis and encephalopathy. Death is usually a result of septicaemia with *E coli*.

Diagnosis: detection of adults or rhabditiform <u>larvae</u> ~~not eggs~~ in the stool. Also modified Baermann technique agar plate culture, ELISA, serology, and stool culture using charcoal. Look for infection in the immunosuppressed or those who are about to be (e.g. on steroids).

Management: treat all infected patients, not just the symptomatic.
1. Albendazole 400 mg PO bd for 3 days
   (Alternatives: ivermectin 200 mcg/kg PO as a single dose or tiabendazole 25 mg/kg PO bd for 3 days)
2. Massive infection also responds well to albendazole.

Prevention: requires improving hygiene and education on a community level, as well as monitoring and evaluation.

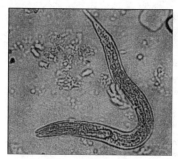

Fig. 2D.6 *S. Stercoralis* larva in stool sample. Size 200–300 ×15μm

Isospora belli
mostly in AIDS pts. + some nl. hosts (months watery diarrhoea
* assoc. c̄ eosinophilia *

diag:- large
Acid fast

tmt: Trimeth-Sulpha

Persistent or chronic diarrhoea

Persistent is the preferred term for episodes starting acutely and associated with gastrointestinal infections. Defined as diarrhoea lasting >2 weeks.

Causes of persistent or chronic diarrhea

1. *Secondary events*
   - Subclinical malabsorption
   - Hypolactasia (1° and 2°)
   - Tropical sprue
   - Cow's milk protein intolerance

2. *Continuing infection*
   - Strongyloidiasis
   - Cryptosporidiosis
   - Enteropathogenic *E. coli*
   - Intestinal flukes
   - Chronic intestinal schistosomiasis

3. *Delayed recovery*
   - Malnutrition
   - Zinc deficiency

4. *Sequential new infections*

5. *Others*
   - HIV enteropathy
   - Chronic calcific pancreatitis
   - Short bowel disease (e.g. recovered pigbel disease)
   - Ileocaecal TB
   - Lymphoma — Burkitt's and Mediterranean
   - Acute and chronic liver disease
   - Inflammatory bowel disease and coeliac disease

Malabsorption and steatorrhoea

May be due to a wide range of causes. The key signs and symptoms are:
- *Diarrhoea:* stool is typically loose, bulky, offensive, greasy, light coloured, and difficult to flush away.
- *Abdominal symptoms:* discomfort, distension, flatulence.
- *Nutritional deficiencies:* e.g. glossitis, pallor, muscle pain bruising, hyper-pigmentation, CNS or PNS signs, skeletal deformity.
- *General ill health:* anorexia, weight loss, lethargy, dyspnoea, fatigue.
- Features related to *underlying cause:* surgical scars, systemic disease.

Investigating malabsorption
Do FBC, U&Es ESR, LFTs, stool culture, and microscopy. Others include faecal fat, INR (deficiency of fat-soluble vitamins), carbohydrate absorption (after glucose or xylose), Schilling test (as measure of ileal function)

Clinical malabsorption
1° hypolactasia (a lactase deficiency of genetic origin) is a common non-infectious cause of watery diarrhoea occurring after consumption of milk . 2° hypolactasia results from brush border damage during GI infection; it may persist afterwards. Incomplete hydrolysis of lactose results in osmotic

diarrhoea, abdominal pain, distension, and flatulence. Colonic bacteria may produce lactic acid by hydrolysing lactose — this can also cause an irritative diarrhoea.

Diagnosis: rests upon detection of worsening symptoms with increased lactose intake (lactose tolerance test), acid stools with positive reducing substances, the hydrogen breath test, or a lactase assay in jejunal biopsy.

Management: consists of reducing lactose in diet, giving only small amounts of lactose at a time. Yogurt may be substituted for milk; cereal-milk mixtures have also been used successfully. In severe cases it may be necessary to eliminate lactose-containing products from the diet. They may be gradually reintroduced after 6 weeks without symptoms. Care should be taken to ensure that reduction or elimination of lactose containing foods does not reduce energy and nutrient intake.

Possible mechanisms for persistent diarrhoea

Different mechanisms may prolong diarrhoea. In areas where sanitation and clean water are lacking and diarrhoea incidence is high, most persistent diarrhoea seems to be attributable to frequent new infections combined with delayed recovery (3 and 4). Delayed recovery is often due to nutrient deficiencies. Persistent diarrhoea is associated with malnutrition and high mortality in children. Dietary management with continued feeding, correction of micronutrient deficiencies, antimicrobial treatment of concomitant infections and dysentery — as well as rehydration if necessary — has been shown to be effective in 80% of children.

Causes of malabsorption

- *Infective:* acute enteritis, intestinal TB, parasitic infections, traveller's diarrhoea, Whipple's disease.
- *Anatomical/motility:* blind loops, diverticulae, strictures, fistulae, small bowel lymphoma, systemic sclerosis, diabetes mellitus, pseudo-obstruction, radiotherapy, amyloidosis, lymphatic obstruction (TB, lymphoma, cardiac disease).
- *Defective digestion:* chronic pancreatitis, cystic fibrosis, food sensitivity (lactose, gluten), malnutrition, gastric/intestinal surgery, Zollinger–Ellison syndrome, pancreatectomy, biliary obstruction, terminal ileal disease/resection (short bowel syndrome), parenchymal liver disease, bacterial overgrowth.
- *Drugs:* antibiotics, cholestyramine, metformin, methyldopa, alcohol, antacids, purgative misuse, paraaminosalicylic acid.

Post-infective malabsorption (PIM or tropical sprue)

A better name for this syndrome of diarrhoea, malabsorption, and weight loss is post-acute infective malabsorption, since a chronicity of at least 2 months is required for the diagnosis. Malabsorption of nutrients is quantitatively more important than that of water or electrolytes in this condition. It produces an estimated 10% deficit of dietary energy. It is therefore obvious that its impact on individuals (particularly children) living on marginal diets is significant and that it will quickly exacerbate malnutrition. PIM is common in central America, northern South America, and Asia; it also occurs around the Mediterranean and in the Middle East.

Aetiology: is thought to involve:
- Genes — an association with certain HLA antigens has been found
- Infection — *Klebsiella pneumoniae*, *Enterobacter cloacae*, and *E. coli* are the organisms most commonly isolated from mucosal biopsy or luminal fluid; they may persist in overgrowth for many months
- Jejunal morphology — partial villous atrophy, crypt hyperplasia, elevated jejunal surface pH, and changes in gut hormones and colonic function have been found.

Clinical features: chronic diarrhoea of >2 months duration with large, pale, fatty stools and often flatulence. Other features include weight loss, glossitis, megaloblastic anaemia, fluid retention, depression, lethargy, amenorrhoea, and infertility. Serum folate and vitamin B12 may fall to very low levels. Hypoalbuminaemia and oedema are late signs.

Investigations: 1-hr blood xylose concentration following a 5g or 25g loading dose; 72-hr faecal fat estimation; Schilling test; serum B12; RBC folate; serum globin; and albumin. Exclude faecal parasites. Barium meal and follow-through will show dilated loops of jejunum with clumping of barium. Jejunal biopsy may show a ridged or convoluted mucosa, depending on the duration of the disease, with T lymphocyte infiltration.

Management
1. Eliminate bacterial overgrowth with tetracycline 250 mg PO qds for at least 2 weeks.
2. Aid mucosal recovery by providing folate supplements.
3. Provide a suitable diet to promote weight gain.
4. Give symptomatic relief in the acute stages:
   - Codeine phosphate 30 mg PO tds **or**
   - Loperamide 4 mg PO initially, then 2 mg after each loose stool. Usual dose 6–8 mg od; maximum dose 16 mg od.

Tropical enteropathy and subclinical malabsorption
Repeated low-grade viral, bacterial, and parasitic infections may also cause damage to the small intestinal mucosa of individuals living in the tropics. Concurrent systemic infections (e.g. TB, pneumococcal pneumonia), malnutrition, and pellagra have also been implicated in causing subclinical malabsorption. Xylose, glucose, and vitamin B12 are most commonly malabsorbed.

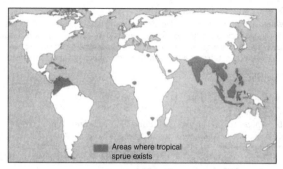

Fig. 2D.7 Distribution of post-infective malabsorption.

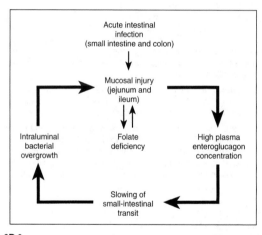

Fig. 2D.8

Other causes of malabsorption

Whipples disease: a rare malabsorptive condition characterized by transient migratory polyarthritis, fever, lymphadenopathy, and cardiac and neurological complications. It is caused by *Tropheryma whippelii*. Treatment is with penicillin, tetracycline, or co-trimoxazole; many patients relapse.

Lymphangiectasia: either 1° or following an abdominal malignancy, it results in lacteal dilatation. Clinically there is peripheral oedema secondary to hypoproteinaemia owing to a protein-losing enteropathy. Diagnosis requires small bowel biopsy. Treatment is with a low-fat diet.

Abetalipoproteinaemia: a rare AR disorder, usually presenting in childhood due to defective triglyceride transport from the liver and gut. Eventually neurological dysfunction (peripheral neuropathy, cerebellar ataxia) may follow. Diagnosis is by small bowel biopsy and symptomatic treatment is with low-fat diet and vitamin supplementation.

Other causes of chronic diarrhoea

1. Chronic calcific pancreatitis
A syndrome of pancreatic calcification associated with both exocrine and endocrine impairment, commonly encountered in the tropics, especially equatorial Africa, southern India, and Indonesia. Its aetiology is unknown, although childhood kwashiorkor, gastroenteritis, excessive alcohol consumption, dehydration, and ingestion of cassava (*Manhiot esculenta*) have all been implicated.

Clinical features: are of chronic malabsorption with weight loss, often associated with DM (10% of diabetes in E&W Africa) and (sometimes severe) pain. There is an association with pancreatic malignancy.

Management: consists of diabetic control, a low-fat diet, and enzymatic supplementation (e.g. pancreatin BP 6g orally with food).
Pancreatic dysfunction may also result from schistosomiasis, trichinellosis, cysticercosis, clonorchiasis, opisthorchiasis, and hydatid disease. Obstruction is commonly a complication of *A. lumbricoides* infection.

2. Intestinal lymphoma
Wide varieties of lymphomas affect the GI tract, originating in either intestinal lymph nodes (e.g. Hodgkin's lymphoma) or mucosa-associated lymphoid tissue (MALT lymphomas). Weight loss is a common feature and nodal disease may be confused with intestinal TB, as X-ray changes appear similar. Diagnosis requires biopsy.

3. Intestinal parasites
Many parasites such as *Giardia, Cryptosporidium, Trichuris,* and *Strongyloides* cause diarrhoea and have been described above. Other intestinal parasites are described below.

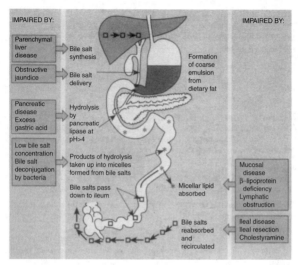

Fig. 2D.9 Mechanisms of Steatorrhoea.

Intestinal flukes

These pathogens are common throughout Asia (particularly S.E. Asia), where their prevalence may reach 30% in certain populations. Children are more heavily infected and prone to symptoms.

1. Fasciolopsiasis

Caused by *Fasciolopsis buski*, infection is via consumption of metacercaria attached to the seed pods of water plants contaminated by human and pig faeces.

2. Echinostomiasis

At least 15 *Echinostoma* spp. infect humans via the consumption of raw or undercooked freshwater snails, clams, fish, and tadpoles. In N.E. Thailand, it is commonly associated with *Opisthorchis* infection.

3. Heterophyasis

Numerous species of the small (2.5mm) *Heterophyes* flukes infect humans following consumption of raw aquatic foods and/or insect larvae.

Clinical features: the attachment of parasites to the intestinal mucosa results in inflammation and ulcer formation. Infections are frequently asymptomatic; when symptoms do occur, they are usually mild and non-specific — diarrhoea, flatulence, mild abdominal pains, vomiting, fever, and anorexia. Fasciolopsiasis may produce severe disease with ascites, oedema, anaemia, and symptomatic malabsorption. Eggs (and sometimes adult worms) of *Heterophyes* spp. may enter the lymphatics after mucosal penetration and be transported to other sites (notably heart, spinal cord, brain, lungs, liver, and spleen) where they cause granulomatous reactions. Myocarditis and neurological deficits may result.

Diagnosis: faecal examination for eggs, after concentration. Differentiation between *F. hepatica, F. buski,* and echinostomes is often difficult. Similarly, heterophydiae eggs closely resemble those of *Clonorchis* and *Opisthorchis*. Recovery of adult worms from post-treatment faeces allows a definitive diagnosis, although in the case of the heterophyids this is difficult owing to their small size. Extraintestinal cases of heterophyiasis are also difficult to diagnose — they are often only revealed during surgery or autopsy.

Management

1. Praziquantel is the drug of choice, with high efficacy at 25 mg/kg as a single dose.
2. Mebendazole or albendazole may be used for echinostomiasis although praziquantel is recommended in areas where other trematodes are present, due to its broad efficacy.

Prevention: should concentrate on breaking the faeco-oral cycle (e.g. stopping the use of human and pig excreta as fertilizer) possibly combined with community-based praziquantel treatment and education regarding the consumption of raw/undercooked foodstuffs.

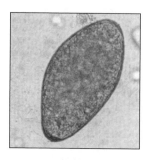

Fig. 2D.10 Eggs of *Fascilopsis buski* (top, 140×85μm) and *Heterophyes heterophyes* (below, 25×15μm)

General management of dehydration

The volume of fluid lost in the stool in 24 hrs can vary from 5 ml/kg to 200 ml/kg or more. The loss of electrolytes also varies. The total body sodium defect in young children with severe dehydration owing to diarrhoea is usually about 70–110 mmol per litre of water lost. The degree of dehydration is graded according to the signs and symptoms that reflect the amount of fluid lost.

In the early stages of dehydration, there are no signs or symptoms. As dehydration increases, these develop, including thirst, restless or irritable behaviour, decreased skin turgor, dry mucous membranes, sunken eyes, sunken fontanelle (in infants), and absence of tears when crying.

In severe dehydration, these effects become more pronounced and the patient may develop signs of hypovolaemic shock, including decreased consciousness, anuria, cool moist extremities, rapid and feeble pulse, low blood pressure, and peripheral cyanosis. Death may follow swiftly if rehydration is not started at once.

Types of dehydration

1. **Isotonic dehydration:** is the most frequently encountered type of dehydration and occurs when the net losses of water and sodium are in the same proportion as is normally found in the extracellular fluid (ECF). The principal features of isotonic dehydration are: a balanced deficit of water and sodium; normal serum sodium concentration (130–150 mmol/l); normal serum osmolality (275–295 mOsmol/l); hypovolaemia because of excess ECF losses. Clinical features are those of hypovolaemic shock (i.e. thirst, reduced skin turgor, dry mucous membranes, sunken eyes, oliguria, and a sunken fontanelle in infants). This progresses to anuria, hypotension, a weak pulse, cool extremities, and eventually coma and death.

2. *Hypertonic (hypernatraemic) dehydration:* reflects a net loss of water in excess of sodium and tends to occur in infants only. It usually results from attempted treatment of diarrhoea with fluids that are hypertonic (e.g. sweetened fruit juices/soft drinks, glucose solution) combined with insufficient intake of water and other hypotonic solutes. Hypertonic solutions cause water to flow from the ECF into the intestine, leading to decreased ECF volume and hypernatraemia. The principal features are: a deficit of water; hypernatraemia (>150 mmol/l); serum osmolality >295 mOsmol/l; severe thirst; irritability; and convulsions (especially if serum Na^+ is >165 mmol/l).

3. *Hypotonic (hyponatraemic) dehydration:* occurs in patients with diarrhoea who drink large amounts of water or other hypotonic fluids containing very low quantities of salt and other solutes. It also occurs in patients who receive IV infusions of 5% glucose in water. It occurs because water is absorbed from the gut while the loss of salt continues, producing a net excess of water and hyponatraemia. The features are: dehydration with hyponatraemia (serum Na^+ <130 mmol/l); low serum osmolality (<275 mOsmol/l); lethargy; and, rarely, convulsions.

Assessment of dehydration in patients with diarrhoea

1. Look at:

Condition	Well, alert	Restless, irritable	Lethargic[1] or unconscious
Eyes[2]	Normal	Sunken	Sunken
Thirst	None	Drinks eagerly, very thirsty	Drinks poorly, unable to drink

2. Pinch the skin[3]:

	Goes back immediately	Goes back slowly	Goes back very slowly

3. Decide:

	No dehydration	**Some dehydration**	**Severe dehydration**

4. Treat:

	Plan A (see p. 156)	Plan B (see p. 158)	Plan C (see p. 160)

Plans B and C require at least two of the four signs to be positive

Notes:

1. A lethargic patient is not simply asleep; the patient's mental state is dull and the patient cannot be fully awakened. The patient may appear to be drifting into unconsciousness.
2. In some infants, the eyes normally appear a little sunken, so ask the mother if the child's eyes appear normal to her.
3. Pinch the abdominal skin in a longitudinal manner with thumb and bent forefinger. 'Goes back slowly' means that it is visible for more than 2 seconds.

Estimation of fluid deficit

Children with dehydration should be weighed without clothing, as an aid to estimating their fluid requirements. If weighing is not possible, the child's age may be used to estimate the weight. Treatment should never be delayed because scales are not readily available.

A child's fluid deficit may be estimated as follows:

Assessment	Fluid deficit as % of body weight	Fluid deficit ml/kg body weight
No signs of dehydration	<5%	<50 ml/kg
Some dehydration	5–10%	50–100 ml/kg
Severe dehydration	>10%	>100 ml/kg

Suitable fluids

Many countries have designated recommended home fluids which should be used in the *prevention* of dehydration only (i.e. treatment plan A – see p. 156). Whenever possible, these should include at least one fluid that normally contains salt (e.g. oral rehydration solution — ORS; salted drinks such as salted rice water or salted yoghurt; vegetable or chicken soup with salt). Other fluids should be recommended that are frequently given to children in the area, that mothers consider acceptable for children with diarrhoea, and that the mothers would likely give in increased amounts if advised to do so. Such fluids should be safe and easy to prepare.

If there are signs of dehydration, ORS should be used as per treatment plans B and C (see pp. 158, 160)

- Teaching mother to add salt (about 3 g/l) to unsalted drinks or soups during diarrhoea is beneficial, but requires education and (initially) supervision.
- A home-made solution containing 3 g/l salt and 18 g/l of common sugar (sucrose) is effective, but the recipe is often forgotten and/or the ingredients hard to obtain.

Unsuitable fluids

A few fluids are potentially dangerous and should be avoided during episodes of diarrhoea. Especially important are drinks sweetened with sugar that can cause osmotic diarrhoea and hypernatraemia (e.g. soft drinks, sweetened fruit drinks, sweetened tea).

Oral rehydration solution (ORS)

The formula for ORS recommended by WHO and UNICEF is given in the box opposite. Where bulk preparation is required, multiply the amounts shown by however many litres of solution you wish to make. ORS should be used within 24 hrs of preparation.

When given correctly, ORS provides sufficient water and electrolytes to correct the deficits associated with acute diarrhoea. For children with severe malnutrition a solution containing 45–60 mMol sodium is preferred.

To make a litre of ORS solution from bulk ingredients

1. Sodium chloride   2.6g
   plus
2. Glucose   13.5g
   plus
3. Trisodium citrate, dihydrate   2.9g
   plus
4. Potassium chloride   1.5g

If glucose and trisodium citrate are not available; use:
   Sucrose   27g
   Sodium bicarbonate   2.5g

- Completely dissolve the sugar and salts in one litre of clean water — boiled or chlorinated water is best.
- ORS solution should be used within 24 hrs, after which time it should be discarded and fresh solution prepared.
- To make 1 litre of rice-based ORS, boil 50g of rice powder in 1.1 litres of water. Mix in sugar and salt in the quantities stated above. Use within 12 hrs.

Treatment plan A

To treat diarrhoea without signs of dehydration at home
Use this plan to teach the mother to:

- Continue to treat her child's current episode of diarrhoea at home
- Give early treatment for future episodes of diarrhoea

Explain the 3 rules for treating diarrhoea at home

1. *Give the child more fluids than usual to prevent dehydration*
   Use recommended home fluids (see above) and ORS as described below. Note: if the child is <6 months old and not yet taking solid foods, give ORS solution rather than a food-based fluid. Give as much of these fluids as the child will take. Use the amounts shown below for ORS as a guide. Continue giving these fluids until the diarrhoea stops.

2. *Give the child plenty of food to prevent malnutrition*
   Continue to breastfeed frequently. If the child is not breastfed, give the usual milk. If the child is >6 months, or already taking solid foods, also give cereal or another starchy food mixed, if possible, with pulses, vegetables, meat, or fish. Add 1 teaspoon (5 ml) of vegetable oil to each serving. Give fresh fruit juice or mashed banana to provide potassium. Give freshly prepared foods. Cook and mash/grind food well.
   Encourage the child to eat; offer food >5 times per day. Give the same foods after diarrhoea stops and give an extra meal each day for 2 weeks.

3. *Take the child to a health worker if the diarrhoea does not improve within 3 days or the child develops any of the following:*

- Many watery stools
- Fever
- Repeated vomiting
- Eating/drinking poorly
- Marked thirst
- Blood in the stool

Children should be given ORS at home if:

1. They have been on treatment plans B or C.
2. They cannot return to the health worker, but the diarrhoea gets worse.
3. It is national policy to give ORS to all children who see a health worker for diarrhoea.

How to give ORS

- Give a teaspoon every 1–2 mins for a child <2 yrs.
- Give frequent sips from a cup to older children.
- If the child vomits, wait 10 mins then give fluid more slowly.
- If diarrhoea persists after all ORS is used, use food-based fluids (see above), or return to the health care centre with the child.

Amount of ORS to give according to child's age

Age	After each loose stool	At home
<2yrs	50–100 ml	500 ml/day
2–10yrs	100–200 ml	1 litre/day
>10yrs	As much as tolerated	2 litres/day

When oral rehydration therapy fails or is inappropriate

In about 5% of patients the signs of dehydration do not improve or worsen after starting treatment with ORS. The usual causes are:
- Continuing rapid stool loss (>15–20 ml/kg/hr), as may occur in cholera
- Insufficient intake of ORS due to fatigue, lethargy, or lack of supervision
- Frequent severe vomiting.

Such patients should be admitted to hospital and given ORS by NG tube or Ringer's lactate solution 75 ml/kg IV over 4 hrs. Look for other signs of cholera infection and take necessary precautions. In most instances, it will not be cholera and the patient will improve.

When not to give ORS

Rarely, ORS should not be given. This is true for children with:
- Abdominal distension due to paralytic ileus (often owing to opiate drugs such as codeine or loperamide, or to hypokalaemia).
- Glucose malabsorption, indicated by a marked increase in stool output as ORS is started. There is no improvement and the stool contains large amounts of glucose.

In these situations, rehydration should be given intravenously until diarrhoea subsides.

Treatment plan B

To treat some dehydration

Approximate amounts of ORS to give in the first 4 hrs of treatment

Age	Weight (kg)	ORS (mls)
<4 mths	<5	200–400
4–11 mths	5–8	400–600
1–2 yrs	8–11	600–800
2–4 yrs	11–16	800–1200
5–14 yrs	16–30	1200–2200
>14 yrs	>30	2200–4000

- Use the patient's age only when you do not know the weight. The required amount of ORS in ml can also be calculated approximately by multiplying the patient's weight by 75.
- If the patient wants more ORS than the dose shown, give more.
- Encourage the mother to continue breastfeeding the child.
- For infants <6 months who are not breastfed, give 100–200 ml of clean water in addition to these ORS amounts within these 4 hrs.

N.B. During the initial stages of therapy, whilst still dehydrated, adults can consume up to 750 ml per hour if necessary and children up to 20 ml per kg body weight per hour.

Observe the patient carefully and help mothers to give ORS

1. Show the mother how much solution to give to her child.
2. Show the mother how to give it — a teaspoon every 1–2 mins for a child under 2 years, frequent sips from a cup for an older child.
3. Check from time to time to see if there are problems.
4. If a patient vomits, wait 10 mins and then continue giving ORS.
5. If the child's eyelids become oedematous, stop ORS and give plain water or breast milk. Give ORS according to plan A once the oedema has subsided.

After 4 hours, reassess the patient using the chart on p. 153 and continue plan A, B, or C as appropriate

- If there are no signs of dehydration, shift to plan A. When dehydration has been corrected, urine will start to be passed and children may become less irritable and fall asleep.
- If signs indicating some dehydration are still present, repeat plan B, but start to offer food, milk, and juice as in plan A.
- If signs indicating severe dehydration are present, treat according to plan C.

If the mother must leave the health post or hospital before completing treatment plan B

1. Show her how much ORS to give to finish the 4-hr treatment period at home.
2. Give her enough ORS packets to complete rehydration and for 3 more days, as in plan A.
3. Show her how to prepare ORS.
4. Explain to her the 3 rules in plan A for treating her child at home: (i) give ORS until diarrhoea stops; (ii) feed the child more to prevent malnutrition; and (iii) bring the child back to the health post/hospital if symptoms persist.
5. Make sure that children receive breastmilk or if >6 months are given some food before being sent home. Emphasize to the mother the importance of continuing feeding throughout the diarrhoeal episode.

Monitoring signs of oral rehydration therapy

Check the patient from time to time during rehydration to ensure that ORS is being taken satisfactorily and that signs of dehydration are not worsening. If at any time the patient develops severe dehydration, switch to treatment plan C. After 4 hrs, reassess the patient following the guidelines in the box on p. 153. Decide what treatment to give next.

- If signs of severe dehydration have appeared, IV therapy should be started immediately, following plan C. This is very unusual, however. It tends to occur in children who drink ORS poorly and continue to pass large volumes of watery stool during the rehydration period.
- If the patient still has signs of mild dehydration, continue oral rehydration therapy following plan B. At the same time start to offer food, milk, and other fluids as described in treatment plan A. Reassess the patient frequently.
- If there are no signs of dehydration, the patient should be considered fully rehydrated. If this is the case: the skin pinch is normal; the thirst has subsided; urine is passed normally; and the child is no longer irritable and may fall asleep.

Teach the mother to treat her child at home using ORS following plan A. Give her enough ORS sachets for 3 days and teach her the signs that indicate she must bring her child back to the health post.

Meeting normal fluid needs

While treatment to replace the existing water and electrolyte deficit is in progress the child's normal daily fluid requirements must also be met. This may be done as follows:

- *Breastfed infants:* continue to breastfeed as often and as long as the infant wants to, even during oral rehydration therapy.
- *Non-breastfed infants <6 months of age:* during rehydration with ORS, give 100–200 ml of plain water by mouth. After completing rehydration, resume full-strength milk or formula feeds. Give water and other fluids normally taken by the infant.
- *Older children and adults:* throughout rehydration treatment, offer as much plain water, milk, or juice as is accepted, in addition to ORS.

Treatment plan C

For patients with severe dehydration in hospital

Can you give IV fluids immediately? If not, see below.

1. Patients who can drink, however poorly, should be given ORS until the IV drip is running. In addition, all children should begin to receive some ORS (5 ml/kg/hr) as soon as they can drink without difficulty, which is usually within 3–4 hrs. This provides additional base and potassium which may not be adequately supplied by the IV fluid.
2. Start IV infusion of 100 ml/kg of Ringer's lactate (Hartmann's solution) as soon as possible. Divide the dose as follows:

Age	First give	Then give
<12 mths	30 ml/kg in 1 hr	70 ml/kg in 5 hrs
>12 mths	30 ml/kg in 30 mins	70 ml/kg in 2.5 hrs

3. Reassess the patient every 1–2 hrs. If the state of hydration is not improving, give the IV fluid more rapidly.
4. After 6 hours (infants <12 months) or 3 hours (>12 months), evaluate the patient using the assessment chart (see p. 153). Follow the appropriate treatment plan to continue treatment.

Notes

- If Ringer's lactate solution is not available, isotonic saline is an acceptable substitute — see box.
- Repeat once if radial pulse is weak or not detectable.

Monitoring IV rehydration therapy

1. Patients should be reassessed every 15–20 mins until a strong radial pulse is present.
2. Thereafter, they should be assessed hourly to confirm that hydration is improving. If it is not, the IV fluid may be run at a faster rate.
3. When the planned amount of IV fluid bas been given (6 hrs for infants, 3 hrs for older patients), the patient's state of hydration should be reassessed using the chart on p. 153.
   - If there are still signs of severe dehydration, repeat plan C. This is unusual, but may occur in cases of cholera and children who pass frequent, watery stools during the rehydration period.
   - If the patient shows signs of mild dehydration, discontinue IV fluid replacement and commence oral rehydration with ORS for 4 hrs according to plan B.
   - If there are no signs of dehydration, discontinue IV therapy and commence ORS treatment according to plan A.
4. Observe the patient for at least 6 hrs before discharging.
5. For children, ensure that the mother is able to continue giving ORS at home and is aware of the signs that indicate she must bring the child back.

Alternative solutions for IV rehydration

- **Ringer's lactate solution with 5% dextrose** — provides glucose to help prevent hypoglycaemia. If available, it is preferred to Ringer's lactate solution without dextrose.
- **Physiological saline (0.9% NaCl, also called normal saline)** — widely available, it is an acceptable alternative to Ringer's lactate solution, but contains neither a base to correct acidosis nor potassium to correct K^+ losses. Sodium bicarbonate or sodium lactate (20–30 mmol /l) and potassium chloride (5–15 mmol/l) may be added.
- **Half-strength Darrow's solution** — is made by diluting full-strength Darrow's solution with an equal volume of glucose solution (50 g/l or 100 g/l). Note that it contains less sodium than is required to replace the sodium lost in diarrhoea.

Plain glucose (dextrose) solution should **not** be used since it does not contain any sodium, base, or potassium and does not correct hypovolaemia effectively.

When no IV fluid is available

1. **Is there the facility for IV infusions within 30 mins' travelling time?**
   If so, transfer the patient, giving ORS as frequently as tolerated.
   If not:
2. **Is there the facility for nasogastric intubation?**
   If so, insert a NG tube and start rehydration with ORS 20 ml/kg/hr for 6 hrs (total 120 ml/kg). Reassess the patient q2h. If there is repeated vomiting or abdominal distension, give the fluid more slowly. If there is no improvement after 3 hrs, send the patient for IV therapy, continuing NG tube rehydration throughout the journey. After 6 hrs, reassess the patient and follow the appropriate treatment plan.
   If not:
3. **Can the patient drink?**
   If yes, start rehydration using ORS, giving 20 ml/kg/hr for 6 hrs (total 120 ml/kg). Reassess the patient every 1–2 hrs. If there is repeated vomiting, give the fluid more slowly. If the patient has not improved after 3 hrs, send for IV therapy, giving oral ORS throughout the journey. After 6 hrs, reassess the patient and follow the appropriate treatment plan.
   If not:
4. **Refer the patient as urgently as possible for IV/nasogastric rehydration.**

Management of persistent diarrhoea

This is diarrhoea, with or without blood, that begins acutely and lasts at least 14 days. Clinically these episodes cannot be differentiated from sequential episodes of acute diarrhoea over a prolonged period but the management is the same. It is usually associated with weight loss and, often, with serious non-intestinal infections. Many children with persistent diarrhoea are malnourished before the diarrhoea starts. Persistent diarrhoea almost never occurs in infants who are exclusively breastfed. Take a careful history and examine the patient well.

The object of treatment is to restore weight gain and normal intestinal function. In most cases, the patient will need to be admitted to hospital for diagnostic tests, treatment, and observation.

Treatment of persistent diarrhoea

1. *Appropriate fluids* to prevent/treat dehydration. (See p. 152.)
2. *Appropriate antimicrobial* therapy to treat diagnosed infections, in particular non-intestinal infections in children (e.g. pneumonia, otitis media, UTI). If there is persistent bloody diarrhoea, look for evidence of *Shigella*, *Entamoeba,* or *Giardia* infection. (See p. 122.)
3. *A nutritious diet* that does not cause worsening of the diarrhoea. Children will require a minimum of 110 calories/kg per day, which may have to be given via a NG tube if the child is too weak or refuses to eat. For infants <6 months, encourage exclusive breastfeeding. Help mothers who are not breastfeeding to re-establish lactation. (See Chapter 15.)
4. *Where possible, replace animal milk* with yoghurt, a lactose-free formula, or a local diet with reduced lactose (<3.5g/kg body weight/day). For older infants and young children, use standard diets made from local ingredients. Two diets are given in the box: the first contains reduced lactose, the second is lactose-free for the 30% of children who do not improve with the first diet.
5. *Supplementary vitamins and minerals.* All children with persistent diarrhoea should receive supplementary multivitamins and minerals each day for 2 weeks. Tablets that are crushed and mixed with food are less costly. One should aim to provide at least two recommended daily allowances (RDAs) of folate, vitamin A, iron, zinc, magnesium, and copper. As a guide, the RDAs for a 1-year-old child are:
   - Folate 50 mcg
   - Zinc 10 mg
   - Iron 10 mg
   - Vitamin A 400 mcg
   - Copper 1 mg
   - Magnesium 80 mg

Diet 1 (low lactose)

83 calories/100g
11% of calories as protein
2.7g lactose in 130 ml/kg
body weight/day

Ingredients

Full fat dried milk 11g
(or 85 ml whole milk)
Uncooked rice 18g
Vegetable oil 4g
Cane sugar 3g
Water to make up to 200 ml
final volume

130 ml/kg provides 110 cal/kg

Boil rice to a slurry with some
of the water, add other
ingredients and rest of water
to make up to 200 ml final
volume.

Diet 2 (lactose-free)

75 calories/100g
15% of calories as protein

Whole egg (without shell) 36g

Uncooked rice 10g
Vegetable oil 5g
Glucose 5g
Water to make up to 200 ml
final volume

145 ml/kg provides 110 cal/kg

Boil rice to a slurry with some of the
water, add the whole beaten egg
and continue to cook for another
minute, stirring well. Add the rest
of the ingredients and the water
to make up to 200 ml final volume.

Malnutrition and diarrhoea

Diarrhoea is as much a nutritional disease as one of fluid and electrolyte loss. Children who die from diarrhoea, despite good management, are usually malnourished — often severely so.

During diarrhoea, decreased food intake, decreased nutrient absorption, and increased nutrient requirements often combine to cause weight loss and failure to grow. The child's nutritional status declines and any pre-existing malnutrition is made worse. Malnutrition itself makes diarrhoea worse, prolonging it and making it more frequent. This vicious cycle may be broken by continuing to give nutrient-rich foods during diarrhoea and giving a nutritious diet, appropriate for the child's age, when the child is well.

When these steps are followed, malnutrition can be either prevented or corrected and the risk of death from a future episode of diarrhoea is much reduced. See Chapter 15 for further information.

Complications of diarrhoea

Electrolyte disturbances
Knowing the serum electrolyte concentrations rarely changes the management of patients dehydrated due to diarrhoea. In most cases, hypernatraemia, hyponatraemia, and hypokalaemia are all adequately treated by oral rehydration with ORS or IV rehydration with Ringer's lactate. In severe dehydration, however, plasma sodium concentrations may reach extremes and hypokalaemia may produce muscular weakness, dangerous cardiac arrhythmias, and paralytic ileus.

Fever
Fever in a patient with diarrhoea may be due to the organism causing the diarrhoea or, particularly in children, a 2° infection (e.g. pneumonia or otitis media). The presence of fever should prompt a search for other infections, particularly if it persists after the patient is fully hydrated.

In an area where *P. falciparum* malaria is prevalent, children with a fever of 38°C or above should be treated with an appropriate antimalarial. High fevers (>39°C) in children should be brought down with an antipyretic drug such as paracetamol. This will reduce irritability and prevent febrile convulsions.

Convulsions
In a child with diarrhoea and convulsions during the illness, the following diagnoses should be considered:
- *Febrile convulsion:* this usually occurs in children <8 yrs old when their temperature exceeds 40°C or rises very rapidly. Treat with paracetamol and tepid water sponging.
- *Meningitis:* needs to be considered in any child or adult following a convulsion. Look for neck rigidity and Kernig's sign. Do a lumbar puncture after checking the retinae for papilloedema (raised ICP) and looking for focal neurological signs.
- *Hypoglycaemia:* this occasionally occurs in children with diarrhoea, due to their small hepatic glycogen reserves and insufficient gluconeogenesis. If suspected, give 1.0 ml/kg of 50% glucose solution or 2.5 ml/kg of a 20% glucose solution IV over 5 mins. If hypoglycaemia is the cause, recovery will usually be rapid. In such cases, Ringer's lactate with dextrose should be given to the child for IV rehydration.

Vitamin A deficiency
Diarrhoea reduces the absorption of and increases the need for vitamin A. In areas where vitamin A deficiency is already prevalent, young children with diarrhoea have an increased risk of developing eye problems.

Doses: 50,000 iu for children <6 months; 100,000 iu for children 6–12 months; 200,000 iu for children >12 months. Give dose on day 1, day 2, and 14 days later or at discharge.

Metabolic acidosis
During episodes of diarrhoea, a large amount of bicarbonate may be lost from the stool. If renal function is normal, this will be replaced. However, renal impairment due to hypovolaemia may result in the rapid development of a base deficit and acidosis. Excess lactate production may also occur. Features of metabolic acidosis are: serum bicarbonate (<10 mmol/l); acidaemia (pH <7.3); with respiratory compensation (look for rapid and deep breathing); vomiting.

Antidiarrhoeal drugs

These agents, though commonly used, have no practical benefit and are never indicated for the treatment of acute diarrhoea in children. Some of them are dangerous.

Adsorbents: (e.g. kaolin, attapulgite, smectite, activated charcoal, cholestyramine) are of no proven value in the treatment of diarrhoea.

Antimotility drugs: (e.g. loperamide, diphenoxylate with atropine, tincture of opium, paregoric, codeine). These drugs reduce the frequency of stool passage in adults, but do not do so appreciably in children. Moreover, they may cause severe paralytic ileus and prolong infection by delaying the elimination of the causative organism/toxin. They may be used cautiously in adults in exceptional circumstances (e.g. required to travel) but should never be used in children or infants.

Other drugs:

- *Antiemetics* (e.g. prochlorperazine, chlorpromazine, metaclopramide). Such drugs should not be given since they often cause sedation and may interfere with ORS treatment. Vomiting will cease as the patient becomes hydrated.
- *Cardiac stimulants* should never be used to overcome shock and hypotension which may occur in severe dehydration with hypovolaemia. Cardiac output will be restored as rehydration fluid is infused IV.
- *Blood or plasma* is only indicated if there is proven shock.
- *Steroids and purgatives* are of no benefit and should never be used.

Dietary management of diarrhoea and zinc supplementation

Diarrhoeal illness is associated with growth faltering and malnutrition. Diarrhoeal infections may cause malabsorption, with increased faecal loss of nutrients, and reduced dietary intake due to anorexia and food restrictions. These adverse consequences can be minimized by correct dietary management.

Children should be encouraged to eat normally if they want to. More frequent 'nutrient dense' (i.e. high energy in small volume) foods such as purees should be offered. If the child is anorexic, food should be offered more frequently and increased food offered as soon as the child will eat. Breastfeeding should continue. High-sugar fruit juices and soft drinks should be avoided as the high osmolar load may exacerbate the diarrhoea. Most children with mild diarrhoea can continue to drink cow's milk. If lactose intolerance occurs reduce the lactose load by mixing milk with cereal such as rice, or using yogurt, and give in small amounts frequently. Give additional food when the child recovers.

Zinc deficiency is common in developing countries and in any population in which there is limited consumption of foods of animal origin, especially red meat or offal. Zinc supplements have been shown to reduce the duration and severity of diarrhoea. Zinc sulfate or gluconate (20 mg elemental zinc) is recommended for 7–14 days. ORS should also be given. Formulations of ORS containing zinc are under trial but it is difficult to ensure a standard dose of zinc. No other micronutrient supplement has shown such consistent and important benefits in diarrhoeal disease as zinc but multivitamin mineral supplements are recommended for children with persistent diarrhoea and/or malnutrition who are especially likely to have multiple nutrient deficiencies.

Prevention of diarrhoea

Proper treatment of diarrhoeal diseases is highly effective in preventing death, but has no impact on the incidence of such diseases. It is every medical professional's responsibility to teach family members and motivate them to adopt preventive measures. Do not overload the mother with technical advice, but emphasize the most important points for each particular mother and child.

1. Measures that interrupt the transmission of pathogen

The various infectious agents that cause diarrhoea are virtually all transmitted by the faeco-oral route. Measures taken to interrupt the transmission of the causative agents should focus on the following pathways:

- Giving only breast milk for the first 6 months of life.
- Avoiding the use of infant feeding bottles.
- Improving practices relating to the preparation and storage of weaning foods (to minimize microbial contamination).
- Using only clean water for drinking.
- Washing hands after defecation, disposing of faeces, and before preparing food.
- Disposing of all faeces in a safe manner.

2. Measures that strengthen host defences

A number of risk factors for frequent or severe diarrhoea reflect impaired host defences. Measures may be taken to improve this:

- Continuing to breastfeed for the first 2 years of life.
- Improving a child's nutritional status by giving more nutritious food, including foods of animal origin that contain essential minerals such as zinc and other micronutrients. Giving complementary foods more often, from 3 times per day when first introduced at 6 months to 5 times per day at 12 months.
- Immunizing against measles.

3. How doctors can help to prevent diarrhoea

- Ensure appropriate in-service training of health facility staff.
- *Make sure that all staff are giving consistent messages on diarrhoea prevention and infant feeding.*
- Display promotional material on how to treat and prevent diarrhoea.
- Be a good role model (breastfeeding, handwashing, water hygiene, latrine hygiene).
- Take part in community-based activities to promote health.
- Co-ordinate efforts for disease prevention with those of relevant government programmes.

Some difficulties encountered in home therapy for diarrhoea

1. The mother is disappointed because she is not given a prescription for drugs or the child does not receive an injection.

Explain that the diarrhoea will stop by itself after a few days. Also, explain that drugs do not help to stop diarrhoea, but that fluid replacement and continued feeding will help shorten the illness and maintain her child's strength and growth.

2. The mother believes that food should not be given during diarrhoea.

Ask her to explain her beliefs about how diarrhoea should be treated. Discuss with her the importance of feeding in order to keep her child strong and to support normal growth, even during diarrhoea. There are almost always some foods which are acceptable — find out and encourage these alternatives.

3. The mother does not know what fluids to give her child at home.

Ask her what fluids she can prepare at home and reach an agreement on appropriate fluids for her child.

4. The mother does not have the ingredients to make a recommended fluid.

Ask her if she can obtain the necessary ingredients easily. If she cannot, suggest another home fluid.

5. The child vomits after drinking ORS or other fluids.

Explain that more fluid is usually kept down than is vomited. Tell her to wait 10 mins and then start giving fluid again, but more slowly.

6. The child refuses to drink.

A child who has lost fluid will usually be thirsty and want to drink, even when there are no signs of dehydration. If the child is not familiar with the taste of ORS, some persuasion may be needed at first. When a child drinks well to begin with but then loses interest, it usually means that sufficient fluid has been given.

7. The mother is given some packets of ORS for use at home but is afraid they will be used up before the diarrhoea stops.

Explain that after the ORS has been used up she should give a recommended home fluid (e.g. rice water) or water or she should return to the health facility for more packets of ORS. In any event, she should continue to give extra fluid until the diarrhoea stops.

Acute respiratory infections/pneumonia

Section editor **Beate Kampmann**

Pneumonia

UNICEF estimates that pneumonia kills around 3 million children per year in the developing world, and health care professionals working in resource-poor settings will constantly be confronted with children suffering from various forms of respiratory distress.

While pneumonia may occur as part of a severe systemic viral infection (e.g. measles or influenza), most serious cases are due to bacteria. Few radiological or clinical findings can reliably differentiate between bacterial or viral agents.

In the absence of CXR facilities, the history and clinical examination provide important clues.

Classification

Cases of pneumonia can be classified in a number of ways. The most useful involve determining:

- Where the pneumonia was acquired — community or hospital?
- The previous health status of the patient — previously healthy (*1° pneumonia*) or chronically ill (*2° pneumonia*).

Important risk factors for pneumonia include:

- Malnutrition
- Pregnancy
- HIV infection
- Diabetes
- Underlying chronic disabilities impairing lung function (e.g. cerebral palsy)
- Periods of unconsciousness (alcoholics, surgical patients)
- Absence of a functioning spleen (post-splenectomy or due to sickle cell disease)

These factors will be important for determining the likely causative agent, disease course, and severity, and therefore the patient's management and prognosis. It is important to ascertain the immunization history of the patient.

Aetiology

Relatively little data defines the causative agents in much of the developing world. The list of organisms causing pneumonia is long and depends on the patient's age, season of the year, and the presence of other diseases. A list of the most common organisms per age group is displayed in the box. It is often impossible to obtain microbiological confirmation in resource-poor settings, hence the choice of antibiotics should always cover the 'most likely suspects'.

Clinical features

- The patient is systemically ill with malaise, fever, anorexia, body aches, and headache. Delirium can occur in severe infections. In children, symptoms can be less specific and include abdominal pain, vomiting, refusal of feeds.
- Respiratory signs and symptoms include raised respiratory rate (**note**: this is age-dependent — see box), nasal flaring, intercostal and sub-costal recession, tracheal tug, cough, sputum production, dyspnoea, pleural pain, and, rarely, haemoptysis. Chest movements might be reduced on the affected side; inspiratory crackles, crepitations, and pleural rub may be present on auscultation. Sputum is often initially scanty or absent, becoming purulent later in the infection except in *Legionella* and other atypical pneumonias. Children tend to swallow

their secretions/sputum, so the absence of sputum production does not exclude pneumonia.
- Lower lobe pneumonia may present as an acute abdomen — abdominal pain, ileus, rigidity.
- In the very young, elderly, or debilitated, there may be few signs of systemic illness or respiratory involvement. Look for raised respiratory rate and perform a careful chest examination. Have a high index of suspicion.

Age	Organism
Neonates	Group B *Streptococcus*
	Gram-negative organisms (*E. coli*, *Klebsiella*)
	Less common: CMV, HSV, *Chlamydia*, *Listeria*, *Bordetella pertussis*; also consider maternal infections
<5 years	*Streptococcus pneumoniae*
	Haemophilus influenzae
	Group A *Streptococcus*
	Staphylococcus aureus (severe), especially post measles infection
	Bordetella pertussis
	Viral: RSV, measles, influenza, adenovirus, parainfluenza (always check immunization history)
School age	*Streptococcus pneumoniae*
	Mycoplasma, *Chlamydia*
	Viral pneumonias as above
Adults	*Streptococcus pneumoniae*
	'Atypical' organisms (*Mycoplasma*, *Chlamydia*, *Legionella*)
	H. influenzae
	Viral pneumonias: influenza, adenovirus, Varicella zoster

Guide to respiratory rates (RR) in children of different ages*

Age	Normal RR/min	Severe respiratory distress
Infants <2 months	40–30	>60
2–12 months	40–30	>50
12 months–5 yrs	30–25	>40
>5 yrs	25–20	>30

*Always count RR for 1 min in calm circumstances, as crying will give a falsely elevated RR

Community-acquired pneumonia (CAP)

In a previously healthy person with community-acquired pneumonia, the most likely pathogens are *S. pneumoniae* and, less often, atypical organisms. Post-primary *M. tuberculosis* infection should also be borne in mind and considered early in the differential diagnosis, especially if the response to antibiotics is poor.

In the history, consider whether the patient is:

- Previously healthy or had chronic lung disease. The latter condition predisposes to colonization of the respiratory tract with pathogenic microbes such as *H. influenzae*.
- Generally debilitated, an alcoholic, or an intravenous drug abuser. These patients are commonly infected by microbes that are more typical of nosocomial infection, although they are also at increased risk of pneumococcal infection. The infection may be an aspiration pneumonia.

Common bacterial causes of CAP

1. *Streptococcus pneumoniae* — see p. 174.
2. *Haemophilus influenzae* type B — occurs particularly in children <5 yrs old who often present with lobar pneumonia, pleural involvement, and an effusion. It also occurs in adults both as a primary infection and in previously damaged lungs. The onset is slower than the other bacteria. The pneumonia is often accompanied by infection elsewhere (e.g. meninges, epiglottis). The use of the Hib vaccine in the tropics should markedly reduce its incidence, if the vaccine can be afforded.
3. *Staphylococcus aureus* can cause pneumonia in patients with pre-existing chronic or acute lung disease, particularly following viral infection, usually influenza or especially measles. Note that the influenza infection may be subclinical. Alternatively, haematogenous spread from a distant site of infection (e.g. skin, bones and joints, or heart) may produce pneumonia in a previously healthy lung. In these circumstances, *S. aureus* may be isolated from blood. It is always a serious condition with high fever and cyanosis; common complications include pulmonary abscess formation, cavitation, empyema.

A poor prognosis is associated with:

- Presence of bacteraemia (e.g. the fatality rate increases from 5% in isolated *S. pneumoniae* pneumonia to 25–35% fatality rate when the bacillus is cultured from blood).
- Infections with *S. aureus*, *H. influenzae*, and Gram −ve bacteria.
- Previous illness, either chronic (e.g. COPD, cardiac disease, malnutrition) or acute (influenza, measles).

Clinical features	Investigations
• Confusion/sepsis	• Blood urea >7mmol/l
• Respiratory rate >30/min	• WCC <4 × 10⁹/l or >30 × 10⁹/l
(**Note**: age-dependent (see opposite)	• Arterial O2 <8 kPA
• Diastolic blood pressure <60 mmHg	• Serum albumin <25 g/l
• New atrial fibrillation	• Multilobe involvement on CXR

Differential diagnosis of pneumonia

- TB
- Foreign body inhalation
- Bronchiolitis
- Epiglottitis
- Croup
- Tracheitis
- Asthma
- LIP
- Gastro-oesophageal reflux leading to aspiration
- Parasitic lung infections (e.g. *Paragonimus*, *Echinococcus*)
- Structural lung abnormalities

Lymphocytic interstitial pneumonitis (LIP)

This condition occurs in HIV +ve children and represents lymphocytic lung infiltrates as a sign of immune activation in response to HIV. It is usually bilateral and often accompanied by parotid enlargement. LIP does not cause respiratory distress and can be an accidental finding on the CXR. It can be confused with miliary TB or PCP, but the clinical condition of the patient should allow the distinction. LIP on its own does not need any therapy, is self-limiting, and carries a good prognosis for the patient. It is a diagnosis of exclusion.

Pneumococcal pneumonia

Although the pneumococcus is an important cause of disease worldwide, the developing world's children are at greatest risk of dying. It causes 25–50% of ARIs in children admitted to hospital and, each year, at least 1 million children die from pneumococcal pneumonia. The disease is worse in crowded communities with poor living conditions. Adults with debilitating diseases (e.g. DM, AIDS, alcoholism, asplenia, hypogammaglobinaemia) are also at increased risk of invasive pneumococcal disease.

Historically, *Streptococcus pneumoniae* was extremely sensitive to common antibiotics such as penicillin. However, 1967 saw the identification of pneumococcus isolates with reduced sensitivity to penicillin in Australasia. 10 years later, children in southern Africa died from isolates that were clinically resistant to penicillin. This trend has continued, driven by indiscriminate use of penicillin antibiotics. Now, >50% of pneumococcal isolates in some areas of the world have reduced sensitivity to penicillin. Many also have reduced sensitivity to other common antibiotics such as tetracycline. The increase in resistance has worrying implications for the management of invasive pneumococcal disease. Currently, the prevalence of penicillin-resistant pneumococci in many parts of the developing world is unknown.

Transmission: assumed to be person–person via droplet spread. Many people become long-term carriers of the infection in their nasopharynx. Local spread to ear or meninges (particularly after head trauma) can produce *otitis media* or meningitis.

Clinical features: the onset is sudden (sometimes following an URTI) with fever, rigors, malaise, headache, and myalgia. (Onset is often less clear at the extremes of age — children show tachypnoea in addition to fever and cough, while the elderly may have little fever and present with confusion.) Chest pain (pleuritic, sometimes referred to shoulder if diaphragm is involved) and cough (initially painful and dry → blood-tinged → purulent) commonly follow. Lower lobe involvement can result in abdominal pain and guarding. The WCC is often raised; leucopenia is a poor prognostic sign.

Complications: Pneumococci in the lungs may spread directly to the pleura producing an empyema. Haematogenous spread can result in infection of meninges, joints, eyes, or abscess formation in distant organs. Rare complications include: acute septicaemia in patients with underlying conditions, such as asplenia; endocarditis; peritonitis in patients with lowered immunity; and ascites (nephrotic syndrome, cirrhosis).

Diagnosis: is most often made on clinical grounds. Bacteria can be cultured from sputum or blood; or by aspiration of abscesses in distant organs.

Management: see p. 180. It is essential to follow local guidelines for antibiotic use that are based on knowledge of local antibiotic sensitivities.

Prevention: general improvements in living conditions and reduced air pollution; new vaccines have been developed but are not widely available and do not cover all strains and all age groups.

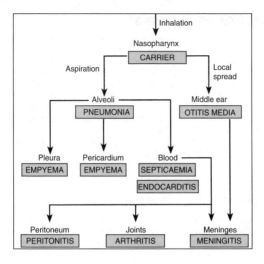

Locally recommended antibiotics for pneumococcal pneumonia

-
-
-

Atypical pneumonia

This type of pneumonia often occurs in previously healthy children and young adults and starts with a mild sore throat followed by dyspnoea, an often non-productive cough, fever, and malaise. Pleuritic chest pain, splinting, and respiratory distress are rare. The CXR picture is often worse than signs would suggest; the WCC can be normal. The clinical course is normally benign; occasionally it is severe and requires ICU admission.

'Atypical' organisms cause probably less than 10% of all pneumonias in the tropics. Of those, common causes are *Mycoplasma pneumoniae* and *Chlamydia pneumoniae*. Others include *C. trachomatis* and *C. psittaci*, *Coxiella burnetti*, *Legionella pneumophila*, and viruses such as influenza and adenovirus. These organisms are difficult to culture and diagnosis is by serology or nasopharyngeal aspirate, if available.

Legionnaires' disease

The importance of *Legionella pneumophila* in the tropics is unknown. It is transmitted by inhalation of aerosolized water droplets from air conditioning systems, water storage tanks, showerheads, and medical equipment such as nebulizers.

Clinical features: vary from subclinical or mild infections to severe pneumonia. In severe infection, after 2–10 days, there is abrupt high fever, rigors, myalgia, and headache followed by the onset of a dry cough, dyspnoea, and crepitations on auscultation. The patient becomes very ill quickly, appearing toxic, sometimes with delirium or diarrhoea. During the toxic phase, complications include respiratory failure, pericarditis, myocarditis, and acute renal failure. CXR shows homogeneous shadowing, often basal initially, subsequently widespread with deterioration.

Diagnosis: Gram -ve slender rods of variable length in biopsy or sputum samples; bacterial antigen in urine for first 1–3 weeks.

Management: erythromycin 0.5–1 g/6h IV or PO for up to 2–3 weeks (adding rifampicin 600 mg bd or a quinolone if patient is deteriorating) is recommended.

Prevention: treatment and maintenance of stored water and tanks to prevent bacterial colonization and spread.

Rare causes of severe CAP include:

- Meliodosis
- Tularaemia
- Typhoid
- Anthrax
- Pneumonic plague
- Paragonimiasis
- Fungi — such as histoplasmosis and blastomycosis
- SARS

Nosocomial pneumonia

Definition: pneumonia that occurs more than 48 hours after admission to hospital.

Signs: development of fever, increased WCC, purulent sputum, lung infiltrate on CXR.

Risk factors: ITU patients, increasing age, obesity, smoking, long preoperative stay, prolonged anaesthesia, intubation, abdominal/thoracic operations, plus risk factors for aspiration pneumonia (see below).

Aetiology

- *Aspiration of nasopharyngeal secretions* — particularly of Gram –ve bacteria and anaerobic bacteria that may colonize nasopharynx during hospital stay. Broad-spectrum antibiotics and serious illness predispose to such colonization.
- *Inhalation of bacteria from contaminated instruments* — such as ventilators, nebulizers, intubation and nasogastric tubes.
- *Haematogenous spread* — e.g. from abdominal infection, infected cannulae, or catheters left *in situ* for too long.

Prevention: prevent smoking pre-operatively, encourage early mobilization. Good hospital staff and respiratory equipment hygiene, and good general infection control measures should decrease the risk. Chest physiotherapy postoperatively may help decrease nosocomial pneumonia.

Aspiration pneumonia

Risk factors: impaired consciousness (e.g. alcoholics, epileptics), dysphagia, being bed-bound, neuromuscular diseases, decreased ability to clear bronchial secretions or cough after general anaesthesia or abdominal/thoracic surgery.

Aetiology

- *In the community* — anaerobes from oropharynx and teeth crevices (normally penicillin-sensitive).
- *In hospital* — aerobic bacteria become more important, particularly Gram –ve enterobacteria and *P. aeruginosa*.

It may be possible to diagnose anaerobic infection from a *history* of poor dental hygiene, aspiration, or impaired consciousness. In children, also consider gastro-oesophageal reflux and underlying neurological/neuromuscular disorders. As the infection proceeds, tissue necrosis results in foul-smelling purulent discharge.

Recurrent pneumonia

Defined as more than two episodes of pneumonia, it may be caused by:
- *Localized respiratory disease* — bronchiectasis, bronchial obstruction (foreign body, bronchial stenosis, bronchial carcinoma, lymphadenopathy), intrapulmonary sequestration.
- *Generalized respiratory disease* — COPD +/− bronchiectasis, impaired local defences.
- *Non-respiratory problem* — recurrent aspiration (see above), immuno-suppression.
- *Acquired immunodeficiency* (recurrent pneumonia is a frequent finding in HIV-infected children)

Management of pneumonia

1. Oxygen — monitor saturation whenever possible; use paediatric probes for children.
2. Antimicrobials: see below and box.
3. Analgesia for pleuritic pain.
4. Fluids (IV if necessary) to rectify dehydration and maintain an adequate urine output (>1.5 litres/24h). Remember that losses are increased if the patient is febrile. If however there is renal impairment, beware of overhydration. In children, calculate volume replacement carefully in ml/kg according to age and state of hydration. Hyponatraemia secondary to SIADH is a common feature of severe pneumonia.
5. Bed rest. The patient should sit up rather than lie flat — except in cases of severe pneumonia where this may exhaust the patient.
6. Treat empirically for sepsis if very ill — see Chapter 3.
7. Physiotherapy is no longer recommended in the early acute stages of pneumonia.

Antimicrobial use: general points

- If the patient is very ill, obtain culture specimens then immediately begin empirical IV antibiotic therapy. Be aware of local guidelines and, if possible, seek advice from a senior colleague. Antibiotic choice in this situation (blind therapy) depends upon the clinical picture/patient history — see box.
- Empirical therapy may be appropriate in outpatient clinics; think of the 'usual suspects' and cover for them.
- Only give IV therapy if the patient is very ill, cannot swallow/vomits, or if the GI tract is not functioning. Have a lower threshold in very young children though, as disease progresses more rapidly. It is often appropriate to give a few doses IV and then switch to PO antibiotics.
- Calculate antibiotic dosages according to weight in children, as adult dosages do not necessarily apply.
- Therapy can be given for 3–7 days in mild pneumonia. For those with severe pneumonia, duration needs to be judged according to the clinical response. In the presence of cavitation and abscesses, treatment might need to be continued for up to 3–4 weeks.

Change the guidelines given in the box to reflect the most common pathogens, and their antimicrobial sensitivities, in your region.

Chest X-rays in pneumonia

CXRs are expensive and their interpretation subject to wide variation. Therefore, the value of an CXR for each patient should be carefully considered before ordering one. In particular:

- Is the diagnosis already clear from the clinical features?
- Will the CXR change the patient's management?

Note: CXR changes in pneumonia may take weeks to resolve following successful treatment and clinical improvement by the patient.

Empirical treatment of pneumonia

Clinical picture	Organisms to be covered	PO	Antibiotic route IV
1. 1° CAP			
(mild to moderate)	S. pneumoniae	Ax	A
	If 'atypicals' likely	Add E	
2. 2° pneumonia			
• Previous lung disease (e.g. COPD)	S. pneumoniae H. influenzae	Co C + E	Co + E or
• If following flu or associated with URTI	S. aureus	Add F to above regimen	
• Aspiration	S. pneumoniae, Klebsiella spp, anaerobes, Gram –ve organisms	P + M + G	
• Immunosuppression (e.g. leukaemia)	Pseudomonas spp	×	Cz + G
• Nosocomial (especially if 2° disease)	Gram –ve	×	Ct + G
• Sepsis elsewhere	Treat as for sepsis	×	F + G + M
3. Severe pneumonia	Widest possible range	×	Ct + E + G

For treatment of an HIV +ve patient, see Chapter 2B.

Key to antimicrobials (dose indicated is for adults)

A   Ampicillin 500 mg q6h IV
Ax   Amoxicillin 500 mg tds PO
C   Cefuroxime 750 mg q8h IV
Co   Co-amoxiclav 1 tablet (500mg/125mg) tds PO or 1.2 g (1000 mg/200 mg) q8h IV
Ct   Cefotaxime 1g q8h IV
Cz   Ceftazidime 2g q8h IV
E   Erythromycin 500 mg qds PO or 500 mg q6h slowly IV
F   Flucloxacillin 500 mg qds PO or 250–1000 mg q6h slowly IV
G   Gentamicin 3–5 mg/kg od IV
M   Metronidazole 500 mg PO q8h (for up to 7 days)
P   Benzylpenicillin 1.2–1.8 g q6h IV (dose may be increased)
×   Oral therapy is inappropriate in these situations

A, Ax, and oral Co doses can be doubled in severe infections; the IV Co dose can be increased in frequency to q6h.

Viral respiratory infections

Many cases of bacterial pneumonia appear to be preceded by a relatively harmless viral infection of the upper or lower airways. These infections damage the epithelial cells that line the airway, possibly inhibiting their ability to remove debris with their cilia. The viral infection may also debilitate the person, making them more susceptible to subsequent bacterial superinfection. Bacterial pneumonia that follows acute respiratory tract infections (ARI) is a major cause of childhood death in the developing world. Their importance is recognized in the WHO's 'Integrated Management of Childhood Illness' (see Chapter 1).

Aetiology — the viral agents of respiratory infections include:
- Measles
- Influenza virus
- Parainfluenza virus
- Adenovirus
- Respiratory syncytial virus (RSV)
- Rhinovirus
- Coronavirus

The viruses are transmitted either in small droplets after sneezing or coughing (e.g. measles, influenza) or by contact with infected secretions (e.g. RSV, rhinoviruses). There is seasonal variability.

Upper respiratory tract infections

A group of infections which are normally self-limiting and do not require specific treatment. They include the 'common cold' (coryza), pharyngitis (sore throat), and laryngitis. Signs of coryza include nasal stinging, a watery nasal discharge, and a blocked nose — signs that are similar to the prodrome of measles and influenza but without the systemic upset.

Acute bronchitis

A condition that is characterized by mild malaise (the patient does not look ill), retrosternal soreness, and a dry, tickly cough which becomes more prominent as the infection progresses and, with 2° bacterial infection, mucopurulent. It may be characterized as a 'common cold that has gone into the chest' and is often still accompanied by signs of an URTI. The severity of the attack is possibly increased by exposure to cigarette smoke, cooking and heating fumes, and air pollution both inside houses and in the outside environment.

Aetiology: most cases are due to viral infection. Superinfection with *H. influenzae* or *S. pneumoniae* is a common complication. Much more rarely bacteria such as *Bordetella pertussis*, *Mycoplasma pneumoniae*, and *Chlamydia pneumoniae* give rise to a 1° bronchitis.

Diagnosis: is one of exclusion — more serious conditions such as pneumonia and cardiovascular or thromboembolic disease must be ruled out. If the cough and wheeze persist, consider the diagnosis of asthma and the use of bronchodilators and steroids.

Management: The uncomplicated viral respiratory infections require supportive treatment only. Bacterial superinfections of the trachea or bronchi on the other hand require specific antimicrobial therapy as described above. Antibiotics according to local guidelines are also warranted for 2° bacterial infection affecting the sinuses or middle ear.

Severe acute respiratory syndrome (SARS)

In the first half of 2003, viral pneumonitis caused by a newly identified coronavirus caused outbreaks in Asia, North America, and Europe.

Transmission: SARS virus appears to spread by inhalation of aerosols of infectious droplets, and possibly by contact with infected faeces, skin contact, or contact with objects contaminated with droplets.

Clinical features

The incubation period for SARS is typically 2–7 days (max. 10 days). The illness begins generally with a prodrome (viraemia): fever >38.0°C, sometimes with rigors, headache, malaise, and myalgia. At the start of illness, respiratory symptoms may be mild; some patients have diarrhoea during the febrile prodrome. Rash and neurological findings are generally absent.

After 3–7 days, a lower respiratory phase begins with a dry, non-productive cough, and/or dyspnoea which may progress to hypoxia. In 10–20% of cases, respiratory failure requires intubation and mechanical ventilation. The severity is probably highly variable, ranging from mild illness to death. Some close contacts report a mild febrile illness without respiratory signs or symptoms. The case-fatality rate among patients meeting the WHO case definition of SARS is approximately 3%, with patients >60 yrs having a high mortality.

Diagnosis: CXR is usually normal during the febrile prodrome. In many patients focal interstitial infiltrates develop and progress to generalized, patchy, interstitial infiltrate, ARDS, or areas of consolidation. WCC are usually normal or low, and lymphocyte counts often decreased. Thrombocytopenia or low to normal platelet counts are typical. Elevated CK, LDH, and hepatic transaminase levels have been noted; renal function usually remains normal.

Management: give antibiotics (e.g. erythromycin 500mg IV/PO q6h) to cover atypical pneumonia. Antiviral agents such as ribavirin and steroids have been used but are of unproven benefit.

Prevention: isolation of cases and contacts, and routine use of universal precautions.

Public health

- Isolation of SARS cases and early identification of cases among contacts quickly brought recent outbreaks under control.
- SARS patients should not leave home until 10 days after the resolution of fever, provided respiratory symptoms are absent or improving. During this time, infection control precautions should be used to minimize the potential for transmission.
- All members of a household with a SARS patient should follow frequent handwashing or use of alcohol-based hand rubs, particularly after contact with body fluids (e.g. respiratory secretions, urine, or faeces).
- Use disposable gloves for direct contact with body fluids of a SARS patient.
- Patients with SARS should cover his/her mouth and nose with a facial tissue when coughing or sneezing.
- Use face masks within the home of a patient.
- Avoid sharing eating utensils, towels, and bedding between SARS patients and others.
- Household waste soiled with body fluids of SARS patients, including facial tissues and surgical masks, may be discarded as normal waste.
- Close contacts of SARS patients should be actively monitored by the local health department for illness for 10 days after the last contact. If fever or respiratory symptoms develop, follow the same precautions recommended for SARS patients.
- In the absence of fever or respiratory symptoms, close contacts of SARS patients need not limit their activities outside the home.

Multi-system diseases and infections

Section editors   **Michael G Jacobs**
Tania Araujo-Jorge (Chagas disease)
Anneli Bjöersdorff (rickettsial infections)
François Chappuis (African trypanosomiasis)
David Dance (plague, melioidosis)
David Goldblatt (measles)
Monir Madkour (brucellosis)
Chris Parry (typhoid)

Differential diagnosis of fevers

Fever is a common presentation of illness and may be the only manifestation of serious disease. Infections are much the more common but not the only cause of fever. Fever is often intermittent and may be absent at presentation.

A history of drenching sweats or *rigors* (uncontrollable shaking lasting for minutes) is always significant. Rigors are particularly, but not exclusively, associated with (i) malaria or (ii) bacterial sepsis. The fever pattern does not reliably distinguish bacterial, viral, parasitic, fungal, or non-infectious causes of fever.

In view of the wide range of possible diagnoses, a detailed history and complete physical examination are essential. During the assessment, ask yourself:

- Where is the site of infection?
- Which are the likely infecting organisms?
- Is this presentation unusual or has it become more numerous recently? Might an epidemic be occurring?

Immunocompromised patients: if you know or suspect that the patient is immunocompromised, aim to formulate two differential diagnoses — 1st for an immunocompetent and 2nd for an immunocompromised individual.

Common examples of infections with localizing features

• Breathlessness, cough, sputum, pleurisy	Pneumonia
• Prolonged cough, haemoptysis	Pulmonary TB
• Urinary frequency, dysuria, haematuria, loin pain	UTI
• Vomiting, diarrhoea, abdominal pain	Infective enterocolitis
• Red, hot skin	Cellulitis
• Painful, swollen joint	Septic arthritis
• Bone pain	Osteomyelitis
• Headache, confusion, neck stiffness	Meningitis
• Sore throat, exudate over tonsils/pharynx	Streptococcal or EBV infection
• Prominent cervical lymphadenopathy	TB lymphadenitis

Serious infections such as meningococcal sepsis and malaria may present with 'false localizing' symptoms and signs such as headache, breathlessness, vomiting, or diarrhoea.

- In the presence of localizing features, investigations are targeted towards the presumed cause. Specimens (blood, urine, CSF, etc.) for microscopy and culture, if available, are most useful.
- Treatment with antibiotics can be started based on a clinical diagnosis. From the available antibiotics, one or more should be chosen that treat the likely infecting organisms. Are there local guidelines for choosing antibiotics?

Causes of fever

- Infections (bacterial, viral, parasitic, fungal)
- Malignancy (e.g. lymphoma, renal cell carcinoma)
- Inflammatory conditions (e.g. autoimmune rheumatic diseases, granulomatous diseases)
- Drug reactions
- Endocrine (e.g. hyperthyroidism)

Fever without localizing features

This is a challenging clinical problem. The following investigations are most helpful in making an initial assessment of the likely cause:
1. Blood smears for microscopy for malaria
2. Total and differential white cell counts
3. Platelet count

The importance of malaria

In many tropical areas, malaria is the most common cause of fever and should be the first consideration when assessing a patient with fever. In endemic areas, low-grade parasitaemia without symptoms is common in adults and older children (due the development of partial immunity to malaria – see Chapter 2A). It follows therefore that the finding of low-grade parasitaemia in an individual with fever does not prove that the fever is caused by malaria. In endemic areas, one approach is to treat all patients with fever and an illness compatible with malaria with antimalarial chemotherapy, while considering other diagnoses.

Blood counts in a patient with fever (see opposite)

Simple blood tests, especially white cell counts and platelet count, may give useful clues to the cause of fever, although this is not an absolutely reliable guide and the information must be considered in the context of careful clinical assessment of the patient.

Treatment of fever of unknown cause

1. Quite commonly, a positive diagnosis cannot be made after the initial clinical assessment and tests. The management then depends on:
   - Your judgement of the most likely diagnoses
   - How severely ill the patient is
   - Available resources
2. Patients who you judge to be (or at risk of becoming) seriously unwell should be given 'best guess' empirical antimicrobial therapy. Are there local guidelines for empirical therapy?
3. Admission to hospital, if possible, is the best course if you are worried about the patient's condition. In time, the diagnosis is likely to become apparent, particularly if the patient is fully reassessed on a regular basis.

Persistent fever despite antimicrobial therapy

- Antimicrobials chosen do not treat the infecting organism
- Infecting organism has developed resistance to chosen antimicrobials
- Inadequate drug concentration at site of infection — think about compliance, dose, absorption, drug penetration into special sites (e.g. CSF)
- Non-infectious cause of fever
- Antibiotic-induced (drug) fever

If the total white cell count is raised, look at the differential counts

Differential white cell count	*Common or important causes*
Neutrophilia	Bacterial infections (sepsis, focal infection, deep-seated abscess, leptospirosis, *Borrelia* infections)
	Amoebic abscess
Lymphocytosis	Infectious mononucleosis (EBV)
	Whooping cough
Eosinophilia	Invasive helminth infections (e.g. acute schistosomiasis)

If the total white cell count is normal or low, then look at the platelet count

Platelet count	*Common or important causes*
Normal	Viral infections (including the prodrome of acute viral hepatitis)
	Typhoid
	Richettsial infection
Low	Malaria
	Dengue and other viral infections
	Patient with established HIV infection

Sepsis

Sepsis is a heterogeneous syndrome resulting from a complex interaction between the invading pathogen and host defences. Bacterial infections are much the more common cause, but other infections (e.g. falciparum malaria) can cause an identical clinical syndrome.

Definitions of sepsis and related disorders

Sepsis: Clinical evidence of infection, plus evidence of a systemic response manifested by 2 or more of:

- Temperature >38°C or <36°C
- Heart rate >90 beats/min
- Respiratory rate >20 breaths/min
- WBC >12 or <4, or >10% immature forms

Severe sepsis: Sepsis associated with organ dysfunction:

- Hypotension
- Lactic acidosis
- Oliguria
- Confusion
- Hepatic dysfunction

Septic shock: Severe sepsis with hypotension despite adequate fluid resuscitation

A variety of non-infectious insults can produce an identical clinical syndrome (e.g. pancreatitis, chemical toxins, and burns).

Management

The cornerstones of treatment are:

- Intravenous fluid resuscitation
- Antimicrobial therapy — 'best guess' empirical treatment should be started immediately (after blood cultures, if available)

In severely ill patients, a wide range of supportive measures (e.g. vasopressor therapy, mechanical ventilation, haemofiltration) might be indicated if available.

However, despite intensive treatment, mortality from sepsis remains high — overall, about 20–30% in sepsis, rising to 50% in patients with severe sepsis or shock, and over 80% in patients with multi-organ failure.

Pregnancy-related infections

The risk of maternal death varies from 7/100,000 in Scandinavia to 1000/100,000 in some parts of Africa and Middle East. The major causes of maternal death are:

- Sepsis
- Hypertensive disorders of pregnancy
- Haemorrhage
- Complications of obstructed labour

General principles of management

- Emptying the uterus is essential for a cure — deliver the baby or evacuate any retained products
- Antibiotics should be started as soon as the diagnosis is made
- A wide range of bacteria may cause these infections and there is often more than one organism — broad-spectrum antibiotic therapy should be used that includes cover for streptococci, Gram –ves, and anaerobes.

Prevention

Are there any simple measures that could be introduced to prevent some pregnancy-related infections? Consider the major risk factors listed in the box. However, the most effective ways to reduce post-abortion infections are to make available:

- Contraceptives to prevent unwanted pregnancies
- Medical abortions

	Major factors increasing risk	**Clinical features**
Intrapartum chorioamnionitis	Pre-term labour Prolonged rupture of membranes Multiple vaginal examinations	Fever Maternal tachycardia Uterine tenderness Fetal tachycardia
Postpartum endometritis	Caesarean section (particularly after onset of labour or rupture of membranes) Use of unwashed hands or unsterilized instruments during delivery	Fever (usually 1–2 days postpartum) Tachycardia Lower abdominal pain Uterine tenderness
Post-abortion	Non-medical abortions Retained products of conception Operative trauma	Fever (usually within 4 days of procedure) Abdominal pain and tenderness Vaginal bleeding High risk of severe sepsis

Cancer

Cancer is a common condition worldwide, although there is wide geographical variation in the prevalence of particular cancers. About 6 million people are estimated to have died from cancer during 1990 — 3.6 million in the developing world. Lung cancer was the most common cancer worldwide, followed by stomach, liver, colon and rectum, oesophagus, and breast. Breast cancer was the most common fatal cancer in women.

Cancer requires early intervention for therapy to be effective. Bearing this in mind, basic rules include:

- Cancer should be suspected with any unexplained illness, particularly in the elderly.
- Every attempt should be made to get a histological or cytological diagnosis as soon as possible.
- Once diagnosed, patients should start a planned regimen of treatment within days, not weeks. Tumours grow exponentially and there is no room for delay.

Signs and symptoms common to many forms of cancer

- ***Pain:*** due to direct effect of tumour (e.g. infiltration of nerves or compression), its treatment, or metastatic spread to the bones. Any patient with unexplained persistent pain should be suspected of having malignant disease.
- ***Weight loss:*** due to involvement of GI tract (obstruction, metastatic liver involvement) or a poorly understood general cachexia syndrome with anorexia and malaise (? due to factors released by the tumour). May be exacerbated by treatment.
- ***Tumour mass:*** often ignored by doctors but requiring early diagnosis by biopsy, preferably by fine needle aspiration.
- ***Fever:*** while normally caused by superimposed infection, fever may itself be a feature of particular cancers such as lymphomas, renal CA, and tumours metastasizing to the liver. Frequently occur as drenching night sweats without rigors.
- ***Anaemia:*** normocytic normochromic (sometimes hypochromic) due to bleeding or malabsorption.
- ***Hypercalcaemia:*** due to widespread metastases to the skeleton or, more commonly, to paraneoplastic syndromes.

Paraneoplastic syndromes

Diverse syndromes which, while individually uncommon, are common when taken together. They are due to tumour-derived cytokines or hormones or to a tumour-induced immune response cross-reacting with normal tissue. The range of syndromes is wide and includes endocrine, neurological, dermatological, musculoskeletal, and haematological syndromes. However, unless obviously paraneoplastic in character, symptoms from cancer should initially be considered direct effects of the tumour since this will have important implications for therapy. Most neurological problems are due to metastases, and most endocrine problems due to the endocrine tumours themselves, not paraneoplastic syndromes.

WHO performance status

This is useful for grading the status of cancer patients and determining prognosis.

0 Able to carry out normal activity without restriction
1 Restricted in physically strenuous activity but walking about and able to carry out light work
2 Walking about and capable of self-care but unable to carry out any work; up and about >50% of waking hours
3 Capable of self-care; confined to bed or chair more than 50% of waking hours
4 Completely disabled; cannot carry out self-care; totally confined to bed or chair

Complications with some tumours

- Spinal cord/cauda equina compression.
- Cerebral metastases and raised intracranial pressure.
  Management of either requires immediate administration of dexamethasone 8mg bd IV. Neurological symptoms should settle quickly. Delay in the treatment of spinal cord compression will result in paraplegia.
- Carcinomatous meningitis — leads to headache and increased ICP.
- Pleural and pericardial effusions.

General rules of cancer management

Whenever you see a patient known to have cancer, think of the following points:

1. ***Could the patient have neutropenia?*** Infection in a neutropenic patient often presents atypically (e.g. without fever or without chest consolidation). Have a high level of suspicion — anyone who is feeling run down must have their WCC done immediately and NOT be sent home. Such patients can deteriorate quickly and be dead within hours.

2. ***Could the patient have hypercalcaemia?*** Unlike 1° parathyroid disease, the onset is rapid and there are none of the classical 'stones, bones, or groans'. Instead clinical features include: polyuria, thirst, confusion, fatigue, coma. Treatment of hypercalcaemia will produce a marked improvement in the patient's condition.

3. ***Is the patient's pain controlled?*** Use morphine — it is a very effective drug. The following regimen is useful:
   - Give quick-acting morphine 10 mg q4h at 07.00, 11.00, etc., until 23.00 at which point give a double dose so that the 03.00 dose can be missed out, offering the chance of a good night's sleep.
   - If pain breaks through at any time, always give an extra dose of morphine 10 mg (even if the next q4h dose is only 10 mins away), continuing the q4h dose as normal.
   - As more breakthrough doses are required, increase the regular q4h dose AND the breakthrough dose (e.g. to 20 mg).
   - (If using long-acting morphine (e.g. MST 80 mg bd), take total daily dose (160 mg) and divide by 6 (q4h doses) to give size of the breakthrough dose — here 160/6 = ~26 mg)

4. ***Could the patient have early cord compression?***
   Ask: Can you walk? When was the last time you walked? Have you been incontinent of urine and/or faeces?
   Do a neurological exam including anal tone and sacral sensation. Missing spinal cord compression may result in the patient spending their last few weeks or months in a miserable paraplegic state.

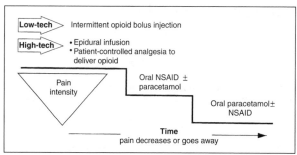

Fig. 3.1 Overview of the management of acute pain

Management of acute pain in hospital

1. Effective relief can be achieved with oral non-opioid and non-steroidal anti-inflammatory drugs (NSAIDs). Studies indicate that ibuprofen 400 mg is very effective; paracetamol 1g and the combination of paracetamol with codeine are also highly effective. Ibuprofen is associated with fewer gastrointestinal bleeds than some other NSAIDs.
2. Initial management of moderate pain, such as in post-surgical patients, should ideally be an oral NSAID such as ibuprofen, supplemented if necessary with paracetamol. In the elderly, paracetamol may be preferred, although it is less effective. There is no evidence that giving the drug by routes other than orally is beneficial.
3. Opioids are the first-choice treatment for severe acute pain. Additional, often smaller, doses can be given if the patient is still in pain and you are sure that all the previous dose has been delivered and absorbed. More drug can be given 5 mins after IV injection, 1 hr after IM or SC injection, and 90 mins after an oral dose. The route of administration can be changed to achieve faster control if there is no response to the repeated dose.
4. The key principle for safe and effective use of opioids is to titrate the dose against the degree of pain relief. If the patient is asking for more opioid then it usually signals inadequate pain control resulting from too little drug, too long between doses, too little attention being paid to the patient, or too much reliance on rigid regimens.
5. It is very important to set up a q4h regimen which prevents the occurrence of pain
6. It may be safer to use only one opioid in routine practice. Morphine is the most appropriate choice and it is popular amongst pain specialists. It has an action which lasts a reliable 4 hrs and is easier to titrate than opioids with a longer half-life. (See previous text for an example of a q4h morphine regimen.)
7. As the pain decreases, the patient can be switched over to ibuprofen and paracetamol (see Fig. 3.1). Supplementation of morphine with an NSAID allows the morphine dose to be reduced.

Rheumatoid arthritis (RA)

A chronic, inflammatory polyarthropathy, with systemic complications. Onset is usually in the fourth decade (can be earlier — Still's disease) with joint ache, swelling and stiffness, progressing in some cases to severely disabling arthropathy. It is usually symmetrical; however, single joints can be affected.

It is more common in women, and in temperate climates, although it is well described in Africa (especially East and South), Asia, and the Caribbean. Both genetic (HLA DR4) and environmental factors are important, the latter since the disease tends to be more severe in urban areas in the tropics.

Clinical signs: joint swelling (often MCP, wrist, knees) progressing to the typical lesions of: ulnar deviation of digits, subluxation at MCPs and wrist, swan-neck and Boutonniere's deformity of fingers, Z-thumb, small muscle wasting, and tendon rupture. Atlanto-axial disease may cause neurological symptoms and be life threatening.

Extra-articular disease: anaemia (see box); subcutaneous nodules (usually extensor); lymphadenopathy; nerve entrapment (e.g. carpal tunnel syndrome); mononeuritis multiplex; splenomegaly (may be Felty's syndrome: rare combination of RA, splenomegaly, leucopenia, and lymphadenopathy); episcleritis; Sjogrens syndrome; pericarditis; and lung fibrosis.

Diagnosis: X-rays of hands, feet, and other affected joints show typical changes (see box). Immunology where available for: rheumatoid factor (usually IgM against *self* IgG) which is +ve in 75% in the West (false +ves: old age, endocarditis, chronic liver disease, fibrotic lung disease). FBC (anaemia); ESR (approximates to disease activity).

Management: continued exercise/physiotherapy. Wrist splints may give symptomatic help and improve function.

- Oral NSAIDs regularly and, if tolerated (asthma, GI bleeding), at high doses, give symptomatic relief but will not affect overall outcome or reduce the ESR.
- Disease-modifying anti-rheumatoid drugs (DMARDs) may be added if NSAIDs are insufficient, but may take months to work and need specialist supervision. Most widely used is sulfasalazine (build up from 500mg od to max 2–3 g in divided doses; monitor LFTs and FBC regularly for the first few months for hepatitis and leucopaenia). Penicillamine at 125–250 mg od increased monthly to a max of 500–750 mg in divided doses is an alternative. FBC (thrombocytopaenia) and urine (proteinuria) need to be closely monitored when initiating or increasing treatment. Gold salts and chloroquine are also used.
- Steroids are widely used with good initial results, although the high doses required with time lead to Cushingoid complications (e.g. weight gain, hypertension, diabetes, and osteoporosis). Methotrexate, azathioprine, ciclosporin, and leflunomide are successfuly used as steroid-sparing agents, though have specific contraindications and monitoring requirements.

Causes of anaemia in RA

- Anaemia of chronic disease
- NSAID-related GI blood loss
- Myelosuppression due to gold/penicillamine
- Folate deficiency due to methotrexate
- Felty's syndrome
- Concurrent illness (e.g. malaria, sickle cell)
- Phlebotomy

X-ray changes in RA

- Soft tissue swelling
- Joint subluxation
- Joint space narrowing
- Juxta-articular osteopenia
- Bony erosions

Differential diagnosis of RA

- Septic arthritis (sudden onset, unwell, fever, WCC, synovial culture +ve)
- Osteoarthritis
- Gout/pseudo gout
- Rheumatic fever
- Juvenile RA (Stills' disease — young onset, RhF+ve)
- Gonorrhoea
- TB
- Drug allergy

Osteoarthritis

A non-erosive arthropathy, usually 2° to 'wear and tear', that is uncommon in the tropics. The knees are most commonly affected. Osteophytes are characterisitic, leading to bony swelling around a joint — quite unlike the 'boggy' feeling of active synovitis in RA. There may be Heberden's and/or Bouchard's nodes (bony osteophytes) at the distal and proximal interphalangeal joints respectively. X-ray changes include: joint space narrowing, juxta-articular osteosclerosis, and soft tissue swelling. There are no diagnostic blood tests and treatment relies upon paracetamol, NSAIDS, and possibly glucosamine. Cod liver oil may be beneficial in 25%.

Systemic lupus erythematosus (SLE)

A multi-system, relapsing and remitting connective tissue disease characterized by facial rash (classically butterfly distribution), vasculitis, nephritis, and fever. It is found in the Caribbean, South Asia, and the Far East, but is uncommon in Africa. Women are more commonly affected and onset is usually in the 2nd–3rd decades.

Clinical features
In decreasing frequency:
- *Musculoskeletal:* arthralgia, myositis, proximal myopathy. Arthritis is usually non-erosive but may be similar to RA (Jaccouds).
- *Skin:* malar rash (photosensitive), scarring alopecia, livido reticularis, Raynaud's phenomenon, purpura, oral ulceration, conjunctivitis, bullae.
- *Renal:* proteinuria, glomerulonephritis, uraemia.
- *CNS:* depression, psychosis, fits, mononeuritis multiplex, cerebellar ataxia, chorea.
- *Pulmonary:* pleurisy/effusion, pneumonia, fibrosis, bronchiolitis.
- *Cardiovascular:* hypertension, pericarditis, sterile endocarditis (Libman–Sachs).
- *Blood:* normocytic anaemia, haemolysis (Coombs +ve), thrombocytopaenia, B-cell lymphoma, thrombosis (especially miscarriage, which may be part of the antiphospholipid syndrome).

Diagnosis: where available, anti-nuclear antibody (ANA) 80% +ve. Anti-double-stranded DNA antibodies are highly specific. ESR, CRP, FBC.

Drugs (see box) may cause a reversible Lupus-like syndrome, whilst OCPs and sulfonamides may exacerbate idiopathic SLE.

Management: sun avoidance, NSAIDS, hydroxychloroquine, short-term (high-dose) steroids for acute exacerbations, occasionally low-dose maintenance in severe cases. Cyclophosphamide, cyclosporin, and methotrexate are used under expert guidance.

Causes of drug-induced lupus
- Chlorpromazine
- Penicillamine
- Hydralazine
- Procainamide
- Isoniazid
- Anti-epileptic drugs

Typhoid and paratyphoid fevers

These conditions, also called enteric fever, follow infection with *Salmonella* spp. (*S. typhi* — typhoid; *S. paratyphi* types A, B, C — paratyphoid). They are endemic and important causes of morbidity across the developing world. Typhoid is the most severe; paratyphoid B the mildest, with types A and C falling somewhere in between. ***Early antibiotic treatment*** is essential to decrease mortality — start empirically if clinical suspicion is strong.

Following 1° multiplication in the mesenteric lymph nodes, bacteria infect cells of the reticuloendothelial system where multiplication occurs again. This produces a 2° bacteraemia, infection of multiple organs, and clinical illness. If untreated, 20% die from overwhelming toxaemia or 2° organ involvement, particularly encephalopathy, toxic myocarditis, or GI haemorrhage and peritonitis. Importantly for infection control, chronic infection of the gall bladder is common — asymptomatic carriers have highly infectious stools.

Transmission: via ingestion of food or water contaminated by infected faeces/urine. Gastric acid is protective so any condition that decreases its production increases an individual's susceptibility to infection. (ie ☓pylori)

Clinical features: The incubation period is normally 10–20 days; untreated illness typically lasts 4 weeks but may be shorter in severe infections (and vice versa).

- *1st week:* non-specific features of malaise, headache, rising remitting fever with mild cough, constipation.
- *2nd week:* patient becomes toxic and apathetic; sustained high temperature with <u>relative bradycardia</u>; rose spots (2–4 mm pink papules on central torso, fading on pressure) may transiently occur; distended abdomen; hepatomegaly and/or splenomegaly.
- *3rd week:* increasing toxicity with persistent high temp; the patient becomes delirious and weak with feeble pulse, tachypnoea (+/– basal creps); ?abdominal distension, ?bowel sounds, profuse 'pea soup' diarrhoea; neurological complications may occur at this stage (may rarely be the presenting complaint). Death occurs during week 2, 3 or 4.
- *4th week:* if the patient survives, fever, mental state, and abdominal distension gradually improve. GI complications occur at any time, most commonly in weeks 2–4.

Expensive used mus- Typhidot-M Tubex

Diagnosis: culture of bone marrow (best), blood, stool, or rectal swab.
NOT USED IN DEV. WORLD   *nested PCR (100% sens.)*   *cult →40-81% sens.*   ↗ 30% sens.   *serology: Vidal test*

Management:
- Give antibiotics — see box.   *can use string test*
- Give dexamethasone (3 mg/kg IV stat, then 1 mg/kg q6h for 2 days) — reduces mortality in patients with shock or reduced consciousness. *severe*
- Toxic patients must be observed carefully for signs of GI haemorrhage (treat conservatively) or peritonitis (treat with surgery).

Relapse: up to 20% of treated patients relapse after treatment and initial recovery. Relapses are generally milder and shorter than 1° illness; 2nd and 3rd relapses have been reported, therefore follow up if possible. Co-infection with schistosomes may result in chronic/recurrent fever since the bacteria survive within parasites, protected from antibiotics.

Prevention: improved sanitation, vaccination.

First-choice antibiotics vary due to local resistance

In Africa and the Americas

Alternatives:
- Chloramphenicol 1g PO qds for 10–14 days
- Amoxicillin 250 mg PO tds for 10–14 days
- Co-trimoxazole 960 mg PO bd for 3 days

In Asia

Although chloramphenicol, amoxicillin, and co-trimoxazole remain effective in some areas, in most areas MDR strains (resistant to chloramphenicol, amoxicillin, co-trimoxazole) and strains with reduced susceptibility to fluoroquinolones are common.

Alternatives:
- Ciprofloxacin 500–750 mg PO bd for 10–14 days
- Ceftriaxone 60 mg/kg IV od for 7–14 days
- Azithromycin 500 mg PO od for 3 days, then 250 mg od for 4 days

In severe disease

Dosages for each drug can be increased 1.5× initially and given IV.

[handwritten margin notes: Cipro = lowest # days con't fever (4 days) + least # relapses]

[handwritten margin note: now 10% resist. to cipro in Asia]

Rickettisoses (typhus fevers)

These are caused by rickettsias — small obligate intracellular microbes that resemble Gram −ve bacteria. Different rickettsia species produce different forms of typhus. These range from subclinical infections to the potentially fulminant louse-borne epidemic typhus or tick-borne Rocky Mountain spotted fever (RMSF). Most patients, except those with mild infections, show a macular petechial rash that is caused by endothelial cell destruction. Typhus fever even if rare can occur as large epidemics. All typhus fevers respond rapidly to tetracycline or doxycycline therapy. Immunity to *Rickettsia* species is solid and longstanding. Treated patients occasionally relapse but respond to therapy.

Transmission: *Rickettsia* are transmitted by lice, fleas, ticks, or mites. The natural hosts often include the vectors themselves. Humans (occasionally flying squirrels) are important hosts of *Rickettsia prowazekii* and rodents are hosts of *R. typhi*. The rickettsioses are normally grouped according to their mode of transmission.

1. **Typhus fever (transmitted by lice and fleas)**
   * *Epidemic or louse-borne typhus* (*R. prowazekii*): a potentially severe disease in conditions of winter, war, natural disasters, non-changed clothing, and crowding. Overcrowded populations in mountainous areas of Asia, Africa, and the Americas may also be at risk.
     Brill–Zinsser disease is a late reactivation of dormant *R. prowazekii* infection.
   * *Endemic murine typhus* (*R. typhi*): occurs in people in close contact with the rodent host and flea vector in temperate and subtropical regions. 50% of the patients develop a rash. Presentation is non-specific with high fever, headache, and myalgia.
   * *Neither form* of typhus fever shows an eschar at the site of infection.

2. **Spotted fevers or tick typhus (transmitted by ticks)**
   * *American spotted fevers* (RMSF and South American tick typhus; *R. rickettsii*)
   * *Old World spotted fevers* (Fièvre Boutonneuse, African tick typhus, tick typhus fevers of Asia, Queensland tick typhus, Japanese spotted fever; *R. conorii, R. siberica, R. africae, R. australis, R. honei*).
     The different fevers follow a similar clinical course with a developing rash on trunk and extremities. An eschar is present except in RMSF. Long-term complications are rare.

3. **Rickettsialpox (transmitted by mouse mites; *R. akari*)**
   Occurs worldwide in urban areas. An eschar is formed at the infection site followed by generalized symptoms and a papulo-vesicular rash. May be confused with varicella lesions.

4. **Scrub typhus (transmitted by larval stage mites — chiggers; *Orientia tsutsugamushi*)**
   A severe infection, indigenous to south and east Asia and northern Australasia. Mortality rate 7% in untreated patients. Life-threatening manifestations are meningoencephalitis, pneumonia, and myocarditis. An eschar may develop at the site of infection. Because of many serotypes, protective immunity may not develop.

Diagnosis: the diagnosis of rickettsial infection is often clinical and epidemiological. It can be verified by serology, PCR, or isolation of rickettsia in cell-culture from samples early in infection.

Management:
1. *Give antibiotics*
   - Doxycycline 100 mg PO bd or 200 mg od for 7 days is standard therapy for all rickettsial infections. In some situations, doxycycline 200 mg PO in a single dose is as good as 7 days.
   Alternatives:
   - Chloramphenicol 0.5–1 g PO qds for 7 days
   - Tetracycline 500 mg PO qds for 7 days
   In severe cases, drugs can be given IV. Continue treatment for 2–3 days after the patient is afebrile to prevent recrudescence.
2. *Prednisolone* have been used. Give 40 mg PO loading dose, then 20 mg od, tailing off over several days.
3. *Delousing:* louse-borne typhus-infected patients must be washed and clothes disinfected by washing in hot water (or autoclaved/burnt). Patient can then be deloused weekly with malathion 0.5% lotion or permethrin 1% lotion. Regular treatment of medical/nursing staff is recommended.
4. *Nursing* involves cold sponging for temp. >40°C; replacement of fluids; mouth toilet; and prevention of bed sores.

Prevention: reduction of vector populations and improvements in hygiene (including delousing) are most important. Use tick repellants and protective clothing to avoid contact with vectors. If a tick is found attached to the skin, remove it by grasping its anterior parts and pulling steadily until it comes away.

Ehrlichia, Bartonella, and *Coxiella* infections

1. **Human ehrlichiosis:** transmitted by ticks, a disease caused by infection with coccobacilli *Ehrlichia* spp. Ehrlichiosis occurs worldwide in two forms — monocytic and granulocytic. Patients present with flu-like symptoms; complications include pneumonitis, encephalopathy, renal failure, and sepsis. Thrombocytopenia and leukopenia are common.

2. **Trench fever:** transmitted by the human body louse; a usually mild systemic illness caused by *Bartonella quintana*. The fever may be self-limiting, recurrent (lasting ~5 days), or prolonged with bacteraemia and endocarditis. Disseminated tissue infection may be manifested by bacillary angiomatosis (cutaneous haemangiomas) or lytic bone lesions.

3. **Cat scratch disease:** is caused by *Bartonella henselae* and usually presents as a self-limiting regional lymphadenopathy with fever following contact with cats, particularly kittens. Many cats have asymptomatic bacteraemia, and infection is by their claws or fleas. Complications occasionally occur (e.g. infection of bones, meningoen-cephalitis). Bacilliary angiomatosis and liver disease (peliosis hepatis) can occur.

4. **Bartonellosis:** *Bartonella bacilliformis* is transmitted by *Lutzomyia* sandflies in Peru and Ecuador and produces several forms of infection:
   - An acute febrile haemolytic illness (Oroya fever)
   - Subclinical illness
   - Cutaneous hemangiomatous lesions (verruga peruana) and internal vascular proliferative lesions which develop several weeks after recovery from the 1° illness (or without any apparent 1° illness if this was subclinical).

   Without treatment, Oroya fever is commonly fatal due to massive haemolytic anemia or co-infection with TB or salmonellae. Bartonellosis can be treated successfully with penicillin and other antibiotics; blood transfusions may be given to relieve the anaemia.

5. **Q fever:** a worldwide disease caused by *Coxiella burnetti*. Transmission is from inhaling aerosolized organisms from placental products or from ingesting contaminated cattle or goat's milk; very occasionally via tick bite. Most infections produce a mild fever without rash; pneumonia is common. Hepatitis occurs occasionally. Some patients have a chronic course with cardiac involvement.

Diagnosis
- Serology or PCR
- Examination of peripheral blood films for morulae within neutrophils or monocytes (ehrlichiosis) or bacilli within or adherent to erythrocytes (Oroya fever).
- For cat scratch disease, large rods can be seen in tissue sections stained with Warthin–Starry silver stain (not Gram or ZN stains).

Management

Give antibiotics

- Doxycycline 200 mg PO stat, then 100–200 mg od for 7–14 days.
- Bacteraemia with *B. quintana* or *B. henselae* requires 4 weeks doxycycline therapy, longer in HIV +ve patients. Bacillary angiomatosis requires 8–12 weeks of oral therapy.
- Bartonellosis (Oroya fever) responds well to penicillin, streptomycin, chloramphenicol, or tetracycline.

Endocarditis with *C. burnetti* requires long-term combination therapy. Rifampin 300 mg bd plus ciprofloxacin 750 mg bd, or doxycycline plus co-trimoxazole, or doxycycline plus rifampicin, continued for 3 years.

Relapsing fever

Two forms are recognized. Epidemic louse-borne relapsing fever is caused by *Borrelia recurrentis* and is most common in the horn of Africa. Endemic tick-borne relapsing fever is a less severe disease caused by one of eight *Borrelia* spp; its distribution is much wider — cases occur on all continents. Both diseases are caused by spirochaetes that multiply in the blood. The antibody clearance of spirochaetes coincides with defervescence but fever recurs because the bacilli have genes that encode around 50 variable membrane proteins that are expressed in sequential broods of spirochaetes.

Louse-borne relapsing fever

Transmission: is human–human via body and head lice. Humans are the only host. Lice become infected by feeding on human blood during a febrile period and infect other humans by being crushed onto the skin, not via a bite. Transmission often occurs during the rainy season when people gather indoors. The disease is also associated with displacement (e.g. due to war or famine).

Clinical features: high fever (100%), severe headache (73%), jaundice (50%), splenomegaly (50%), arthralgia (45%), cough (23%), confusion (14%). Bleeding may occur into the skin (petechial rash), mucous membranes (epistaxis), or conjunctivae. Initial fever lasts 3–5 days at which point it falls with relief of symptoms. Subsequent attacks tend to be less severe.

Death: is due to DIC, myocarditis, or hepatic encephalopathy during the first febrile period, or hyperpyrexia with shock, heart failure, and cerebral oedema during the first crisis. Death may also occur after antibiotic treatment due to a Jarisch–Herxheimer reaction.

Tick-borne relapsing fever

Transmission: via the bite of *Ornithodoros* soft ticks. Rodents may constitute an animal reservoir, although ticks tend to feed on just one type of animal during their lifetime. Transmission is associated with thatched or mud houses.

Clinical features: after an incubation period of up to 14 days (possibly as few as 2), there is severe fever and headache (rarely this continues to coma and death). Splenomegaly and splenic infarction are common (hepatomegaly less so; jaundice rare), as are diarrhoea, bronchitis, pneumonia, and haematuria. Neurological involvement without long-term sequelae are common: cranial and spinal nerve involvement, meningitis +/– subarachnoid haemorrhage, encephalitis, hemiplegia. Other rare complications include bronchitis, liver failure, arthritis. Fever may recur up to 11 times, separated by a gap of a few days to 3 wks.

Diagnosis: definitive diagnosis of relapsing fever rests on the detection of spirochaetes in a Giemsa-stained thick blood film. Culture is complex and serology insufficiently specific.

Prevention: control of ticks and rodent vectors (tick-borne relapsing fever); use of insecticides and improved personal hygiene (louse-borne relapsing fever).

Management
1. Single-dose antibiotic therapy is adequate for louse-borne relapsing fever:
   • Tetracycline 500 mg PO stat *or*
   • Erythromycin 500 mg PO stat *or*
   • Doxycycline 100–200 mg PO stat
2. For tick-borne relapsing fever, longer courses of the same agents (500 PO mg qds for 10 days) are routine.
3. A severe Jarisch–Herxheimer reaction can occur shortly after the first dose of treatment, especially in louse-borne relapsing fever. This can be reduced in severity by prior infusion of anti-TNF antibodies; adequate hydration, and antipyretic and oxygen therapy also probably help.
4. Louse-infected patients must be washed and disinfected, and then deloused weekly, with 1% malathion (0.5% lotions or 1% shampoos). Regular treatment of medical/nursing staff is recommended. The patient's clothes should be autoclaved or burnt.

Leptospirosis

Pathogenic leptospires all belong to the species *Leptospira interrogans*; serovar *canicola* is most frequent in the USA and Europe, while *ictero-haemorrhagiae* most commonly causes the severe form (Weil's disease). Following infection, the spirochaetes spread to multiple organs and cause direct damage to parenchymal and endothelial cells. Further damage in the form of immune complex glomerulonephritis and vasculitis then results from the host's immune response. Leptospirosis is primarily a disease of wild and domestic animals, which may asymptomatically pass large numbers of leptospires in their urine.

Transmission: *Leptospira* enter the body through cut or abraded skin, mucous membranes, and conjunctivae, following contact with contaminated water (pools, canals, rivers) or through close animal contact. Rats are the most common source of human infection in developing countries, and dogs and livestock in industrialized countries.

Clinical features: Vary from mild, low-grade chronic febrile illness, with or without meningitis, to the classical Weil's disease with hepatitis and nephritis. Travel-associated leptospirosis is often seen in febrile travellers.

- *Subclinical infection* — many infections are subclinical and in endemic areas seroprevalence is 5–10%.
- *Clinical disease* — 1–3 weeks post-infection there is sudden onset of fever, headache, myalgia, anorexia, N&V, eye discharge, subconjunctival haemorrhage, and sore throat. In severe infections, the patient becomes prostrate with high fever and marked myalgia, cough, haemoptysis, dyspnoea, persistent vomiting, abdominal pain, constipation, mild hepatomegaly, and jaundice. Other features include meningism, a transient non-specific rash, and purpura (indicative of underlying endothelial damage and 2° thrombocytopenia). In mild cases, a 2-day remission occurs after 4–7 days but this may usher in a second immunopathologic phase. If this is severe, the patient's condition worsens with the development of persistent high fever, myocarditis, widespread haemorrhage (into lungs, GI, skin), renal failure, and shock.
- *Severe leptospirosis* — jaundice, renal failure, haemorrhage, and shock. Recent epidemics in Central America have presented with pulmonary haemorrhage. Death in leptospirosis is due to hepatorenal failure or haemorrhage (2° to endothelial damage rather than consumption of clotting factors).

Diagnosis: during days 1–4, it is possible to culture *Leptospira* from the blood and visualize it on blood films under dark field microscopy. They can also be seen after day 10 in fresh alkaline urine. Look for motile, viable, fine spiral bacteria with hooked ends. Serology.

Prevention: education of at-risk groups to reduce exposure; control of rodent population and vaccination of domestic animals; chemoprophylaxis in very high risk groups (e.g. sewerage workers) — doxycycline 200mg weekly (has a prophylactic efficacy of 95%).

Treatment

1. *Antibiotics* — should be used at any stage of leptospirosis:
   - Doxycycline 100 mg bd for 7 days, started within 3 days of the onset of symptoms, will hasten recovery from mild disease.
   - In moderately or severely ill patients, use benzylpenicillin 1.2–2.4 g IV q6h for 5–7 days, even if the patient has been ill for several days.
   - (Alternatives for severe disease: ampicillin 1 g IV q6h *or* cefotaxime 1–2 g IV q12h *or* ceftriaxone 1–2 g IV od.)
   - Chloramphenicol is ineffective in human infections.
   - Severe disease may warrant ICU care. Haemodialysis is often required.
2. The Jarisch–Herxheimer reaction may occur 4–6 hrs after initiation of IV antibiotics in some patients.

Brucellosis

A classic zoonotic disease of worldwide distribution. It is caused by Gram −ve bacilli of the genus *Brucella*. Four species affect humans: *B. melitensis* (the most common), *B. abortus*, *B. suis*, and *B. canis*. Neutrophils and activated macrophages migrate to the site of entry of the organisms. Humoral (complement-mediated) and cell-mediated immune responses play an important role in eliminating the intracellular bacteria. Surviving organisms multiply and spread via the lymphatics to organs rich in reticuloendothelial cells and via the blood to other organs.

Transmission: is from infected goats, sheep, camels, cows, pigs, and dogs to humans via ingestion of unpasteurized milk, inhalation of infected dust (in animal barns), or animal contact. Human to human transmission (sexual, congenital, and breastfeeding) is rare.

Clinical features: Incubation period is 1–3 weeks and may be as long as several months. Brucellosis simulates other diseases and has no specific clinical features.

- A 'flu-like' illness is the most common presenting feature at onset of disease. The fever has no distinctive or characteristic pattern but may be high in the afternoon. Hepatosplenomegaly and lymphadenopathy occurs in up to 30% of patients.
- Alternatively, localization of infection leading to orchitis, septic arthritis, spondylitis, meningitis, endocarditis, or abscess formation may be the presenting clinical feature at the outset.

Diagnosis: of active brucellosis with or without localization of infection in body organs depends on the detection of raised (>1/160) or rising antibody titre in symptomatic patients. High IgG indicates active disease and high IgM indicates recent infection. Positive culture of blood, bone marrow, body fluid, or tissue occurs in ~50% of patients but may take as many as 6 weeks to be available. Serology is most important diagnostically, since it is quicker. Blood count and biochemical tests are often normal.

Management: Give antibiotics in combination. A treatment duration of at least 8 weeks is recommended; the presence of localized infection (e.g. in bone) requires hospitalization and longer duration of treatment.

- Start with streptomycin 1 g (0.5–0.75 g in patients >45 yrs) IM od *plus* doxycycline 100 mg PO bd for 2 weeks, followed by
- Doxycycline 100 mg PO bd *plus* rifampicin 600–900 mg PO od, both for 4–8 wks
- Netilmicin or gentamicin can be used in place of streptomycin, as a single daily dose of 5 mg/kg
- Children <8 yrs and women who are pregnant or lactating should receive rifampicin and co-trimoxazole

Prevention: animal vaccination, control and eradication programmes, and pasteurization (boiling) of milk in endemic areas.

Plague

An acute disease caused by the Gram −ve coccobacillus, *Yersinia pestis*, that can be rapidly fatal. It thus requires empirical antibiotic therapy when clinical suspicion is high. It is common among animals and occasionally among humans in many countries.

- The commonest clinical form is ***bubonic plague***, in which bacteria spread to lymph nodes and then to every organ including the lungs, liver, spleen, kidneys, and, rarely, CSF. Severe illness follows. Bubonic plague has a 1–15% death rate in treated cases and a 40–60% death rate if not treated.
- ***Pneumonic plague:*** occurs after inhalation of plague bacteria, resulting in a fulminant pneumonia and sepsis which is uniformly fatal if not treated within 24 hrs. Pneumonic plague might occur as a result of biological warfare or terrorism; or from inhalation of infective droplets coughed from a patient with pneumonic plague.
- ***Septicemic plague:*** may be primary, or as a complication of bubonic or pneumonic plague. The mortality is ~40% in treated cases and ~100% in untreated cases.

Transmission: of bubonic plague is via the bite of infected rodent fleas. Plague is a zoonosis, maintained in wild rodents. Most sporadic human infection comes from sylvatic rodents (e.g. ground squirrels, prairie dogs), occasionally from domestic cats. Outbreaks however are associated with urban rats, and spectacular die-offs of rats may herald an outbreak.

Clinical features:
Bubonic plague: the first specific sign is often local lymphadenitis in the nodes draining the site of the flea bite. After 2–7 (always <15) days, a bubo forms in these nodes. There is typically a short prodrome of fever, malaise, headache, and, in some cases, a dull ache in the nodes for up to 24 hrs before the bubo is apparent. The enlarged nodes are extremely painful and swollen, the overlying skin warm, red, oedematous, and adherent. The mass is non-fluctuant and immobile.

Pneumonic plague: initially, intense headache, malaise, fever, vomiting, prostration. Later, cough, dyspnoea, bloodstained sputum with few chest signs, ↓consciousness. Patient soon dies from respiratory failure. CXR shows multilobar consolidation or bronchopneumonia — paucity of chest signs compared with the CXR is characteristic. This picture needs to be distinguished from ARDS which may occur in bubonic and septicaemic forms of plague.

Septicaemic plague presents with fulminant sepsis, multi-organ failure, and skin bleeding.

Diagnosis: fever plus localized lymphadenopathy in endemic area (Africa, Asia, South-West USA); aspiration of a bubo for culture and Giemsa/ Gram-stained smear (bipolar coccobacillus); blood, sputum, CSF for culture; acute and convalescent serology. Antigen detection if available.

Prevention: flea and rodent control (fleas must be dealt with before rodents during outbreaks); public education; vaccination (currently not available); surveillance.

- Suspected cases should be reported to both local health authorities and the WHO.
- Pneumonic plague patients are highly contagious and must be isolated until after >3 days of antibiotics *and* clinical improvement. Prophylaxis with tetracycline may be considered for contacts and medical staff.

Management of plague

For severe disease: antibiotics must be given without delay.
- Most clinical experience is with streptomycin 15mg/kg IM bd for 7–10 days.
- Alternatives (good activity in vitro, but little clinical experience): gentamicin 5 mg/kg IV od; ceftriaxone 2–4 g IV od; ciprofloxacin 750 mg PO bd; chloramphenicol 1 g IV qds.

For milder cases:
- Tetracycline 500–1000 mg PO qds or doxycycline 100 mg PO bd.

For meningitis:
- Chloramphenicol 25 mg/kg IV stat as a loading dose then 25 mg/kg IV qds (PO when clinical condition permits).

All regimens are for 7–10 days.

Melioidosis

A disease caused by the bacterium *Burkholderia pseudomallei* that is endemic in S. and S.E. Asia, N. Australia, the Caribbean, and probably elsewhere in the tropics. It is a major cause of septicaemia in N.E. Thailand. The bacterium is present in mud and surface water (rice paddy); people in regular contact with either are probably infected by inoculation or inhalation. **Glanders** is a similar disease caused by *Burkholderia mallei* that normally occurs in horses but may be transmitted to humans.

Clinical features: infection is often subclinical; clinical illness commonly presents as septicaemia or infection localized to lung (cavitating pneumonia with profound weight loss), bone, or (in children) parotid glands (although any organ may be affected). Septicaemia causes rapid deterioration with metastatic abscesses in lung, liver, and spleen. A failure to respond to empirical regimens for sepsis (e.g. penicillin plus aminoglycosides) may suggest this diagnosis in endemic regions.

Anthrax

Anthrax is a disease of wild and domestic herbivores caused by *Bacillus anthracis*. There are ~4000–8000 human cases worldwide annually, with occasional epidemics. Humans acquire anthrax via contact with diseased animals (e.g. eating or skinning livestock such as cattle or sheep). The bacterium produces spores which can survive almost any environmental condition (except 5–10% formalin for 4 hrs or boiling for >10 mins). The spores may be transported around the world in hides and wool, infecting people and initiating disease in non-endemic areas. Animals which have died from the disease are highly infectious.

Clinical features: Human anthrax has three major clinical forms: cutaneous, inhalation, and gastro-intestinal. If untreated, anthrax in all forms can lead to toxaemia and death. Early treatment of cutaneous anthrax is usually curative, and early treatment of all forms is important for recovery

Cutaneous anthrax: results from introduction of a spore through the skin in industrial or agricultural settings. A rapidly growing papule occurs which ulcerates, becoming a dry black scab (eschar) — the anthrax sore. It is of variable size and surrounded by purple vesicles, sometimes massive local oedema, and lymphadenopathy. Pus indicates 2° infection or a different aetiology. There is usually little pain. The lesion should not be incised; most sores resolve with or without treatment in 2–6 wks; oedema and lyphadenopathy may take longer. Neck sores with extensive oedema may lead to laryngeal obstruction — consider early tracheotomy.

Inhalational or gastro-intestinal anthrax: are life-threatening. Spores may be inhaled to give a pneumonia with toxaemia or ingested to give a severe intestinal infection, with rapid development of haemorrhage, shock, and death in 2–3 days if untreated.

Diagnosis: visualization of capsulated, dark, square-ended bacilli in short chains using the McFadyean stain in smears made from vesicular fluid; fluid from under the eschar (lift edge and extract fluid with capillary tube); blood; lymph node biopsy; or CSF.

Diagnosis and management of melioidosis

Diagnosis: culture blood, pus, sputum, etc; immunofluorescence; serology (problems of specificity and sensitivity).

Management
Treat sepsis with:
- Ceftazidime 40 mg/kg (max 2g) IV q8h for 10–14 days or until clinical improvement
- (Alternatives: imipenem 20 mg/kg q8h (or meropenem) or co-amoxiclav 1.2 g IV q6–8h)

Then give oral therapy to prevent relapse:
- Co-trimoxazole 960 mg (child 480 mg) PO bd *plus* doxycycline 100mg PO bd for 20 wks *plus* chloramphenicol 500 mg PO qds for the first 4 wks
- Co-amoxiclav 625 mg tds *plus* amoxicillin 500 mg tds for 20 wks

Resistance to these drugs may develop during treatment.

The oral regimen can be used IV for sepsis in beta-lactam allergic patients (or if beta-lactams not available), but it is not as effective as ceftazidime.

Management of anthrax

- Give benzylpenicillin 2.4 g IV q4–6h for 10 days. Patients who are allergic to penicillin should be treated with erythromycin, tetracycline, or chloramphenicol.
- Surgical debridement of the black, necrotic eschar is contraindicated. The eschar becomes sterile in <2 days.
- Systemic steroids have been used for the extensive oedema but their efficacy is unproven.
- In late presentations, bacterial toxins may cause severe shock and death even with use of antibiotics.

Prevention of anthrax

- Veterinary public health measures — disposal of infected carcases; disinfection of contaminated areas; vaccination of herds after single cases. Mass vaccination of animals should also be effective.
- An anthrax vaccine has been licensed for use in humans — see <www.cdc.gov/mmwr/preview/mmwrhtml/rr4915a1.htm> for guidelines on its use. It is reported to be 93% effective in protecting against anthrax and has been offered in some countries to military personnel.
- Ciprofloxacin 250–500 mg PO bd is used following aerosol exposure to B. anthracis spores to prevent development or progression of inhalation anthrax in humans.

African trypanosomiasis

Human African trypanosomiasis (HAT), more commonly known as sleeping sickness, is a protozoan disease caused by *Trypanosoma brucei* spp. that is confined to sub-Saharan Africa. Two forms exist — see box.

Transmission: the disease is transmitted to humans by the bite of tsetse flies, genus *Glossina*. Humans are usually infected by *T.b. gambiense* around waterholes or rivers and by *T.b. rhodesiense* in areas of savanna or recently cleared bush. Humans are the principal reservoir of *T.b. gambiense* but are incidental hosts of *T.b. rhodesiense*, which is a zoonosis that affects game animals and cattle.

Pathogenesis: after inoculation, a local inflammatory reaction results in an itchy, painful chancre (for *T.b. rhodesiense* only) and regional lymphadeno-pathy (both *T.b. rhodesiense* and *T.b. ganbiense*). Invasion of the blood-stream and lymphoreticular system follows — the haemolymphatic (early) stage. Trypanosomes then invade the CNS, producing the meningo-cephalitic (late) stage of the disease. Trypanosomes escape the host immuno-logical response by changing their surface antigens (antigenic variation).

Clinical features: *T.b. gambiense* HAT is a chronic disease that develops insidiously. Evolution towards the late stage of the disease and death gen-erally takes months or years. By contrast, *T.b. rhodesiense* HAT is an acute, sometimes fulminant, disease. Both forms are almost invariably fatal if left untreated.

Gambian trypanosomiasis

A chancre is rarely seen at the site of inoculation. After an asymptomatic period of mths–yrs, the early stage of infection is characterized by irreg-ular fevers with fatigue, arthralgia, myalgia, pruritus, and headaches. Lymphadenopathy, often in the posterior cervical triangle (Winterbottom's sign), is common; lymph nodes are soft and non-tender; splenomegaly is rare. Trypanosome invasion of the CNS is manifest by continual headaches, changes in personality, apathy, and forgetfulness; psychosis (abnormal behaviour, agitation, delusions) may also occur. A variety of CNS signs may be seen: pyramidal (focal motor weakness), extra-pyramidal (a resting tremor is common), and cerebellar (ataxia). Late features include daytime somnolence progressing to coma and seizures. Patients ultimately die of starvation, intercurrent bacterial infections, or convulsions.

Rhodesian trypanosomiasis

An area of painful induration — the 1° chancre — often develops at the bite site, subsiding by 2–3 wks. After a 1–3 wk incubation period, trypanosomes entry into the blood causes an acute severe illness with high fever, chills, malaise, severe headaches, weight loss, myalgia, and arthralgia. An erythema-tous rash that may be macular, papular, or circinate sometimes occurs. The disease often runs a fulminant course with multiple-organ failure and early death. CNS involvement produces a meningoencephalitis that progresses rapidly and is fatal within 1–3 mths if untreated. Myocarditis, resulting in atrial or ventricular dysrhythmia or heart failure, may precede meningoen-cephalitis. Infection during pregnancy causes abortions and stillbirths.

Two forms of HAT exist with different clinical and epidemiological features: *T.b. gambiense* is present in Central and West Africa, and *T.b. rhodesiense* in East Africa. An estimated 300,000 people are thought to be currently infected. The incidence of *T.b. gambiense* HAT has increased sharply during the past decades in war-torn countries of Africa because of the collapse of disease control measures. Human infections with *T.b. rhodesiense* are sporadic but outbreaks occur. Travellers to game parks in East Africa have a significant risk of being infected.

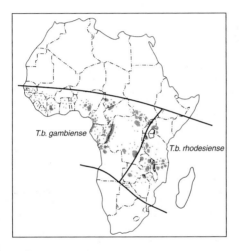

Fig. 3.2

Diagnosis: in most Gambian HAT control programmes, initial screening for infection relies on the card agglutination trypanosoma test (CATT), a very sensitive and practical serological test. No such serologic assay exists for Rhodesian HAT. The direct microscopic observation of trypanosomes in lymph node aspirates, blood (Giemsa-stained thick smear, quantitative buffy coat (QBC) or hematocrit centrifugation technique) or CSF (double centrifugation) confirms the diagnosis. The sensitivity of blood examination is higher for *T.b. rhodesiense* because circulating trypanosomes are more numerous.

Clinical staging of disease: by lumbar puncture is mandatory before considering the use of the toxic drugs for CNS involvement. CSF findings indicating trypanosomal meningoencephalitis are the presence of:

1. Trypanosomes
2. Increased number of leucocytes (> 5 per mm³) *and/or*
3. Specific anti-trypanosomal IgM in the CSF

Management

Treatment and follow-up of HAT require specialist knowledge. The choice of treatment depends on the stage of the disease and whether the disease is Gambian or Rhodesian. **Note:** following a recent agreement between the pharmaceutical industry and WHO, drugs for HAT are being donated to WHO until 2006.

Gambian HAT

1. *Early stage:* pentamidine isethionate 4 mg/kg IM od for 7 days.
2. *Late stage: either*
   - Eflornithine 100 mg/kg IV q6h for 14 days, diluted in normal saline and infused over 2 hours (for children, infuse 150 mg/kg q6h) **or**
   - Melarsoprol by slow IV injection (using a glass syringe, or drawing up and injecting with a plastic syringe as quickly as possible since the drug binds to plastic). Strictly IV (risk of soft tissue necrosis). Several treatment regimens exist. The most frequently used is 3 cycles of 3 daily injections of 3.6 mg/kg with a resting period of 7–10 days between each cycle. A more practical regimen of 2.2 mg/kg/day for 10 consecutive days has been shown to be of similar efficacy and toxicity in Angola. **Note:** resistance to melarsoprol (up to 30% treatment failure) is increasing in parts of Angola, Uganda, and southern Sudan.

Eflornithine is likely to be a safer treatment than melarsoprol.

Rhodesian HAT

1. *Early stage:* suramin 5 mg/kg by slow IV injection on day 1, followed by 20 mg/kg on days 3, 10, 17, 24, and 31.
2. *Late stage:* melarsoprol as described above. The new 10-day regimen has not been evaluated for *T. b. rhodesiense.* Eflornithine is ineffective.

Prevention: Gambian HAT control programmes rely on active case finding through systematic screening of communities and treatment of all those infected (human beings are the only significant reservoir). Vector control by tsetse fly trapping is cumbersome but effective, particularly in Rhodesian HAT control programs.

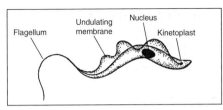

Fig. 3.3 *T. brucei* as seen on a blood film

Adverse effects of drugs used for HAT

- ***Eflornithine:*** leucopenia, anemia, thrombocytopenia, diarrhoea, and convulsions.
- ***Melarsoprol:*** acute reactive encephalopathy (see below), polyneuropathy, severe (sometimes bloody) diarrhoea, and rash.
- ***Pentamidine isethionate:*** hypoglycemia (frequent), hypotension, sterile abscess, and pancreatitis (rare).
- ***Suramin:*** anaphylactic shock, fever, neurological, haematological, and/or renal toxicity.

Melarsoprol-induced acute reactive encephalopathy (ARE)

- Occurs in 5–10% of treated patients, producing status epilepticus and coma. Mortality is ~50%.
- May be partially prevented by oral prednisolone 1 mg/kg PO od given during melarsoprol treatment.
- Onset of fever, tachycardia, headache, tremor, and conjunctival suffusion during melarsoprol treatment should be considered as a warning. ***Melarsoprol treatment should be stopped immediately***; it can be restarted once symptoms subside.
- Some authorities recommend the use of high-dose dexamethasone IV (e.g. 30 mg loading dose followed by 15 mg every 6 hrs for adults) for treatment of ARE or impending ARE.

American trypanosomiasis

A parasitic disease of south and central America, also called Chagas' disease, that is caused by the protozoa *Trypanosoma cruzi*. It may result in fatal cardiomyopathy and GI tract dilatation. The acute infection is often subclinical in adults and children, although potentially severe and fatal in the latter.

Pathogenesis: parasites invade mesenchymal tissues such as heart muscle and intestinal smooth muscle where they persist in their amastigote form, without necessarily re-entering the blood, making detection and chemotherapy difficult. In ~70% of adults, an adequate immune response controls infection, producing a benign chronic phase ('indeterminate form'). Persistent infection and immune dysregulation causes chronic disease in 30% of cases: destruction of the GI autonomic ganglia leading to chronic dilatation of hollow viscera and, in the case of the heart, arrhythmias.

Transmission: through contamination of mucous membranes, conjunctivae, and skin by the faeces of nocturnal house-dwelling reduviid bugs. Domestic and wild animals are reservoirs for the infection; however, repeated infection of humans and vector in the absence of natural hosts can occur. It may may also be congenital, via blood transfusion or organ graft.

Clinical features:

Acute disease: most cases are subclinical with non-specific symptoms. Parasites invading the bite site cause a local swelling, the chagoma, and lymphadenopathy. If close to the eye, unilateral eyelid oedema may occur, a characteristic feature (Romaña's sign) that remains for about 2 mths. 2–4 wks post infection, parasite entry into the blood coincides with the onset of fever. Other features include: a non-pruritic rash of sharply-defined, small macules on the trunk which fades after 7–10 days; swelling, particularly of the face; hepatosplenomegaly; cardiac dysrhythmia or insufficiency; meningoencephalitis (often mild, but fatal in ~10% children).

Chronic disease: includes:
Cardiomyopathy with cardiomegaly, dysrhythmias, conductance disorders, heart block (→sudden death). Valvular incompetence (tricuspid and/or mitral) may occur as a mechanical consequence of ventricular dilatation and dysfunction.

- Megaoesophagus, late dysphagia, oesophagitis, and regurgitation of food.
- Parotid hypersalivation.
- Recurrent aspiration pneumonia.
- Megacolon, chronic constipation, abdominal pain, and, rarely, acute obstruction.

Diagnosis: Serology for anti-*T. cruzi* IgG is the main diagnostic tool; detection of parasites in wet mount or Giemsa-stained blood films or CSF precipitate. Parasite DNA may be detected by PCR. *T. rangeli*, which is not a cause of human disease, may be mistaken for *T. cruzi*.

Prevention: improve the construction of, and chemically disinfect, houses so that the vector cannot live in close contact with humans. Screen blood. Promote the use of mosquito nets.

Management

Acute phase: current treatment is effective at this point. Give either:
- Benznidazole 2.5–3.5 mg/kg (children 5mg/kg) PO bd for 60 days *or*
- Nifurtimox 2.6–3.6 mg/kg PO tds (children 3–5 mg/kg PO qds) for 90 days

Chronic phase: benznidazole is also indicated in this phase but it may be not so effective.

Symptomatic treatment: is often necessary for later omplications: CCF, arrhythmias (see Chapter 00), AV block, and sick-sinus syndrome.

Surgery: may be required for megaoesophagus or megacolon.

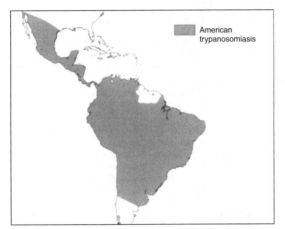

Fig. 3.4 Distribution of American trypanosomiasis

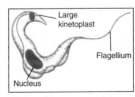

Fig. 3.5 *T. cruzi* as seen in a blood film

Visceral leishmaniasis (kala-azar)

An endemic parasitic disease caused by infection with *Leishmania donovani* or *L. infantum* (called *L. chagasi* in S America) that is increasing in incidence and causing major epidemics with high mortality. The disease is seasonal and geographically focal.

Pathogenesis: at infection, promastigotes invade macrophages, becoming amastigotes which spread to spleen, bone marrow, liver, lymph nodes, and other tissues. Infection may be subclinical, controlled by an efficient cell-mediated immune response. Latent infections are reactivated during immunosuppression, especially HIV. In clinical disease, the immune response is ineffective and the parasite continues to multiply, producing pancytopenia and immunosuppression. The patient dies from malnutrition, bleeding, or intercurrent infection.

Transmission: is by the evening or nocturnal bite of female *Phlebotomus* and *Lutzomyia* sandflies. Dogs are the major reservoirs of *L. infantum* (=*L. chagasi*) a zoonotic form of VL. Humans are the hosts of Indian and E. African *L. donovani* parasites, sandflies spreading infection human to human. Patients with post kalar dermal leishmania (PKDL) can be long-term reservoirs of infection.

Clinical features: Incubation is typically 2–6 months, but the onset can be more sudden with high afternoon fevers that persist. Initially, the patient appears well, is ambulant, and has a good appetite. Dry cough and epistaxis are common. The spleen enlarges and can reach the RIF, though a modest splenomegaly is more common. Anaemia causes fatigue.

Endemic areas: patients present sub-acutely with wasting, weakness, low-grade fever, and abdominal distension or pain due to the splenomegaly. Other features: diarrhoea, moderate hepatomegaly, lymphadenopathy (in Africa), pedal oedema, darkened skin, zoster, and cough. Dysentery, pneumonia, and TB may develop due to immunosuppression; malaria, measles, or influenza can be severe or fatal. Death may follow epistaxis or anaemic heart failure.

During treatment: 3–10% of patients will succumb to the complications above. The risk of death during treatment is much higher in those aged >45 yrs or <4 yrs, or with the following features: severe anaemia (Hb <8 g/dL), severe malnutrition (BMI <13 kg/m^2), inability to walk unaided, and symptoms for >5 months.

Diagnosis: serology — most patients have very high titres. Confirm by finding parasites in Giemsa-stained smears of spleen aspirates (best, but requires training) or lymph node/bone marrow aspirates. Culture of aspirate improves diagnostic yield; cultures on other media can eliminate differential diagnoses (e.g. typhoid, brucellosis, miliary TB). In HIV co-infected patients, parasites are often numerous in skin, gut, liver, and on bronchoalveolar lavage.

Prevention: spraying to reduce sandfly vectors (in urban areas) and culling canine/rodent reservoirs. Deltamethrin-impregnated dog collars reduce transmission of *L. infantum/L. chagasi*. In areas of human to human spread, case identification and treatment of visceral leishmaniasis and PKDL cases reduces transmission. Bednets are ineffective but may provide some personal protection.

Management

1. *The parasite is usually responsive* to IM or IV pentavalent antimony (Sb^v) — 20 mg/kg IM od for 30 days. Meglumine antimoniate (85 mg Sb^v/ml) or sodium stibogluconate (100 mg Sb^v/ml) are equivalent; good quality generic stibogluconate is as effective as brand-name preparations. There is no upper limit on the daily dose. 1° Sb^v resistance is a major problem in India; 2° resistance occurs in relapsed patients.

2. *Patients who relapse* following the 1st course can be retreated with the same daily dosage of Sb^v for a longer course, ensuring that at least 2 test-of-cure aspirates are parasite-free before the patient is discharged. Alternative: give infusions of amphotericin B 0.5 mg/kg/day (or 1 mg/kg on alternate days) to a total dose of 20 mg/kg, or liposomal amphotericin B 2–4 mg/kg/day to a total of >20 mg/kg over 7–10 days.

3. *Second-choice drugs* include paromomycin (also called aminosidine) 15 mg/kg/day IV/IM for 21 days. Miltefosine 25 mg/kg/day (for patients weighing 8–20 kg); 50 mg/kg/day (20–25 kg); or 100 mg/kg/day (>25 kg), for 28 days. It is teratogenic; do not give to women of childbearing age unless pregnancy can be entirely prevented during treatment and for 2 mths thereafter; unsafe in lactating mothers.

4. *Drug combinations* are logical developments for the future, to prevent resistance. Sb^v 20 mg/kg/day plus paromomycin 15 mg/kg/day, both for 17 days, is a safe combination.

5. *Clinical improvement should be evident in 7–10 days.* Response can be monitored by fever, haemoglobin, and spleen size. A parasitological response can be verified by a negative splenic aspirate (bone marrow or lymph node if spleen now small) at the end of treatment. Clinical follow-up is important after 3 and 6 months to detect relapse; by 12 months the person can be considered cured. Relapse rates should be <5%, except in HIV +ve patients, almost all of whom will relapse.

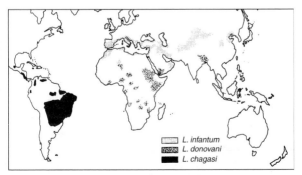

Fig. 3.6 Distribution of viceral leishmaniasis: 400,000 cases annually, 90% in Indian, Sudanese, and Brazilian regions.

L. infantum
L. donovani
L. chagasi

Influenza

Influenza viruses serogroups A, B, and C are RNA viruses that cause respiratory tract infections in humans. Influenza causes disease sporadically, in epidemics, and in pandemics. The virus evolves through small mutations ('drift') and, infrequently, reassortment of its segmented genome ('shift'), thereby evading existing population immunity. Influenza is spread from person to person in respiratory secretions.

Clinical features: the illness starts abruptly. Characteristic features are fever, chills, headache, coryza, dry cough, and myalgia. The symptoms are worst in the first 24–48 hours and thereafter improve in uncomplicated illness. In most cases, the patient recovers fully after 4–7 days. The most common and important complication is 2° bacterial pneumonia, usually due to pneumococcus or *Staph aureus*. This accounts for the significant mortality associated with influenza infection in the elderly and those with underlying lung disease.

Diagnosis: is usually clinical.

Management: in uncomplicated cases, is supportive. Early treatment with antibiotics that are active against pneumococcus and *Staph aureus* (e.g. amoxicillin plus flucloxacillin) is indicated if there is any clinical suggestion of 2° pneumonia (e.g. breathlessness, discoloured sputum, or clinical signs of pneumonia). Failure to improve as expected after the first 24–48 hours of the illness is a warning sign of complications or perhaps that the initial diagnosis of influenza was wrong. In these cases, the patient needs careful reassessment.

Prevention: immunization against known circulating strains. Recommended annually for individuals at high risk of developing complications.

Infectious mononucleosis

Infectious mononucleosis is caused by Epstein–Barr virus (EBV) infection.

Clinical features: fever, sore throat, headache and malaise, lymphadenopathy, and splenomegaly. The typical white exudate on the tonsils is easily confused with streptococcal infection. Rash is uncommon except in patients treated with amoxicillin (for the sore throat) who develop a rash in >90% of cases. Clinical course may be prolonged, with fevers for 2 weeks. In most cases, the illness resolves spontaneously; serious complications are rare. Tonsillar enlargement may cause impending upper airway obstruction — this is an emergency that is treated with corticosteroids and supportive measures. Autoimmune haemolytic anaemia can be severe; spontaneous splenic rupture has occurred.

The acute clinical syndrome may, however, be closely mimicked by some other infections, notably HIV seroconversion illness, acute cytomegalovirus (CMV) infection, and, rarely, acute toxoplasmosis. EBV is also a co-factor (with malaria) in the pathogenesis of Burkitt's lymphoma.

Diagnosis: the WCC often provides supporting evidence — the typical finding is lymphocytosis with atypical (enlarged and polygonal) lymphocytes visible on the blood film (whereas streptococcal infection usually results in neutrophil leucocytosis). Blood tests frequently show mild hepatitis and thrombocytopaenia. If available, the Paul–Bunnell or Monospot test provides a rapid diagnosis in most cases.

Management: there is no specific antiviral treatment; treatment is supportive. Avoid giving amoxicillin for empirical treatment of sore throat if infectious mononucleosis is a possibility since it will cause a rash.

Prevention: there is no vaccine. Infectious mononucleosis evokes lifelong immunity to further clinical attacks with EBV although the virus continues to intermittently shed from tonsils.

Measles

This paramyxovirus is a major cause of childhood illness and death in the developing world. In addition to sporadic disease with a fatality rate of ~5%, it also occurs in devastating epidemics that kill up to 40% of infected children in unvaccinated populations. In contrast, it tends to be a self-limiting infection in industrial societies. Although the reasons for the severity of infection in the developing world are still debated, two possible reasons stand out:

1. *Overcrowding:* measles is very contagious: up to 90% of non-immune people who come into contact with a case will be infected. Transmission rates are therefore high in areas of overcrowding. 2° cases resulting from household contact are also more severe — in one epidemic, case fatality was 23% for 2° cases vs. 1% for the first household case; 85% of deaths were due to 2° household infections.
2. *Malnutrition:* cellular immunity is important for the host's response to the measles virus. Since this is impaired in the severely malnourished child, poverty and malnutrition predispose to severe and persistent infections.

Pathogenesis: the virus infects and lyses epithelial cells of the respiratory and GI tracts, leading to 2° bacterial pneumonia and enteropathy that produces further malnutrition. It also attacks and depresses the immune system itself, encouraging the 2° infections and reactivation of dormant pathogens. Death occurs from chest and CNS complications. Infection of pregnant women is associated with a marked increase in infant and child death.

Immunity: an infant receives passive immunity from an immune mother in the form of maternal antibody. Once this immunity wanes between 6–9 months, a live vaccine can be given — it is highly effective in protecting infants and children. Non-immune infants <16 months old have a high mortality rate. Vaccination limits both the extent of epidemics and mortality by increasing herd immunity and decreasing the number of children susceptible to 2° infection.

Transmission: is directly from humans via inhalation of virus in respiratory droplets following face to face exposure. Exposure to airborne virus may also be important in areas of high density. Medical clinics are recognized sources of infections. There is no animal reservoir or vector.

Clinical features: after 10–14 days, fever and coryza develop over 24 hrs followed by severe conjunctivitis and cough. During this prodromal phase, infants often lose a lot of weight. By day 3, Kopliks spots (bright red blobs with bluish/white centre) become visible on the buccal mucosa. 24–48 hrs later, a rash appears on the forehead and neck, spreading to the trunk over 2–4 days. On dark skin, the maculopapular rash is deep red or purple and ultimately desquamates; on pale skin, it is initially reddish, becoming brown. The patient is most ill during the first day or two of the rash; if the infection is uncomplicated, the fever abates several days after the rash's appearance.

Measles

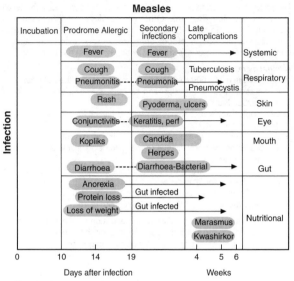

Fig. 3.7 Timecourse of measles infection

Complications

- Laryngitis (both 2° bacterial and viral) ? upper airway obstruction.
- 2° bronchopneumonia (normally ? bacterial) — may be difficult to recognize since patients already have fever, cough, raised RR.
- Sore mouth (decreases feeding by infant); otitis media.
- Corneal ulceration and keratomalacia (+ 2° HSV infection) leading to blindness (exacerbated by vitamin A deficiency).
- Diarrhoea (+/– tenesmus, blood) → dehydration and malnutrition
- Haemorrhagic measles with purpuric rash and mucosal haemorrhage (very rare but has a high mortality rate).

CNS complications: febrile convulsions are the most common. Encephalitis is a rarer manifestation, occurring in three forms:
1. *Acute post-infectious measles encephalitis:* occurs in older children (>2 yrs) 4–7 days after the rash's appearance; it has a 10–20% fatality rate and many survivors have neurological sequelae.
2. *Acute progressive encephalitis:* occurs in immunosuppressed patients; manifests with lethargy, seizures, motor and sensory defects.
3. *Subacute sclerosing panencephalitis (SSPE):* very rare late complication of 5–15 yr olds, M > F. Slow progressive disease develops over months with subtle changes in personality and intellect due to continuing infection; later: myoclonic jerks, chorioathetosis; ataxia; coma; focal retinitis → ? blindness. There is no specific treatment.

Diagnosis: the clinical features of cough, conjunctivitis, coryza, and morbil-liform rash are often diagnostic. Otherwise: serology (rarely, multinucleate giant cells in Giemsa-stained smears of urine/sputum by light microscope). The virus is present in blood, urine, respiratory secretions, and on conjunctivae from onset of symptoms until ~4th day of the rash.

Management:
1. *Give vitamin A 200,000 IU PO immediately* and repeat the next day. It may save the child's eyesight and decrease the severity of the disease. See Nutrition section.
2. Give topical antibiotics to patients with conjunctivitis or corneal dryness to prevent 2° bacterial infection.
3. *Chloramphenicol eyedrops,* preferably q2h, but at least q6h.
4. Eye problems are normally due to the child being unable to close eyelids adequately.
5. Give symptomatic care, with particular regard to hydration and nutrition.
6. Give antibiotics for 2° infections.
7. Studies from Senegal have suggested that prophylactic antibiotics markedly decrease mortality during an epidemic.

Control: active immunization. Passive immunization with human γ-globulin (750 mg for adults and children >3 yrs; 500 mg for children 1–3 yrs; 250 mg for children <1 yr) is effective up to 5 days post exposure.

Hospital admission

During an epidemic, decide which clinical signs should determine whether a patient is ill enough to warrant admitting to hospital. The following criteria were used by Lamb in a Gambian epidemic to grade severity of illness.[*]

	Degree of severity of infection			
	Severe	Mod/Sev	Moderate	Mild
Oral lesions				
Buccal mucosa	+	+	+	+
Gingiva	+	+	+/−	−
Tongue/palate	+	+	−	−
Haemorrhagic	+	−	−	−
Rash				
Haemorrhagic	+	−	−	−
Confluent	+	+	−	−
Desquamating	+	+/−	−	−
Widespread	−	−	+	−
Scattered	−	−	−	+
Systemic upset				
Bronchopneumonia	+	+	−	−
Cough	+	+	+	−
Coryza	+	+	+	+
Diarrhoea	+	+	+	−
Bloody diarrhoea	+	−	−	−

Other signs that may warrant admission include:
- Severe mouth or skin ulceration
- Corneal ulceration
- Convulsions/LOC
- Laryngeal obstruction
- Marked dehydration

If the child is malnourished or underweight, these signs should be considered with greater seriousness.

[*]Lamb WH (1996) Rev Infect Dis, **10**, 457

Arboviruses

Arboviruses are transmitted to man by arthropod vectors — insects (mosquitoes, sandflies) and ticks. A large number cause clinical disease:

- Arboviruses occur throughout the world, although the geographical range of individual viruses is limited.
- Most are zoonoses — infection in man is incidental (but may become epidemic).

The illnesses caused by arbovirus infections can be broadly classified into four, overlapping syndromes:

1. Acute benign fever, with or without rash
2. Acute encephalitis
3. haemorrhagic fever (see later)
4. Polyarthritis and rash

Overall, dengue causes more illness and death than any other arboviral infection. Locally, other viruses may be more important. What are the local arboviruses? — see box. Yellow fever has the potential to cause disasterous epidemics. Japanese encephalitis — a common and important arboviral infection in parts of Asia — is considered elsewhere (see Chapter 8).

Dengue and dengue haemorrhagic fever

Dengue is transmitted from infected to susceptible humans by day-biting *Aedes aeqypti* mosquitoes — a domestic mosquito that breeds in human-made containers. There are four viral serotypes (1, 2, 3, and 4). Infection with one serotype does not induce solid immunity to the other serotypes, and so an individual may be infected with dengue more than once. Dengue is not transmitted directly from one person to another, and therefore special infection control measures are not required for suspected cases in hospital.

The most intense transmission occurs in S.E. Asia, but in recent years there have been dramatic increases in dengue transmission in other areas of the world including the Indian subcontinent and the Western hemisphere. An estimated 40–80 million people are infected with dengue each year. In established areas of intense dengue transmission (such as S.E. Asia) almost all infections occur in children, and adults are immune to locally circulating serotypes of dengue virus. In contrast, if a particular serotype of dengue is newly transmitted in a geographical area, both adults and children will become infected.

Clinical features. Infection may be subclinical. Symptomatic infection may present as an undifferentiated febrile disease, with maculopapular rash, particularly in infants and young children. Dengue syndromes range from a benign febrile illness (dengue fever — DF) to a severe, life-threatening syndrome characterized by disordered haemostasis and shock (dengue haemorrhagic fever/dengue shock syndrome — DHF/DSS).

Local arboviruses

This box can be used to list the arboviruses that are known to occur in the local area.

- *Acute fever with or without rash*

- *Acute encephalitis*

- *Haemorrhagic fever*

- *Polyarthritis and rash*

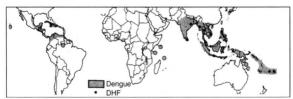

Fig. 3.8 Distribution of dengue fever.

DF

Begins abruptly 3–15 (usually 5–8) days after an infected mosquito bite. Fever is often accompanied by severe headache, retro-orbital pain, and intense myalgia and arthralgia (hence name 'break bone fever'). A blanching rash typically appears after a few days; it is a useful clue to diagnosis if present. DF usually lasts for 4–7 days, followed by complete recovery. Severe complications are uncommon; they include: bleeding without evidence of vascular leak (therefore not fulfilling case definition of DHF/DSS) in particular of GI tract and menorrhagia; encephalopathy; encephalitis.

Management: is symptomatic. Avoid aspirin because of bleeding risk.

DHF/DSS

Is initially usually clinically indistinguishable from DF. After 2–7 days, more serious manifestations of disease become apparent, reflecting disordered haemostasis and increased vascular permeability. Diagnostic criteria for DHF/DSS are based on clinical observation and simple laboratory tests – see box. The presence of vascular leak is the key feature that distinguishes DHF from DF.

   Without treatment, mortality may be as high as 50%, but this is reduced to less than 1% by simple supportive care. Adequate plasma expansion with simple crystalloid solutions is the cornerstone of therapy. The vascular leak syndrome typically resolves within 24 to 48 hours, and careful monitoring is required to avoid fluid overload during the recovery phase.

Prevention: there is currently no vaccine. Vector control is effective but difficult to sustain. Insecticide spraying may help control an outbreak.

WHO case definition of DHF

The following must all be present:
1. Fever, or history of acute fever
2. Haemorrhagic tendencies, evidenced by at least one of:
   - Positive tourniquet test
   - Petechiae, ecchymoses, or purpura
   - Bleeding
3. Thrombocytopaenia
4. Evidence of plasma leakage
   - Haematocrit >20% above average
   - Drop in haematocrit >20% after volume replacement
   - Clinical signs (e.g. pleural effusion, ascites)

WHO case definition of DSS

All of the above, plus evidence of circulatory failure:
- Rapid and weak pulse
- Narrow pulse pressure
- Hypotension
- Cold, clammy skin and restlessness

Laboratory diagnosis

Usually performed in specialist laboratories and is not routinely available in many parts of the world where the disease is most prevalent. Rapid, bedside tests for dengue infection are currently under development. Dengue viraemia correlates highly with temperature. It follows that virus isolation (or antigen detection or genome amplification) is usually successful in a patient with dengue and a fever. Conversely, once the fever has resolved, serology is a more useful diagnostic test.

Yellow fever

Yellow fever is a flavivirus that is transmitted by several different species of mosquito. Yellow fever occurs mainly in sub-Saharan Africa; there are far fewer cases in tropical South America and it does not occur in Asia (see Fig. 3.9). Accurate incidence data is lacking — there are ~200,000 cases each year and >30,000 deaths.

Transmission: the primary transmission cycle involves non-human primates, but humans may be accidentally infected when they are bitten by an infected mosquito. The disease may then be spread by mosquitoes from infected human to susceptible human, causing explosive epidemics in urban environments.

Clinical features: illness begins abruptly 3–6 days after the bite of an infected mosquito. Characteristic features are fever, chills, headache, widespread myalgia, conjunctival congestion, and relative bradycardia (Faget's sign). After several days, the majority of patients recover. Others deveop a life-threatening illness with increasing fever, jaundice, renal failure, and bleeding (due to thrombocytopaenia and coagulopathy). Death is preceded by shock, agitated delirium, stupor, and coma.

Diagnosis: can be confirmed by virus isolation from blood in the first 4 days of illness or by detection of specific IgM. WHO will advise on availability of laboratory diagnostic services.

Management: there is no specific anti-viral therapy and treatment is supportive. Direct human to human transmission, without the agency of a mosquito vector, has not been reported. The case fatality rate is not accurately known — perhaps 20% of patients with jaundice will die.

Prevention: the disease is statutorily notifiable to WHO. Immunization is the cornerstone of prevention — protective immunity is probably lifelong after a single dose of live-attenuated vaccine. Universal immunization in endemic areas would be effective but has not been achieved. Insecticide spraying may help control an urban outbreak.

Chikungunya

Chikungunya is a mosquito-borne alpha virus that has a wide geographical range — sub-Saharan Africa, India, much of S.E. Asia — and can cause explosive urban outbreaks of disease. The illness begins abruptly 2–4 days after the bite of an infected mosquito and is characterized by fever, chills, headache, photophobia, vomiting, and a predominantly truncal rash. A striking feature is severe arthralgia/arthritis affecting single or multiple joints. Recovery in 5–7 days without serious complications is usual. Prolonged joint pain and stiffness may occur.

Overview of haemorrhagic fevers

Infections that cause haemorrhagic fever (HF) evoke great fear. The term defines a clinical syndrome, not a specific cause.

Viral haemorrhagic fevers (VHF) occur in most parts of the world — see p. 240. Knowledge of local HF viruses is essential in assessing the risk to an individual patient. Acute bacterial infections (especially meningococcal disease, leptospirosis, rickettsial infection) and falciparum malaria may produce a similar clinical picture and require specific treatment.

The management of HF always includes general support. Infection control measures to protect medical, nursing, and laboratory personnel should be instituted until more information becomes available. If a VHF that can be spread from person to person (in particular Ebola, Marburg, Crimean–Congo HF, but also Lassa fever, Bolivian HF, and Argentine HF) is plausible, based on time and place of exposure, then local experts, WHO, or CDC should be consulted immediately to advise on infection control and to help expedite diagnosis.

Viral haemorrhagic fevers (VHF)

Viruses belonging to four different families of RNA viruses cause HF (see p. 241).

Clinical features: VHF typically begin with a non-specific illness — fever, myalgia, and malaise. Within a few days, the illness progresses with increasing prostration, specific organ involvement, and evidence of vascular damage (injected conjunctivae, oedema, organ dysfunction, haemorrhage). Severe cases develop shock, CNS involvement, or extensive bleeding.

Diagnosis: the particular clinical features associated with different viruses are listed on p. 241 but, in general, accurate diagnosis requires virological confirmation in a specialist laboratory.

Management: in addition to supportive therapy, antiviral therapy with ribavirin has been shown to be effective in reducing mortality in severe cases of Lassa fever. Ribavirin is probably also effective in other arenavirus infections, Crimean–Congo HF, and HF with renal syndrome if administered early in the course of infection. If available, ribavirin could also be considered for treatment of severe Rift Valley fever.

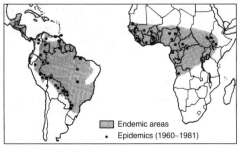

Fig. 3.9 Distribution of yellow fever

Important HF viruses and their distribution in tropical and subtropical regions

Africa
- Crimean–Congo HF
- Dengue
- Ebola
- Lassa
- Marburg
- Rift Valley fever
- Yellow fever

Asia
- Crimean–Congo HF
- Dengue
- Kyasanur forest disease
- HF with renal syndrome (Hantavirus)

Americas
- Argentine (Junin) HF
- Bolivian HF (Machupo virus)
- Dengue
- HF with renal syndrome (Hantavirus)
- Venezualan HF (Guanarito virus)
- Yellow fever

Table 3.1 Taxonomic classification of HF viruses and modes of transmission

	Important examples	Modes of transmission
Arenaviruses	Guanarito	All have rodent reservoir
	Junin	Humans infected by aerosols of rodent
	Machupo	excreta or other close contacts
	Lassa	with rodents
Bunyaviruses	Rift Valley Fever	Mosquito bite
		Aerosol or contact with blood of domestic animals
	Crimean–Congo HF	Tick bite
		Aerosol or contact with slaughtered cattle or sheep
	Hantaan	Aerosols of rodent excreta or other close contacts with rodents
Filoviruses	**Ebola**	Index case probably infected from non-human primates
	Marburg	Person to person spread by contact with body fluids (? aerosol) is most important route of transmission to humans
Flaviviruses	Yellow fever	Mosquito bite
	Dengue	Mosquito bite
	Kyanasur forest disease	Tick bite

Viruses listed in bold may spread from person to person and necessitate special attention to infection control

Table 3.2 Clinical features of VHFs*

Disease	Incubation period (days)	Case infection ratio	Case fatality rate	Features of severe disease
Arenaviridae				
South American HFs	7–14	>50%	15–30%	Overt bleeding and shock; CNS involvement (dysarthria, intention tremor) common
Lassa fever	5–16	Mild infection common	2–15%	Prostration and shock; fewer haemorrhagic or neurological manifestations cf. South American HF
Bunyaviridae				
Rift Valley fever	2–5	1%	50%	Bleeding, shock, anuria, jaundice; encephalitis and retinal vasculitis occur but are distinct from HF syndrome
Crimean–Congo HF	3–12	20–100%	15–30%	Most severe bleeding and bruising of all the HFs
HF with renal syndrome (Hantavirus)	9–35	>75%	5–15%	Febrile stage followed by shock and renal failure; bleeding at all stages
Filoviridae				
Marburg or Ebola	3–16	High	25–90%	Most severe of HFs; marked prostration; maculopapular rash common
Flaviviridae				
Dengue				See p. 234
Yellow fever				See p. 238
Kyasanur Forest disease	3–8	Variable	0.5–9%	Typical biphasic illness — fever and haemorrhage followed by CNS involvement

*Adapted from Peters and Zaki, in *Tropical Infectious Diseases* (eds. Guerrant, Walker, and Weller)

Universal precautions

The purpose of these guidelines is to ensure that the accidental exposure of patients and health care workers to potentially infectious blood is reduced to a minimum. They are based on the assumption that
ALL BODILY FLUIDS ARE POTENTIALLY INFECTIOUS
 (i) regardless of whether they are from a patient or a health worker and
(ii) regardless of whether laboratory tests are positive, negative, or not done.

Principles of infection control

- *Handwashing:* hands and other parts of the body that have been contaminated with blood or body fluids should be washed immediately after removal of protective gloves.
- *Gloves and other attire:* health workers should wear gloves of suitable quality for all direct contact with blood and bodily fluids. When gloves are unavailable, other methods should be used to prevent direct contact with blood (e.g. forceps, a towel, gauze, or, if these are unavailable, even a leaf may be employed) to hold a blood-stained needle or syringe). If gloves are not disposable they should be changed, washed, and disinfected or sterilized after contact with each patient. When injuries from sharp instruments are possible (e.g. when they are being cleaned), extra-heavy-duty gloves are recommended and the instruments should be handled with extreme caution. During procedures in which there may be splashing or suspensions of blood (e.g. during surgery or childbirth), the eyes, nose, and mouth should be protected with a face shield or mask, and glasses and gowns or aprons worn.
- *Needlestick and other sharp injuries:* methods should be devised to reduce the risk of needlestick and other injuries from sharp instruments, which should always be handled with extreme care. The handling of anything sharp should be reduced to a minimum. To prevent needlestick injuries, needles should not be recapped, bent, broken, removed from disposable syringes, or otherwise manipulated by hand. After use, needles and other sharp instruments should be placed in puncture-proof containers located as close as possible to where they are used and then handled as infected material.
- *Mouth to mouth resuscitation:* although HIV has been recovered from saliva, there is no conclusive evidence that saliva is involved in HIV transmission. Nevertheless, to reduce occupational exposure to HIV, mouthpieces, resuscitation bags, or other ventilation devices should be used if available when resuscitation is necessary. Resuscitation equipment should be used once only and discarded, or be thoroughly cleansed and disinfected. Mouth to mouth mucus extractors should be replaced, if possible, by electrical hand-operated or foot-operated suction machines.

Injections and skin piercing

- Injections and other procedures in which the skin or mucous membranes are pierced for preventive, diagnostic, cosmetic, or therapeutic purposes play an important role in both traditional and modern care.
- It is important to restrict injections and other skin-piercing procedures to situations in which the indications are clearly and appropriately defined. In many situations drugs given by injection would be equally effective if given orally. Reducing the number of unnecessary injections and procedures, such as episiotomies, is important in protecting both health workers and patients.
- To avoid person to person transmission of HIV, single-use (disposable) instruments should be used once only. To prevent reuse, they should then be destroyed under careful supervision. Multiple-use (reusable) instruments should always be washed and appropriately sterilized (or disinfected) according to existing guidelines. Chemical disinfection must not be used, however, for needles and syringes. If these procedures are always strictly observed, the risk of HIV transmission through injections and other skin-piercing procedures can be eliminated.

Invasive procedures

- An invasive procedure may be defined as a surgical entry into tissues, cavities, or organs, whether for an operation or for repair of injury. Strict precautions for infection control should be observed in relation to blood and other bodily fluids.

In addition:
- Health workers who perform or assist in vaginal or Caesarean deliveries should wear gloves and gown or apron when handling the placenta and until the blood has been removed from the infant's skin and post-delivery care of the umbilical cord is complete.
- If a glove is torn or a needlestick or other injury occurs, the glove should be changed and the hands washed carefully as soon as the safety of the patient permits. The needle or instrument involved in the accident should be removed from the sterile field.

Postmortem procedures

Health workers performing procedures should follow the precautions outlined above and the standard guidelines for the health care setting involved.

Disposal of infected wastes

- Needles and other sharp instruments or materials should be placed in a puncture-proof container immediately after use and should preferably be incinerated.
- Liquid wastes such as bulk blood, suctions fluids, excretions, and secretions should be carefully poured down a drain connected to an adequately treated sewer system, or disposed of in a pit latrine.
- Solid wastes, such as dressings and laboratory and pathology wastes, should be considered as infectious and treated by incineration, burning, or autoclaving. Other solid wastes, such as excreta, may be disposed of in a hygenically controlled sanitary landfill or pit latrine.
- Solid waste materials in the home (dressings, diapers, menstrual pads) should be considered infectious. They should preferably be burned; if this is not possible, they should be deposited in a domestic or public hygienically-controlled sanitary landfill or pit latrine.

Laundry

- Soiled linen should be bagged where used and not sorted or rinsed where patients are being cared for. Linen soiled with blood or other body fluids should be placed and transported in leak-proof bags. If such bags are not available, the linen should be folded with the soiled parts inside. When handling soiled linen, gloves and protective apron should be worn.
- Linen should be washed with detergent and water at a temperature of at least 71°C/160°F for 25 mins. If low-temperature laundry cycles are used (less than 70°C/158°F), chemicals suitable for low-temperature washing should be used at the appropriate concentration as recommended by the manufacturer.

Laboratory specimens

- Gloves should be worn by anyone handling and processing specimens of blood.
- All open wounds on hands and arms should be covered with a watertight dressing. Hands should always be washed with soap immediately after exposure to specimens.
- Specimens should be placed in containers with a secure lid to prevent leakage during transport. Care should be taken to avoid contamination of the outside of the container. When samples are mailed or otherwise transported, they should be placed inside unbreakable plastic containers.
- Working surfaces should be covered with a non-penetrative material that is easy to clean thoroughly (e.g. plastic film). Any spillage of blood or other bodily fluid should immediately be decontaminated with a disinfectant such as sodium hypochlorite 0.5% before disposal. Gloves should preferably be worn during disposal.
- Hands must be carefully washed after laboratory activities.

Isolation precautions

Ethleen Lloyd, Special Pathogens Branch, Centers for Disease Control and Prevention, USA.

These guidelines have been developed by the CDC and WHO following their experience with VHFs in central Africa. Isolation precautions are based on the principle of establishing a physical barrier to prevent the transmission of disease from an infectious patient. Protection of skin and mucous membranes from fomites and droplets is a major consideration. The barrier can be in many forms, from wearing protective clothing to the use of isolation rooms. As in earlier outbreaks, patient isolation was critical in the management of the Ebola HF outbreak in Kikwit during 1996 and it is therefore advised in the management of all suspected VHF patients. The guidelines replace universal precautions.

- Reinforce and ensure the use of universal precautions in non-isolation areas of the health facility.
- Isolate the patient.
- Wear protective clothing (enhanced by use of two sets of gloves, two sets of clothing, plastic apron, boots, eyewear, bonnet, and mask) in the isolation area, cleaning and laundry area, laboratory, or when in contact with the patient. (Because of experimental infection of primates by aerosols, the observed high mortality among health care workers, and the desire to provide the maximum protection, masks which meet the US HEPA or N series standards are recommended.)
- Handle needles and other sharp instruments safely. Do not recap needles. Dispose of non-reusable needles, syringes, and other sharp patient-care instruments in puncture-resistant containers.
- Avoid sharing equipment between patients. Designate equipment for each patient, if supplies allow. If sharing equipment is unavoidable, make sure it is not reused by another patient until it has been cleaned, disinfected, and sterilized properly.
- Disinfect all spills, equipment, and supplies safely (this is enhanced by using disinfectant sprayers and 0.05% hypochlorite solutions).
- Dispose of all contaminated waste by incineration or burial (including safe disposal of corpses).

Appropriate information should be provided to the families and community about the prevention of VHF and the care of infected patients.

Cardiology

Section editors   **Ian Ternouth**
                  James Hakim

Cardiology in the tropics

In tropical countries, heart disease was previously dominated by rheumatic heart disease, congenital heart disease, cardiomyopathies, and hypertensive heart disease. As populations increasingly urbanize and 'Westernize', there is an increase in ischaemic heart disease, obesity, the insulin resistance syndrome (also known as the metabolic syndrome), and cerebrovascular and peripheral vascular disease. The incidence of acute rheumatic fever is decreasing, but we will be left with patients with terrible sequelae for very many years. HIV infection has led to a large increase in TB pericarditis.

Chest pain

Central chest pain

Nature:
- A constricting pain suggests angina, oesophagitis, or anxiety.
- A sharp pain may be from the pleura or pericardium (both may be exacerbated by deep inspiration, particular movements or positions, postures — i.e. pleuritic pain).
- A prolonged, crushing, tight ('like an elephant sat on my chest') intense pain not related to position or breathing suggests myocardial infarction (MI).

Pains that are unlikely to be cardiac in origin include:
- Short, sharp stabbing pains.
- Pains lasting <30 secs, however intense.
- Well-localized left submammary pain ('In my heart, doctor').
- Pains of continually varying location.

Ask about:
- Radiation (to shoulders, neck, jaw, or arms — especially left: suggests ischaemia).
- Precipitating and exacerbating factors (exercise, emotion, or palpitations suggest ischaemia, whereas food, lying flat, hot drinks, or alcohol suggest oesophagitis).
- Alleviating factors (N.B. glycerol trinitrate relieves both cardiac pain and oesophageal pain, but acts much more rapidly in the former). Pericardial pain classically improves on leaning forward.
- Associations (e.g. dyspnoea and/or palpitations, pallor, sweating, feeling of impending doom, nausea and vomiting — can be present with both an inferior MI and GI pathology).

Non-central chest pain

May still be cardiac in origin, but other conditions enter the differential diagnosis (see box). The more common conditions include:
- Pleuritic pain, including pneumonia
- Musculoskeletal pain
- Gall bladder disease
- Varicella zoster infection (shingles)
- Pancreatic disease

Causes of chest pain

Cardiovascular
Myocardial ischaemia
Myocardial infarction
Aortic dissection
Aortic aneurysm
Large pulmonary embolus

Pleuro-pericardial
Pericarditis
Infective pleurisy
Pneumothorax
  Pneumonia
Autoimmune disease
Tumours (primary)
Metastatic tumour

Airway
Intubation
Central bronchial carcinoma
Inhaled foreign body
Tracheitis

Chest wall
Rib fracture
Muscular strain
Thoracic nerve compression
Rib tumour
Thoracic varicella zoster
Coxsackie B infection

Mediastinal
Oesophageal spasm
Oesophagitis
Mediastinitis
Sarcoid lymphadenopathy
Lymphoma

Angina

This, classically, is central, crushing chest pain that may radiate to the jaw, neck, or one or both arms. It may only be felt in the jaw or arm, or be felt as tightness across the chest. It represents myocardial ischaemia and may be precipitated by exertion, anxiety, cold or a heavy meal and be associated with dyspnoea, pallor, and faintness. It is relieved by rest and nitrates. In most cases, it is caused by coronary artery disease, but may be due to aortic stenosis, hypertrophic obstructive cardiomyopathy, and hypoperfusion from dysrhythmias, arteritis, or anaemia. Indigestion is the most common differential diagnosis.

Ischaemic heart disease is particularly common in people of Asian, Melanesian, Polynesian origin (who also have high incidence of NIDDM). The incidence is also higher in black than in white Americans.

Diagnosis: on the ECG look for ST depression, flattened (or inverted) T waves, and evidence of old infarcts (Q waves). If available, do an exercise ECG 48 hrs after the angina settles. Take bloods for FBC and ESR to exclude non-atheromatous causes (see above), U&Es, and cardiac enzymes as available to exclude infarct.

Management:

1. Encourage the patient to give up smoking, improve diet to reduce lipids, salt, and weight, and exercise more.
2. Improve diabetic control.
3. Start with glycerol trinitrate (GTN) either sublingually, or as a spray at 0.5 mg per dose, used for anginal symptom prn up to every hour. When this is no longer adequate, work up to a functioning dose of quadruple therapy:
   - **Aspirin**: 75–150 mg od.
   - **Beta-blockers**: e.g. Atenolol 50–100 mg PO od. CI: asthma, significant LVF, bradycardia.
   - **Slow-release calcium antagonists**: e.g. nifedipine MR 20 mg–60 mg PO od; felodipine 2.5–10 mg/day, diltiazem 60 mg PO 2–3 times od, increasing to max 360 mg od. CI: fertile women. Short acting Ca^{2+} blockers increase cardiac events.
   - **Isosorbide mono or dinitrate**: (as available) od/bd for mono, 10–40 mg/d, 10–20 mg tds for di NB: need nitrate free interval of 7 hrs/24 hrs.
4. When drugs fail to control angina, surgical options are available. Coronary artery bypass grafts (CABG) improve the overall prognosis, but pain returns to 25–50% of patients in 5 yrs. It carries a 2% mortality risk. Angioplasty where available/appropriate is often a suitable alternative.

Unstable angina is new onset angina, or angina that is rapidly worsening and present on minimal exertion or at rest.

Management: aspirin, beta blockers, oxygen, and bed rest. Give unfractionated heparin 7500–10,000 IU IV q4h to keep APTT twice control if monitoring is available. (If available, low molecular weight heparin does not require monitoring.) If pain/ECG does not resolve, refer for specialist assessment/angiography/revascularization.

Preventing ischaemic heart disease (IHD)

Hypercholesterolaemia, smoking, diabetes, and hypertension are the main risk factors for IHD. Others include male sex, family history, excess alcohol, obesity, and use of the OCP. Geographic, environmental, and social factors are also clearly involved.

1. *Stop smoking*
2. *Check for and manage diabetes*
3. *Check for and manage hypertension*
4. *Check for and manage hypercholestrolaemia*
   - Dietary manipulation can lower lipids; aim for a body mass index (see Chapter 15) of 20–25, on a diet which has <10% of calories derived from saturated fats and is high in fibre.
   - If the plasma cholesterol is raised, look for a cause: alcohol abuse, DM, hypothyroidism, cholestasis, renal failure, nephrosis, and oestrogen use.
   - Encourage a reduced alcohol intake. Small amounts of alcohol can raise HDL and reduce cardiac risk. Recommend <2 units/day for women, <3 units/day for men.
   - Encourage exercise (increases HDL).

Drug treatment should begin if the cholesterol remains >6 mmol/l (or triglycerides >2.3 mmol/l) after 3 months of diet and exercise, or if total : HDL cholesterol ratio is <5. In patients with known cardiovascular disease risk factors, aim for even lower cholesterol levels.

Statins, fibrates, nicotinic acid (preferably slow release: aspirin taken 30 mins before often blocks side-effects) or resins may be used. The diet should continue. Statins are expensive but highly effective drugs for treating hyperlipidaemia. There is no lower limit, the lower the ratio of total:HDL cholesterol, the better. Maximum benefit of treatment is in those with highest cholesterol (most cost effective).

Myocardial infarction (MI)

This is the irreversible necrosis of part of the heart muscle, almost always due to coronary artery atherosclerosis. Although not as common in the tropics as it is in the West (5/1000/yr in England), the mortality in the tropics is probably higher.

Clinical features: the pain is usually of greater severity and duration (>30 mins) than angina, though similar in nature and usually associated with nausea and vomiting, sweating, pallor, and distress. In the elderly and diabetics, small MIs may be painless. There may be tachycardia, tachypnoea, cyanosis, mild pyrexia (<38.5°C). The BP may be increased, normal, or decreased. There may also be features of the complications (e.g. dyspnoea, basal lung crepitations, pericardial rub, or the pan-systolic murmur of mitral incompetence or VSD).

Diagnosis: an ECG is essential. Absence of Q-waves in a proven infarct is associated with a higher risk of subsequent infarcts and a poorer long-term prognosis. CXR — heart failure, change in cardiac size (ventricular aneurysm); aortic dissection. Monitor FBC, U&E, glucose, and ESR (may be up to 80 mm/hr; returns to normal over weeks). Lipids may be raised for several weeks. Cardiac enzymes are useful in the diagnosis of MI. Diagnosis is based on 2 out of 3 of (i) history (ii) ECG changes, and (iii) cardiac enzymes. Troponins where available are the investigations of choice.

ECG changes in myocardial infarction

An initially normal ECG progresses to tall T waves and ST elevation (>2 mm in two chest or >1 mm in two adjacent limb leads for a diagnosis of MI). Alternatively, patient may develop new onset LBBB. Within 24 hrs, the T wave inverts as ST elevation begins to resolve. Pathological Q waves (>1 small square in width and >2 mm in length) form within a few days. These may persist, or completely resolve in 10%. T-wave inversion may or may not persist. ST elevation rarely persists, unless there is a ventricular aneurysm.

Site of infarct

- *Anterior:* changes occur in V2–5
- *Septal:* changes in V3–4
- *Inferior:* changes in II, III, and VF
- *Lateral:* changes in I, VL, and V6
- *Posterior:* look for the reciprocal (i.e. inverted) changes in the anterior leads V1–5; dominant R wave (= inverted Q wave); and ST depression (= inverted ST elevation) with the clinical features of an infarct. Always ask for posterior leads (V7–9) if you suspect a posterior infarct. May be associated RV infarct — ask for V4 R

Non-Q-wave infarcts: (formerly called subendocardial infarcts) do not involve the whole thickness of the myocardium and thus have the ST changes but not the Q waves.

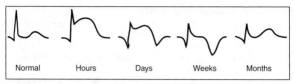

Fig. 4.1 ECG changes following MI

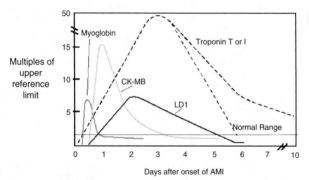

Fig. 4.2 Release patterns of cardiac markers (Wu, A.H., *Journal of Clinical Immunoassay* 1994, **17**, 45–8.)

Immediate management of MI

The greatest risk of death is in the first hour — prompt action can save lives.

1. Relax and reassure the patient.
2. Give 100% O_2 via face mask (if you suspect COPD, give less concentrated O_2 and check ABGs).
3. Insert an IV line and give pain relief (morphine 10 mg by slow IV injection, followed by further 5–10 mg doses as necessary. Half the dose in elderly or frail patients).
4. Give glycerol trinitrate 0.5 mg sublingual or spray.
5. Give aspirin 300 mg PO stat, then 75–150 mg od thereafter.
6. If possible, refer to a centre where streptokinase may be given within 16 hrs.
7. Give a beta-blocker (e.g. atenolol 5 mg IV over 5 min, 50 mg PO 15 mins later, then 50 mg bd) unless the patient has heart failure or asthma. It will decrease cardiac O_2 demand, infarct size, and risk of dysrhythmias and septal rupture.
8. Give heparin 5000 units SC then 5000 units tds until mobilized (as prophylaxis against DVT) and to keep open recanalized coronary arteries. (Low molecular weight heparin can be used instead.)
9. Start the patient on an oral ACE inhibitor 24 hrs after the infarction. Titrate against BP.
10. Discontinue any pre-infarction cardiac drugs.
11. Prohibit smoking.
12. At least 24 hrs bed rest with continuous ECG monitoring and q4h temp, pulse, RR, BP. Perform frequent checks for complications.
13. Daily ECG, cardiac enzymes, U&Es (and CXR if there is worsening lung function) for the subsequent 2–3 days.

Post-infarct management

If the post-MI period is uncomplicated, the patient may be mobilized by day 2 or 3 and the SC heparin stopped on day 3–5. If there are no complications, the patient can usually be discharged by day 3–6 and gradually increase the amount of exercise done over 1 month. The patient should not drive during this period. Strongly discourage smoking and advise about diet. If MI is uncomplicated, especially inferior MI, patients can often go home by day 3.

Prognosis: depends upon the degree of LV dysfunction, presence of significant dysrhythmias, heart size on CXR, presence of post-MI angina, and the presence of pulmonary oedema. In the UK, mortality rates for the first year after discharge are 6–8% with over half these deaths occurring in the first 3 months.

Long-term treatment: patients with no complications and good prognostic indices should be discharged and followed ideally by a specialist physician or cardiologist. All patients should be advised to modify their risk factors and have a follow-up appointment at 6–8 weeks for CXR, ECG, and exercise treadmill test if there is post-infarct angina.

All patients should ideally take (if they have had a Q-wave MI) aspirin, beta blocker (for >18 months), an ACE inhibitor, and a statin.

Contraindications to streptokinase therapy

Streptokinase should not be given if the patient:
- Has had a stroke or active bleeding (e.g. peptic ulcer) within the last 2 months
- Has systolic BP>200 mmHg
- Has had surgery or trauma in the past 10 days
- Has a bleeding disorder or uses anticoagulants
- Is pregnant
- Is menstruating
- Has had previous streptokinase treatment between 4 days and 1 year previously.

tPA, rPA, tNK thrombolytics are **much** more expensive than streptokinase, but slightly more effective and cause less hypotension.

Complications of MI

1. **Infarct extension:** occurs in ~10% (in both Q- and non-Q-wave infarcts) in the first 10–14 days, with varying severity. Treat as a new infarct. Angiography is indicated.

2. **Post-infarct angina:** is associated with increased mortality and occurs in up to 30%. Can occur post non-Q-wave infarct. Treat vigorously with nitrates, beta-blockers, Ca^{2+} channel blockers, heparin, and aspirin. Again angiography is indicated.

3. **Arrhythmias:** see ALS protocols below.
   - *Sinus bradycardia* — may be due to infarct or medication (beta-blocker). May require atropine and, rarely, temporary pacing.
   - *Supraventricular tachycardia* — a sinus tachycardia is common post-MI. Atrial fibrillation (AF) occurs in ~10% and should be rapidly controlled to avoid the onset of ventricular tachycardia (VT) and infarct spread. Use beta blockade or digoxin after excluding hypokalaemia (0.5 mg initially, then 0.25 mg every 90–120 mins up to 1–1.25 mg as a loading dose; followed by 0.125–0.25 mg PO od — assuming normal renal function; loading dose of digoxin in children is 20–30 mcg per kg. The daily dose is 5–10 mcg per kg per day). AF is usually transient, but if necessary conversion back to sinus rhythm can be achieved by DC cardioversion (if AF <48 hrs old, presence of heart failure, hypotension, or refractory to other treatments), IV sotalol, or IV amiodarone.
   - *Ventricular arrhythmias* are most common in the first few hours post-MI and may be heralded by ventricular premature beats. VT >120 bpm may progress to ventricular fibrillation (VF). Treat early with amiodarone or lignocaine IV, or synchronized cardioversion. VF may occur in the first few hours or days and needs emergency treatment. It carries a poor prognosis in the presence of cardiogenic shock or failure. Accelerated idioventricular rhythm can occur after any MI and is usually benign, not affecting cardiac output. Treat expectantly.
   - *Nodal rhythms:* have a narrow QRS complex, normal axis usually, but have no associated P wave (or it may come after the QRS). They are usually intermittent and self-limiting, but in a large MI may decrease both cardiac output and BP. Treat with atropine or a temporary pacemaker.

4. **Conduction disturbances:** all degrees of AV block may occur, most commonly in inferior MIs (20%). First-degree block needs no treatment. Second-degree block is usually Wenckebach and only requires treatment if there is symptomatic bradycardia. Third-degree block often follows second-degree block and is usually temporary. Again, treat with atropine or isoprenaline if symptomatic. In extensive anterior MIs, damage to the conducting system will cause complete and progressive AV block that will require pacing, possibly permanently. Heart block in inferior MIs is usually temporary, lasting <5 days.

5. **Myocardial dysfunction:**
   - *Left ventricular failure* (see below).
   - *Cardiogenic shock:* severe failure causing hypotension, tachycardia, oliguria, distress, and peripheral shutdown. It may be due to: acute MR, severe LV dysfunction, cardiac rupture, VSD, arrhythmias, RV infarct. Treatment is with 100% O_2, IV diuretics (if LVF), fluids (if RVF), GTN, inotropes.

6. *Right ventricular infarct:* occurs in one-third of inferior infarcts but is clinically significant in less. There is reduced BP and raised JVP with clear lungs. Lead V4 right on the ECG may show ST elevation. Treatment is with IV fluids to increase LV filling. Inotropes may be useful.

7. *Mechanical defects* (MR and VSD): papillary or septal rupture occurs in <1% of all MIs and may occur 1–7 days after an anterior or inferior MI (MR most commonly after infero-lateral MIs, VSD after septal MIs). Listen for new murmurs and basal crepitations, and watch for clinical deterioration. Need surgical assessment.

8. *Left ventricular aneurysm:* occurs in 10–20% of anterior MIs. The apex beat is diffuse and there may be atypical/stabbing chest pain, accompanied by ST elevation lasting 4–8 weeks. They rarely rupture but are associated with emboli, arrhythmias, and CCF. Patients may require lifelong anticoagulation.

9. *Cardiac rupture:* usually results in rapid death 2–7 days post-MI. It occurs in <1% of MIs. A small or incomplete rupture may be sealed by the pericardium, forming a pseudoaneurysm that needs prompt surgical repair.

10. *Pericarditis:* 20% of patients have a pericardial rub after 24 hrs. There is chest pain, relieved by sitting up and varying with respiration. It is usually self-limiting but may require analgesia.
    - *Dressler's syndrome:* is an autoimmune pericarditis occurring 1–10 weeks post-MI in 5% of patients. There is fever, leucocytosis, and occasionally pericardial or pleural effusion. Treatment is with NSAIDs +/− corticosteroids. Watch for signs of constrictive pericarditis.

11. *Mural thrombus:* is common in large MIs and may cause arterial emboli, leading to strokes, gut/limb/renal infarcts. Usually diagnosed by echocardiography; needs warfarin for 3 months minimum.

Advanced life support (ALS) protocols

The majority of sudden deaths result from dysrhythmias associated with acute MI or chronic ischaemic heart disease. Successful resuscitation following a cardiopulmonary arrest is most likely if:

1. The arrest is witnessed
2. Basic life support is started promptly *and*
3. Defibrillation (if appropriate) is carried out as early as possible.

Basic life support (BLS)

The purpose of BLS is to maintain adequate ventilation and circulation until a means can be obtained to reverse the underlying cause of the cardiac arrest.

Remember **A**, **B**, and **C** — **A**irways, **B**reathing, and **C**irculation. Ensure that it is safe to approach the patient.

A. Remove foreign bodies from the *airways* (including false teeth); use suction if necessary. Tilt the head back (unless a neck injury is suspected) or do jaw thrust.

B. Is the patient *breathing*? If not, assist via a mask (with 100% O$_2$) and bag ventilation if available, or mouth to mouth resuscitation until intubation is possible. If there is upper airway obstruction, a cricothyrotomy may be needed. If there is a tension pneumothorax, relieve it before proceeding further.

C. *Circulation*: is there a pulse in the carotid arteries? If not, begin external cardiac massage until defibrillation under the guidelines below is possible.

If you are alone and the patient is unconscious, assess whether going/calling for help would be of more benefit than attempting resuscitation alone. It is hard to leave an injured/unconscious person, but their only realistic hope of survival may be if you go straight for help.

ALS treatment algorithms for cardiopulmonary arrest

The algorithm in Fig. 4.3 is merely a summary of the methods used in the ALS training scheme. The methods involve skilled procedures which should only be attempted by qualified staff, since improper use of defibrillators could result in more harm being done to the patient, as well as harm to those carrying out the resuscitation. It is strongly recommended that all medical staff read the ALS (or equivalent) course book and practise arrest protocols in 'mock' arrest scenarios.

Note: If at any stage a pulse is felt, defibrillation should stop and the patient be ventilated. Watch for peri-arrest dysrhythmias (see below). Intubation and IV access should take no longer than 30 secs. If difficult, they should be delayed until the next loop of the cycle. If defibrillation remains unsuccessful, consider changing the paddle positions or the defibrillator.

All ALS protocols are presented with the kind permission of the Resuscitation Council (UK) Ltd.

Ventricular fibrillation

Ventricular tachycardia at 235 beats/min

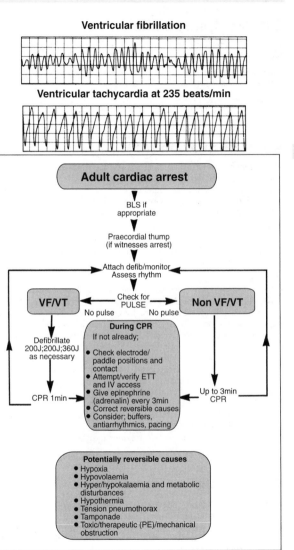

Adult cardiac arrest

BLS if appropriate

Praecordial thump (if witnesses arrest)

Attach defib/monitor
Assess rhythm

Check for PULSE

VF/VT — No pulse — — No pulse — **Non VF/VT**

Defibrillate 200J;200J;360J as necessary

CPR 1min

During CPR
If not already;
● Check electrode/ paddle positions and contact
● Attempt/verify ETT and IV access
● Give epinephrine (adrenalin) every 3min
● Correct reversible causes
● Consider; buffers, antiarrhythmics, pacing

Up to 3min CPR

Potentially reversible causes
● Hypoxia
● Hypovolaemia
● Hyper/hypokalaemia and metabolic disturbances
● Hypothermia
● Tension pneumothorax
● Tamponade
● Toxic/therapeutic (PE)/mechanical obstruction

NB: Each successive step is based on the assumption that the one before has been unsuccessful

Fig. 4.3

Cardiac dysrhythmias

These most commonly occur in the setting of an acute MI, but may also occur during chronic ischaemia.

Clinical features: are usually of 'funny turns', collapse, and palpitations. Distinguish from epilepsy — a witness may help in this.

Investigations: FBC, U&E, Ca^{2+}, glucose, TFTs, CXR, ECG. Arrange echocardiography if cardiomyopathy or valvular disease is suspected.

Atrial fibrillation (AF)

AF is an ineffective, irregular atrial tachycardia, which results in irregular ventricular contraction. Common causes are MI, ischaemia, MV disease, hyperthyroidism, hypertension, and excess alcohol intake. Also: cardiomyopathy, pericarditis, sick sinus syndrome, Ca bronchus, endocarditis, atrial myxoma, and haemochromatosis. It is a significant risk factor for stroke.

Clinical features: an irregularly irregular pulse with a first heart sound of varying intensity and the apex rate greater than the radial rate. The patient may be breathless. ECG shows a chaotic baseline with no P waves and irregularly irregular QRS complexes of normal shape.

Management:
- *Acute AF:* if <48 hrs, DC cardiovert then anticoagulate with warfarin for 1/12; if >48 hrs or uncertain, give warfarin for 1/12 then attempt DC cardioversion followed by warfarin for another 1/12 (if in sinus rhythm).
- *Chronic AF:* the aim is to control the ventricular rate, not the atrial rhythm. Give 3 doses of digoxin 0.5 mg PO over 2 days as a loading dose, then continue on maintenance of 0.25 mg PO od for life (if renal function is normal). Use half these doses in the elderly; reduce further if renal impairment. If still tachycardic, assess compliance, check serum level, and if subtherapeutic cautiously increase digoxin dose. If this fails, add in a low-dose beta-blocker (e.g. propranolol 10–20 mg tds po) or use diltiazem/verapamil. Give warfarin anticoagulation (INR 2–3) to reduce the risk of embolic stroke. The loading dose of digoxin in children is 20–30 mcg per kg. The daily dose is 5–10 mcg per kg per day.
- *Paroxysmal AF:* refer for specialist treatment; requires oral amiodarone or other antiarrhythmic.

Bradycardia

If the bradycardia is acute and symptomatic (usually post-MI):
- Treat or remove the underlying cause (e.g. beta-blockers, nb eye drops).
- Give atropine 0.3–0.6 mg slowly IV, repeating to a max. of 3 mg in 24 hrs.
- Alternatively, try isoprenaline 0.5–4 mcg/min IV (increasing to 10 mcg/min if necessary).
- Temporary pacing may be needed for unresponsive bradycardia. Chronic bradycardia necessitates permanent pacing.

Other causes of arrhythmias and conduction disturbances

- Drugs (mostly those used to *treat* arrhythmias)
- Cardiomyopathy
- Myocarditis
- Cardiac dilatation
- Thyroid disease
- Electrolyte disturbances

Heart failure

Heart failure occurs when the heart fails to maintain sufficient circulation to provide adequate tissue oxygenation in the presence of a normal filling pressure. It may be classified as right, left, or biventricular failure. Heart failure is a syndrome and not a diagnosis — i.e. the patient may have features consistent with heart failure, but what is the *cause*?

1. **High output failure:** occurs when the heart fails to maintain a normal or increased output in the face of grossly increased requirements. It can occur with a normal heart, but will occur earlier if there is cardiac disease. Causes: anaemia, hyperthyroidism, Paget's disease, AV malformation, pregnancy. Features are usually of RVF before LVF.

2. **Low output failure:** occurs when the heart fails to generate adequate output or only does so with increased filling pressures. Causes:
   - *Intrinsic heart muscle disease* — ischaemia, infarction, myocarditis, cardiomyopathy, Chagas disease, beriberi, amyloid.
   - *Chronic excessive afterload* — aortic stenosis, hypertension.
   - *Negatively inotropic drugs* — e.g. antiarrhythmic drugs.
   - *Chronic valvular regurgitation/stenosis.*
   - *Restricted filling* — constrictive pericarditis, tamponade, restrictive cardiomyopathy.
   - *Inadequate heart rate* — beta-blockers, heart block, post-MI.

3. **Fluid overload** involves pushing the myocardium too far over the Starling length–tension relationship (initially, stretching results in increased contractile force, but beyond the apex of the curve, further stretch results in decreased force), resulting in a lower cardiac output. Clinical features are of LVF and do not normally occur unless there is renal impairment leading to fluid retention or gross overhydration.

4. **Left ventricular failure (LVF):** is dominated by pulmonary oedema, resulting in exertional dyspnoea, orthopnoea, paradoxical nocturnal dyspnoea, wheeze, cough, haemoptysis, and fatigue.
   - *Signs:* tachypnoea, tachycardia, basal lung crackles, third heart sound, pulsus alternans, cardiomegaly, peripheral cyanosis, pleural effusion, reduced peak expiratory flow.
   - *CXR signs* — see box.
   - *ECG* will show changes according to the specific cause.
   - *Echocardiography* may differentiate between valvular and pericardial lesions.

5. **Right ventricular failure (RVF):** causes dependent oedema (i.e. in the legs if standing, in the sacrum if supine), abdominal discomfort, nausea, fatigue, and wasting. Usually 2° to chronic lung disease or LVF.
   - *Signs:* increased JVP, hepatomegaly (may be pulsatile), pitting oedema, peripheral cyanosis.

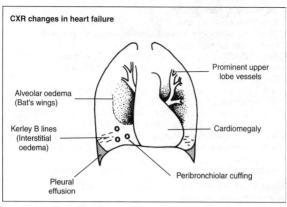

Fig. 4.4

Peripartum cardiac failure

Cardiac failure beginning in pregnancy or up to 6 months postpartum, of up to 6 months' duration, with no other history of heart failure, and with no discernible cause for the failure other than anaemia or hypertension, presumed to be acute.

Aetiology: commonest in multiparous, hypertensive black women. Myocarditis was found in 50% of cases in some series, but the mechanism is unclear. Cultural practices such as eating Na^+ and K^+-rich foods in hot climates during pregnancy may have a role. One theory is that the combination of increased circulatory demands (+/− anaemia), heat (→ peripheral vasodilatation), and high salt load lead to a high output dilated cardiac failure, with accompanying systematic and pulmonary symptoms.

Investigation and management: as for other forms of heart failure. In a few cases, there is permanent cardiac damage. Do not use an ACE inhibitor, so that the mother can continue breastfeeding. A poor prognosis is heralded by any dysrhythmia, a persistently dilated heart, and systemic or pulmonary emboli. In those with myocarditis, if there is no improvement after one week of a diuretic, a course of steroids may be helpful.

Management of heart failure
1. Treat the cause if possible.
2. Treat reversible exacerbating factors (e.g. anaemia, hypoxia).
3. Restrict salt and alcohol intake.
4. Avoid NSAIDs as they cause fluid retention. They may also interact with diuretics and ACE inhibitors to cause renal failure.
5. Drug treatment:
   - Start with a diuretic (usually loop sealing) — monitor U&Es.
   - Once stabilized, begin an ACE inhibitor (see box).
   - If this is inadequate, add a vasodilator such as isosorbide dinitrate 30–160 mg daily in divided doses (not in RVF).
   - Consider low-dose spironolactone (12.5–25 mg od) if available and the patient is not hyperkalaemic *and/or* adding an inotrope such as digoxin.
   - Beta blockers: Introduce cautiously, starting low dose and uptitrating.

Treatment of resistant heart failure: search for other causes and check patient compliance with drug regimes.
- Admit to hospital for bed rest, anti-thromboembolic stockings, heparin 5000 units SC tds, and furosemide IV up to 4 mg/min.
- Increase the ACE inhibitor or venodilator dose to the maximum tolerated; consider metolazone where available. Often adding in a thiazide to a loop diuretic will cause synergistic diuresis.
- In extreme circumstances, consider using IV inotropes for a short time (e.g. dobutamine, starting at 2.5–10 mcg/kg/min, or dopamine starting at 2.5–5 mcg/kg/min; increasing both according to response up to a maximum of 40 mcg/kg/min (dobutamine) or 50 mcg/kg/min (dopamine)), though these should not be used long term.

Sometimes the patient must accept mildly swollen ankles and exercise limitation in order to avoid unacceptable symptoms of low output.

Starting an ACE inhibitor

- Watch for hypotension after the 1st or 2nd doses.
- Check the BP. If <100 mmHg systolic, give the first doses in hospital.
- Ensure the patient is not salt or volume depleted (e.g. due to D&V).
- Check for AS, MS (relative contraindication), and renal artery stenosis.
- Stop or reduce all diuretics and hypotensive drugs a few days before. If there is symptomatic hypotension, give 0.9% sodium chloride infusion (plus atropine if the patient is bradycardic).
- Start with captopril 6.25 mg PO bd (short $T_{1/2}$) building up to 25 mg bd or tds.
- Consider changing to other ACE inhibitors once stabilized (longer acting → better compliance) according to price/availability, or if side-effects occur (cough, D&V).

Contraindications: significant hypotension, angioedema, renal artery/ aortic stenosis, pregnancy, collagen disease, porphyria.

Other precautions:

- Check U&Es and creatinine routinely and stop the ACE inhibitor if there is significantly worsening renal function. However, urea and Cr will often rise when ACE inhibitors or diuretics are first used. This is not necessarily a reason to stop — levels will usually plateau and drop later. Monitor closely; stop if Cr/Urea increase >20% or continue to rise.
- Weigh the patient regularly to monitor the response.
- Monitor WCC and urine protein if there is co-existent connective tissue disease.
- Beware of other interactions: Li^+ (levels increase), digoxin (levels may increase), NSAIDs (urea and K^+ rise), anaesthetics (BP decrease).
- Watch for K^+ derangement (usually decreased) through diuretic action. Mild hypokalaemia is well tolerated without the need for K^+-sparing diuretics as long as: (i) the K^+ is >3.5 mmol/l, (ii) there is no predisposition to dysrhythmias, and (iii) there are no other K^+-losing conditions (e.g. cirrhosis, chronic diarrhoea).

However, do not be put off trying a patient on ACE inhibitors by these cautions. Most patients tolerate ACE inhibitors very well and gain a significant benefit from them.

Shock

Shock is inadequate perfusion of vital organs due to hypotension.

Clinical features: are of tachycardia (unless on beta blockers or in spinal shock), hypotension (although in fit adults there may be ~10% blood loss before any BP change, which is often an initial *rise* in diastolic pressure — i.e. a narrowing of the pulse pressure), pallor, faintness, sweating, and cold peripheries with poor capillary refill.

Causes of shock

1. **Cardiogenic shock**

   Failure of the heart to pump sufficient blood around the circulation. It may occur rapidly or after progressive heart failure. It carries a high mortality and may be due to dysrhythmias, tamponade, pneumothorax, MI, myocarditis, endocarditis, PE, aortic dissection, drugs, hypoxia, sepsis, and acidosis.

   Management: treat the cause if known. Give morphine 10 mg by slow IV injection (half the dose in elderly and frail) and O_2 mask. Monitor ECG, urine output, ABGs, U&Es, CVP. Consider inotropic agents (see previous page) adjusted to keep the systolic BP >80 mmHg. Refer to a specialist if possible.

2. **Anaphylactic shock** — see box.

3. **Endocrine failure** — see Addison's disease (p. 544) and hypothyroidism (p. 540).

4. **Septic shock** — see p. 192.

5. **Hypovolaemic shock**

   Due to for example to trauma, ruptured aneurysm, or ectopic pregnancy.

   Management: prevent further blood loss and aim to restore circulatory volume as quickly as possible until the pulse rate falls and the BP starts to rise. Give whole blood where possible (crossmatched if there is time, otherwise use Rh -ve blood). Whilst waiting for blood to arrive, give warmed crystalloids such as Hartmann's solution or a synthetic colloid.

For the last two causes of shock, the immediate need is rapid IV fluid replacement.

Points on fluid resuscitation

- Use the largest vein and largest cannula possible.
- Add pressure to the fluid bag to speed the infusion.
- If access is difficult it may be necessary to cut down to a vein (e.g. 2 cm above and anterior to the medial malleolus).
- If this fails, intraosseous infusion is possible using specific cannulae below and medial to the tibial tuberosity; especially useful in children.
- Give extra fluid if there are fractures: ribs ~150 ml, tibia ~650 ml, femur ~1500 ml, pelvis ~2000 ml.
- Double these estimates if there are open fractures.
- Remember to splint fractures and apply traction to reduce blood loss.

Anaphylaxis

Anaphylactic shock requires prompt energetic treatment of laryngeal oedema, bronchospasm, and hypotension. It may be caused by exposure to insect venom (bee stings), food (eggs, peanuts), drugs (antibiotics, aspirin; especially if given IV) and other medicinal products (e.g. vaccines, antivenom).

Management

1. Stop infusion if this has caused the anaphylaxis.
2. Secure the airway, give oxygen.
3. Give epinephrine/adrenalin 0.5 mg (0.5 ml of a 1:1000 solution) IM.
4. Repeat every 5 mins until BP and pulse both increase.
5. (Patients on non-cardioselective beta-blockers may not respond to epinephrine in usual doses; they may need salbutamol IV for 48 hrs.)
6. Give an antihistamine (e.g. chlorphenamine 10–20 mg by slow IV injection). Continue this PO for 48 hrs.
7. Continuing deterioration requires additional treatment with IV fluids, and IV aminophylline or nebulized salbutamol. Assisted ventilation and emergency tracheostomy (for laryngeal oedema) may be required.
8. Give hydrocortisone 100–300 mg IV slowly; may need oral steroids tapered for a few days depending on the antigen.
   - If there is doubt about the adequacy of the patient's circulation, it may be necessary to give the epinephrine/adrenalin IV as a dilute solution.
   - Anaphylactic reactions require prior exposure to the antigen. Anaphylactoid reactions appear clinically similar but occur when large quantities of allergen are infused IV (e.g. antivenoms rich in Fc antibody portions). Prior skin testing does not exclude the possibility of a subsequent anaphylactoid reaction since the reaction is dependent on the quantity of antigen injected. Always have epinephrine already drawn up when injecting antivenoms.

Hypertension

Hypertension (HT) is an increasing problem in the tropics, particularly in urban areas, where lifestyles are becoming similar to those in the West. Environmental factors are chiefly involved in this process, since in these same countries HT is virtually unheard of in rural populations, living traditional lifestyles. It is a major risk factor for MI, stroke, renal and heart failure, and peripheral vascular disease. Treatment aims to reduce incidence/progress of complications.

Clinical features: people are usually asymptomatic until irreversible damage has occurred. **Symptoms:** dizziness, fatigue, headache, palpitations. **Signs:** raised BP (although BP may be normal with heart failure); if 2° HT, there may be signs of the 1° disease; end-organ damage (e.g. LV hypertrophy, heart failure, retinopathy, proteinuria, uraemia).

BP should be checked with the correct sized cuff, sitting (erect and supine in the elderly/suspected postural drop) after at least 5, preferably 15 mins, relaxing, and checked twice.

Who to treat?

All patients with hypertension should be advised to lose weight, exercise, reduce Na intake/increase K intake, and address co-risk factors (e.g. smoking).

1. Where the BP is systolic (>180 mmHg) or diastolic (>95 mmHg), treat if these values are confirmed on 3 separate occasions over 1–2 days. If severe or in the presence of associated conditions (e.g. heart failure), treat immediately — see box.
2. Where the initial BP is >140/90 over several weeks:
   - If there are no vascular complications, no end-organ damage, and no diabetes, advise non drug Rx, and reassess in 3 months. If still high, start drug therapy.
   - If there are vascular complications, end-organ damage, or diabetes, start drug therapy.
3. Isolated systolic hypertension (systolic >160 mm Hg, diastolic <90 mm Hg) in persons >60 yrs should be monitored over 3 months and then treated, preferably with a low-dose thiazide diuretic +/− low-dose beta-blocker.
4. Hypertension during pregnancy can be treated with methyldopa; beta-blockers and Ca^{2+} channel blockers can be used during the third trimester.

In diabetics and patients with vascular risk factors, aim should be BP<125/85

Investigations: recheck the BP on at least 3 separate occasions. Search for a cause (particularly in the young). U&E, Cr, glucose, plasma lipids, MSU (twice), renal USS, urinary VMA, ECG, CXR, fundoscopy.

Specific indications/agents

- *Diabetes* — ACEI
- *CHF* — ACEI, beta-blockers
- *IHD* — beta-blockers, Ca channel blockers (not short-acting ones)
- *PVD* — beta-blockers exacerbate

- *Gout* — diuretics exacerbate/trigger
- *Black patients* — ACEI as monotherapy not useful, but work well with diuretics/CCBs. Beta-blockers less effective.
- *Reserpine* — still used; cheap, effective, keep dose <1.25mg/day

Accelerated HT

Rapidly increasing BP with end organ damage. It is heralded by sudden onset heart failure, renal failure, encephalopathy (convulsions/coma), or a diastolic BP >140 mmHg. Untreated, mortality is ~90%; treated, it carries a 5-yr survival of only 60%. See box for Rx.

Management of HT

Aim to reduce the incidence of stroke, heart and renal failure, and MI.
1. **Non-drug therapy**
   - Stop smoking (not itself a risk factor for HT; only for MI/stroke)
   - Reduce sodium, alcohol intake, weight if obese
   - Increase intake of potassium, fresh vegetables, and fruit
   - Increase exercise
2. **Drug therapy:** explain that the patient may need to be on tablets for life, even though had no symptoms, and may even feel worse on the medication. Encourage patient to return to a doctor if there are unacceptable side-effects and not simply to stop taking the medication.

Suggested approach:
- Start with a thiazide diuretic (e.g. bendroflumethiazide 2.5 mg od PO). Use lowest possible dose; check plasma K 4 wks after starting therapy).
- If not controlled, add a beta-blocker (e.g. atenolol 50 mg PO od).
- If still uncontrolled, start either an ACE inhibitor (e.g. captopril 6.25 mg tds) or a Ca^{2+} channel blocker (e.g. modified-release nifedipine 20mg PO bd).
- If the HT is still not resolved (<10% will not respond to one or a combination of these drugs) seek expert help before starting centrally acting α-agonists, peripheral α-antagonists, or hydralazine.

Always try to stop ineffective drugs — this helps patient compliance.

Management of accelerated HT

- Bed rest, use of IV furosemide 40–80 mg, IV glyceryl nitrate 5–10 mcg/min, nifedipine 5 mg.
- Drugs noted above for Rx of HT should be used.
- Patients need close monitoring; may need specialist evaluation/opinion. Dihydralazine should be used with caution.
- Aim is drop in BP over hrs or days, not mins (which will increase the risk of stroke).
- Do not lower BP in acute stroke unless >220/120. If so, lower by 15–20% every 24 hrs.

Rheumatic fever

Rheumatic fever (RF) is an important cause of cardiovascular mortality throughout the developing world. Group A beta-haemolytic streptococcal (*Streptococcus pyogenes*) pharyngitis leads in ~0.3–3% of cases to rheumatic fever, due to an immune cross-reactivity between the bacteria and connective tissue.

It is a disease of the poor, the overcrowded, and the poorly housed, with children being chiefly affected. The disease is often more severe in the developing world than in the West. This severity reflects a failure of health services to prevent recurrences of acute rheumatic fever. If these recurrences can be prevented, many patients who have carditis in their first attack will eventually lose their murmurs and have normal or near normal hearts.

Clinical features
- *Arthritis:* occurs in 80% of cases. Typically an asymmetrical and migratory 'flitting polyarthritis', affecting large joints; the pain is severe while swelling is often modest. Onset is acute and subsides over a week; as one joint improves, a second gets worse. This process may continue for 3–6 weeks. There is a dramatic response to aspirin.
- *Carditis:* occurs in 40–50%. It is the most serious manifestation of acute RF, causing death acutely in <1% of cases. It may affect only the endocardium (valvulitis, often MR +/– AR, 'mild carditis'), or the myocardium and pericardium may also be involved ('severe carditis').
- *Chorea:* occurs in ~10% after a longer incubation period. Sydenham's chorea is emotional lability and involuntary movements (face, limbs, esp. hands). More common in girls; one-third have no cardiac involvement.
- *Erythema marginatum:* <5% cases.
- *Subcutaneous nodules:* now rare.

Diagnosis: is based upon the revised Jones criteria (see box) and requires (i) evidence of recent streptococcal infection *plus* (ii) either two major criteria *or* one major and two minor criteria.

Management:
1. Bed rest for at least 2 weeks, *and* until the child feels better.
2. Anti-inflammatory drugs to suppress the inflammatory process:
   - Aspirin 20–25 mg/kg PO qds. Continue for 3–6 weeks if heart is not involved; 3 months in mild carditis; 4–6 months in severe carditis.
   - In severe carditis, give prednisolone 0.5 mg/kg qds for 2 weeks.
3. Treat as for heart failure from other causes.
4. Sodium valproate 7.5–10 mg/kg PO bd for 3 months for chorea (alternative haloperidol 0.05 mg/kg od).

Secondary prophylaxis is essential for all patients

Give benzathine benzylpenicillin 900 mg (children <30 kg, 450 mg) IM every 4 weeks for:

- >5 yrs after last episode and at least until age 21 (sometimes for life) for patients with carditis and residual heart (valvular) disease.
- >5 yrs or until age 21, whichever is the longer, for patients with carditis but no residual heart disease.
- 5 yrs or until age 21 yrs, whichever is the longer, for patients who did not have carditis.

(Alternative for penicillin-allergic patients is erythromycin 250 mg bd PO.)

Revised Jones criteria

A. Evidence of recent group A streptococcal infection
- Positive throat culture or rapid streptococcal antigen test
- Elevated or rising streptococcal antibody titre

B. Major manifestations
- Carditis
- Polyarthritis
- Chorea
- Erythema marginatum
- Subcutaneous nodules

C. Minor manifestations

Clinical findings
- Arthralgia
- Fever

Laboratory findings
- Elevated acute-phase reactants (ESR or C-reactive protein)
- Prolonged PR interval

Any effort that will make the IM injection less painful, and therefore less frightening for the child, will make 2° prophylaxis more successful. Painful monthly IM injections for a young child can be a very frightening prospect that could make the child unwilling to take this life-saving treatment.

Prevention of rheumatic fever: requires improvements in housing conditions, as well as better methods of 1° prevention. These can include early detection of streptococcal sore throats and their selective treatment or treatment of all children with pharyngitis with a single IM dose of benzathine penicillin.

Infective endocarditis

Fever + regurgitant murmur = endocarditis until proven otherwise.
50% of endocarditis in the UK is on normal valves. When it is caused by highly pathogenic bacteria like staphylococci, pneumococci, and beta-haemolytic streptococci, endocarditis follows an acute course, often with serious emboli, heart failure, and death. The course is subacute if *Streptococcus viridans* affect valves previously damaged by RF or other causes. Endocarditis often occurs on prosthetic valves (~2%), in which case the involved valves usually need replacing.

Pathogenesis: any bacteraemia, especially following dental procedures, GU manipulation, or surgery may expose the valves to colonization. In the UK, *Strep. viridans, Enterococcus faecalis,* and *S. aureus* are common. Rarely fungi, *Coxiella,* or *Chlamydia* species infect valves; other rare non-infective causes include SLE and malignancy. Right-sided disease is more common in IV drug users, leading to pulmonary abscesses.

Clinical features include evidence of:
- *Infection:* fever, malaise, night sweats, finger clubbing, splenomegaly, anaemia.
- *Heart murmurs:* especially regurgitation of aortic or mitral valves; sometimes murmurs change from day to day. There may be intermittent fever; occasionally regurgitation improves when vegetations get smaller, but usually the murmurs deteriorate until treatment is effective.
- *Embolic events:* vegetations on valves may cause embolic events (e.g. strokes or acute limb ischaemia). Occasionally, embolic abscesses or mycotic aneurysms form.
- *Vasculitis:* microscopic haematuria, splinter haemorrhages, Osler's nodes (painful lesions on finger pulps), Janeway lesions (painful red patches on the palms), Roth's spots, and renal failure.

Diagnosis: take 3 blood cultures from different sites at different times when febrile. Take blood cultures before starting antibiotics — a delay of a few hours is seldom critical. At least one culture will be positive in 99% of cases. ESR, FBC, U&E, Cr, echocardiography may show the vegetations on valves. Perform urinalysis for haematuria.

Management:
1. For fully sensitive streptococcal infection, give benzylpenicillin 1.2 g IV q4h (or vancomycin) *plus* synergistic doses of gentamicin 60–80 mg IV bd for 2 weeks, then if there is a good clinical response switch to amoxicillin 1g PO tds for 2 weeks. Less sensitive organisms require 4 weeks of penicillin *plus* gentamicin.
2. For *S. aureus* infections, give flucloxacillin 2 g IV q4–6h and gentamicin as above for 2 weeks, then IV flucloxacillin for 2 weeks.
3. For *S. epidermidis* infections, use vancomycin and rifampicin for at least 4 weeks.
4. If 'blind' empirical therapy is required, give benzylpenicillin and gentamicin and add in flucloxacillin if the endocarditis is acute in onset. Wait for blood culture results. This recommendation is based on streptococcal infections being the most common cause of endocarditis. Alter these recommendations according to the local circumstances.

Prognosis: 30% mortality in the UK from staphylococcal endocarditis, 14% with anaerobic infection, and 6% with sensitive streptococci.

Prevention:

Prophylaxis required
- Previous history of endocarditis
- Prosthetic valves
- Congenital heart disease except secundum ASDs
- All acquired valvular heart disease
- Hypertrophic cardiomyopathy, mitral valve prolapse with regurgitation
- Surgically corrected shunts/conduits

Prophylaxis not required
- Previous CABG
- Pacemakers/ICD
- Mitral valve disease without regurgitation
- Previous RhHD without valve defects
- 'Innocent' murmurs

Procedures requiring prophylaxis
- Any dental procedure that causes bleeding from gingiva, mucosa, or bone
- Tonsillectomy
- Rigid bronchoscopy
- Incision of abscess
- Vaginal delivery with chorioaminonitis
- 'Dirty' surgery/procedure

Procedures not requiring prophylaxis
- Natural shedding of teeth
- Caesarian section
- Vaginal delivery without infection
- 'Clean' procedures

Antibiotics
- Amoxicillin 3 g PO 1 hr before procedure under local anesthetic.
- If allergic to penicillin or >1 course of penicillin in last month, give clindamycin 600 mg PO 1 hr before procedure.
- For procedures under general anaesthetic, give amoxicillin 3 g PO 4 hrs before the procedure and again as soon as possible after the procedure.
- For procedures under general anaesthetic in patients at high risk (antibiotics in the previous month, prosthetic valve, or allergic to penicillin), refer all procedures to hospital. Amoxicillin plus gentamicin (or vancomycin in penicillin-allergic patients) can be used for such patients.

Cardiomyopathies

Diseases of heart muscle are classified as follows:

1. Congested (dilated) cardiomyopathy

Common throughout the tropics, there is often no identifiable cause, although contributing factors may include heart failure, alcohol, thiamine deficiency, or previous myocarditis.

Cardiomyopathy is seen in association with HIV infection, either caused by HIV itself or by toxoplasma, other viral infections, anti-retroviral drugs (e.g zidovudine), and nutritional deficiencies.

Clinical features: are those of heart failure, although there is a poor response to treatment. The apex beat is diffused and displaced and there is often functional valvular incompetence giving rise to murmurs. There may be AF (especially in alcoholics) and associated embolic events. Typically, the patient is a man of 40–50 years. HIV cardiomyopathy is seen in young individuals, often in their twenties or thirties.

Diagnosis and management: echocardiography shows a dilated hypokinetic heart. However, in an HIV-associated cardiomyopathy, the left ventricle may be of normal size but severely hypokinetic. The cause may be difficult to ascertain but include hypertension, mitral and tricuspid incompetence in rheumatic heart failure, and endomyocardial fibrosis. The distinction is academic however, since treatment is for the underlying heart failure. Mortality is high ~40% by two years.

2. Restrictive cardiomyopathy

Due to endomyocardial stiffening, it clinically resembles constrictive pericarditis. It is often due to endomyocardial fibrosis in which hypereosinophilia (possibly triggered by helminthic infection, especially filariasis) damages the myocardium. This in turn causes mural thrombus formation, producing a fibrotic mass. It may rarely be caused by amyloid or carcinoid.

Clinical features: may begin with a febrile illness, facial oedema, and dyspnoea that may be progressive and fatal within a few months. However, most patients are seen in the chronic stage, presenting with features of heart failure. The clinical features may be those of predominantly LV disease or RV disease, or a combination similar to other causes of congestive heart failure. LV disease consists of MR (never MS or AR — cf. RF) with an S_3, and progressive pulmonary hypertension. RV disease (usually TR) results in gross ascites and markedly elevated JVP but often minimal peripheral oedema. There may be exophthalmos, central cyanosis, delayed puberty, markedly reduced pulse pressure, pericardial effusion, and AF. Murmurs may be heard (cf. pericardial disease). Pericardial effusion is a common manifestation of endomyocardial fibrosis.

Diagnosis: CXR findings vary from a massive cardiac shadow (aneurysmal of right atrium, vaguely resembling the shape of Africa, or pericardial effusion) to an almost normal film. Echocardiography and Doppler studies show fibrosis in the inflow tracts with involvement of left or right or both ventricles and regurgitation of mitral and tricuspid valves. Pericardial effusion and thrombi in the atria or ventricles are also seen.

Management: in the acute stage, treatment is purely supportive. If there is hyper-eosinophilia, look for and treat the cause. In established disease, resist the temptation to drain the ascites, since it may cause the patient to lose a lot of protein. Digoxin may control the ventricular rate if there is AF.

3. Hypertrophic (obstructive) cardiomyopathy (HOCM)

There is asymmetrical hypertrophy of ventricular muscle (50% are inherited as autosomal dominant — screen other family members).

Clinical features: are of dyspnoea, angina, syncope, palpitations. There may be a double impulse at the apex, jerky pulse, S_3/S_4, late systolic murmur. The ECG may show LBBB or RBBB; the echocardiography is sometimes diagnostic.

Management: give beta-blockers for angina and treat the dysrhythmia. Uncontrolled AF should prompt lifelong anti-coagulation.

4. Acute myocarditis

Inflammation of the myocardium may present like an MI. Causes are: viral (coxsackie virus), diphtheria, RF, drugs, and other infections. There is angina, dyspnoea, arrhythmia, tachycardia, and heart failure. Exclude MI and pericardial effusion.

Management: is supportive or for heart failure if it ensues.

5. Left atrial myxoma

A rare benign primary tumour, developing from the inter-atrial septum presenting with left atrial obstruction (as in mitral stenosis), systemic emboli, AF, fever, weight loss, and raised ESR. There may be a family history. Rarely, one may hear a tumour 'plop' on auscultation. Atrial myxoma is twice as common in females as in males. Differentiate from mitral stenosis by the occurrence of emboli in the absence of AF or on echocardiography (investigation of choice). Treatment is by surgical excision. Atrial myxoma may recur.

Pericardial disease

Pericarditis

In the tropics, this is commonly due to TB or pyogenic infection.

- **Tuberculosis pericarditis** is especially important in the areas of high HIV prevalence. Spread is probably from the adjacent lymph nodes and pleura. The effusion may be massive in HIV; echocardiogram may show strands of fibrin floating in the effusion.
- **Acute pyogenic pericarditis** results from generalized bacteraemia derived from, or associated with, a 1° focus elsewhere.
- **Other causes:** any infection (especially coxsackie virus), malignancy (such as KS in HIV +ve individuals), uraemia, MI, Dressler's syndrome, trauma, radiotherapy, connective tissue diseases, and hypothyroidism.

Clinical features

Pericarditis: a sharp constant sternal pain, which may radiate to the left shoulder, down the left arm, or to the abdomen. It is relieved by sitting forward, and worse by lying on the left, coughing, inspiring, or swallowing. Auscultation may reveal a scratchy superficial pericardial rub, loudest at the left sternal edge. In a large effusion the rub is generally lost, and heart sounds are heard faintly.

Pericardial effusion: depends on the speed at which it is formed. If formed quickly, the pericardium cannot stretch and so pressure rises and the heart is compressed to produce cardiac tamponade. There is a fall of cardiac output (reduced BP), elevated JVP, Kussmaul's sign (JVP rises with inspiration), tachycardia, impalpable apex, pulsus paradoxus, peripheral shut down, and quiet heart sounds. In more chronic effusions, signs of heart failure predominate with severe ascites and hepatomegaly. Percussion reveals an increased area of cardiac dullness, and the apex beat is impalpable or felt within the area of dullness. Impending tamponade or restriction is first indicated by elevated JVP; however, the JVP may be so high that the patient must be examined sitting or standing upright. Patients with pyogenic pericarditis are extremely unwell with signs of severe sepsis.

Diagnosis: ECG classically shows upwardly concave (saddle shaped) ST segments in all leads except lead AVR, with no reciprocal changes. In pericardial effusions, CXR shows a large globular heart (and may show pleural effusions). ECG has low voltages and changing QRS complexes (electrical alternans = a changing axis beat to beat). Echocardiography is diagnostic with an echo-free zone showing the heart surrounded by effusion. In exudative effusions, fibrinous stands are clearly seen within the fluid. Differentiate from an MI and PE.

Constrictive pericarditis

Encasement of the heart in a non-expansive pericardium, usually following TB infection. Features are as for chronic effusion, however the heart is small on CXR and may show calcification, especially on the lateral CXR. The onset is usually insidious, with ascites, oedema, hepatomegaly, proteinuria being found. The patient may or may not be breathless. Often the JVP is so far elevated that it is missed on routine inspection of the neck.

Management

1. *Pericarditis:* find and treat the cause.
   - Give analgesia and consider systemic steroids for unresolving cases (prednisolone up to 2 mg/kg od for 11 weeks).
   - For TB pericarditis, commence anti-TB treatment plus steroids for the first 6–8 weeks and consider an HIV test.
2. *Pericardial effusion:* find and treat the cause (e.g. antibiotics for bacterial infections; anti-TB drugs and steroids for TB).

   Tamponade requires urgent drainage. Aspirate with a 50 ml syringe, fitted with a long needle and two-way tap, inserting upwards and to the left of the xiphisternum. Patient should be propped up 45°. Watch the ECG monitor to know when the myocardium is touched. Recurrent pericardial effusion, especially of pyogenic origin, requires surgery draining through a pericardial window or pericardiotomy.
3. *Constrictive pericarditis:* requires surgical excision of the pericardium.

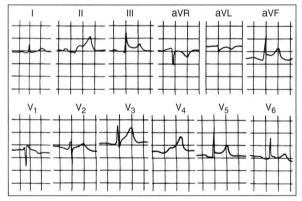

Fig. 4.5 ECG changes in pericarditis

Chest medicine

Section editor   **Benjamin G. Marshall**

Cough

A cough in isolation is common. It is often due to mild viral infection and needs only symptomatic relief or more often no therapy. In contrast, a productive cough or one associated with dyspnoea may be more ominous and requires further investigation. A careful search for cardiac or pulmonary causes should be started.

A cough without associated signs or symptoms may be due to diphtheria or tuberculosis (TB). Both require specific management.

- A cough by itself does not warrant a CXR.
- TB, pertussis, smoking, lung cancer, and a foreign body can each cause a chronic cough.
- A change in cough habit is significant, particularly in a smoker.

Pulmonary causes of cough

- Smoking
- Lung cancer
- Bacterial pneumonia
- Drugs (e.g. ACE inhibitors)
- Asthma
- TB
- Reflux
- COPD
- Bronchitis
- Post-nasal drip (sinusitis/ rhinitis)

Other infective causes include: Typhoid, *P. falciparum* malaria (due to respiratory distress syndrome), measles, bronchiectasis (post-measles or pertussis), amoebic liver abscess, pulmonary hydatid disease, AIDS, rickettsial infections, paragonimiasis, tropical pulmonary eosinophilia, Loeffler's syndrome, *Yersinia pestis*, *Neisseria meningitidis*.

Nocturnal coughing is characteristic of asthma.

Haemoptysis

- Consider TB in anyone with a chronic cough and haemoptysis.
- Be careful to distinguish haemoptysis from haematemesis or blood from the gums, throat, or nose.

Causes

- **Acute:** pneumonia, bronchitis, pulmonary embolism.
- **Chronic:** TB, lung cancer, bronchiectasis (including cystic fibrosis).

Other causes include

- **Lung infection:** parasitic disease (e.g. paragonimiasis), bronchitis, lung abscess, fungal disease (e.g. aspergillosis, paracoccidioidomycosis).
- **Trauma:** contusion, foreign body, post-intubation.
- **Vascular disease:** vasculitis.
- **Parenchymal disease:** diffuse parenchymal diseases, haemosiderosis.
- **Cardiovascular disease:** pulmonary oedema, mitral stenosis, aortic aneurysm.
- **Bleeding diatheses:** sepsis, DIC, viper bites, haemorrhagic fevers.

Whooping cough

The Gram −ve bacteria *Bordetella pertussis* causes whooping cough. It commonly affects infants aged 2–4 yrs but can cause illness and death at any age. Vaccination has markedly reduced incidence in the West, but it is still a major problem in some developing countries.

Clinical features: the incubation period is 6–20 days. The first clinical phase is indistinguishable from the common cold, and lasts 1–2 weeks. Fever is not usually prominent.

Paroxysms of severe coughing with a 'whoop' are the classical feature of the disease. The 'whoop' is caused by forced inspiration against a closed glottis and can result in cyanosis and hypoxic unconsciousness. Infants <6 mths do not whoop but become apnoeic. The child commonly drools and vomits after coughing, and may become exhausted. Wheezing does not occur. After 1–3 weeks of whooping, a more tolerable chronic cough may persist for several weeks; adults and older children may have a chronic cough throughout.

Many cases are uncomplicated and self-limiting; however, illness can persist for weeks to months and result in bronchiectasis and malnutrition. Prolonged coughing may produce petechiae, conjunctival haemorrhages, and rectal prolapse. Death is usually due to severe infection, 2° pneumonia, or encephalopathy — reduced consciousness that is *not* due to hypoxia, seizures, or brain damage.

Diagnosis: is normally made clinically. The WCC shows a lymphocytosis. Culture is difficult — a per-nasal swab is taken.

Management: erythromycin is recommended, but its effect in modifying whooping cough is weak. Nebulized beta-agonists and steroids are sometimes used, but generally have little effect because wheezing is not a prominent feature.

Prevention: routine immunization.

Diphtheria

The Gram +ve *Corynebacterium diphtheriae* causes infection of the naso-pharynx and occasionally skin and mucous membranes. Its endotoxin has potentially fatal effects on the heart, kidney, and peripheral nerves. Death occurs in ~50% without treatment, and in 5–10% despite treatment. Children <5 yrs and adults >40 yrs have a worse prognosis. Although its incidence is falling worldwide, it remains a significant problem in some developing countries.

Transmission: is by droplets or secretions from infected humans (the only reservoir). Incubation is 2–5 days. Patients are infectious for ~1 mth; however, some become carriers.

Clinical features
The incubation period is ~2–5 days (7 days for cutaneous diphtheria). The patient may present with general non-specific symptoms, including: fever and chills, malaise, sore throat, hoarseness and dysphagia, cervical oedema and cervical lymphadenopathy, nasal discharge, cough, stridor, wheezing, nausea and vomiting, headache.
Local: mucosae are initially red and oedematous; this progresses to necrosis of epithelium. An inflammatory grey-white pseudo-membrane forms at the site of infection (commonly the tonsils and oropharynx); it is adherent. There is fever, malaise, sore throat (may cause dysphagia), cervical lymphadenopathy, and bad breath. The neck is often swollen with oedema and enlarged lymph nodes. Palatal paralysis by toxin produces a 'nasal' quality to the speech.
Tracheo-laryngeal: hoarseness, dry cough and, rarely, airways obstruction.
Cutaneous: is rare. There are pustules and ulcers with a grey membrane.
Systemic effects of toxin: myocarditis (10%), heart block (often >1wk after acute infection; can cause death up to 8 wks after), murmurs, heart failure. Neuronal demyelination causes peripheral neuritis (often ~6 wks after initial illness), paralysis (soft palate, ocular, and intercostals muscles). There may be renal failure (tubular necrosis) and pneumonia.
Malignant diphtheria: indicates rapid spread of membranes, neck oedema and adenitis, stridor, and shock.

Diagnosis: treat on suspicion — do not wait for confirmation. Arrange for throat swabs of membrane, ECG (look for ectopics, ST and T wave changes, RBBB, CHB), U&Es, FBC.

Treatment: give antitoxin as soon as possible. Give 10,000–30,000 units IM for mild-moderate disease, and 40,000–100,000 for severe disease. For doses >40,000, give a portion of the dose IM and then the bulk of it IV 0.5–2 hrs later. Antitoxin is made from horse serum, so **beware anaphylaxis** which is rare but potentially fatal. Have adrenaline drawn up. Tracheostomy may save life; do not delay if there are signs of respiratory distress. Give high-dose antibiotics IV (penicillin, erythromycin, cephalosporin, tetracycline are all effective).

Prevention: routine childhood vaccination prevents disease. Recovering patients should also receive vaccine as a booster dose, as well as close contacts. Immunity can be assessed by the Shick test.

Causes of sore throat

- *Streptococcus pyogenes* (rheumatic heart disease and glomerulonephritis)
- Mild viral infections
- *Corynebacterium diphtheriae*
- Epstein–Barr virus
- *Neisseria gonorrhoeae*
- 2° syphilis
- Herpes simplex virus — especially in AIDS patients
- Lassa virus
- *Fusobacterium necrophorum*

Dyspnoea/breathlessness

A subjective sensation of difficulty with breathing.

Causes
- **Cardiac:** left heart failure (e.g. due to ischaemic heart disease, anaemia, myocardial infarction, cardiomyopathy, myocarditis, pericarditis). Normally occurs on exertion, associated with orthopnoea and paroxysmal nocturnal dyspnoea. A dry cough may be present.
- **Pulmonary diseases:** asthma, COPD, effusions, pneumothorax, pulmonary embolism (PE), foreign body, parenchymal disease, pulmonary hypertension.
- **Diseases of the chest:** wall and muscles, spine, diaphragm, or pleura.
- **Miscellaneous:** thyrotoxicosis, acidosis, gross ascites, hyperventilation syndrome.

Of value in finding a cause for the breathlessness is determining the rate of onset. Dyspnoea has an acute onset in PE, pneumothorax, pulmonary oedema, pneumonia, asthma, and LVF. Dyspnoea with a more chronic or insidious onset may be due to pleural effusions, lung cancer or metastases, and subacute pulmonary infiltrations. COPD, diffuse fibrosing diseases, and anaemia may come on over months. Try to determine any initiating and resolving factors.

Both asthma and LVF tend to cause intermittent dyspnoea.

Sudden onset or exacerbation of dyspnoea
Immediately sit the patient up and give O_2. In COPD give O_2, but monitor ABGs for signs of CO_2 retention.

Causes
- Pulmonary oedema
- PE
- Pneumonia
- Cardiac tamponade
- Pneumothorax
- ARDS
- Asthma

- Exacerbation of COPD
- Acute toxin inhalation
- Pulmonary haemorrhage
- Allergic airways disease
- Pulmonary effusion
- Acute large airway obstruction (e.g. foreign body)

Take a Hx (looking for pre-existing disease; exposure; travel; operations; chest pain) and investigate to exclude particular conditions.

Treat pulmonary oedema, asthma, and tension pneumothorax before continuing to do CXR or blood gas analysis if these are indicated.

Wheezing/stridor

Stridor is the harsh inspiratory sound that arises from obstruction in the larynx or major airways. Wheezes are sounds that may occur during inspiration and/or expiration. They can be heard externally and are of polyphonic nature in patients with asthma, obstructive bronchitis, and cardio-vascular dyspnoea. Forced expiration may reveal wheezes when tidal breathing is silent.

A foreign body or tumour mass in a major airway produces a wheeze with a single pitch (monophonic). This wheeze cannot be altered by coughing to shift mucus.

Pneumothorax

Rupture of an alveolar bulla (sp) or traumatic chest injury may produce a pneumothorax — air entering the pleural space. Part of the lung subsequently collapses, reducing the vital lung capacity and ventilation of the affected lung. Where there is pre-existing pulmonary disease, this additional insult may be sufficient to cause respiratory failure. In many cases, however, there is little functional impairment.

- **1° pneumothorax:** occurs spontaneously in previously healthy individuals, often tall, young men. It is commonly small with little functional deficit. There is ~20% risk of recurrence (ipsilateral) after a first episode, which increases to 65% after a second pneumothorax.
- **2° pneumothorax:** is a consequence of pre-existing lung disease, often COPD, necrotizing infections such as *S.aureus*, TB, PCP, or anaerobic bacteria; less often, asthma or malignancy.
- **Traumatic pneumothorax:** common complication of road traffic injuries and assault.
- **Iatrogenic pneumothorax:** common complication of percutaneous lung biopsy or CVP line insertion. Also occurs during mechanical ventilation and after transbronchial lung biopsy.

Clinical features: a small pneumothorax may be asymptomatic. Otherwise, common features include pleuritic chest pain of sudden onset; dyspnoea (partly due to ventilatory deficit but also due to the pain of breathing → small breaths; in 2° disease, it may be an acute exacerbation on top of pre-existing respiratory distress); reduced breath sounds; percussive resonance; reduced chest movements.

A tension pneumothorax will present with trachea deviated away from the side of pneumothorax and marked respiratory distress.

Management

- A 1° pneumothorax, if small, does not require aspiration — watch and wait. A large pneumothorax should be aspirated through the second intercostal space in the midclavicular line with a cannula and 50 ml syringe. If >2 litres of air is aspirated, it is likely that there is a continuing air leak. Where there are significant symptoms or simple aspiration fails, a chest drain can be inserted with underwater seal.
- For a pneumothorax complicating pre-existent lung disease, attempt simple aspiration even for a small pneumothorax. Symptomatic pneumothoraces require insertion of chest drain.
- A pleurodesis may be required once the lung is fully inflated again — see box. Surgery may be indicated for patients with air leakage that continues for >1–2 weeks.

Tension pneumothorax

Loose tissue at the site of a penetrating chest injury may act as a flap, allowing air to enter during inspiration but preventing it leaving during expiration. As air accumulates in the pleural space, mediastinal shift across into the opposite hemithorax results in lung compression and respiratory compromise. Unless relieved quickly, cardiorespiratory arrest will occur. If suspected, insert a wide bore needle into the affected side (2nd intercostal space, midclavicular line; opposite side to direction of tracheal deviation) before doing anything else. There should be rapid relief of the respiratory distress. Obtain a CXR both before and after going on to insert a chest drain.

Pleurodesis

Give the patient 10mg morphine IM. This will take effect as you instil 20 ml of 1% lidocaine into the chest drain and clamp it off. Ask the patient to roll from side to side. After 20 mins, instil 0.5–1 g of tetracycline dissolved in 30–50 ml of normal saline and leave clamped off for 2–3 hrs, again with the patient rolling intermittently to spread the solution around the pleura. This can be very painful; so don't hesitate to provide strong analgesia quickly. After 3 hrs max, unclamp and allow fluid to drain through the underwater seal. Once no longer bubbling, remove the drain after 12 hrs and recheck CXR to see whether the lung has remained inflated.

Pleural effusion

The accumulation of fluid in the pleural space. The fluid may be a transudate, exudate (protein content >35 g/l), blood, pus, or lymphatic fluid (chyle).

- **Transudates** are serous fluids, low in protein, that form when the capillary hydrostatic pressure forcing fluid out of the capillaries is not balanced by the colloid osmotic force drawing the fluid back in (Starling's equation). Transudates may also occur if fluid passes across the diaphragm in patients with ascites.
- **Exudates** are serous fluids that flow into the pleural space because of leaking capillaries — their protein content is the same or increased by comparison with the plasma level.
- **Chylothorax** results from leakage of lymphatic fluid from the thoracic duct.

Clinical features: pleuritic chest pain (worse if 'dry pleurisy', decreases as fluid accumulates); dyspnoea (often only apparent if patient has low reserve or as the fluid accumulates); decreased chest movement on affected side; stony dull percussion-decreased breath sounds on auscultation (although there may be signs of consolidation at the top of the effusion).

Diagnosis: is confirmed by CXR and/or ultrasound. Aspiration of 50–100 mls of pleural fluid across the thoracic wall (thoracocentesis) may indicate the underlying cause — see box. Best site: 10 cm lateral of the spine and one intercostal space below the top level of the effusion as determined by percussion. If this fails to draw fluid, the effusion may be loculated or the aspiration too high — ultrasound may help. Note macroscopic appearance of the fluid and stain for organisms and cells; culture. If neoplasm or TB is suspected a pleural biopsy (open or closed) is often useful.

Management: treatment of the underlying condition (e.g. heart failure, RA) will often resolve the effusion. Aspiration of 1–2 litres provides at least temporary relief from dyspnoea. With recurrent effusion, an intercostal drain may be useful. In malignant disease, the effusions will continue to recur unless prevented with pleurodesis — see above and box. *N.B. no more than 2 litres should be drained in 24 hrs, as this increases the risk of reactive pulmonary oedema.*

Empyema

An infected pleural effusion that is normally 2° to bacterial pneumonia, pulmonary TB, or lung abscess. Empyema should be suspected if a patient with pneumonia has persisting fever after adequate antibiotic therapy. Ultrasound may guide aspiration with a wide-bore needle for both drainage and culture/microscopy of pus. Treat with antibiotics — high-dose ampicillin plus metronidazole 400 mg PO or per rectum q6h until antibiotic sensitivities are known. If antibiotic treatment is unsuccessful, fibrin deposition leading to fibrosis of the interpleural space may require thoracotomy and surgical removal of pus.

Rarely a TB empyema present as pulmonary TB plus pleuritic pain and dyspnoea, but most pleural TB characteristically presents in the absence of active pulmonary lesions.

Causes of pleural effusion

Transudate:
- Cardiac failure
- Peritoneal dialysis
- Hepatic cirrhosis
- Myxoedema
- Nephrotic syndrome
- Hepatic/renal failure

Exudate:
- Infections (e.g. pneumonia, TB)
- Lymphomas
- Collagen vascular diseases
- Pancreatitis
- Subphrenic abscess, infection
- Metastatic CA
- Drug reactions
- PE
- Mesothelioma

Chylothorax:
- Trauma
- Metastatic CA
- Lymphatic filariasis
- Lymphomas

Haemothorax:
- Trauma
- Rarely, spontaneous PTX
- Tumour (e.g. mesothelioma or metastatic lung cancer)

Diagnostic features of pleural effusions

Neutrophils = Pyogenic infection
Lymphocytes = TB, lymphoma, malignancy
Malignant cells = Malignancy
>30 g/l protein = Exudate
<4 mmol glucose = RA, infection, malignancy
High amylase = pancreatitis

Asthma

Asthma is a chronic inflammatory disorder of the airways, with reversible airflow obstruction. It is caused by a combination of genetic susceptibility and a triggering factor:

• Allergens (e.g. food, dust, house dust mite in an atopic individual)
• Infections (particularly viral in children e.g. RSV, or aspergillus)
• Environmental or occupational pollutants, particularly cigarette smoke

Each of these stimuli will also trigger acute exacerbations of asthma. Severe asthmatic attacks can be provoked by β-blockers (including eye drops) and NSAIDS.

Pathology: a triggering factor elicits chronic mucosal inflammation. This has two consequences that result in asthmatic attacks:

1. It makes the bronchi more prone to constrict in response to irritants such as cold dry air, pollen, fumes, paints — termed bronchial hyper-responsiveness.
2. The inflammation produces mucosal oedema and intraluminal mucus that block or reduces the calibre of the airway during this bronchoconstriction.

Current treatment for asthma therefore aims primarily to control the inflammation.

Clinical features: polyphonic wheeze on both inspiration and expiration (often only present during exertion or forced expiration); chest tightness; cough (often producing mucoid sputum); dyspnoea; difficulty breathing in.

Asthma has diurnal variation — it is worse in the early hours of the morning. If the asthma is severe, the patient may wake up between 3.00 a.m. and 5.00 a.m. If less severe, sleep is uninterrupted but symptoms are worse on waking — morning cough. The patient gradually gets better through the day. Into this daily rhythm are interspersed episodic attacks, the stimulus for which may not be recognized. These attacks can be acute and over in mins to hrs, or drawn out, initiating a deterioration in symptoms that lasts days.

Diagnosis: from characteristic clinical features and >15% change in peak expiratory flow (PEF) either on exercise or stimulus challenge or, if PEF normally <80% of predicted value, after therapy with β2-agonists or steroids. Serial PEF measurements are also extremely valuable in following the course of the condition and its response to therapy.

Management: involves identification of and subsequent avoidance of allergens and triggers, prophylaxis, and relief of symptoms during an acute attack. Most attacks will respond to adequate doses of β2-agonists, steroids, and O_2.

Aims of treatment
• Freedom from symptoms, particularly nocturnal awakening
• Lung function within the normal range, varying by <20% during 24 hrs
• Normal quality of life

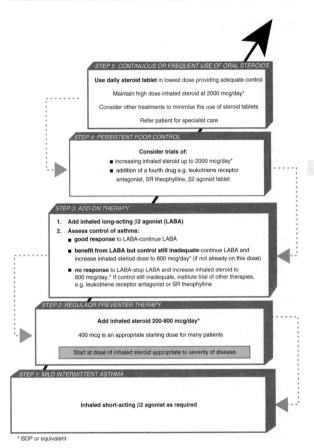

Fig. 5.1 Summary of stepwise management in adults. Reproduced with kind permission from the British Thoracic Society, BMJ Group.

Acute severe asthma[1]

Find out what the normal PEF is, what the current medication is, and when the last severe attack was.

Features of severe asthma
- Unable to finish sentences in one breath
- PEF <50% normal
- Pulse >110 beats/min
- RR>25 breaths/min

Life-threatening features
- Silent chest or cyanosis
- PEFR <33% normal
- Exhaustion, confusion, or decreased consciousness,
- Bradycardia or hypotension
- Arterial blood gases: PaO_2 <8kPa, $PaCO_2$ normal or increased, low pH

Rule out respiratory obstruction from — inhaled foreign body, epiglottitis, mediastinal/neck lumps.

Immediate management
1. Sit the patient up and give 100% O_2
2. Give salbutamol 5mg by O_2-driven nebulizer
3. Give hydrocortisone 200 mg IV
4. Do ABGs, CXR, PEF (may be too breathless), pulse oximetry

If there is no improvement or there are severe signs:
1. Contact an anaesthetist concerning possible emergency intubation
2. Add ipratropium 0.5 mg to the nebulized salbutamol
3. Give aminophylline 250 mg by IV infusion over 20 mins or salbutamol 250 mcg IV over 10 mins. **Do not give** aminophylline (unless plasma concentration known to guide dosing) to patients already taking theophyllines
4. Give prednisolone 30–60 mg PO

Subsequent management
If patient is improving, continue:
1. 100% O_2
2. Prednisolone 30–60 mg PO od or hydrocortisone 200 mg IV q6h
3. Salbutamol 5 mg by O_2-driven nebulizer q4h

If patient is not improving:
1. Continue 100% O_2 and steroids
2. Give nebulized salbutamol more frequently, up to every 15–30 mins
3. Repeat ipratropium q6h
4. If still no improvement, give aminophylline 750–1500 mg IV over 24 hrs = 500 mcg/kg/hr (monitor blood concentrations if continued over 24 hrs). Salbutamol infusion can be given as an alternative.

Monitoring treatment
1. PEF 15–30 mins after starting treatment, then at least q6h
2. Maintain SaO_2 >92% by oximetry
3. Repeat ABG within 2 hrs of starting treatment if initially abnormal

---

1 British Thoracic Society Guidelines (1997), *Thorax*, **52** (Suppl. 1), S12.

On discharge from hospital, a patient should have:

1. Been on discharge medication for 24 hrs and have had inhaler technique checked and recorded.
2. PEF >75% of predicted or best and PEF diurnal variability <25%, unless discharge is agreed with a respiratory physician.
3. Treatment with oral and inhaled steroids in addition to bronchodilators.
4. Their own PEF meter and written self-management plan.
5. Follow-up arranged within 1 week.

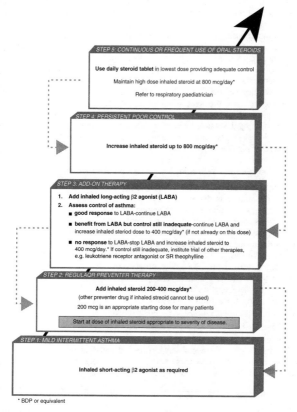

STEP 5: CONTINUOUS OR FREQUENT USE OF ORAL STEROIDS

Use daily steroid tablet in lowest dose providing adequate control

Maintain high dose inhaled steroid at 800 mcg/day*

Refer to respiratory paediatrician

STEP 4: PERSISTENT POOR CONTROL

Increase inhaled steroid up to 800 mcg/day*

STEP 3: ADD-ON THERAPY

1. **Add inhaled long-acting β2 agonist (LABA)**
2. **Assess control of asthma:**
   - **good response** to LABA-continue LABA
   - **benefit from LABA but control still inadequate**-continue LABA and increase inhaled steroid dose to 400 mcg/day* (if not already on this dose)
   - **no response** to LABA-stop LABA and increase inhaled steroid to 400 mcg/day.* If control still inadequate, institute trial of other therapies, e.g. leukotriene receptor antagonist or SR theophylline

STEP 2: REGULAOR PREVENTER THERAPY

Add inhaled steroid 200-400 mcg/day*
(other preventer drug if inhaled streoid cannot be used)
200 mcg is an appropriate starting dose for many patients

Start at dose of inhaled steroid appropriate to severity of disease.

STEP 1: MILD INTERMITTENT ASTHMA

Inhaled short-acting β2 agonist as required

* BDP or equivalent

Fig. 5.2 Summary of stepwise management in children aged 5–12 years. Reproduced with kind permission from the British Thoracic Society, BMJ Group.

Chronic obstructive pulmonary disease (COPD)

This chronic, progressive, predominantly irreversible condition variably affects both intra-thoracic airways and terminal alveoli of much of the lungs. It is mostly a disease of smokers, ex-smokers, and people who live or work in smoke-filled, poorly ventilated buildings.

Pathology: inhaled smoke elicits an inflammatory response with recruitment of neutrophils. An imbalance between neutrophil-derived proteinases and lung-derived proteinase inhibitors (which control and dampen the inflammatory response) is believed to predispose towards chronic inflammation and lung damage. The disease process also impairs lung defences, leading to recurrent infection and colonization of the normally sterile central airways.

- *Airways disease:* inflammation and mucosal gland hyperplasia results in mucous hypersecretion into the central conducting airways, producing a chronic productive cough (previously termed chronic bronchitis) and narrowing of the peripheral airways (due to fibrosis, stenosis, gland hyperplasia, and intraluminal mucus). Both chronic cough and airways obstruction can exist without the other.

- *Alveolar disease:* the alveolar walls become destroyed, probably due to chronic inflammation — a process termed emphysema. Macroscopic emphysema (i.e. visible by imaging) is associated with a loss of lung function since perfusion and ventilation of these areas is decreased. In microscopic disease, the attachments between terminal bronchioles and alveoli are lost. The bronchioles are then no longer held open as the lung expands, producing further airways obstruction.

Clinical features: occur after a period of gradual decline in lung function. The first feature is decreased FEV1 but this is often asymptomatic — dyspnoea on exertion may not develop until FEV1 is <50% of normal.

Patients often present with recurrent bronchial infections, chronic productive cough, and/or dyspnoea on exercise. Lung function deteriorates during acute infections and takes some weeks to recover. Increased dyspnoea at this time may bring the patient to medical attention. The lung fields are normal on CXR. With progression, the chest shows signs of hyperinflation (barrel-shaped; laryngeal prominence lower than normal; loss of cardiac/hepatic dullness to percussion; typical CXR). There may also be tachypnoea; use of accessory muscles; wheeze; and later, cyanosis, pursed lip breathing ('auto-PEEP'), ankle oedema, left- or right-sided heart failure, and respiratory failure.

Management: **stop smoking**.
Give a trial (assessing reversibility by pre- and post-trial pulmonary function tests) of (i) bronchodilators and (ii) steroids: prednisolone 30–40 mg PO od for 2–3 weeks, at least six weeks after an acute exacerbation. Continue at lowest maintenance dose if effective. Physiotherapy to increase respiratory muscle strength can benefit some patients.

Prevention of COPD: stop patients smoking and actively dissuade people from starting. Decrease smoke in the workplace and house.

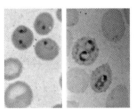

Plate 1 *P. falciparum* trophozoites. Several may be present in one cell. Note Maurer's dots present in late trophozoites (right).

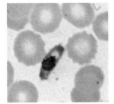

Plate 2 *P. falciparum* gametocyte, note crescent-shaped.

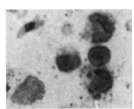

Plate 3 *P. falciparum*. Several trophozoites and one gametocyte (top left). Thick blood film.

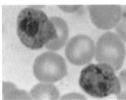

Plate 4 *P. vivax* trophozoites. Infected red cells are enlarged and may contain Schuffner's dots.

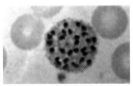

Plate 5 *P. vivax* schizont. Enlarged cell containing many merozoites.

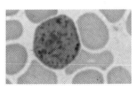

Plate 6 *P. vivax* gametocyte. Large cells, often irregular in shape. Note Schuffner's dots.

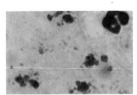

Plate 7 *P. vivax*. Trophozoites and one leucocyte (top right). Thick blood film.

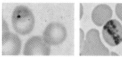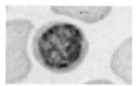

Plate 8 *P. malariae* trophozoites. Usually few and band forms (right) may be seen.

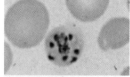

Plate 9 *P. malariae* schizonts. Neat and may contain up to 10 merozoites.

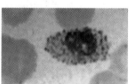

Plate 10 *P. malariae* gametocytes. Small and oval or round.

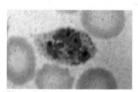

Plate 11 *P. malariae*. One early schizont (right) and one trophozoite (left). Thick blood film.

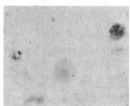

Plate 12 *P. ovale* trophozoites contain James' dots and may be oval.

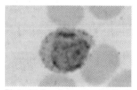

Plate 13 *P. ovale* schizonts. Contain up to 10 merozoites and James' dots.

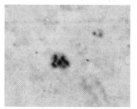

Plate 14 *P. ovale* gametocyte. Small and contains James' dots.

Plate 15 *P. ovale*. One trophozoite (upper right) and one schizont (centre). Thick blood film.

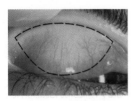

Plate 16 Normal tarsal conjunctiva. The dotted line is the area to be examined.

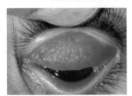

Plate 17 Follicular trachomatous infiltration (>5 follicles in upper tarsal conjunction).

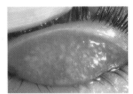

Plate 18 Intense trachomatous infiltration. Inflammatory thickening partially obscures numerous follicles.

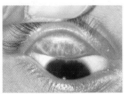

Plate 19 Trachomatous scarring - white bands/sheets in the tarsal conjunctiva.

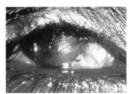

Plate 20 Trachomatous trichiasis and corneal opacity: eyelashes rub on cornea, which eventually clouds.

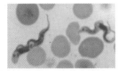

Plate 21 *Trypanosoma b. rhodesiense* in Giemsa stained thin blood film. 100x objective.

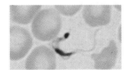

Plate 22 *Trypanosoma cruzi* (Chagas' disease). Leishman or Giemsa stained. 100x objective.

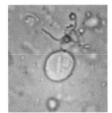

Plate 23 *Entamoeba histolytica*, faecal slide in saline. 40x objective.

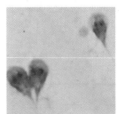

Plate 24 *Giardia lamblia* flagellates in modified Field's stain. 40x objective.

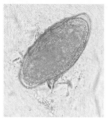

Plate 25 *Schistosoma mansoni* egg (faecal) in saline. 40x objective. Note lateral (side) spine.

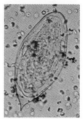

Plate 26 *S. haematobium* in urine (note terminal spine and red cells from haematuria).

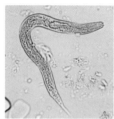

Plate 27 *Strongyloides stercoralis* larva in saline prepared faecal slide. 40x objective.

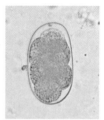

Plate 28 *Ancylostoma duodenalis* egg. Size ~65x45μm (x40 objective).

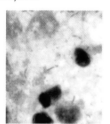

Plate 29 *Mycobacterium tuberculosis* in Ziehl-Neelsen sputum smear. AFBs are usually scarce.

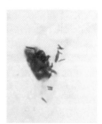

Plate 30 *Mycobacterium leprae* in Ziehl-Neelsen skin smear. AFBs present in macrophages.

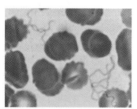

Plate 31 *Borrelia duttoni* spirochaetes in a blood film. 40x objective.

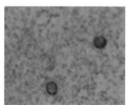

Plate 32 Cryptosporidium oocysts in Ziehl-Neelsen stained faecal smear.

Advice to smokers regarding smoking cessation*

- **Preparation:** make a positive decision and list reasons for quitting. Get the support of family/friends. Set a target date. Have realistic expectations of the difficulty. Know that most relapses occur in the first week after quitting.
- **Switch brands:** to one that is distasteful and low in tar/nicotine prior to the target date.
- **Cut down the number of cigarettes:** smoke only half of each cigarette. Postpone the first cigarette of each day by 1 hr. Smoke only during odd or even hrs of the day. Remember that cutting down is not a substitute for quitting.
- **Don't smoke automatically:** smoke only the cigarettes you really want. Don't empty ashtrays. Make yourself aware of each cigarette you smoke by using the opposite hand or putting the cigarettes in an unusual location.
- **Make smoking inconvenient:** buy one packet/cigarette at a time. Stop carrying them on your person.
- **Make smoking unpleasant:** only smoke alone, if used to smoking in company. Whilst smoking, isolate yourself from others and focus on the negative effects of smoking. Collect all butts in a large glass container.
- **Prepare for the target day:** practise going without cigarettes. Think of quitting in terms of one day at a time.
- **On the day of quitting:** throw away all cigarettes and matches, and hide ashtrays and lighters. Make a list of things you want to buy, price them in terms of cigarettes, and put the money aside to buy them. Keep very busy on the target day. Remind family/friends about the day. Buy yourself a treat or do something special.
- **Immediately after quitting:** develop a clean, fresh, non-smoking environment around you. Go to places where smoking is not allowed.
- **Avoid temptation:** avoid situations you associate with smoking; socialize only where smoking is not allowed.

*From Dilworth and Baldwin (2001) *Respiratory medicine specialist handbook*, Harwood.

Oxygen therapy

If the patient has a PaO_2 <8 kPa on air, give a trial of oxygen at 2 l/min via a mask. Recheck ABG after 1 hr. If there is no rise in $PaCO_2$, increase the oxygen to 4 l/min and recheck ABGs after another hour. If there is still no rise, the patient is not CO_2 retaining, and may have oxygen therapy without risk. If CO_2 does rise, reduce oxygen delivery to the level before which CO_2 was retained. At this point, if available, it is worth considering non-invasive ventilation via mask (e.g. BiPAP).

Bronchiectasis

A condition characterized by chronic dilatation of bronchioles and inflammation of airways +/− parenchyma. The normally sterile airways may become persistently infected with bacteria such as *H. influenzae*, *S. pneumoniae*, *Mycoplasma catarrhalis*, or *P. aeruginosa*. Lung pathology is normally widespread but may be localized (e.g. distal to bronchial obstruction, or in a lung apex following TB).

Aetiology: appears to be due to defects in the lungs' defence systems → chronic self-perpetuating inflammation after an initial trigger. 1° inherited causes include Kartagener's syndrome and cystic fibrosis. Immunosuppression in AIDS or hypogammaglobulinaemia also predispose to bronchiectasis. 2° disease can follow TB, pneumonia, whooping cough, a foreign body, aspergillosis.

Clinical features: patients may be asymptomatic except during exacerbations — purulent cough; fever; chest pain; dyspnoea; haemoptysis. Hx may suggest a trigger for these episodes (e.g. infection or other lung injury). Between exacerbations, patient may produce mucoid sputum; in more severe disease, the sputum is continuously purulent and there may be clubbing. Other features include: recurrent or chronic sinusitis; otitis media; post-nasal drip.

Complications: include cor pulmonale, respiratory failure; brain abscesses; 2° amyloidosis; arthropathy.

Diagnosis: CXR shows a variety of changes including cysts, atelectasis, and tram-lining. Because of persistent airway infection, sputum culture is rarely valuable but Gram stain of the sputum may indicate a likely causative agent. Also, check immune status, neutrophil function.

Management

1. Treat any underlying condition that can be identified. Surgery may be contemplated for focal disease or severe persistent haemoptysis.
2. Regular physiotherapy, particularly during exacerbations, can offer symptomatic relief.
3. Check for airflow obstruction — treat if reversible.
4. Give antibiotics — amoxicillin 500 mg PO tds either for a minimum of 10 days for an acute exacerbation or continually as prophylaxis for recurrent disease (>6 episodes/year).
5. Persistent purulent sputum or unresponsive exacerbations may require higher doses — amoxicillin up to 3 g PO bd. If unresponsive, attempt to culture *Pseudomonas* spp. from sputum. If positive, this may respond to oral fluoroquinolones or IV antipseudomonal antibiotics.

Prevention: reduce smoking; reduce infections (education, better housing, antibiotics); vaccinate against *Pneumococcus, H. influenzae*, and influenza.

Lung cancer

Bronchial carcinoma is related to tobacco smoking in the majority of cases (95%). While once an uncommon disease in much of the developing world, the recent epidemic of cigarette smoking in these areas will soon make it an all too common diagnosis. Importantly:
1. It is preventable by reducing exposure to tobacco smoke, and
2. It is often a condition that presents late with a very poor prognosis (7/8ths of a lung tumour's life may have passed before it is diagnosed; the vast majority will be disseminated at time of diagnosis).

Clinical features
1. *Pulmonary features:* cough; sputum (often grey and viscous if there is no infection; contains malignant cells in <30% of cases); dyspnoea; haemoptysis; chest pain/discomfort; wheeze; stridor; pleural effusion; pneumonia due to proximal airway obstruction.
   Cough and haemoptysis may be early signs of lung cancer. If the cancer is recognized at this stage, there may be some hope of a cure.
   However, lung cancer is a 'silent' cancer and, in the majority of cases, the disease has metastasized and is therefore inoperable by the time the patient presents with first symptoms.
2. *Due to local invasion:* Horner's syndrome; vocal cord paralysis; unilateral diaphragmatic paralysis; pain due to brachial root involvement; superior vena cava obstruction; dysphagia; cardiac dysfunction; bone pain (ribs/spine).
3. *Due to metastatic spread:* signs relate to the organs which are involved: lymph node enlargement (particularly scalene and supraclavicular); bones (especially ribs, vertebrae, femora, humeri); brain; liver; adrenal gland; skin (blue umbilicated lesions).
4. *Systemic effects:* tiredness; lack of energy; weight loss; fever and night sweats (normally due to 2° infection).
5. *Endocrine and metabolic abnormalities:* caused by secretion of a variety of hormone-mimicking peptides by the tumour. They include SIADH; ectopic ACTH secretion; hypercalcaemia (mostly due to bone metastases; sometimes secretion of a parathyroid-like hormone); gynaecomastia; testicular atrophy. Other endocrine effects are uncommon.
6. *Other complications:* including neuromyopathy; finger clubbing; hypertrophic pulmonary osteoarthropathy; dermatomyositis.

Diagnosis: lesions or 2° consolidation/collapse may be seen on CXR. Lateral CXRs are often useful. Normal CXRs do not exclude the diagnosis since the tumour may be central. Microscopy of sputum (particularly if induced with warm saline aerosol) may reveal malignant cells — take at least 3 early morning samples to increase diagnostic yield. Bronchoscopy (with biopsies, brushings and washings) and a thoracic CT (+/- percutaneous lung biopsy), if available, are valuable for diagnosis and staging.

Prevention: decrease active and passive smoking; decrease exposure to smoke and chemicals in workplace and home environments.

Management

Depends on the performance status of the patient (see Chapter 4) and the tumour type.

1. Patients with ***performance status 3 or 4*** require palliative treatment.
2. Other patients should be referred for specialist treatment.

- *Non-small-cell tumours,* if localized (~20%), respond well to surgery. Many other patients gain symptomatic relief from palliative radiotherapy for haemoptysis, cough, dyspnoea, chest wall pain, dysphagia, superior vena cava obstruction, and, less often, bone pain. Palliative chemotherapy improves quality of life and gives modest gains in life expectancy.
- *Small-cell tumours:* careful staging almost always rules out surgery since most are disseminated. Chemotherapy is worthwhile for most patients, markedly increasing median survival from ~6 wks to 9–12 months in extensive disease. Radiotherapy has a useful palliative role and may have an additive effect in a few patients. Prophylactic cranial irradiation appears to reduce the risk of cerebral metastases.

Different tumour types

- ***Squamous cell carcinoma:*** tumours with a medium rate of growth that often present with obstruction. Metastatic spread is common (80% of tumours at presentation).
- ***Small-cell (oat-cell) carcinoma:*** fast-growing tumours that often present with disseminated disease. They may secrete hormones.
- ***Adenocarcinoma:*** (includes bronchoalveolar cell carcinoma) the most common peripheral tumour, it may produce mucin and will surround associated bronchi, stenosing the lumen. May not be smoking related.
- ***Large-cell carcinoma:*** large, necrotic, pleomorphic, mucin-producing tumours. They are frequently peripheral and locally invasive; while metastatic spread is common, survival rates post-surgery are good.
- ***Carcinoid tumours:*** a group of tumours that are unrelated to smoking and occur in a younger age group. They may be malignant and metastasize to distal organs. Most occur in proximal airways.
- ***Metastases:*** often from primaries in the breast, colon, kidney, prostate, and lung. Less often choriocarcinoma, testicular cancer, sarcomas, melanoma.

Lung abscess

A suppurative infection with necrosis of lung parenchyma. See box for the main causes of lung abscesses.

Clinical features: acute onset of fever, shivers, cough, and pleuritic pain often followed >1 week later by production of large quantities of blood-stained sputum as the abscess discharges into a bronchus. Finger clubbing occurs rapidly, the patient remaining febrile and ill. Empyema develops in 20–30% of cases. If the abscess is formed because of septicaemia, the clinical features of this condition will predominate. The onset may also be chronic over months. Short courses of antibiotics will result in only temporary improvement if the diagnosis is not suspected.

Diagnosis: a cavitating opacity with fluid level on CXR. Location of the abscess may suggest its aetiology (see box). Take blood cultures. Examine sputum for anaerobes, mycobacteria, fungi.

Management: give antibiotics — benzylpenicillin 1.2–1.8 g IV q6h, changing to penicillin V 500 mg qds or amoxicillin 500 mg tds as the patient's condition improves. Continue for 4–6 weeks. Metronidazole can be added if anaerobes are considered unlikely to respond to penicillin alone. Abscesses 2° to bac-teraemia require broad-spectrum antibiotics. The possibility of a lung CA should be explored where this is considered a possible cause.

Pulmonary embolism (PE)

Most PEs consist of thrombi that have formed in the deep veins of the legs and pelvis, or uncommonly from mural thrombi post-MI or infected thrombi from right-sided endocarditis. Rarely, they may be due to material from tumours, amniotic tissue, fat, and parasites. Conditions that predispose to the formation of deep vein thrombi (DVT) therefore also predispose to the occurrence of PEs.

Clinical features: vary greatly

- Acute minor embolism will cause dyspnoea, pleuritic pain if the damaged tissue lies close to the pleura, and in ~30% of cases haemoptysis. Heparin therapy is required for 4–5 days; warfarin should be started at least 2 days before stopping heparin. Aim for INR 2.5–3.5 and continue for 3 mths (6 mths or more if there is no obvious cause/recurrent PE).
- Acute massive embolism is less common. It follows obstruction of >50% of the pulmonary vascular tree in a previously well person. The person collapses, becoming severely breathless, +/– central chest pain. In contrast to LVF, dyspnoea is not relieved by sitting the patient up and there are no crackles on auscultation. The patient requires heparin; thrombolysis with streptokinase (1.5 megaunits IV) if the circulatory state worsens, or surgery should be urgently considered. Long-term anticoagulation may be needed.
- In many cases, the PEs occur without clinical manifestations as small thrombi pass deep into the pulmonary vasculature. Over time, however, repeated damage from these silent PEs results in pulmonary hypertension and cor pulmonale.

Causes of lung abscesses

- **Pulmonary aspiration:** most occur in the right lung; aspiration while supine results in abscesses in apical segment of the lower lobe or posterior segment of the upper lobe. Often caused by anaerobes, *Actinomyces* spp.

- **Bronchial obstruction:** due to lung CA or inhaled foreign body. Caused by mixed anaerobes.

- **Bacteraemia/septicaemia:** often multiple abscesses from sites such as right-sided endocarditis, infected IV cannulae, IV drug abuse. Common causes are *S. aureus, Streptococcus milleri*.

- **Primary infection with cavitation:** TB or as a complication of severe pneumonia with *S. aureus, Klebsiella pneumoniae, Nocardia asteroides*.

- **Spread from subphrenic or hepatic abscess:** produces 2° abscess, often in the right lower lobe. Due to *Entamoeba histolytica*, coliforms, *Streptococcus faecalis*.

- **Immunosuppression:** such as malignancy, AIDS. Predisposes to unusual infections.

Cavitating lesions seen on CXR may be caused by — lung abscess; TB; paragonimiasis; fungal infection; cavitating squamous cell CA; pulmonary infarct; pulmonary vasculitis (e.g. Wegener's granulomatosis).

Fungal pulmonary infections

Some fungi infect the lung after inhalation of their spores. The infections manifest in a variety of ways, depending on the immune status of the individual and the level of exposure. While many cases are asymptomatic, others may present as:

- **Self-resolving pneumonitis (acute pulmonary form):** cough, chest pain, fever, joint pains, malaise, occasionally erythema nodosum or multiforme. Specific therapy may be required in addition to bed rest.
- **Localized cavitation:** may be asymptomatic and found on CXR for other reasons. No treatment is required. However, since they can be similar to lung tumours, they may be diagnosed only at surgery.
- **Persisting or spreading cavitation:** producing chest pain, cough, and sometimes haemoptysis (which can be heavy). Surgery and antifungal therapy may be required. These manifestations look similar to, and can be mistaken for, pulmonary TB.
- **Acute or chronic systemic dissemination:** to organs characteristic of each infection. Patients present with fever, often marked weight loss, skin lesions. If acute, there may be signs of lung disease and purpura due to thrombocytopenia. Disseminated disease is fatal in the absence of systemic antifungal therapy.

Moderate immunosuppression associated with DM predisposes to spreading cavitation in some infections. Immunosuppression or neoplasia predispose to acute disseminated disease. The elderly, pregnant women, and children are also at increased risk of disseminated disease.

Aspergillosis

Most infections are caused by *Aspergillus fumigatus*, *A. flavus*, or *A. niger* in predisposed hosts. The fungus is ubiquitous; infection and disease occur sporadically throughout the world.

Transmission: via inhalation of fungal spores. The spores occur in the environment in the soil and, in the case of histoplasmosis, bat faeces. Human–human transmission does not appear to be a problem. Accidental transmission may occur through the skin.

Clinical forms and management

- *Allergic bronchopulmonary aspergillosis (APBA):* persistent endobronchial infection/colonization elicits a chronic Type 1 hypersensitivity response in atopic individuals. This produces asthma and, with time, a chronic cough (producing mucoid plugs) and dyspnoea. CXR may show shadowing in the peripheral fields. Manage with steroids. May lead to proximal bronchiectasis.
- *Aspergilloma:* a fungal ball that develops in a pre-existing cavity (commonly due to TB). Intermittent cough is often the only sign but haemoptysis may develop. If this is severe, the aspergilloma should be surgically excised.
- *Invasive disease:* occurs in brain, kidney, liver, and skin of the severely immunocompromised (e.g. bone marrow transplant recipients). Attempt to reduce immunosuppression, if possible. Give amphotericin B 1–1.5 mg/kg IV od, to a total dose of 2–2.5 g. This is a toxic drug; check local formulary.

Diagnosis
This is often difficult. Microscopic analysis of skin lesion scrapings, sputum, or pus for evidence of fungal infection. Serology (*Aspergillus* precipitins), culture. In disseminated disease, yeasts may be seen in Giemsa-stained bone marrow. Skin prick tests to *Aspergillus* and *Aspergillus* RAST test useful in ABPA. In acute 1° lung infection, the radiographic appearances may give a clue, being typically more severe than expected from clinical examination. Isolated chronic lung lesions (mycetomas) may only be distinguished from lung tumours at surgery.

Other fungal infections

Histoplasmosis

A disease which occurs in two forms:
1. Small-form histoplasmosis (caused by *Histoplasma capsulatum* var. *capsulatum*) which occurs in the Americas plus Africa and Asia.
2. Large-form or African histoplasmosis (*H. capsulatum* var. *duboisii*.) which occurs in central Africa.

- Acute disseminated **small-form histoplasmosis** particularly affects bone marrow, spleen, liver, lymph nodes, and skin (papules, ulcers). A chronic form in immunocompetent patients presents with persistent painful oral ulceration and/or hypoadrenalism. Complications include laryngeal ulceration, endocarditis, and meningitis.
- **African histoplasmosis** is either a focal disease affecting bone, skin, and lymph nodes or a progressive disseminated disease affecting mucosal surfaces, particularly the GI tract and lungs.

Blastomycosis

A systemic infection caused by *Blastomyces dermatitidis* that occurs in northern America, Africa, India, and Middle East. It causes chronic pulmonary or disseminated disease (involving both lung and skin of face and forearm). Skin lesions are commonly an initial single nodule, then crusted plaques, ulcers, and abscesses. Complications include lytic bone lesions (particularly axial skeleton) and GU tract disease (particularly epididymitis).

Coccidioidomycosis

A disease of semi-arid regions of the Americas, caused by the fungus *Coccidioides immitis*. It is inhaled into the distal airspaces, where it rounds up and divides to form a large spherule with thick outer wall. The clinical features are typically varied with dissemination occurring particularly to meninges, joints, and skin.

Paracoccidioidomycosis

A granulomatous disease caused by the fungus *Paracoccidioides brasiliensis*. It occurs sporadically in south and central America where it is the most common systemic mycosis. An acute form of the disease occurs in children and adults <30 yrs, while a chronic form is more common in 30–50 year olds, particularly agricultural workers living in endemic areas. The M : F ratio is ~10 : 1.

- **Acute form:** presents with generalized lymphadenopathy, moderate hepatosplenomegaly, fever, and weight loss over several months. The nodes are hard but may become fluctuant. Involvement of mesenteric and hepatic perihilar nodes may produce an appendicitis-like picture or obstructive jaundice. Complications include lytic bone lesions, small bowel disease, multiple mucocutaneous lesions (lymphatic/ haematogenous spread). Pulmonary involvement is uncommon. Immunosuppression can lead to severe superinfection (e.g. TB, cryptococcus, pneumonia).
- **Chronic disease:** normally presents with lung disease: dyspnoea, cough, (rarely haemoptysis and fever), with extensive involvement

on CXR. Mucocutaneous lesions are common on skin (face, limbs); painful lesions in the mouth, pharynx, or oesophagus inhibit eating, producing marked weight loss. Other features: ulcerated tongue, hypoadrenalism. Chronic inflammation and fibrosis may result in tracheal/laryngeal fibrosis, pulmonary fibrosis, and bowel obstruction due to enlarged lymph nodes. Tumours may arise in the skin or lung lesions.

Management

Follow local guidelines
- Amphotericin B 0.6 mg/kg IV od for 7 days, then 0.8 mg/kg every second day, up to a total of 15 mg/kg
- (Alternative: fluconazole 200–400 mg PO od for 6–18 months depending on specific fungus)
- Meningitis due to coccidioidomycosis requires fluconazole 400–600 mg PO od for 9–12 months
- Surgery may be required for management of chronic sequelae in paracoccidioidomycosis

Paragonimiasis (lung fluke disease)

A persistent lung disease, occurring widely around the globe, which is caused by >15 different species of *Paragonimus* trematodes.

Transmission

Humans are infected by eating undercooked crustaceans infected with the metacercariae. The flukes pass out of the intestine into the peritoneum, where they mature and tunnel their way into the lungs. Here they cause inflammation, haemorrhage, and necrosis of the lung parenchyma. Turbid fluid accumulates in the pleural cavity, and abscesses, later becoming encapsulated, form in the lungs. Ova are released from cysts that lie close to bronchi and are expelled out of the body either in expectorated sputum or in the faeces after being swallowed. Flukes that miss the lungs produce extra-pulmonary symptoms (due to cysts, granulomas, and abscesses) in muscles, abdominal viscera, brain, genitalia.

Clinical features

A few days to weeks after eating infected food, migration of the flukes within the peritoneal and pleural cavities causes signs of inflammatory and allergic responses — fever, rashes, urticaria, abdominal, and chest pain or discomfort.

The classic feature of chronic pulmonary disease is a persistent cough with production of a thick brownish-red sputum (due to the presence of ova and flukes). While diverse lesions can be found on CXR (including infiltration, consolidation, effusion, cysts +/− calcification), physical examination of the chest often reveals little and the patients appear quite well.

Aberrant migration of the flukes may produce signs of a cerebral SOL (epilepsy, raised ICP, psychiatric syndromes, meningeal irritation) or spinal SOL, necrosis of abdominal viscera, transitory subcutaneous swellings. Extrapulmonary disease may occur in the absence of pulmonary signs, but this is uncommon.

Diagnosis: presence of ova or adult flukes in the sputum, faeces, or effusion; serology.

Management: is contentious.
1. Follow local guidelines.
2. Praziquantel 25 mg/kg PO tds for 2–3 days often produces rapid symptomatic improvement, although radiological changes may take some months to improve.
3. However, treatment of cerebral infection may result in neurological deterioration, in some cases producing seizures and coma. Beware of raised ICP due to dying parasites. Treat cautiously and consider using dexamethasone 4 mg IV q6h as cover.

Prevention: improve health education to decrease consumption of undercooked crustaceans; mass treatment of persons in endemic areas.

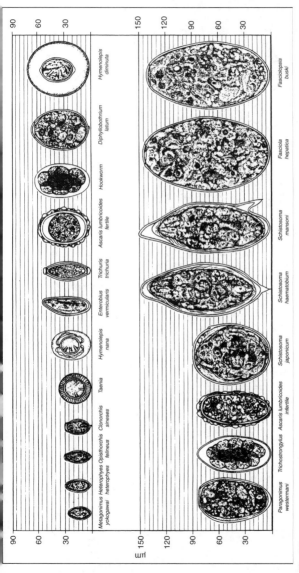

Fig. 5.3

Chapter 6

Renal medicine

Section editor **Sita Nanayakkara**

Assessing renal function

The kidney regulates fluid, electrolyte, and acid base balance; eliminates many substances; and produces renin, erythropoietin, and 1,25-dihydroxycholecalciferol.

Glomerular filtration rate (GFR): is the best index of overall renal function. It is estimated by:
1. Measuring the concentration of creatinine and urea, which are inversely proportional to the GFR, and
2. Calculating the creatinine clearance (CCr)

Serum Cr and blood urea: are simple to measure and widely available (unlike the CCr). Both urea and creatinine concentrations remain in the normal range until the GFR has fallen by approximately 60% and hence do not detect early renal impairment.
- Blood urea is affected by non-renal factors: it is elevated by dehydration, increased dietary protein intake, GI bleeding, and accelerated catabolism, and reduced by over hydration and liver disease.
- Serum Cr is elevated in muscle damage and reduced in people with a low muscle mass.

CCr: a measure of the GFR — the volume of fluid filtered by the glomeruli per minute. It can be expressed as follows.

$$[\text{Creatinine}]_{\text{in plasma}} \times \text{GFR} = [\text{Creatinine}]_{\text{in urine}} \times \text{urine flow rate}$$

$$\therefore \text{GFR} = \frac{[\text{Creatinine}]_{\text{in urine}} \times \text{urine flow rate}}{[\text{Creatinine}]_{\text{in plasma}}}$$

The urine flow rate is obtained by a 24-hr urine collection (important: start with an empty bladder and end with an empty bladder). A blood sample for plasma creatinine is taken during the 24-hr period.
- GFR varies with body size – normal CCr for an adult is ~100 ml/min
- Major sources of error are use of incorrect units and failure to collect all urine. If urine collection is unreliable use the following formula:

$$\text{CCr} = \frac{(140 - \text{age in years}) \times \text{weight (in kg)}}{72 \times \text{creatinine (in mg/dl)}}$$

(For women multiply result by 0.85)

This formula is unreliable if there is unstable renal function or the patient is obese or oedematous.

Urine analysis

1. **Colour:** see Table 6.1.
2. **Transparency:** cloudiness may be due to infection, blood, pus, chyle, crystals of phosphate (white) or urate (yellow).
3. **Smell:** an unpleasant smell is characteristic of a UTI. Antibiotics may also cause a smell.
4. **Specific gravity (SG):** normally 1.002–1.025; a low SG suggests diabetes insipidus. A high SG suggests dehydration or DM (large amounts of dissolved glucose).
5. **Chemical analysis:** Dipsticks are used to detect pH, protein, glucose, ketones, blood, urobilinogen, bilirubin, and nitrites in the urine.
   If dipsticks are not available, simple lab tests can be used detect urine abnormalities (e.g. heat coagulation test for protein and Benedict's test for reducing substances).
   - *pH:* the urine is normally acidic (range 4.5–8).
   - *Protein:* see proteinuria (p. 314).
   - *Glucose:* modern dipstix are specific for glucose. The Benedict's test detects reducing substances in the urine (glycosuria, salicylates, ascorbic acid, and galactose). Renal glycosuria is an impaired ability of the kidney tubules to reabsorb glucose, and may be due to normal variation or be part of tubular disease (e.g. Faconi's syndrome).
   - *Ketones:* are found in diabetic ketoacidosis and in starving patients.
   - *Nitrites:* their presence suggests a UTI, but their absence does not exclude it. False positives may be seen after a protein-rich meal or vitamin C ingestion.
   - *Blood:* dipsticks rely on the peroxidase activity of haemoglobin. Intact red cells give a punctuate staining, while free haemoglobin or myoglobin give a homogeneous colour. Confirm by urine microscopy — intact red cells will be seen in haematuria, but not in haemoglobinuria or myoglobinuria.

Abnormal urinary sediment

The urine is centrifuged, supernatant poured off, and the sediment then microscoped.

Cells

- *Red cells:* see haematuria.
- *Leucocytes:* usually indicates a UTI. May also occur in glomerulonephritis and interstitial nephritis. If a sterile pyuria persists, consider TB of the urinary tract.

Casts

- *Hyaline casts or fine granular casts:* consist of mucoprotein, and are a non-specific finding. Found in normal urine, febrile illnesses, after exercise, in concentrated urine, and in renal disease.
- *Coarse granular casts:* granules derive from degeneration of embedded cells. They are more usually pathological and are seen in glomerulonephritis.

- *Red cell casts:* indicate glomerular bleeding, and are a sign of glomerulonephritis.
- *White cell casts:* indicate an acute pyelonephritis.

Table 6.1 Urine analysis by colour

Pale/colourless	Yellow/orange	Red	Brown	Black
Overhydration Diabetes insipidus	Dehydration Bilirubin	Haematuria Haemoglobin	Bilirubin Haemoglobin	Severe haemoglobinuria
Post-obstructive diuresis	Rifampicin Tetracycline	Myoglobin Porphyrins	Myoglobin Nitrofurantoin	Methyldopa Melanoma
Excessive beer consumption	Sulfasalazine Riboflavine Clofazimine	Beetroot	Metronidazole Phenothiazines	Ochronosis

Proteinuria

Normal protein excretion is <150 mg/day and includes albumin (<30 mg/day), Tamm–Horsfall protein, and other small proteins.

- Microalbuminuria: is daily excretion of between 30–300 mg albumin/24 hrs. It is not detected by dipsticks; special methods are needed for detection. It is abnormal and an early feature of diabetic nephropathy.
- Dipsticks become positive for protein when albuminuria >300mg/24 hrs (macroalbuminuria).
- Dipsticks are very sensitive to albumin but are insensitive to Bence–Jones protein and light chains found in urine in myeloma.

If persistent proteinuria is present, the next step should be a measurement of the 24-hr urine protein excretion.

Causes of persistent proteinuria

- *Postural (orthostatic) proteinuria:* absent proteinuria after overnight rest, but the presence of mild proteinuria after 2 hrs of standing and quiet walking. Patients are asymptomatic; have no haematuria; other investigations are normal. A renal biopsy is not indicated and the long-term prognosis excellent.
- *Renal disease:* glomerular disease is likely when proteinuria is >2 g/day; when proteinuria is >3 g/day, the nephrotic syndrome results (see later). In tubular/interstitial disease, protein loss is <2 gm/day.
- *Other causes:* exercise-induced, CCF.

Chyluria

Presence of chyle in the urine makes it resemble milk or rice water. Caused by the rupture of lymphatic varices, resulting in a fistula between lymphatic system and urinary tract. It is relatively common in the tropics, especially where filariasis is common. Must be differentiated from pyuria, phosphaturia, and lipuria. A rose/pink colouration to the urine may mean that there is also haematuria.

- Common cause is parasites blocking the lymphatics, usually *W. bancrofti.*
- Non-parasitic chyluria is rare and usually involves stenosis or obstruction of the thoracic duct (eg. neoplastic infiltration, trauma, TB).

Clinical features: usually relapse and remit over a long period. Main symptom is passage of milky white urine; there may be loin pain, ureteric colic, passage of clots (may cause retention), and fever.

Investigations: urine microscopy reveals chylomicrons and fat globules. IVU, cystoscopy (2 hrs after a fatty meal) to detect site of lesion; lymphography may be required. Look for a cause. Measure 24-hr urine protein excretion and serum proteins (to assess albumin loss).

Management: treat filariasis, though lesions often irreversible; >50% resolve spontaneously. A low-fat diet and a high fluid intake helps reduce the risk of urinary stasis and clot formation. If the chyluria is severe and/or accompanied by episodes of dysuria, colic, retention, and/or weight loss, surgical repair should be considered.

Haematuria

Blood in the urine always requires investigation. It may be:

- **Microscopic:** with =5 red blood cells per high-powered field, or
- **Macroscopic:** (i.e. seen with the naked eye) if >0.5 ml of blood is present per litre of urine.

While almost half of patients presenting with haematuria in the West have neoplastic lesions, in the developing world a large number of other diseases present with bleeding from the urinary tract.

Causes

- **Surgical:** renal stone disease; transitional cell or squamous carcinoma of the bladder, ureter, or pelvis; renal cell carcinoma; trauma; benign prostatic hyperplasia; AV malformations.
- **Medical:** UTI, schistosomiasis, TB, glomerular disease (IgA nephropathy, glomerular nephritis, SLE), polycystic kidneys (PCK), infarction, bleeding diatheses.

Investigating haematuria

Focus on stones, urological malignancy, and UTIs before considering the rarer medical causes.

Ask the following questions:

- **Is it true haematuria?** Check other causes of red urine (see p. 313).
- **What is the timing** of the red colouration in relation to micturition? Early haematuria suggests a low (urethral/genital) bleeding site, while late haematuria (i.e. at the end of voiding) suggests a bladder site; red colouration throughout micturition implies a ureteric or renal lesion.
- **Is the haematuria painful?** Carcinoma and schistosomiasis tend to be painless, whilst cystitis, obstruction (e.g. stones), and infection are commonly painful.
- Is there dysuria and fever (UTI), poor stream (urethral /bladder neck lesion), loin pain (ureteric obstruction due to tumour, stone, or clot), family history (PCK), or a history of trauma.

Investigations: urine microscopy (red cell casts and dysmorphic red cells suggest glomerular bleeding), culture, and cytology of a midstream urine sample; renal USS; IVU; cystoscopy, FBC, blood urea.

Haemoglobinuria: caused by intravascular haemolysis due to toxins/venoms, falciparum malaria, incompatible blood transfusions, G6PD deficiency, paroxysmal nocturnal haemoglobinuria, chronic cold agglutinin disease, microangiopathic haemolytic anaemia, march haemoglobinuria,

Myoglobinuria: is caused by rhabdomyolysis (muscle destruction) after muscle injury, excessive contraction (convulsions, hyperthermia, very heavy exercise), viral myositis (influenza, legionnaires' disease), and drugs/toxins (alcohol, snake venoms). Myoglobinuria may also be idiopathic.

Urinary schistosomiasis

Schistosoma haematobium causes urinary schistosomiasis in Africa and parts of the Middle East *S. intercalatum* and hybrid species between *S. haematobium* and other species *can* produce atypical clinical pictures, with ectopic localization of worms. For distribution and life cycle, see p. 377.

Transmission: depends on:

- Human (definitive host) availability and water-contact activities
- *Bulinus* snails (intermediate host)
- *S. haematobium* strain
- The host-parasite relationship
- The host's immune response

Prevalence increases to a peak at 15 yrs, after which there is a plateau until ~30 yrs, at which point it begins to decline (age-related changes in water-contact, increased immunity, the death of adult worms).

Pathology: eggs of the worm stimulate a T-cell-mediated immune response, resulting in eosinophilic granulomata in the bladder, uterus, and genitals. They may also involve the GI tract, lungs, liver, skin, and CNS.

Clinical features

- *Egg deposition:* begins ~3 months after infection; it is often accompanied by painless haematuria which may persist for months–yrs. It may be accompanied by dysuria, pain, lassitude, and mild fever.
- *Established infection:* haematuria often decreases in the chronic stage, unless there is 2° infection, ulceration, or malignancy. Fibrosis and calcification of the bladder reduce its volume, producing frequency and dribbling. Other complications include perineal fistulae and 2° bacterial infection. In severe cases, there may be urinary retention, stasis, stone formation, and renal failure. In men, involvement of the seminal vesicles causes eggs to shed in semen ('lumpy' semen); prostate, epididymis, and penis are uncommonly affected. In women, ulcerating, polypoid, or nodular lesions may be seen in the vulva, vagina, and cervix. The ovaries, fallopian tubes, and uterus are rarely affected. *S. haematobium* infection may be associated with ectopic pregnancies and infertility.

Diagnosis: visualization of parasite eggs in the urinary sediment, bladder biopsies, or rectal mucosal snips. Schistosome antigens may also be detected immunologically. Antibodies to *Schistosoma* develop 6–12 weeks post exposure and serology can be performed at this time (ELISA). Radiologically, one should look for bladder calcification on AXR; IVU may be useful, and ultrasound can show bladder wall thickening or hydronephrosis.

Treatment: see p. 379. Praziquantel is effective against all species of schistosomes, a single dose of 40–60 mg/kg usually being curative. The patient should be followed up at 2 and 6 months for urinalysis and clinical assessment of improvement.

S. haematobium and bladder cancer

The association between bladder cancer and chronic, heavy *S. haematobium* infection is well-recognized. There is a lag period of at least 20 yrs between infection and the development of cancer. 75% of patients in Egypt are <50 yrs old; in contrast most patients are >65 yrs in non-schistosome areas. It is more common in men, smokers, and those working with aromatic amines (e.g. in the rubber industry).

Clinical features: haematuria, cystitis, and obstruction. Spread is local to pelvic structures, via the lymphatics to the iliac and paraaortic nodes, and via the blood to liver and lungs.

Investigation: urinalysis, FBC. AXR may show a calcified bladder wall. IVU, cystoscopy, and biopsy. Staging is as follows:

- T1 — tumour in mucosa or submucosa. Not felt at EUA.
- T2 — superficial muscle involved. Rubbery thickening at EUA.
- T3 — deep muscle involved. Mobile mass at EUA.
- T4 — invasion beyond bladder. Fixed mass at EUA.

Management: T1 & T2 — cystoscopic diathermy. Consider intra-vesicular chemotherapy or BCG administration. T3 — radical surgery and radiotherapy. T4 — palliation (long-term catheterization).

Kidney lumps

Enlarged kidneys tend to bulge forwards, whilst perinephric abscesses or collections tend to bulge posteriorly. A tender loin mass may suggest an obstructed kidney, but, if there is evidence of psoas muscle spasm, a perinephric abscess is more likely. With acute obstruction, or development of a pyonephrosis, guarding is common and the mass difficult to define. With chronic obstructed states and tumours, the mass is usually better defined and less tender. Bilateral, irregular kidneys suggest polycystic renal disease. A horseshoe kidney may present as a central abdominal mass, whilst ectopic kidneys may be felt lower in the loins, in the iliac fossae, or even suprapubically.

Kidney tumours

There are three main types of renal tumours:

1. **Nephroblastoma (Wilm's tumour):** is an undifferentiated mesodermal tumour of children which may be sporadic or familial; 95% are unilateral.
2. **Urothelial tumours:** may arise in the renal pelvis, ureters, urethra, or bladder. In the West, transitional cell carcinoma account for 90% of urothelial malignancies, whilst in Africa, squamous carcinoma predominates due to the high incidence of urinary schistosomiasis (see above). Tumours may lead to chronic urethral strictures, obstruction, and recurrent infection.
3. **Renal carcinoma (hypernephroma):** spread is direct to nearby tissues and via the blood to lung, liver, and bone. *Clinical features:* include haematuria, flank pain, abdominal mass, and fever (PUO may be the presentation). There may be polycythaemia due to increased erythropoietin secretion.

Diagnosis: urinalysis, renal ultra sound scan, IVU (shows renal pelvis distortion and hydronephrosis), CT scan, and CXR (for metastases).

Management: surgical excision (usually nephrectomy) is the only successful treatment for localized tumours. For patients with metastatic renal carcinoma, use of immunotherapy (e.g. interferon alpha and interleukin-2) has shown promising results. Radiotherapy and chemotherapy have limited value.

Genitourinary hydatid disease

After passage through the portal system, right heart, and pulmonary circulation, eggs of the tapeworms *Echinoccocus granulosus* and *E. multilocularis* may come to rest in the genitourinary system. Cysts form in the kidney, bladder, prostate, seminal vesicles, and epididymis, in descending frequency. For details, see p. 382.

Renal masses

Unilaterally palpable
Renal cell carcinoma
Hydro/pyonephrosis
Acute pyelonephritis
Polycystic kidneys
(asymmetrical enlargement)
Hydatid disease

Bilaterally palpable
Polycystic kidneys
Bilateral hydro/pyonephrosis
Bilateral renal cell carcinoma
Amyloid, lymphoma, acromegaly

Polycystic kidney disease

In adults, this is an autosomal dominant condition (on chromosome 16). Cysts develop in the kidney, causing a gradual decline in renal function and CRF in the 4–6th decades.

Clinical features: haematuria, abdominal mass (~30% also have cysts in the liver or pancreas), loin pain and abdominal pain, hypertension, and UTI. Aneurysms of intracerebral arteries and subarachnoid haemorrhages are a recognized association. A family history is often present.

Diagnosis: USS and IVU show characteristic multiple cortical cysts in both kidneys. Polycythaemia may be a feature. Features of CRF and hypertension present later.

Management: supportive. Treat hypertension, UTI. CRF is the usual cause of death unless there is access to dialysis or transplantation. Check family members for asymptomatic disease.

Urinary tract infection (UTI)

A UTI may progress more rapidly in the tropics and complications are common, especially in the malnourished. Infection is commonly due to gut bacteria, chiefly *E. coli* (70%), *Proteus* spp., *Klebsiella*, and *Strep. faecalis*.

Clinical features
- **Cystitis:** abrupt onset of frequency, dysuria, urgency, supra pubic pain, and tenderness; occasionally haematuria, incontinence, retention.
- **Acute pyelonephritis:** features of cystitis, plus high fever ± rigors, loin pain, nausea and vomiting, D&V (in children).

Ask about: previous infections, recent urinary instrumentation, diabetes, childhood UTI, known urinary tract abnormalities, renal colic, stone disease, obstructive uropathy.

Examine for: loin tenderness, renal mass, large prostate, meatal ulcers, vaginal discharge, pelvic mass on vaginal exmination, hypertension, signs of CRF.

Is it a complicated UTI?
The following should cause concern: UTI in a male or pregnant female; acute pyelonephritis; urinary tract abnormalities (e.g. congenital, calculi, obstruction); neurogenic bladders; recent urinary instrumentation; frequent attacks; history of childhood UTI; associated diabetes; kidney transplant; immunosuppression.

Diagnosis
If the urine looks clear, it probably is clear. Sterile bags are useful in infants and children — a negative culture rules out infection, while a positive culture requires repeating the culture. Suprapubic bladder aspiration is a reliable technique but invasive. Two clean-catch, mid-stream urine specimens will give ~95% sensitivity. Specimens should be sent for microscopy and culture, and if there is a delay in reaching the laboratory the specimen should be kept in the refrigerator.

On microscopy of centrifuged urine, =10 white cells/high power field (or >100 per microlitre of uncentrifuged urine) suggests a UTI; there should be few or no epithelial cells in a clean sample; bacteria may be visible. A growth >10^5 colony forming units per mL of urine confirms UTI.

Perform further investigations if recurrent UTI, first UTI in men, UTI in children, overt or persistent haematuria, sterile pyuria.

Further investigations include: abdominal X-ray, ultrasound, IVU, cystoscopy, micturiting cystourethrogram, and DMSA scan for scars in children.

Treatment of a UTI

Advise the patient to drink plenty of water; provide analgesia

- *Lower tract infection (cystitis):* 3–5 days of any of the following, being guided by the prevalence of resistant coliforms in your area — trimethoprim 200 mg bd; nitrofurantoin 50 mg qds, nalidixic acid 500 mg–1 g qds; ciprofloxacin 250–500 mg bd; cefalexin 500 mg tds.
- *Upper tract infection (pyelonephritis) or complicated UTI:* 2 weeks of antibiotics. Start with IV 3rd generation cephalosporin (e.g. ceftriaxone 1 g daily), or ampicillin 1–2 g q6h plus IV gentamicin 5 mg/kg/day, or ampicillin plus ciprofloxacin; when clinical improvement, change to one of the oral agents used for lower tract UTI but continue for 2 weeks total. If the urinary tract is obstructed (urethral valves/stricture, prostate, stones) urgent decompression is required (urinary catheter; suprapubic catheter; nephrostomy — be guided by ultrasound).
- *Recurrent UTIs:* nitrofurantoin 50–100 mg, trimethoprim 100 mg, or cephalexin 125 mg at night, or cefalexin 500 mg after sexual intercourse. Investigate children under 5 years for reflux nephropathy etc.

Sterile pyuria: consider partially treated UTI, TB, or other atypical organisms; calculi; bladder tumour; prostatitis; papillary necrosis (the elderly, NSAID overuse); polycystic kidneys; appendicitis.

Renal calculi and renal colic

Urinary stones are common in the tropics, due to dehydration and high vitamin D levels (pale skinned people). Congenital renal abnormalities (e.g. polycystic disease, horseshoe kidney), GU schistosomiasis, and GU TB also predispose to stone disease.

Clinical features: stones in the kidney cause loin pain; stones in the ureter cause renal colic — typically radiating loin to groin (pain may be felt at the tip of the penis). Renal colic often relieved by curling up; some patients cannot lie still. There is abdominal or loin tenderness with haematuria. Symptoms do not always correlate with stone size. Bladder stones cause strangury — urgent desire to pass something which will not pass; attacks of pain may occur with exercise. Urethral stones may obstruct.

Diagnosis: on plain AXR, look down the line of the ureters for calculi (90% of urinary stones are radio opaque). Dipsticks for blood. Look for a UTI. Ultrasound or IVU to look for stone and obstruction. Blood tests: U&E, uric acid, Ca^{2+}, bicarbonate.

Management

1. **Increase fluid intake.** Treat any UTI.
2. **Give pain relief:** NSAIDs (beware in patients with poor renal function) or opiate analgesia for severe pain during acute ureteric colic.
3. **Most stones will pass spontaneously:** >70% of ureteric stones <4 mm wide will pass spontaneously in 1 year while <10% of stones >8 mm wide will pass. Stones likely to pass and not complicated can be managed conservatively.
4. **If there is obstruction, infection, or bilateral involvement:** seek urgent urological advice; decompress renal tract before renal failure occurs. Stones can sometimes be removed by extracorporeal shock-wave lithotripsy or surgery.
5. **Avoid** oxalate-rich foods (spinach, beetroot, green peppers, almonds, cashew nuts, cocoa, grapefruit juice, orange juice, black tea, cola drinks); lower protein intake since protein increases uric acid excretion.

Glomerular disease

Glomerulonephritis (GN) is common in the tropics and nephrotic syndrome is 100× more common in some countries than it is in the West. In many cases, infection is the underlying cause and the GN resolves after treating the infection. However, the damage associated with chronic parasitic infections such as malaria may be permanent.

Clinical features: GN may present with:

- Urinary abnormalities: microscopic haematuria and/or asymptomatic proteinuria
- Acute nephritis
- Nephrotic syndrome
- Rapidly progressive renal failure/acute renal failure (ARF)
- Chronic renal failure (CRF)

Acute nephritis

In the tropics, this is most often due to post-streptococcal glomerulonephritis, occurring 2–3 weeks after a beta-haemolytic streptococcal throat, ear, or skin infection (impetigo, infected scabies, or infected eczema).

Clinical features: haematuria, oliguria, fluid retention (with mild oedema, elevated JVP), hypertension, and variable uraemia. **Complications** include hypertensive encephalopathy, pulmonary oedema, acute renal failure; rarely, rapidly progressive glomerulonephritis and CRF.

Diagnosis: haematuria, ± red cell casts, proteinuria, elevated blood urea and Cr, reduced CrC, and elevated ASOT. Culture throat and skin for streptococcus. CXR may show pulmonary oedema.

Management

1. Strict bed rest if there is severe hypertension or pulmonary oedema.
2. Restrict fluid intake if oliguric to 500 ml plus urine output over past 24 hrs.
3. Restrict salt and potassium in diet.
4. Give diuretics (e.g. frusemide) IV or PO and anti-hypertensive treatment (beta-blockers may precipitate pulmonary oedema).
5. To eradicate residual streptococcal infection give penicillin V 500 mg PO qds for 10 days, *or* benzathine benzylpenicillin 900 mg IM stat, *or* erythromycin 500 mg PO qds for 10 days if allergic to penicillin.

Acute renal failure and pulmonary oedema requires specialist treatment and/or dialysis.

Prognosis: usually good. Proteinuria and urinary sediments may persist for up to 2 years — if persists longer, consider biopsy.

Renal oedema

Renal oedema is often the presenting feature in both nephrotic syndrome and acute nephritis. It can also occur in ARF and CRF.

- **Nephrotic syndrome:** glomerular damage → large protein loss in urine → hypoalbuminaemia → reduction of colloid osmotic pressure → oedema due to transudation of fluid from capillaries to the extracellular fluid compartment → reduced intravascular volume → activation of the renin-angiotensin-aldosterone system → 2° hyperaldosteronism with retention of salt and water → increase in oedema.
- **Acute nephritis:** glomerular inflammation → reduction in glomerular filtration → retention of sodium and water → increased intravascular volume → increased hydrostatic pressure within capillaries → oedema due to transudation of fluid into extra cellular fluid compartment.
- **Renal failure:** oedema occurs in ARF or CRF due to volume overload: Na^+ and water intake exceeds the kidney's capacity to excrete them due to the loss of glomerular filtration.
- **Other causes of generalized oedema:** CCF, cirrhosis of the liver, malnutrition, hypothyroidism, drugs (NSAIDS, calcium channel blockers, oestrogens, and steroids), pregnancy, and idiopathic oedema.

Table 6.2 Clinical differentiation of nephrotic syndrome and acute nephritis

	Nephrotic syndrome	Acute nephritis
Oedema	Gross (± ascites & pleural effusion)	Mild (periorbital & ankle oedema)
Oliguria	±	+
Haematuria	±	+
Hypertension	±	+ (with dysmorphic red cells & RBC casts in urine)
Intravascular volume expansion	No (↓ intravascular volume seen)	Yes (oedema, raised JVP, pulmonary oedema)
Uraemia	±	+ (plus variable ↑ in Ur & Cr, and ↓ GFR)

Nephrotic syndrome

The nephrotic syndrome occurs when there is glomerular basement membrane damage causing severe loss of protein into the urine. The resulting proteinuria (>3.5 g/24 hrs) causes hypoalbuminaemia (serum albumin <35 g/L), oedema, and often hypercholesterolaemia. Milder damage causes asymptomatic proteinuria, detected most often on routine urine analysis.

Causes: nephrotic syndrome may be caused by 1° (idiopathic) glomerulonephritis (see below), or be 2° to:

- Infections including malaria and SBE
- Diabetic nephropathy
- Drugs: penicillamine, gold
- Autoimmune diseases: SLE, systemic vasculitis
- Neoplasia (especially lymphoma and carcinoma) — consider in older patients
- Other: amyloid (leprosy, myeloma), sickle cell disease

Clinical features: There is marked facial and peripheral oedema. In severe cases, there is ascites and pleural effusions. The urine may be frothy. **Complications** include: venous thrombosis and PE. Renal vein thrombosis occurs in >15% of patients with nephrotic syndrome, GN, and children with severe dehydration Suspect it if there is sudden loss of renal function with haematuria, especially if some back pain. Treat with anticoagulants; consider streptokinase.

- Infection: especially pneumococcal peritonitis. Immunize if the nephrotic state is chronic; give penicillin V 500mg PO bd as prophylaxis during oedematous state; treat infections.
- Hypercholesterolaemia — treat in chronic cases.
- Hypovolaemia and ARF.
- Loss of specific binding proteins, causing iron-resistant hypochromic anaemia.

Investigations

- **Urine:** 3^+ or 4^+ proteinuria; dysmorphic RBCs (and RBC casts in proliferative GN) on urine microscopy; 24-hr urine collection for 24-hr protein excretion ahnd CrC.
- **Blood:** albumin, lipid profile, U&E, FBC, ESR; *to determine cause* ANA, αDsDNA, C3 & C4 complement (SLE); HBsAg, ASO titre, HepC antibody (infections); in RPGN — ANCA (vasculitis), anti-GBM Ab (Goodpasture's disease). Look for chronic malaria.
- **Radiology:** renal USS.
- **Renal biopsy:** not needed in children unless unusual features; renal biopsy is indicated in adults.

Treatment

1. *Give adequate protein diet:* protein 1 mg/kg/day.
2. *Restrict salt intake.*
3. *Diuretics:* relieve oedema but do not treat the underlying disorder. Avoid diuretics in children. Use cautiously in adults since volume depletion may already be present (postural drop in BP, low urine output — use frusemide 40–80 mg PO od, with spironolactone 100 mg PO od or amiloride as K^+-sparing agents).
4. *Monitor U&Es and weight daily:* aim to lose 1 kg/day.
5. *Use ACE inhibitors* to reduce proteinuria.
6. *Treat hypercholesterolaemia* with statins if nephrotic syndrome chronic.
7. *Consider anticoagulation* in severe cases.
8. *Penicillin prophylaxis* during oedematous state (risk of pneumococcal peritonitis).
9. *Treat the cause:*
    - 1° GN: use immunosuppresive drugs, usually prednisolone +/− other agents such as azathioprine, cyclophosphamide, or cyclosporin A.
    - 2° GN: treat the underlying disease.

Acute renal failure (ARF)

ARF complicates a variety of diseases in the tropics; if part of multiple organ dysfunction it carries a poor prognosis. The prognosis is better, however, when the ARF is isolated (e.g. following snake bite or malaria).

Clinical features

- Raised blood urea and creatinine in all types of ARF.
- Oliguria with <15 ml urine/hr or anuria leading to fluid retention ($\uparrow$ JVP, pulmonary oedema). Nonoliguric ARF can occur.
- Anorexia, N&V, confusion, pericarditis.
- Raised serum K^+ is usually asymptomatic — but check height of T waves on ECG, as cardiac dysrhythmias can be fatal.
- Acidosis — usually obvious deep, sighing breathing. Arterial blood gases (ABG) show low pH, low HCO_3^-.
- Bruising, GI bleeding.

Pre-renal ARF: ARF is 2° to dehydration, shock, blood loss, hypotension, or septicaemia. Postural drop in BP is an important clue. Urine is concentrated. Treat by giving fluids to prevent ARF from becoming established.

Intrinsic renal disease: (e.g. leptospirosis, falciparum malaria, snake bite, post-streptococcal GN, history of drugs, toxins, IV contrast, etc.)

Post-renal ARF (obstruction): look for anuria if both kidneys affected, distended bladder, palpable kidneys (hydronephrosis), pelvic mass, large prostate. USS diagnostic.

Investigation of ARF

Examination of urine: a urinary $Na^+ < 20$ mmol/L and little sediment suggest a pre-renal cause; proteinuria, red cells, and red cell casts suggest glomerulonephritis.

Blood: urea, creatinine, electrolytes, ABG, FBC, ESR.

Radiology: US scan of kidneys to exclude obstruction; CXR for pulmonary oedema.

Renal biopsy: if cause is not clear.

Course and progress: most patients with ARF have acute tubular necrosis (ATN): the oliguria lasts 2–3 wks with rising urea and Cr, followed by a polyuric phase. Recovery is usual. If oliguria lasts >3 wks, consider glomerulonephritis or interstitial nephritis, and a biopsy may be needed.

ARF in pregnancy: common causes are post-abortion septicaemia, pre-eclampsia and eclampsia, antepartum and postpartum haemorrhage, abruptio placentae, and puerperal sepsis.

Management of ARF

1. Search for and correct causes (particularly pre- and post-renal).
2. Optimize fluid balance (examine: postural drop in BP; jugular venous pressure). Try to establish a urine output by fluid challenge ± frusemide (see below)
3. ***While anuric, remove urinary catheter to prevent infection.***
4. Record fluid input and output, daily weight.
5. Check urea and electrolytes daily.
6. Limit fluids to 500 ml + previous days losses.
7. Diet: give plentiful calories; restrict protein to 0.5 gm/kg/day; low potassium intake.
8. Drugs: avoid nephrotoxic or K^+ sparing drugs; adjust doses of other drugs.
9. Treat sepsis.
10. Watch IV access sites and temperature for signs of infection.
11. Prevent GI bleeding (e.g. with ranitidine 150 mg bd).
12. Dialysis is indicated for pulmonary oedema, hyperkalaemia, acidosis, pericarditis, uraemic encephalopathy.
13. During the polyuric recovery phase: avoid dehydration and hypokalaemia by ensuring adequate fluids and giving K^+ supplementation.

Management of complications of ARF

1. *Pulmonary oedema:* urgent dialysis is needed for removal of fluid. Consider removing 500 mL of blood as emergency measure before dialysis, if very severe. Sit upright, lower legs, give oxygen.
2. *Hyperkalaemia:* serum K^+ can rise rapidly in patients who are hypercatabolic and/or acidotic. Look for ECG changes. See box for management.
3. *Acidosis:* most patients with ARF have a metabolic acidosis. If pH 7 or less, give bicarbonate starting with 50 ml of an 8.4% solution by slow IV injection.
4. *Optimize hydration* and attempt to establish a urine output.

Management of hyperkalaemia

- If ECG changes are present, cardioprotection is needed. Treat with 10 ml of 10% calcium gluconate IV slowly.
- Then give soluble insulin 10 units IV along with 50 ml of 50% glucose by IV infusion (effective within 30 mins), followed by 100 ml of 5% dextrose in next 1 hr to prevent late hypoglycaemia. Alternatively, give according to blood glucose if this can be monitored.
- Give nebulized salbutamol 2.5 mg. Salbutamol also shifts K^+ intracellularly and is additive with insulin/dextrose.
- If K^+ level is >6.0 mmol/l, dialysis is urgently required. The above measures are used until dialysis is available.
- Cation exchange resins (polystyrene sulfate) 15 g/6 hr PO or as enema increase faecal K^+ excretion and are used to prevent hyperkalaemia.

Dialysis

Dialysis is often needed in severe ARF.

- Where facilities exist, daily or alternate day haemodialysis is preferred, since it is more effective and confers a greater survival benefit.
- In acute situations (e.g. unstable patients), where facilities exist, use either continuous arterio-venous or venous-venous haemodiafiltration.
- Intermittent peritoneal dialysis (PD) is effective in patients with mild ARF. Instill 1–2 litres of dialysate over ~10 mins into the peritoneal cavity via a peritoneal dialysis catheter. The dialysate remains for 20–30 mins within the peritoneal cavity and is then allowed to drain out by gravity over ~30 mins. Up to 60 cycles can be carried out. The risk of peritonitis increases when >60 cycles of PD are used.
- Continuous PD may be done for longer periods. Insert a tunnelled PD catheter into the peritoneal cavity (reduces risk of peritonitis). Up to 5 litres of dialysate is exchanged, up to 5 times a day.
- Complications of PD include peritonitis, catheter blockage, leakage of dialysate from peritoneal cavity, and pleural effusions.

Chronic renal failure (CRF)

CRF results from progressive and irreversible loss of renal function.

Causes: diabetic nephropathy, untreated hypertension, chronic GN (eg. malaria, SLE), chronic pyelonephritis, obstructive uropathy, renal calculi, schistosomiasis, polycystic kidneys, amyloid, myeloma, hyperuricaemia.

Clinical features: some patients rapidly progress into CRF from ARF (e.g. rapidly progressive glomerulonephritis; following a snake bite). Most patients with CRF present with a gradual deterioration caused by loss of various functions of the kidney.

- *Uraemia:* malaise, weakness, anorexia, N&V, hiccups, sallow skin pigmentation, itching, breathlessness (due to anaemia and heart failure), pericarditis, drowsiness, confusion, epilepsy.
- *Loss of fluid regulation:* polyuria and nocturia in early stages; oliguria with fluid retention in end-stage CRF.
- *Loss of electrolyte and acid base regulation:* hyperkalaemia, hyperphosphataemia, acidosis.
- *Loss of erythropoietin production:* anaemia.
- *Hypertension:* raised renin, fluid retention.
- *Bone disease:* see box.

Signs: pallor, sallow colour of skin; uraemic frost on skin, peripheral oedema, hypertension, pericarditis, pulmonary oedema, pleural effusions, flapping tremor, peripheral neuropathy. Look for any reversible factor: infection, dehydration, drugs, hypertension.

Investigation of CRF

- *Blood:* serum urea and Cr, electrolytes, Hb, FBC, Ca^{2+}, PO_4, urate, glucose, ESR, serum proteins, and electophoresis (if myeloma suspected).
- *Urine:* analysis, microscopy, culture, 24-hr collection for proteinuria and CrC.
- *Imaging:* AXR or USS (for renal size, obstruction).
- *Renal biopsy:* especially in patients who have normal sized kidneys with mild to moderate CRF, when the cause of CRF is unknown.

Management of CRF

1. ***Treat the cause and reversible contributing factors:***
   - Relieve obstruction
   - Avoid nephrotoxic drugs
   - Treat infections
   - Obtain good glycaemic control in DM

2. ***Prevent progression:***
   - Control blood pressure — aim for BP 120/80
   - Use ACE inhibitors to slow progression of CRF — **but** requires regular K^+ checks
   - Control hyperlipidaemia

3. ***Conservative management*** is effective in patients with stable CRF (GFR >10 ml/min).
   Diet
   - *Fluids:* during the polyuric phase, free fluid intake is possible. In end-stage renal failure, oliguria develops, with oedema and hyponatraemia. Fluid restriction may become necessary: 500 ml + previous days losses.
   - *Protein:* limit to 0.5 g/kg per day
   - *Potassium:* limit K^+ intake (e.g. avoid fruits, fruit juices, coconut water)
   - *Sodium:* restrict if hypertensive or oedematous
   Anaemia
   - If human erythropoietin (EPO, e.g. Epoetin alfa) is available, give 25–50 units/kg IV three times weekly. Aim for Hb >10 g/dl. Adjust EPO to a maintenance dose of 75–300 units/kg/week as single or divided doses. If EPO is not available, blood transfusions may be needed — but may precipitate pulmonary oedema. Give blood slowly with IV frusemide. Give oral iron and vitamins.
   Fluids and electrolytes
   - Weigh the patient often and check plasma electrolyte levels
   - Manage hyperphosphataemia by low PO_4 diet; give oral calcium carbonate
   - Manage hypocalcaemia by giving vitamin D (1,25-dihydroxy-cholecalciferol or calcitriol)
   - Monitor CRF-associated bone disease

Gastroenterology

Section editor   **Clement Kiire**

Mouth and pharynx

Viral, bacterial, and mycotic infections may all give rise to oropharyngeal pathology. It is often more pronounced in malnourished children.

Gingivostomatitis and aphthous ulcers

HSV, EBV, and many of the enteroviruses can cause gingivostomatitis. Oral ulceration is also found in Behcet's syndrome (common in the Middle East and Japan), Crohn's disease, coeliac disease, and Stevens–Johnson syndrome. Malignancy should be excluded (e.g. by biopsy) in any ulcer which does not heal after 3 weeks since typical features of a rolled edge and induration may be absent.

Treatment: often not needed. Hydrocortisone 2.5 mg lozenges or tetracycline mouth wash (125 mg/5ml) held in the mouth for 3 mins, 3 times a day for 3 days, may help.

Oral candidiasis

Appears as small, white mucosal flecks surrounded by a ring of erythema, often in AIDS patients. Treat with nystatin or amphotericin lozenges sucked q6h. Severe infection should be treated with fluconazole.

Hairy leukoplakia

Associated with a rapid progression of HIV infection/AIDS. It appears as a poorly demarcated, slightly raised, and corrugated white patch on the side of the tongue or on the buccal mucosa. Unlike candida, it cannot be scraped off. High-dose aciclovir may sometimes cause the lesions to regress, although the condition may be premalignant.

Other diseases with buccal manifestations

Any acute bacterial infection, TB, leprosy, syphilis, yaws, histoplasmosis, blastomycosis, and coccidioidomycosis may all produce buccal lesions. Cancrum oris is a gangrenous condition involving the gums and cheeks following infection by *Borrelia vincenti* or *Fusiformis fusiformis*, most commonly in malnourished W. African children. Angular stomatitis is a feature of iron-deficiency anaemia and ariboflavinosis.

Tongue

Glossitis is a feature of the post-infective malabsorption syndrome (tropical sprue), vitamin B deficiency (a raw, red, and fissured tongue), amyloid-osis, and iron deficiency. The tongue may be furred and dry in dehydration and Sjogren's syndrome. Overgrowth of papillae and *Aspergillus niger* result in a black, hairy tongue. Carcinoma of the tongue typically appears as a raised ulcer with firm edges and surrounding induration. Check the draining lymph nodes for spread.

Gingivitis and gingivorrhoea

Gingivitis may occur with certain drug treatments (phenytoin, cyclosporin, or nifedipine), AML, Vincent's angina, and pregnancy. In the latter stages of vitamin C deficiency (scurvy), it may be accompanied by haemorrhage. Massive gingivorrhoea may follow envenoming by certain snake species. Periodontal disease and caries are a major problem in developing countries; oral hygiene should be encouraged at all times.

Acute necrotizing ulcerative gingivitis

This is characterized by swelling and gingivorrhoea, severe pain, and an ulcerated, foul-smelling mouth. It is commonly found in malnourished children in poor housing and should be managed with warm saline mouth washes, metronidazole 200 mg PO tds and penicillin V 500 mg qds for 5–7 days. Any underlying malnutrition should be treated.

Buccal mass

Buccal carcinoma and Burkitt's lymphoma are numerically the most important, especially in India, S.E. Asia, and tropical Africa (buccal carcinoma possibly due to betel nut consumption; Burkitt's lymphoma due to EBV infection). Nasopharyngeal carcinoma is common in the Far East and S. China. Malignant change may be preceded by fibroelastosis of the submucous tissues and epithelial atrophy. Salivary gland hypertrophy is common in malnourished children but may also be associated with *Ascaris lumbricoides* infection and chronic calcific pancreatitis. A **rannula** is a bluish salivary retention cyst to one side of the frenulum.

Pigmented buccal lesions

Blue/brown patches in the mouth suggests Addison's disease; a dark line below the gingival lining suggests heavy metal poisoning; brown spots on the lips suggest Peutz–Jeghers' syndrome. Malignant melanoma should also be borne in mind — particularly with raised, painless, pigmented lesions. Lead, bismuth, and iron poisoning may all cause pigmented lesions on the palate.

Pharyngitis

Typically due to Streptococci, viral infection, or overgrowth of normal commensual bacterial fauna — the classical 'sore throat'. *Fasciola hepatica* (ingested in raw sheep or goat liver) causes acute pharyngitis. Lassa fever, diphtheria, and rabies can all have pharyngeal involvement.

Dysphagia

A difficulty in swallowing food or liquid. Unless associated with a sore throat it is a serious symptom and merits further investigation, including ESR, FBC, barium swallow, endoscopy with biopsy. In severe cases it may lead to malnutrition. Dysphagia for fluids implies severe narrowing of the oesophageal lumen and may indicate imminent complete obstruction. The five questions presented in the box will supply many diagnoses.

Reflux oesophagitis

Heartburn and regurgitation are the hallmarks of gastro-oesophageal reflux. It is due to lower oesophageal sphincter malfunction (smoking, fatty meals, pregnancy, gastric surgery, hiatus hernia); intra-abdominal pressure (obesity, big meals); drugs (e.g. tricyclics, anticholinergics); irradiation and ingestion of corrosive agents (including tablets taken without water). It is regarded as a precursor to Barrett's oesophagus and hence important in the aetiology of oesophageal carcinoma. It may also cause anaemia. Symptoms may closely resemble those of ischaemic heart disease.

Diagnosis: history (worse with hot drinks and stooping). CXR (fluid level in hiatus hernia), barium studies, endoscopy.

Management: minimize precipitating factors, raise the bed head at night. Antacids (e.g. magnesium trisilicate mixture 10 ml PO tds with water) or alginates (e.g. Gaviscon 10–20 ml PO after meals and at bedtime) may be used. Severe cases may require H_2 receptor antagonists or proton pump inhibitors +/– prokinetic agents (e.g. metoclopramide).

Oesophageal carcinoma

Oesophageal CA is common in C. and E. Africa, N.E. Iran, S.E. Asia, and N. China, affecting adults in their 4th and 5th decades. In most areas, the M:F ratio is 3:1, although the incidence amongst females in S. Africa is rising.

Aetiology: alcohol and smoking (? eating commercial maize or drinking maize-brewed beers); malnutrition; vitamin A, C, or riboflavin deficiency; consumption of Chinese pickled vegetables. Pre-malignant associations include Barret's oesophagus (columnar replacement of squamous oesophageal epithelium), achalasia, and Plummer–Vinson syndrome.

Clinical features: dysphagia, weight loss, retrosternal pain, hoarseness, or lymphadenopathy. Disease progression is usually rapid. Extensive oesophageal carcinoma can result in Horner's syndrome, recurrent laryngeal nerve palsy (hoarse voice), and coughing. Episodes of coughing when swallowing may also be due to oesophago-tracheal fistulae, 2° to CA or traumatic perforation.

Management and prognosis: long-term survival is poor (4% 5-yr survival in UK) since many patients present late. Treatment is mainly palliative, consisting of nutritional and respiratory support, pain relief, and occasionally intubation. Surgical resection may increase survival to 8–22% at 5 yrs. Adjuvant trials with chemotherapy are underway. Radiotherapy may cause strictures and fistulae.

5 key questions for dysphagia

1. *Can fluid be drunk normally, except if food is stuck?*
   Yes: suspect a stricture (benign or malignant).
   No: possible motility disorder (achalasia, neurological).
2. *Is it difficult to make the swallowing movement?*
   Yes: suspect bulbar palsy, especially if there is coughing upon swallowing.
3. *Is the dysphagia constant and painful?*
   Yes: suspect a malignant stricture.
4. *Does the neck bulge or gurgle upon swallowing?*
   Yes: suspect a pharyngeal pouch.
5. *Are there signs of systemic infection or illness?*
   Yes: oesophageal symptoms may be a local manifestation of a systemic disease.

Causes of dysphagia

Neoplastic
- Oesophageal CA
- Gastric CA
- Pharyngeal CA
- Extrinsic pressure (e.g. lung CA, goitre)

Neurological
- Bulbar palsy
- Lat. medullary syndrome
- Myasthenia gravis
- Syringomyelia
- Globus hystericus

Others
- Benign strictures
- Chagas disease
- Systemic sclerosis
- Fe-deficiency anaemia
- Pharyngeal pouch
- TB

- Trauma
- Achalasia
- Mucormycosis
- Foreign body (bezoar)
- Candidiasis (HIV)

Upper GI bleeding

Upper GI bleeding manifests as either haematemesis or melaena. A methodical approach to management can result in the successful treatment of most patients.

Resuscitate if signs of shock are present:
1. Give IV fluids, high flow O_2, keep nbm.
2. Take bloods for Hb, group and save (or crossmatch), LFTs, U&Es.
3. Monitor vital signs and watch for signs of fluid overload.
4. Insert a urinary catheter and ensure output is >30 ml/hr.
5. When the systolic BP is >100 mmHg, aspirate gastric contents using a wide-bore NG tube and follow by washing out with ice-cold saline and antacids every 2 hrs. If bleeding persists, instil a solution of noradrenalin (8 mg in 100 ml saline) via the NG tube every 30 mins for 4 hrs. **Do not insert a NG tube if you suspect oesophageal varices to be the cause of the bleed.**
6. Tell the patient what is happening and when haemodynamically stable, proceed towards determining a diagnosis.

Diagnosis — where possible, **endoscopy** is the Ix of choice
- If there is splenomegaly, suspect oesophageal varices caused by portal hypertension.
- If the spleen is not enlarged, check Hb levels:
  If <10 g/100 ml the patient is likely to be bleeding from a peptic ulcer.
  If >10 g/100 ml there is probably erosive mucosal disease.
- Other (less likely) causes include: Mallory–Weiss tear (oesophageal tear owing to repeated vomiting); drugs (NSAIDs, steroids, thrombolytics, anticoagulants); epistaxis (swallowed blood); upper GI malignancy; haemobilia (triad of haematemesis, jaundice, and biliary colic); oesophagitis; angiodysplasia; haemangioma; Ehlers–Danlos syndrome; Peutz–Jeghers syndrome; bleeding disorder; aorto-enteric fistula.

Control of bleeding

Low-risk group — these patients make up ~70% of patients and will normally stop bleeding spontaneously. They have the following characteristics: non-variceal bleeding, <40 yrs old, melaena, no haematemesis, not shocked on admission. They may be treated at home with bed rest, ice-cold antacid sips every 2 hrs, and followed up with a barium meal/endoscopy 1 week later.
High-risk group — contains all patients who are not considered low risk. They should be managed as an inpatient according to the diagnosis made.
Bleeders/rebleeders — patients who continue to bleed, or who rebleed, should be admitted and treated as for the high-risk group. Where available, IV proton pump inhibitors may help in bleeding ulcers.

Indications for surgery in peptic ulcer:
- Continuous bleeding after 4 or more units of blood given.
- Rebleeding in hospital.
- Shocked on admission.
- If blood of required group is in short supply.

Oesophageal varices

In the presence of portal hypertension oesophageal veins may dilate and consequently bleed, with frequently fatal results. Hepatic fibrosis from schistosomiasis is the major cause. Bleeding varices constitute an emergency.

Aetiology: portal hypertension due to:

- *Pre-sinusoidal disease*: schistosomiasis; portal vein thrombosis; pancreatic tumours or pseudocysts; myelofibrosis; Hodgkin's lymphoma; sarcoidosis.
- *Post-sinusoidal disease*: cirrhosis; Budd–Chiari syndrome (hepatic vein thrombosis e.g. during pregnancy or with OCP use).

Assessment: if the patient is bleeding, check for signs of shock. Look for indications of chronic liver disease and schistosomiasis. Endoscopic visualization is better than barium radiography.

Treatment: the treatment of choice is endoscopic ligation or sclerotherapy using absolute or 50% alcohol, or monoethanolamine oleate. Oesophageal compression is possible with a Sengstaken tube. Shock should be treated appropriately. The cause of the underlying liver disease should be sought and treated. Where available, octreotide (50 mcg/hr IV) should be given for 2–5 days. Alternatively, tarlipressin 2 mg IV stat, followed by 1–2 mg q4–6h for up to 72 hrs. Oral beta-blockade (propranolol) may reduce rebleeding and mortality.

Prognosis: In the UK, 40–70% of those bleeding from varices for the first time will die. Signs of a poor prognosis include jaundice, ascites, hypoalbuminaemia, and encephalopathy.

Peptic ulcer and gastritis

Both are common in populations where there is heavy smoking, high alcohol intake, and very spicy foods. Infective causes are *Helicobacter pylori*, TB, *S. typhi*, *Shigella* spp, hookworm and roundworms. *H. pylori* may cause gastric carcinoma as well as ulcers. However, ~100% of people in developing countries are seropositive for *H. pylori* by early childhood. Ulceration normally occurs in the oesophagus, stomach, and duodenum, but may develop in the jejunum (Zollinger–Ellison syndrome) or ileum (Meckels diverticulum with gastric mucosa).

Clinical features: epigastric pain (often worse in the day, cf. duodenal ulcers which are worse at night, radiate to the back, and are relieved by eating); waterbrash (the mouth fills with saliva); haematemesis; melaena.

Diagnosis: endoscopic biopsy is the best method, although barium radiography will show most ulcers. *H. pylori* may be demonstrated. All ulcers visualized on endoscopy must be biopsied to exclude cancer.

Management: is based on three levels:
1. Reduce exacerbating factors, use antacids. If relapse occurs, exclude malignancy (repeat biopsy) and *H. pylori* infection.
2. Give 'triple therapy' for *H. pylori* infection: 1 week of ranitidine bismuth citrate 400 mg bd (a PPI is an alternative) *plus* amoxicillin 1 g bd *and* metronidazole 400 mg bd.
3. Surgery is now rarely necessary. Other drug treatments include PPIs, Sucralfate, H_2-antagonists (e.g. cimetidine), and misoprostol.

Hiatus hernia — a herniation of the stomach through the oesophageal hiatus of the diaphragm; it is rare in the tropics. There are two sorts: sliding and rolling (para-oesophageal). Presentation may be with acute chest pain and/or epigastric pain. A fluid level behind the heart on upright CXR, or on Ba meal, is diagnostic. Management is as for reflux oesophagitis, with surgery reserved for serious complications.

Dyspepsia

Dyspepsia is upper GI pain associated with eating. It can be of four types:
- **Ulcer** — epigastric pain, night waking, and relief by eating food, drinking milk, or taking antacids.
- **Gastro-oesophageal reflux** — retrosternal discomfort, heartburn, and regurgitation/acid. It is worse on lying flat or after large meals.
- **Dysmotility** — early satiety, bloating, and nausea.
- **Idiopathic** — upper GI pain related to meals but without specific features on history or examination.

Diagnosis: stool microscopy, diagnostic trial of antacids, Ba meal or gastroscopy, depending upon the patient's age and symptom severity.

Parasitic infections: are a common cause of dyspepsia in the tropics. They include: hookworm, *Taenia* spp, *Ascaris lumbricoides*, *Giardia intestinalis*, and *Entamoeba histolytica* — see Chapter 2D. However, detection of parasites does not necessarily exclude other causes of GI pain.

Gastric cancer

The incidence of gastric cancer varies throughout the tropics. It is particularly common in certain regions such as Costa Rica and N.E. Brazil.

Aetiological factors: include chronic gastritis, bile reflux from previous gastric surgery, corrosive ingestion, infection with *H. pylori*, pernicious anaemia, and dietary factors such as high salt intake, lack of fresh fruit, and ingestion of toxic nitrosamines from fish.

Clinical features: patients present with dyspepsia, abdominal mass, left supraclavicular lymph nodes (Virchow's node), or metastatic spread (to umbilicus = Sister Mary Joseph's nodule; to ovary = Kruckenberg tumour). There may be melaena, deranged liver function (from metastatic involvement), anaemia, acanthosis nigricans, and peritonism. Occasionally the presenting picture is one of a protein-losing enteropathy.

Diagnosis: definitive diagnosis requires biopsy material for histology and staging.

Management: gastric cancers remain extremely difficult to treat; surgical resection offers the only hope of cure. Palliation should be aimed at relieving pain and obstruction, and controlling haemorrhage.

Acute abdomen

The patient has one or more of: pain, tenderness, vomiting, distension, fever, and constipation. Such symptoms are also features of diseases outside the GI tract so thorough history taking and examination are essential. Abdominal pain may be misinterpreted as body aches and treatment given for malaria, only for generalized peritonitis to be found several days later. Two clinical syndromes may require immediate laparotomy:

1. **Organ rupture** (e.g. spleen, aorta, ectopic pregnancy). Shock and abdominal swelling may be seen. Note any history of trauma (especially if there has been pre-existing splenomegaly — however splenic rupture may occur several weeks after trauma). Peritonism may be surprisingly mild.
2. **Peritonitis** (e.g. due to perforated peptic ulcer, diverticulum, appendix, bowel, or gall bladder). The patient lies still and has signs of shock, abdominal tenderness, guarding, rebound tenderness, board-like abdominal rigidity, and absent bowel sounds. Acute pancreatitis also produces this clinical picture but *does not* require laparotomy, so do not omit doing a serum amylase.

Immediate management consists of:
Resuscitation with saline, colloid, or blood as appropriate
- Taking bloods for analysis and/or culture
- Inserting an NG tube
- Giving broad spectrum antibiotics if infection is suspected, until specific sensitivities are known.

Medical causes of acute abdominal symptoms

- Gastroenteritis
- Typhoid fever
- Malaria

- UTI
- Sickle-cell crisis
- Herpes zoster

- Pneumonia
- TB
- *Yersinia enterocolitica*

Others
- Cholera
- Porphyria
- Heroin addiction

- PAN
- MI
- Thyroid storm
- Lead colic

- Epidemic myalgia
- Pneumococcal peritonitis
- Diabetes mellitus
- Henoch–Schonlein purpura

Causes of painless abdominal distension: large cysts (ovarian, dermoid, pancreatic pseudocyst, or renal), megacolon (Hirschsprung's, anorectal atresia with fistula, idiopathic, Chagas disease), solid tumours (ovarian, fibroids, teratoma), organomegaly (spleen, liver), fluid (ascites, hydronephrosis).

Causes of painful abdominal distension: peritonitis, intra-abdominal abscess, obstruction, paralytic ileus, haematoperitoneum (ruptured ectopic, bleeding hepatoma, ruptured aneurysm, abdominal trauma).

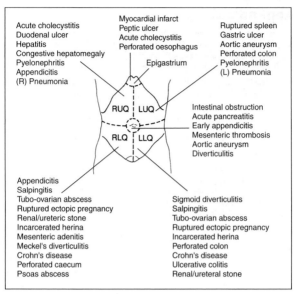

Fig. 7.1 Causes of acute abdominal pain.

Appendicitis

The most common emergency abdominal operation. It may progress to gangrene and perforation with peritonitis in up to 20% of cases. Mortality is highest at the extremes of age, but also in young adults in malaria-endemic areas, where non-specific symptoms may be misinterpreted.

Aetiology: appendicitis follows obstruction of the appendiceal lumen normally due to either lymphoid hyperplasia (hence common in adolescents) or faecolith impaction. Inflammation occurs together with superimposed infection; this is bacterial in the vast majority of cases (although amoebae and helminths such as *S. mansoni*, *S. stercoralis*, *T. trichuria*, *A. lumbricoides*, and *Taenia* spp. have also been implicated). Very rarely, appendiceal tumours may present as appendicitis.

Clinical features: as the inflammatory process begins, there is colicky, central abdominal pain. Once the peritoneum becomes involved the pain shifts to the RIF (classically localized at McBurneys point; two-thirds of the way from the anterior superior iliac spine to the umbilicus). Anorexia is common, but vomiting rarely prominent. The patient lies still, is flushed, and takes shallow breaths (coughing hurts). Common signs include tachycardia, mild fever, RIF tenderness, guarding, rebound tenderness, and Rosving's sign (LIF palpation causes pain in RIF). An appendix mass may be palpable, due to encasement of the appendix in peritoneum, omentum, small bowel, or mesentery. An appendix abscess may form when escaping pus is enclosed by these tissues.

Diagnosis: is made on the clinical picture. Examine the patient often, since the severity may change rapidly. Do ESR, FBC, U&E, urine culture and microscopy, pregnancy test, and thick film if in doubt. AXR and USS are useful only to exclude other pathology and may take up vital time. Do a PR (painful on right side) and a PV in women to exclude pelvic disease.

Differential diagnosis: see box. USS may differentiate between an appendix mass and an abscess.

Management

1. Prompt appendicectomy to avoid perforation unless there is a mass or surgery is otherwise contraindicated. Surgery is well tolerated during pregnancy, but perforation carries a 30% fetal mortality, so prompt assessment is vital.
2. Give metronidazole 500 mg IV or 1 g PR plus cefuroxime 1.5 g IV prior to surgery.
3. If an appendix mass is present try conservative management alone to begin with. Give metronidazole 1 g PR tds plus either gentamicin 3–5 mg/kg IV daily or chloramphenicol 12.5 mg/kg IV q6h.
4. Any abscess should be drained.
5. Surgery is indicated if the patient's condition deteriorates, so monitor vital signs and size of the mass regularly. Elective appendicectomy is carried out once inflammatory adhesions have subsided, usually at ~3 mths.

Mesenteric adenitis

A viral inflammation of the mesenteric lymph nodes affecting children. Suspect it if there is high fever, vomiting, a history of URTI, and cervical lymphadenopathy. Abdominal signs are usually less severe than in appendicitis and usually subside within 48 hrs. Exclude meningitis.

Differential diagnosis of RIF pain

	Clinical features
Inflammation	
Mesenteric adenitis (children)	High fever, vomiting, cervical nodes; improvement with observation.
Meckel's diverticulitis	Usually discovered at appendicectomy; rarely bleeds or causes obstruction.
Caecal diverticulum	May be inflamed, perforate, or bleed; blood PR cannot be attributed to other causes.
Inflammatory masses	?Abdominal mass, weight loss.
TB	Other systemic signs of TB.
Crohn's disease/UC	Caucasian patient with systemic, eye, joint, and/or anorectal manifestations.
Infestation	Worms or ova in stool. Chronic history +/− weight loss; pruritis ani.
Amoebic colitis	Diarrhoea with blood and mucus; cysts in stool; patient may be critically ill.
Malignancy	
Lymphoma	Weight loss; lymphoma elsewhere.
Caecal CA	Anaemia, weight loss, intermittent pain.
Large bowel tumour	Diarrhoea; blood PR; eventually obstruction with caecal distension.
Genital tract pathology	
Salpingitis	Vaginal discharge; pelvic pain.
Ectopic pregnancy	2° amenorrhoea, vaginal bleeding, abdominal distension; may be shocked.
Pelvic abscess	Previous salpingitis; ? history of an illegal abortion.
Torsion/bleeding	Severe pain, minimal signs; requires USS. Ovarian cyst/fibroid.
Testicular torsion	Testis is swollen and very tender +/− referred pain.
Intra-abdominal testis	Torsion/malignancy (teratoma/seminoma).

Peritonitis

Peritonitis in the tropics is most commonly due to appendicitis, perforated duodenal ulcer, tubo-ovarian infection, typhoid perforation, or amoebic colitis.

Clinical features

The patient is immobile, anxious, febrile, and in obvious pain. There may be sweating, tachycardia, and tachypnoea with use of accessory breathing muscles. Septicaemia results in hyperdynamic peripheral circulation initially, but shock may develop as fluid is extravasated into the peritoneal cavity. The abdomen may be rigid and distended, move poorly or not at all with respiration, have signs rebound tenderness, guarding; absent bowel sounds. In chemical peritonitis (bile, gastric acid, or pancreatic enzymes) the pain is intense; the abdomen may be so rigid that distension is minimized. The reaction to blood is more variable and may produce more subtle signs. Signs of peritonism may be vague in the very young or critically ill (e.g. post-op) and present as unexplained renal or respiratory failure, or hypotension. Abdominal signs are also absent in one-third of cirrhotic patients with infected ascites.

Diagnosis

Is usually evident from history and examination. CXR may show gas or fluid under the diaphragm; subphrenic abscesses often have atelectasis or small pleural effusions at the adjacent lung base. Supine AXR may show fluid between thickened loops of bowel if longstanding; an erect AXR with distended bowel and fluid levels at the same level is characteristic of paralytic ileus. USS may show intraperitoneal fluid or abscesses. Paracentesis with a fine (21-gauge) needle, aspirating in all four quadrants, should be reserved for doubtful cases with abdominal distension and suspected free fluid. Do FBC, ESR, U&E, serum amylase, blood cultures. Crossmatch blood if the patient is likely to go to theatre.

Treatment

Resuscitate the patient. Start broad spectrum IV antibiotics immediately (e.g. cefuroxime 750 mg q8h and metronidazole 500 mg q8h). Monitor vital signs and urine output. Give fluid as necessary. Where facilities allow, intra-abdominal/subphrenic abscesses should be drained under ultrasound guidance. If the patient's condition deteriorates or the pus is too thick to aspirate, drainage by laparotomy will be required.

Female genital tract sepsis

In tubo-ovarian sepsis, where peritonitis is localized to the pelvis, a trial of 48 hrs of antibiotic therapy may be indicated in stable patients. Again, if the patient's condition deteriorates, the mass continues to expand, or it is suspected that the uterus is perforated, urgent laparotomy (+/– hysterectomy) should be carried out as soon as the patient is resuscitated. Rupture of tubo-ovarian abscesses carries a high mortality.

Amoebic colitis

Failure to respond within 48 hrs to metronidazole (800 mg tds PO, or 500 mg/8 hrs IV) indicates that transmural disease, with likely ischaemic necrosis, is present and urgent surgery is required. See Chapter 2D.

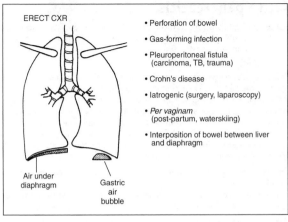

Fig. 7.2 Causes of gas under the diaphragm.

Acute pancreatitis

Acute pancreatitis is rare in most tropical countries and tends to follow trends in alcohol consumption, gallstone incidence, and, more infrequently, roundworm-induced obstruction. It is more common in S.E. Asia, S. Africa, and amongst Australian Aborigines.

Pathology: self-perpetuating acute inflammation of the pancreas (+/− other retroperitoneal tissues) results in fluid sequestration (up to several litres) in the gut, peritoneum, and retroperitoneum. Acute attacks may be isolated incidents, recurrent, or superimposed on chronic pancreatitis. Progression to haemorrhagic, necrotizing disease may be very rapid and mortality is high (see box for Ronson's criteria). Death is from shock, renal failure, sepsis, or respiratory failure, with contributory factors being protease-induced activation of complement, kinin, fibrinolytic, and coagulation cascades.

Causes: alcohol, gallstones, trauma, duct obstruction (e.g. Ascaris, tumour, hydatid cysts in common bile duct), scorpion venom, autoimmune (e.g. PAN), hypercalcaemia, hyperlipidaemia, hypothermia, viruses (mumps, coxsackie, EBV, HAV, HBV), drugs (e.g. thiazides, steroids, tetracycline).

Clinical features: acute epigastric pain (often radiating to the back, especially on the left — sitting forward may give relief); vomiting. Peritonism may develop, but since the pancreas is retroperitoneal, tenderness and rigidity are often not marked. 30% of patients have jaundice due to oedema around the common bile duct. In severe disease there may be discolouration around the umbilicus (Grey Turner's sign) or flank (Cullen's sign).

Diagnosis: serum amylase raised 3–4 fold in the first 48 hrs (though may be normal even in severe disease). AXR may show absent psoas shadow due to retroperitoneal fluid. **Exclude**: other causes of an acute abdomen, myocardial infarction.

Treatment: is as for the acute abdomen plus strong analgesia (e.g. morphine 10 mg/4 hr *plus* prochlorperazine 12.5 mg q8h IM); take blood for Ca^{2+}, Cr, amylase, glucose, and arterial blood gasses. Consider USS to look for gallstones and/or pseudocyst. Antibiotics and peritoneal lavage are of unproven value.

Complications

- *Early:* acute respiratory distress syndrome, acute renal failure, DIC, hypocalcaemia (may require albumin replacement or 10 ml of 10% calcium gluconate IV slowly), transient hyperglycaemia (5% require insulin).
- *Late (>1 week):* pseudocyst (fluid in lesser sac, presenting as a palpable mass, persistently raised amylase or LFTs, and/or fever). It may resolve or require drainage into bowel. If it becomes infected, it requires drainage. A small number of patients have persisting DM.

Ronson's criteria of severity of acute pancreatitis

At presentation	**During the first 48 hrs**
Age >55 yrs	Haemocrit fall >10%
WCC >16 × 109/l	Urea rise >4 mmol/l
Glucose >11 mmol/l	Serum Ca^{2+} <2 mmol/l
LDH >450 IU/l	Base defect >4
AST >60 IU/l	PaO_2 <8 kPa
	Plasma albumin <32 g/l
	Estimated fluid sequestration >6 litres

Prognosis (in UK)

Criteria	Mortality
0–2	2%
3–4	15%
5–6	40%
7–8	100%

Chronic pancreatitis

Destruction of the pancreas with atrophy results in permanent loss of both exocrine and endocrine function, either in part or totally. It is characterized by pain, diabetes, and malabsorption with steatorrhoeic diarrhoea. There are 3 main types: chronic obstructive, minimal change (often post-acute), and chronic calcific.

Ascariasis

Ascaris lumbricoides is a soil-transmitted roundworm, thought to infect ~25% of the world's population. Prevalence reaches 95% in parts of Africa; infection is also common in C. and S.E. Asia, and S. America. Infection is acquired via the faeco-oral route. Eggs are killed by direct sunlight and temperatures >45°C but are resistant to cold and normal detergents.

Clinical features: most infections are asymptomatic. However, heavy infection, especially of children, may produce symptoms roughly proportional in severity to the worm burden.

- *Larval ascariasis:* 1–7 days after infection, larvae cause pulmonary symptoms (Loffler's syndrome or pneumonia). Circulating larvae reaching the CNS cause convulsions, meningism, epilepsy, and insomnia; those reaching the eye cause ocular granulomas similar to those of *T. canis*. Larvae may wander anywhere in the body causing acute symptoms.
- *Adult worms:* in the small intestine cause intestinal colic, vomiting, intussusception, volvulus, obstruction, perforation; plus anaemia and malabsorption. Death of adult worms in the liver causes abscess formation, recurrent cholangitis, or acute biliary obstruction, with fever, RUQ pain, and jaundice. Worm, larva, or egg presence may initiate stone formation; eggs released into the peritoneum may cause granulomas resembling TB peritonitis. High fever and exposure to tetrachloroethylene or anaesthetics can cause adult worms to migrate (e.g. to Eustachian tubes). Hence it is important to deworm patients in such circumstances.
- *Nutritional effects:* a child may lose 10% of dietary protein to parasites. Look for kwashiorkor and vitamin A or C deficiency.
- *Immunopathology:* hypersensitivity conjunctivitis, urticaria, and asthma may occur in presensitized individuals upon re-exposure. It may also occur upon passing worms, producing intense anal pruritis.

Diagnosis: is made by identifying worms or eggs in faeces. There is a marked eosinophilia during larval disease; persistent eosinophilia implies concurrent *Toxocara* or *Strongyloides* infection. Worms may be seen on CXR or contrast AXR (string-like shadows, where the worms take up contrast medium). The differential diagnosis of larval ascariasis includes toxocariasis, hookworm, strongyloidiasis, schistosomiasis, and TPE.

Management is only effective against adult worms.

1. Albendazole 400 mg PO as a single dose (half dose in children <3 yrs). (Alternative for adults and children >1 yr: mebendazole 100 mg PO bd for 3 days.)
2. Pneumonitis is treated with prednisolone, followed by an antihelminthic 2–3 weeks later.
3. Biliary and intestinal obstruction are best managed conservatively (analgesia, NG tube, antispasmodics, IV fluids, liquid paraffin) followed by antihelminthic treatment once the acute phase is over.
4. If symptoms of intestinal obstruction worsen or persist >48 hrs, surgical intervention will be necessary.

Prevention: requires improved hygiene and faecal disposal, education, chemotherapy (since only partial immunity to reinfection is acquired).

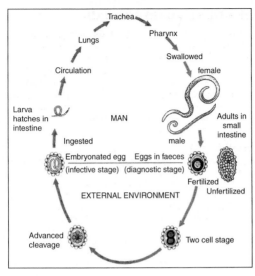

Fig. 7.3 Life cycle of *A. lumbricoides*.

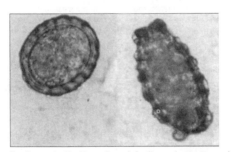

Fertile egg (~ 60 × 40 mcm)   **Infertile egg (~ 90 × 50 mcm)**

Fig. 7.4 Faecal microscopy of *A. lumbricoides* eggs.

Right upper quadrant pain

RUQ pain is normally due to pathology in the liver or gallbladder; occasionally, the heart in congestive cardiac failure or the right lung in R lower lobe pneumonia may be the source.

Biliary 'colic': occurs when a stone impacts in the gallbladder outlet. It is severe, constant pain lasting several hours, with associated N&V, that may radiate to the interscapular region of the back. Treatment consists of strong pain relief +/− antispasmodics (e.g. hyoscine butylbromide 20 mg IV/IM, repeated after 30 min if necessary) until the stone frees itself, which may be during surgery.

Cholecystitis

In nearly all cases, this involves gallstones, although acalculous cholangitis can be a feature of any severe disease, particularly in the malnourished, in typhoid fever, and gas gangrene. Cholecystitis can be acute or chronic:

- *Acute cholecystitis:* follows impaction of a stone in the cystic duct. Features include RUQ pain, vomiting, fever, local peritonism, gallbladder mass, and/or jaundice. The gallbladder may rupture resulting in peritonitis or an abscess. Superimposed infection of the bile ducts produces cholangitis; this classically presents with RUQ pain, fever, and jaundice (Charcot's triad). It is common throughout Asia.
- *Chronic cholecystitis:* intermittent colic and chronic inflammation, with abdominal discomfort, distension, flatulence, nausea, and fat intolerance. Differential diagnosis includes reflux, ulcers, irritable bowel syndrome, pancreatitis, and abdominal masses.

Other complications: mucocoele (when impaction occurs in an empty gallbladder), empyema (gallbladder fills with pus), gallbladder CA, gallstone obstruction (gallstone ileus: stone ulcerates through gallbladder wall into the duodenum, blocking the ileocaecal junction).

Diagnosis: Murphy's sign — pain during deep inspiration when the RUQ is palpated, without pain following the same procedure at the LUQ. Tests include: USS, WCC, AXR, ERCP.

Differential diagnosis: appendicitis, perforated duodenal ulcer, pancreatitis, R basal pneumonia, hiatus hernia.

Management

1. Most will settle on bed rest, fluid, and pain relief, *plus:*
2. Broad-spectrum antibiotics covering Gram −ve bacteria (e.g. cefuroxime 750 mg IV q8h).
3. For cholangitis add metronidazole 500 mg IV (or 1 g PR) q8h.
4. Cholecystectomy is carried out within 48 hrs if the patient's condition allows, otherwise in 6–10 weeks. Without surgery, recurrence occurs in ~18%. Chronic cholecystitis requires elective cholecystectomy.
5. Asymptomatic (silent) gallstones do not require treatment unless the gallbladder wall is calcified, in which case there is a significantly increased risk of gallbladder carcinoma.

Sclerosing cholangitis: a rare condition, frequently associated with UC. It predisposes to cholangiocarcinoma; transplantation is the only cure.

Gallstones

Gallstones are uncommon in the tropics. They are most often encountered when there is a parasitic nidus for their formation (especially *Ascaris* infection) or there is biliary stasis due to pregnancy. Pigment stones occasionally complicate sickle cell disease. **Courvoisier's law** states that a palpable gallbladder in the presence of jaundice is not likely to be due to gallstones.

Features of three stone types

Pigment: small, friable, irregular, radiolucent, female >60, obesity, infection, brown

Cholesterol: large, freq. solitary, 10% radiolucent, haemolysis, black, pregnancy

Mixed: faceted, radio-opaque, clofibrate, OCP use

Other causes of RUQ pain

Include acute hepatitis, liver abscesses, hydatid cyst, hepatoma, Trichuriasis (whipworm), duodenal ulcer, congestive hepatomegaly, pyelonephritis, appendicitis, and right lower lobe pneumonia.

Liver disease, jaundice, and hepatomegaly

Liver disease is common in the tropics due not only to the widespread consumption of alcohol but also, since the organ is in effect a filter of blood coming from the portal circulation, it is far more frequently exposed to bacteria, viruses, parasites, ova, and toxins.

Although the patient will often complain of other symptoms, jaundice and/or hepatomegaly are almost always encountered clinically in hepatic disease. More subtle dysfunction can be demonstrated by liver enzyme abnormalities; such tests are often useful in differentiating between possible diagnoses. Determine the liver size (normally <12 cm) and feel whether it is soft, smooth, non-tender, regular, and non-pulsantile (all normal).

Jaundice (icterus) refers to the yellow pigmentation of the skin, sclerae, and mucosae due to a raised plasma bilirubin (>35 mcmol/l). Examine the sclerae in good light since they are the most sensitive indicators. Jaundice also causes itching, which may be severe (look for scratch marks); the stools may be pale, offensive, or float on the water (steatorrhoea).

Other signs of liver disease
- **Hands:** leuconychia, clubbing, palmar erythema, bruising, asterixis.
- **Face:** scratch marks, spider naevi, hepatic fetor.
- **Chest:** gynaecomastia, loss of body hair, spider naevi, bruising, pectoral muscle wasting.
- **Abdomen:** splenomegaly, ascites, signs of portal hypertension, testicular atrophy.
- **Legs:** oedema, muscle wasting.

Pre-hepatic causes of jaundice

- Falciparum malaria
- Haemolytic-uraemic syndrome
- Sepsis
- Filoviruses
- Pneumococcal pneumonia
- Q fever
- Ineffective erythropoiesis
- Gilberts syndrome
- Drugs
- Crigler–Nagar syndrome
- Haemolytic diseases (G6PD, favism, sickle cell disease)

For haematological and infective causes see the relevant chapters.

Acute systemic bacterial infections: are important tropical causes of jaundice, particularly pneumococcal pneumonia and pyomyositis.

Gilberts syndrome: is an inherited metabolic disorder of bilirubin uptake and conjugation, leading to an unconjugated hyperbilirubinaemia. The prognosis is good.

Crigler–Najjar syndrome: has two forms. In type I disease, the defect lies in the conjugating enzymes and leads to early death; type II disease is a partial lack of the enzyme. It is treated in infants with phototherapy; adults are given phenobarbital to reduce plasma bilirubin.

Hepatitis D

Only exists in the presence of HBV and is spread by similar routes. An estimated 5% of HBsAg carriers are HDV +ve, with dual infection particularly prevalent in the Mediterranean region, parts of E. Europe, Africa, the Middle East, and S. America. Immunofluorescence for the delta antigen (HDAg) signifies infection. The virus is a single-stranded circular RNA virus.

Clinical features: co-infection leads to more severe acute HBV hepatitis or, in chronic HBV infection, accelerated hepatic failure and cirrhosis. HBV vaccination prevents co-infection. Treatment and prevention is as for HBV.

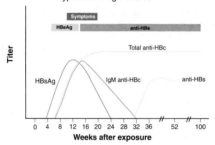

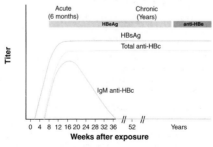

Fig. 7.5 Serological changes in hepatitis infections.

Chronic hepatitis

Chronic passive hepatitis

An inflammatory reaction lasting >6 mths which causes portal fibrosis but not necrosis. In the tropics, it is most commonly due to HBV or HCV, although alcohol and drugs (notably isoniazid and methyldopa) may play significant roles.

Clinical features: may follow acute hepatitis. There is hepatomegaly and tenderness, often with no other symptoms. Serum ALT/AST are raised up to 10-fold. Do a liver biopsy to exclude CAH (see below).

Management: is supportive, since the condition is benign and will remit.

Chronic active hepatitis (CAH)

A slowly progressive condition which may lead to cirrhosis and hepatocellular carcinoma. It is most commonly caused by infection with HBV (particularly if there is co-infection with HDV) or HCV. (~30% of HBV carriers develop CAH; mortality may reach 50% from liver failure or hepatocellular carcinoma — see below.) Chronic alcohol excess and lupoid CAH (ANF positive, IgG markedly increased) are other causes.

Diagnosis: histologically there is piecemeal necrosis and fibrosis with plasma cell and lymphocyte infiltration of the hepatic parenchyma +/− the changes of acute hepatitis and cirrhosis.

Clinical features: jaundice, fatigue, spider naevi (very difficult to see on dark skin), hepatosplenomegaly.

Treatment: strict alcohol avoidance. Steroids and NSAIDs are contraindicated during the viral replication (HBeAg +ve) stage. Interferon α is effective in ~40% of patients, although up to 50% of those with HCV CAH will relapse when treatment is stopped. Almost all of those who relapse will respond to retreatment. ~20% of patients who respond by clearing HBeAg will also clear HBsAg within a year of treatment (65% will clear it within 6 years). New treatment regimes (interferon α and ribavirin) are available but unlikely to be affordable in developing countries.

Primary biliary cirrhosis

A slowly progressive, non-suppurative cholangiohepatitis, with destruction of the small interlobular bile ducts. The aetiology is thought to be autoimmune. 90% of patients are women.

Clinical features: vary widely but include pruritus, hepatosplenomegaly, pale stools, dark urine, clubbing, xanthomata, xanthelasma, arthralgia, fatigue. It is associated with thyroid and pancreatic disease, Sjogren's syndrome, and localized cutaneous scleroderma.

Diagnosis: plasma bilirubin is usually normal, AlkP raised or normal, AST slightly raised. Biopsy and/or ERCP confirm the diagnosis.

Management: is symptomatic, cholestyramine for pruritus, low-fat diet, vitamin supplementation. Monitor for signs of portal hypertension. Death commonly occurs within 5 years in severe disease.

Haemochromatosis

An autosomal recessive inherited disorder resulting in increased iron absorption from the small bowel. Iron is deposited in cells of the heart, pancreas, liver, and joints. If caught early, it is possible to treat and prevent the late complications.

Clinical features: early signs include fatigue, arthralgia, arthritis, gonadal failure, hepatomegaly, and bronze-coloured skin. Late complications include chronic liver disease, diabetes, and cardiomyopathy.

Diagnosis: TIBC is highly saturated (>70%) and ferritin >1 mg/ml. Liver biopsy shows the extent of the disease; >2% iron by weight is diagnostic.

Management: patients require regular venesection until they are iron deficient, which may take months.

In Africa, consider African iron overload (previously Bantu Siderosis) in the differential diagnosis. Treatment is similar.

Wilson's disease

An autosomal recessive inherited disorder of copper metabolism that results in copper deposition in liver and brain.

Clinical features: are those of cirrhosis together with signs of basal ganglia damage — tremor, convulsions, and mental disorientation.

Diagnosis: check serum copper and caeruloplasmin levels; liver biopsy shows copper and is diagnostic.

Management: penicillamine 1.5–2 g od for first year, then 0.75–1 g od for life.

Cirrhosis and alcoholic liver disease

Cirrhosis is the irreversible destruction of the liver's cytoarchitecture by fibrosis, with nodular regeneration of hepatocytes. The cause is unknown in 30% of cases; otherwise, HBV or HCV infection, alcohol, and CAH are common. Inherited chronic liver diseases such as Wilson's disease, Budd–Chiari syndrome, haemochromatosis, and α1-antitrypsin deficiency are rare. Although many of these conditions are associated with hepatomegaly, as cirrhosis progresses, fibrotic contraction causes the liver to shrink.

Clinical features: are variable and depend upon the degree of compensation. When present, they are due to hepatocyte failure and portal hypertension. There may be jaundice, pruritus, palmar erythema, spider naevi, leuconychia, Dupuytren's contracture, hepatic fetor, gynaecomastia, small testes, clubbing, liver flap (asterixis; a slow hand tremor made worse by hand extension which is due to encephalopathy), peripheral oedema (owing to hypoalbuminaemia). Portal hypertension may produce haematemesis or melaena (oesophageal varices), splenomegaly, and ascites. Osteomalacia occurs due to altered vitamin D metabolism.

Diagnosis: USS and/or liver biopsy. Do FBC, INR, platelets, and LFTs before biopsy — if the INR is prolonged, postpone biopsy until normalized. After biopsy, lie the patient on their right side for 2 hrs (bed rest for 24 hrs) and carefully monitor vital signs. The following day check for signs of pneumothorax and blood or bile leaks. Tests may show bilirubin, AST, INR all raised, clotting factors, glucose, albumin all down.

Management: there is none which will reverse the damage.
1. Avoid (or treat) precipitants such as alcohol, dehydration, shock, and hepatotoxic drugs.
2. Give nutritional support if the patient is malnourished.
3. Monitor BP if there is risk of bleeding varices.
4. Aspirate the ascites. Send a sample for cytology to exclude other causes (if diagnosis doubtful). A low-salt diet and fluid restriction may reduce the ascites, but check U&E, plasma Cr, weight, and urine volume daily.
5. Diuretics (spironolactone or frusemide) may be used in severe ascites — monitor for hypokalaemia and stop if encephalopathy occurs.
6. Treat pruritus with colestyramine 4–8 g od taken 1 hr after other drugs.
7. Watch for signs of liver failure (see next page).

Indian childhood cirrhosis

A disease presenting in children age 1–3 yrs from the Indian subcontinent. It may follow a fulminant, acute, or sub-acute course ranging from a viral type acute hepatitis to florid cirrhosis. There is fibrosis with micro- and macronodular degeneration and, although progression to hepatocellular CA is rare, mortality is high. The cause is unknown, although a high copper intake (e.g. from milk stored in copper vessels), possibly coupled with an inherited defect of copper absorption/metabolism is implicated. There is no specific treatment.

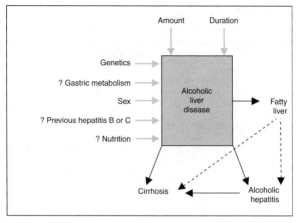

Fig. 7.6 Aetiology and consequences of alcoholic liver disease.

Liver failure

In the tropics, liver failure usually results from viral hepatitis, particularly HBV, and in some areas alcohol. Less common causes are other viruses, bacteria, drugs such as paracetamol, and acute fatty liver of pregnancy. Beware development of renal failure via the hepato-renal syndrome.

Clinical features: presentation is likely to involve one (or more) of:
- Encephalopathy
- Hypoglycaemia
- Bleeding
- Overwhelming infection
- Ascites.

The onset may be acute, with no preceding illness or jaundice (fulminant hepatic necrosis). However, liver failure occurs more commonly in patients with pre-existing cirrhosis. These patients have a chronic deterioration with infection, lethargy, GI bleeds, diuretics usage, and/or electrolyte disturbances.

Hepatic encephalopathy

Early signs are: lethargy, delirium, psychiatric symptoms, amnesia, ataxia, tremor, incontinence, ophthalmoplegia, and extra-pyramidal signs.

Management

1. If signs of encephalopathy, manage as for coma (Chapter 8).
2. Be careful to avoid contamination with blood or secretions.
3. Insert an NG tube, unless oesophageal varices are suspected.
4. Monitor TPR, BP, pupils, urine ouput, blood glucose, INR, U&E, LFTs.
5. Consider haemodialysis if there is water overload.
6. Give cimetidine 200 mg IV q4–6h to keep stomach pH >5.
7. If infection is suspected, give gentamicin 2–5 mg/kg od in divided doses *plus* metronidazole 500 mg IV q8h *plus* benzylpenicillin 1.2 g IV q6h. Otherwise give neomycin or ampicillin (1.5 g IV q6h) to sterilize bowel.
8. Watch for convulsions, treating with diazepam (see Chapter 8).
9. For bleeding, give vitamin K 10 mg IV od for 2–3 days. Beware anaphylaxis; give with caution and have adrenalin close at hand.
10. Give IV glucose and monitor blood sugar levels.
11. Beware hypokalaemia.
12. Control pain with normal dose paracetamol or morphine.

Avoid sedatives, drugs with hepatic metabolism, NSAIDs (risk of GI bleed).

Poor prognosis: is associated with grade IV coma, presence of HBsAg, co-infection with HDV, serum bilirubin >20 mg/100 ml, and sodium <119 mmol/l. Liver transplantation before irreversible CNS damage is the only curative treatment.

Hepatic neoplasia

Hepatic secondaries are rare in the tropics compared with the West. They have a characteristic knobbly feeling. Jaundice is relatively uncommon as a presenting feature; unexplained weight loss is more common.

Investigations: USS is the best means of determining the cause of focal liver lesions.

Hepatocellular carcinoma

This cancer is the most common 1° cancer of men in sub-Saharan Africa, and is also common in parts of Asia and the western Pacific. Its incidence is as high as 100/100,000 in Mozambique males, with an estimated 1 million deaths/year worldwide. It is common in the 20–40 age group.

Aetiology
1. *Hepatitis B* and to a lesser extent HCV are thought to cause ~80% of cases worldwide.
2. *Non-viral factors* which may be involved include:
   - *Aflatoxin B:* a toxin produced by the plant mould Aspergillus flavus. It grows commonly on groundnuts (peanuts) but is also found on maize, millet, peas, and sorghum. Levels of food contamination in Mozambique are the highest in the world and there is a correlation between levels of ingestion and incidence of hepatocellular carcinoma (HCC).
   - *Cigarette smoking:* a significant factor in low-risk areas of the world and increasing in importance in the developing world.
   - *Alcohol:* HCC is 5-fold more common in males who drink >80 g alcohol per day than in non-drinkers.
   - *Oral contraceptive pill use:* some studies suggest a 5-fold increased relative risk for women using the OCP for >5 yrs.

Clinical features: RUQ pain, weakness, and weight loss. Hepatomegaly occurs in 90%, cachexia and ascites in 50%, abdominal venous collaterals in 30%, jaundice in 25%. There may be pathological fractures due to bone metastases and haematemesis from oesophageal varices.

Diagnosis: is clinical. CXR may show a raised R hemidiaphragm. AlkP and α-fetoprotein may be increased. Other Ix: USS, CT scan, biopsy.

Management: is usually palliative. Aim to relieve pain and reduce symptoms (e.g. with drainage of ascites, anti-pruritic agents, transfusions for anaemia). Chemotherapy, radiotherapy, and transplantation are disappointing. Surgical resection provides the only prospect for cure, although this is only possible in ~2% of cases at presentation. HCC may have a fulminant presentation in the tropics; death occurring within weeks of diagnosis.

Prevention: HBV vaccination.

Differential diagnosis of the non-smooth liver

- *Cystic lesions*: amoebic (or other pyogenic) abscess, congenital liver cysts, polycystic liver, or hydatid cyst.
- *Solid lesions*: are likely to be malignant. Surgical resection of small, solitary lesions may be attempted. If the patient is terminally ill, omit all investigations and concentrate on palliation.

Primary sites for liver metastases

Male	*Female*	*Rarer malignancies*
• Stomach	• Breast	• Pancreas
• Lung	• Colon	• Leukaemia
• Colon	• Stomach	• Lymphoma
	• Uterus	• Carcinoid

Post-hepatic causes of jaundice

Cholestatic jaundice: is caused by blockage of the common bile duct. In the industrialized world, it is normally due to gallstones or pancreatic disease. In the tropics, however, most biliary disease is due to parasitic infection — ascariasis, clonorchiasis, or opisthorchiasis.

Intrahepatic biliary obstruction: may be caused by reaction to numerous drugs (e.g. chlorpromazine, isoniazid), primary biliary cirrhosis, the cholestatic phase of viral hepatitis (see above), 1° and 2° cancer, lymphoma, or pregnancy. Liver biopsy may be diagnostic. The condition is usually self-limiting, although it sometimes persists for months or years, mimicking primary biliary cirrhosis.

Fascioliasis

Fascioliasis is an animal disease that follows infection with the trematodes *Fasciola hepatica* or *F. gigantica*. Human infection is relatively rare, although epidemics do occur. Infection occurs after the ingestion of aquatic plants, particularly watercress, grown in water contaminated with animal faeces. Transmission is favoured by high humidity and rainfall, and temp between 10–30°C. The trematode's life cycle is similar to the liver flukes (see p. 372), using a snail intermediate host and attaching to aquatic plants before they are ingested by ruminants or humans. Cercariae excyst in the gut and migrate to the bile ducts, where they can live for years.

Clinical features: are due to the host's immune response against the parasite. Although many infections are asymptomatic, there may be bile duct proliferation, dilatation, fibrosis, and calcification with stone formation. Symptoms begin ~2 months after ingestion and include diarrhoea, upper abdominal pain, urticaria, malaise, fever, and night sweats. In this acute phase, there is hepatomegaly, anaemia, and marked eosinophilia. Obstruction may lead to jaundice, pruritus, and fatty food intolerance. In severe cases, there is ascites, profound anaemia, and haemorrhage into the bile ducts. Migration to other tissues causes nodules, granulomata, and tracts. Mortality, although rare, is highest in children.

Diagnosis: eggs can be seen in the faeces by 2–4 months after infection; USS, FBC, serology, and antigen ELISA are useful. In epidemics, ask about dietary history. The presence of eggs in the stool may simply indicate that the patient has eaten the liver of an infected animal.

Management

1. Bithionol 10–18 mg/kg PO tds on alternate days for 10–15 days. (Alternative: dehydroemetine 1 mg/kg IM od for 10 days may be effective during the acute stage.) Both drugs and multiple courses are often required, sometimes with significant side-effects.
2. Give antibiotics for 2° bacterial cholangitis.

Prevention: improved hygiene, education, and where practicable, treatment of livestock.

Causes of post-hepatic jaundice

- Cholestatic jaundice
- *Ascaris lumbricoides*
- *Fasciola hepatica*
- Opisthorchiasis/clonorchiasis
- HIV infection
- Amoebic liver abscess
- Hydatid disease

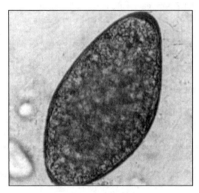

Fig. 7.7 *F. hepatica* egg in a faecal smear ~140×50 mcm size.

Opisthorchiasis and clonorchiasis

An estimated 200 million people are infected by the human liver flukes: *Clonorchis sinensis* (E. Asia), *Opisthorchis felineus* (E. Europe, N. Asia), *O. viverrini* (Thailand, Laos), and *O. guayaquilensis* (Ecuador). Infection of up to 25% of the population in N.E. Thailand with *O. viverrini* is believed to be a major factor in their high incidence of cholangiocarcinoma.

Life cycle and transmission: eggs released by adult worms living in the biliary tree pass into the faeces with bile. The excreted parasites pass through snails before developing in fish into metacercaria which are infective to humans. The parasites are ingested by humans in uncooked fish; they then migrate from the bowel to the biliary system where they mature into adults and can live for many years. Pathology results from inflammation around retained eggs.

Clinical features: asymptomatic hepatomegaly is common, although USS often reveals gallbladder enlargement, sludge, gallstones, and poor function. Symptoms include RUQ pain, diarrhoea, loss of appetite, indigestion, and fullness. In more severe cases, there may be fever, eosinophilia, obstructive jaundice, weight loss, ascites, and oedema. Many patients complain of a feeling of something moving within the liver. Gallstones and intrahepatic stones are common complications of clonorchiasis; the most serious complication is cholangiocarcinoma due to *O. viverrini* infection (5-fold increased risk for mild infection, 15-fold for heavy infection). *O. felineus* can cause **acute opisthorchiasis**, usually soon after exposure to a large dose of metacercaria: presents with fever, hepatosplenomegaly, tenderness, and eosinophilia (up to 40% of WCC).

Diagnosis: requires detection of eggs; however, eggs may not be able to pass into the gut in patients with complete obstruction. Percutaneous bile aspiration is dangerous and not recommended due to the high risk of biliary peritonitis and haemorrhage. Others: serology, antigen/DNA assays.

Management
1. Praziquantel 40 mg/kg PO as a single dose is often effective.
2. Heavy clonorchis infection may require up to 150 mg/kg over 2 days.

Prevention: improved sanitation (preventing eggs from reaching water); education to discourage the consumption of raw fish. Molluscicidal control of snail vectors is not feasible.

Amoebic liver abscess

The most common form of extraintestinal amoebiasis; it may present as a complication of acute amoebic dysentery (~10%) or long after exposure with no history of diarrhoea (up to 70%).

Clinical presentation: either acutely with RUQ +/− R shoulder tip pain and hepatomegaly (abscesses may enlarge upwards into the diaphragm) or chronically with dull RUQ ache, weight loss, fatigue, low-grade pyrexia, and anaemia. The pain of left lobe abscesses often radiates to the left side. There may also be jaundice (usually mild), vomiting, right-sided pleural effusion/collapse, ascites or emphysema.

Diagnosis: USS. Stool microscopy is +ve in 50% (culture =75%). The abscess fluid is odourless and may resemble anchovy paste. Beware misdiagnosis of the acute attack as acute cholecystitis or appendicitis.

Management: almost all amoebic abscesses will heal without scarring if treated with drugs +/− drainage (Chapter 2D). Drainage is indicated if the abscess cavity is >6 cm since there is a risk of perforation and high mortality. ~1% of abscesses, especially those of the left hepatic lobe, involve the pericardium; this requires open drainage (40% mortality).

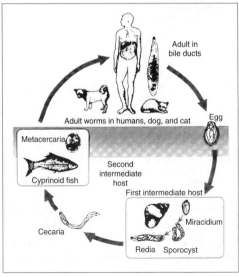

Fig. 7.8 Life cycle of *O. viverrini*.

Hepatomegaly without jaundice

May be due to:
- Portal hypertension
- Schistosomiasis
- Chagas disease
- Sarcoid
- Tricuspid incompetence
- Trypanosomiasis
- Toxocariasis
- Beri beri
- Hydatid disease
- Kwashiorkor
- Fascioliasis
- Plague
- Bartonellosis
- Visceral leishmaniasis

Portal hypertension

Portal hypertension (PHT) can be a sequel to any chronic liver disease, although cirrhosis and schistosomiasis are the most common causes in the tropics. It is useful to split causes according to the level of obstruction:

Causes of PHT

Pre-hepatic	• Hyper-reactive malarial splenomegaly
	• Portal vein occlusion (lymphoma, pancreatic CA)
	• Splenic vein occlusion (following umbilical sepsis)
	• Severe dehydration (cholera, dysentery)
Hepatic (sinusoidal)	• Cirrhosis
	• Schistosomiasis (*S. mansoni* or *S. japonicum*)
	• Hepatocellular CA
	• Veno-occlusive disease
	• Congenital hepatic fibrosis
	• Drugs (e.g. dapsone)
	• Sarcoidosis
Post-hepatic	• Cardiac dysfunction (e.g. due to RF or TB)
	• Constrictive pericarditis (endomyocardial fibrosis)
	• Inferior vena cava obstruction
	• Hepatic vein thrombosis (Budd–Chiari syndrome e.g. during pregnancy).

Clinical features: the most serious complication is oesophageal varices which carry a 70% mortality if they rupture. Signs of PHT include hepatosplenomegaly, caput medusae, haemorrhoids, haematemesis, or melaena.

Management: where possible, treat the cause. Oral beta-blockade (propanolol) can lower portal (as well as systemic) pressure and reduce the incidence of bleeding varices. Neither intensive sclerotherapy nor surgical insertion of porto-systemic bypass shunts have shown benefit.

Veno-occlusive disease: caused by ingestion of pyrrolizidine alkaloids contained in certain herbal teas (e.g. *Helotropium*, *Crotalaria*, and *Senecio*). It is an important cause of thrombosis and PHT in Jamaica, S. Africa, central Asia, and S.W. USA.

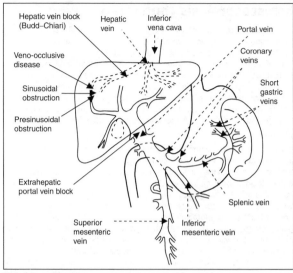

Fig. 7.9 Sites of blockage and veins affected by PHT.

Schistosomiasis (bilharzia)

A common, chronically debilitating and potentially lethal disease affecting ~200 million people worldwide. It is second only to malaria in socioeconomic importance, with ~600 million people at risk.

It is caused in humans by infection with the mammalian blood flukes or trematodes *Schistosoma mansoni, S. japonicum, S. haematobium*, and, occasionally, *S. mekongi* and *S. intercalatum*. In the majority of cases, infections are light or moderate; however, *S. haematobium* and *S. mansoni* infections can be more serious. It is usually a slow insidious disease but may be lethal or potentiate other diseases (hepatitis, cirrhosis, bladder CA).

Life cycle

Transmission occurs when humans are exposed to water infested with the intermediate snail host while swimming, washing, or collecting water. Schistosome cercariae released from the snails penetrate human skin and enter blood vessels, passing via the lungs to the liver where they mature into adults. The adults mate and start producing eggs, which the female will continue to do for the rest of her life. Some of the eggs pass into the urinary tract (*S. haematobium*) or into the bowel (other species) before being passed in urine or faeces to the outside world. Other eggs embolize in the blood to various sites (e.g. lungs, liver, CNS) where they stimulate a strong immune response, causing immunopathological disease.

Adult worms do not multiply in humans, so the level of infection and disease is proportional to the degree of exposure. Usually there is a slow rate of accumulation; presentation occurs only after many years. Infection peaks in early adult life with both sexes equally affected. However, prevalence and intensity of infection decrease in older age groups due to behavioural changes (less water contact) and acquired immunity.

Clinical features

1. *Early reaction (swimmers' itch):* occurs ~1 day after infection. It is a pruritic papular rash with oedema, erythema, and eosinophilia caused by death of cercariae upon skin penetration. It resolves spontaneously within 10 days and is rare in endemic areas.

2. *Katayama fever (acute toxaemic schistosomiasis):* is a rare, but potentially lethal serum-sickness illness (immune complex mediated) occurring 1–3 mths after 1° infection (usually with *S. japonicum*). Features include fever, rash, chills, sweating, anorexia, headache, diarrhoea, cough, hepatosplenomegaly, lymphadenopathy, and urticaria. Ix show eosinophilia, raised IgG, IgA, IgM, +/− immune-complex glomerulopathy. It is more common in non-immunes and usually subsides after several weeks (although egg output may remain high).

3. *Chronic disease:* egg-induced chronic granulomatous inflammation and fibrosis affects many organs. Often asymptomatic, it may present with fatigue, fever, abdominal pain and diarrhoea.
   - *Pulmonary disease:* embolizing eggs cause arteritis and pulmonary blood flow obstruction, leading to pulmonary hypertension. There may be fatigue, syncope, chest pain, raised JVP, tricuspid incompetence, and ultimately cor pulmonale.

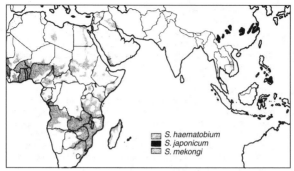

Fig. 7.10 Distribution of S. *haematobium*, S. *japonicum* and S. *mekongi*.

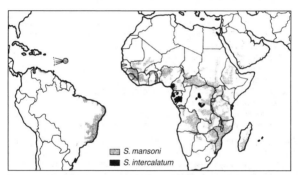

Fig. 7.11 Distribution of S. *mansoni* and S. *intercalatum*.

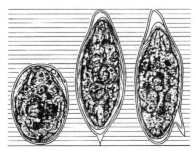

Fig. 7.12 Schematic representation of S. *japonicum*, S. *haematobium*, and S. *mansoni* (from left to right). Total height is 150 mcm, width 170 mcm.

- *Hepatic disease:* often occurs in the left lobe. Features include portal hypertension and portalsystemic collateral circulation, hepatosplenomegaly (often severe), ascites, oesophageal/gastric varices. Liver enzymes are usually normal, with few stigmata of chronic hepatic disease, although in endemic areas hepatosplenic decompensated schistosomiasis may develop in which liver enzymes are abnormal. Hypersplenism may result in pancytopaenia and reduced RBC lifespan.
- *Intestinal disease:* eggs may reach both the superior and inferior mesenteric venous plexi (and superior haemorrhoidal veins in *S. japonicum* disease) and pass through to the intestinal mucosa to involve both small and large bowel. Chronic inflammation of the large bowel may cause intermittent, bloody diarrhoea with tenesmus, pseudopolyp formation, hypoalbuminaemia, and anaemia, giving a clinical picture similar to that of ulcerative colitis/proctitis.
  A 'bilharzioma' is a mass of schistosomal eggs, which may be found in the omentum and/or mesenteric lymph nodes. Other features include protein-losing enteropathy, intussusception, and rectal prolapse.
- *CNS disease:* is a rare but severe complication of *S. japonicum* and *S. mansoni* disease. Eggs of the former may embolize to the brain to cause meningoencephalitis or focal epilepsy. *S. mansoni* eggs embolize to the spinal cord, causing cauda equina, a transverse myelitis-like syndrome, paraplegia, or bladder dysfunction. Both may present as a SOL or encephalitis, although most are asymptomatic.
- *Other sites:* very rarely there is placental, genital, arthropathic, or cutaneous schistosomiasis.
- *Bacterial superinfection:* bacteria (e.g. *Salmonella* spp) may colonize adult worms, providing a source for bacteraemic episodes.

Diagnosis: rests upon a history of exposure (? itch or fever), clinical signs +/– demonstration of eggs in the urine/faeces or rectal biopsy specimen. Collected eggs may be hatched in fresh water to demonstrate miracidia. Other methods include serology; sigmoidoscopy or Ba enema for intestinal disease; liver biopsy, Ba swallow, oesophagoscopy, USS, and splenoportography for liver disease; CT or myelography for CNS lesions.

Prevention: no repellents, vaccines, or prophylactic drugs are yet available. Avoid coming into contact with fresh water (even flowing or deep water), although very fast water with little vegetation (and therefore snails) is likely to be less infective. Beware so-called 'safe lakes' (classically Lake Malawi) or unchlorinated swimming pools. If contact is unavoidable, keep to a minimum (e.g. wear boots) and follow with rapid, vigorous drying which may kill cercariae not fully penetrated. Infectivity of cercariae is lost in water left standing for ~20 hrs.

At a community level, break the human snail cycle by cleaning and isolating water supplies (however, rarely cost-effective). Avoid urination and defecation near open water. Molluscicides are difficult to implement and ecologically destructive. Human treatment and education are the most effective means of prevention.

Management

Total cure is reasonable in non-endemic areas but usually unfeasible in endemic areas due to the high rate of re-infection. Egg-count studies have shown that in cases where appropriate treatment does not achieve a full cure, egg production is nevertheless decreased by over 90%.

1. *Early reaction:* antihistamine ointment or tablets may help although they are usually unnecessary.
2. *Katayama fever:* treatment is difficult since most drugs do not affect the early migratory phase of the immature parasites. Give oral prednisolone to suppress the acute reaction, then praziquantel 75 mg/kg PO as a single dose.
3. *Chronic disease:*
   - **Praziquantel** — is effective against all schistosome species (as well as cestodes and other snail-borne trematodes). For most species, give 40 mg/kg PO as a single dose; for *S. japonicum* give 20 mg/kg PO tds for one day only; *S. mekongi* may require repeated doses. For CNS disease give 75 mg/kg. Paediatric dosage is the same. Cure rate is ~70%. If possible give the single doses after food.
   - **Oxamniquine** — is cheaper but only effective against *S. mansoni*. Give 15 mg/kg PO as a single dose in W. Africa and Brazil. In the rest of Africa, give 20 mg/kg PO od for 3 days.
   - **Metrifonate** — is used to treat *S. haematobium* infections. Give 7.5–10 mg/kg PO on 3 days, each 2 weeks apart.
4. *Surgical treatment is not recommended* — most seemingly irreversible lesions will eventually resolve, especially in the young. Even CNS disease may show resolution after treatment.

Toxocariasis

The canine roundworm — *Toxocara canis* — has a worldwide distribution. Although adult worms do not develop in humans, the larvae may persist for >10 years, causing toxocariasis, visceral larva migrans, and ocular disease.

Life cycle: eggs excreted in dog faeces (particularly from puppies) are ingested by humans. These hatch in the stomach, releasing larvae which penetrate the intestinal mucosa, entering the mesenteric blood vessels. They may remain in the visceral organs or pass into the general circulation and reach the brain, eye, and other organs.

Clinical features: symptoms depend upon the density of infection.
* *Visceral larva migrans:* inflammation and granulomatous reactions in heavy infections of the liver and other organs (e.g. lungs, brain) results in hepatomegaly, fever, or asthma. Severe cases may have cardiac dysfunction, nephrosis, fits, pareses, and transverse myelitis. The condition usually occurs in children. Most resolve within 2 years, although the disease can be fatal, particularly if the brain is involved.
* *Ocular toxocariasis:* subretinal granulomata and choroiditis closely resemble a retinoblastoma in the early stages and tend to occur in older age groups. Symptoms include strabismus and iridocyclitis with posterior synechiae. Toxocariasis is an important cause of decreased visual acuity in the tropics.
* *Infected children* often also harbour *Ascaris* and *Trichrurus* spp; 2° infection with gut bacteria carried by the larvae is common.

Diagnosis: history of exposure (particularly to puppies), eosinophilia, leukocytosis, reduced albumin:globulin ratio, raised IgG, IgM, anti-A and anti-B isohaemagglutinin titres. CXR may show mottling in lung disease. Larval demonstration is very difficult, though they are sometimes present at the centre of granulomatous lesions at biopsy or post mortem. ELISA tests for antigen are now available.

Management
1. Diethylcarbamazine 1 mg/kg PO initial dose, increased to 3 mg/kg PO tds for 3 weeks.
2. (Alternative: tiabendazole 25 mg/kg PO bd for 2 days, repeated after 2 days if necessary)
3. Steroids may be required for ocular disease.

Prevention: centres around elimination of the infective canine reservoir, with human treatment of symptomatic cases and education regarding child hygiene.

Hydatid disease

Echinococcus granulosus and *E. multilocularis* are responsible for causing cystic hydatid disease and alveolar hydatid disease, respectively.

Cystic hydatid disease

E. granulosus is a small (3–6 mm) cestode tapeworm that lives in the small intestine of dogs and occasionally other carnivores. Eggs passed in canine faeces are infective to humans; following ingestion, they develop into larvae which penetrate the intestinal mucosa and pass to target organs such as the liver (50%), lungs, and peritoneal cavity. There the larvae (oncospheres) mature and form an expanding, fluid-filled metacestode vesicle, or hydatid cyst. These may be multiple and reach massive proportions.

Clinical features: are usually due to the expansive growth of cysts and commonly include abdominal pain, hepatomegaly, fever, jaundice, and cholangitis. Rupture can be life-threatening and may be accompanied by anaphylactic shock, although conversely, cysts may disappear or collapse spontaneously.

Diagnosis: USS is usually sufficient. Because of the high risk of spreading protoscolices around the body, aspiration of cysts is not recommended. Serological and molecular tests are also available.

Management: cystectomy offers the best chance of cure. However, spillage of cystic contents at surgery causes disease to recur, so great care is needed. Chlorhexidine, hydrogen peroxide, ethanol, and cetrizamide can be used to sterilize the cyst before operation (formalin or hypertonic saline should no longer be used since they may cause tissue damage, hypernatraemia, and severe acidosis). Albendazole, mebendazole, and praziquantel are believed to be parasitostatic agents, though reliable data are still lacking. Use pre- and post-operatively is thought to give lower recurrence rates, but doses may need to be high (4.5 g/day mebendazole or 20 mg/kg/day albendazole) and for many months. Life expectancy in successfully operated patients is normal, though those presenting with complications (especially cholangitis) have significant mortality.

Alveolar hydatid disease

Alveolar hydatid disease is restricted to the northern hemisphere; it is not a tropical disease. *E. multilocularis* infects humans via their accidental ingestion of faeces from foxes or other canines. After digestion of the eggs, oncospheres penetrate the intestinal mucosa and passes to the liver (a few pass to other sites including the lungs and brain). Maturation produces a characteristic alveolar cyst. Patients present with abdominal pain, hepatomegaly, and sometimes cholangitis. Unlike *E. granulosus*, the cysts expand externally and invade surrounding tissue, resembling a malignant tumour. Metastatic spread occurs in ~10% of patients to CNS, lungs, bone, and eyes. Mortality untreated is high — >60% at 10 yrs. Surgery requires early presentation to be successful; mebendazole and albendazole may be beneficial but the data is not clear as yet.

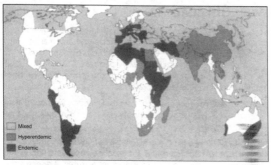

Fig. 7.13 Distribution of cystic hydatid disease.

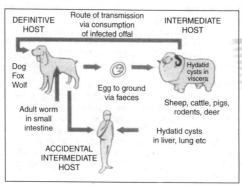

Fig. 7.14 Life cycle of *E. granulosus*.

Lower GI bleeding

Lower GI bleeding is seen less frequently than upper GI bleeding in the tropics, but tends to be more difficult to diagnose and manage. Patients present with haematochezia — red, maroon, or brownish stools — rather than haematemesis or melaena. Always perform a thorough abdominal and PR examination in any patient with rectal bleeding and exclude other pathology, even if haemorrhoids are present.

Causes: the most frequent causes of lower GI bleeding (without diarrhoea) are haemorrhoids, typhoid fever, non-specific ulcer, TB, neoplasms, amoebic ulcer, rarely angiodysplasia, diverticulosis, ulcerative colitis.

Diagnosis and management: initially consist of resuscitation as for upper GI haemorrhage. Then determine if it is acute or chronic (Hb will help). The history and examination may reveal other features of diseases such as typhoid fever or TB. The colour of the stool is the best indicator of the level at which the causative pathology lies; the darker the stool, the higher the cause. Rectal bleeding leaves bright red streaks of blood on the stool surface. Pass a NG tube if small bowel pathology is suspected; a bile-stained aspirate that is free of blood excludes an upper GI source. Use proctoscopy and sigmoidoscopy to examine the rectum and sigmoid colon. In many cases bleeding will cease with bed rest, IV fluid, and 24 hrs nil by mouth. Prolonged bleeding will necessitate further investigation (e.g. colonoscopy). The patient should be transferred to theatre for exploratory laparotomy if >6 units of blood are needed to replace that lost.

Diverticular disease

A diverticulum is a congenital or acquired outpouching of the gut wall. Most develop when raised intra-luminal pressures force the mucosa to herniate through the muscular layers of the gut wall and present with changed bowel habit, colicky RIF pain (relieved by defecation), and painless rectal bleeding. Diverticulae can become infected (diverticulitis), giving fever, raised WCC, ESR. Exclude typhoid fever. Treat with bed rest, high-fibre diet, and (if infected) antibiotics. Watch for signs of perforation (>40% mortality).

Colorectal carcinoma

Remains uncommon in the tropics. Aetiology includes high-fat, low-fibre diet, prolonged colonic transit time, polyposis coli, and ulcerative colitis. Tumours are annular, polypoid, or ulcerous and are staged using Duke's classification. Clinical features are frequently of a change in bowel habit, diarrhoea, blood/mucus PR, and tenesmus. A mass (commonly left-sided) may be felt. Late presentation may be with obstruction or perforation.

Diagnosis and management: faecal occult blood, +/− anaemia, pr, procto-colonoscopy with biopsy, where available. With complete surgical resection, the prognosis of Duke's A carcinoma resection is good.

Common causes of acute confusion/delirium at presentation (they may all progress to coma)

- CNS infection (malaria; meningitis — including TB meningitis; encephalitis; HIV-related infections
- Systemic infections
- Hypoxia
- Metabolic causes (e.g. hypoglycaemia, hyerglycaemia)
- Alcohol — excess or withdrawal
- Drugs
- Head injury/concussion
- Stroke
- Mental illness such as schizophrenia
- Raised intracranial pressure
- Epilepsy (post-ictal)

Coma

A persistent pathological state of unconsciousness. In the comatose patient immediately ensure a clear airway, check that they are breathing, establish haemodynamic stability, and check for life-threatening injuries.

Take a history from relatives or bystanders — did anyone see how the patient became unconscious? Is there any past medical history such as diabetes, alcohol abuse, or drug overdose that might explain the coma?

Examine the patient in an attempt to distinguish metabolic causes of coma from brainstem causes — see below. It is particularly important to identify coma due to brainstem compression since surgical relief of the enlarging mass may be urgently required. Use the Glasgow coma score (GCS) — see below.

Useful clinical features

- Fever   →   Meningitis or encephalitis
                       →   Cerebral malaria
                       →   Metabolic coma of infection
- Hypothermia   →   Hypothyroidism; hypothermic coma
- Hypertension   →   Coma may be due to stroke
- Hypotension   →   Shock
- Pallor, cyanosis   →   Metabolic disease
- Bleeding, bruising →   Head trauma

Progressive deterioration suggests brainstem compression.

Look for focal CNS signs. Search for asymmetry (e.g. in response to pain or in the face during expiration). If the response to pain is different, the side with lower response in the GCS is the side with hemiparesis.

Diagnosis

There are three broad categories.

1. Metabolic
   - Normal pupil responses
   - Normal or absent eye movements depending on the depth of coma
   - Suppressed, Cheyne–Stokes, or ketotic respiration
   - Symmetrical limb signs, usually hypotonic
2. Intrinsic brainstem disease
   From the outset there may be:
   - Abnormal pupil responses and eye movements
   - Abnormal respiratory pattern
   - Bilateral long tract signs
   - Cranial nerve signs
3. Extrinsic brainstem disease due to compression
   Papilloedema and hemiparesis **with progressive**
   - Loss of pupillary responses
   - Loss of eye movements
   - Abnormal respiratory pattern
   - Long tract signs

Management of an unconscious patient

1. **ABC:** ensure adequate airway, oxygenation, and circulation.
2. **Obtain a reliable history:** check for signs of injury or trauma especially to the head. Record the vital signs — temperature, pulse, BP, respiratory rate, O_2 saturations. Do a BM stick to determine blood glucose.
3. **Assess the level of coma:** use the Glasgow coma score (see box). Check for meningism, pupillary light reflex, corneal reflexes, fundi, and focal neurological signs in the limbs. Do brainstem reflexes, Doll's eye movements, and caloric tests if brain death is suspected.
4. **Investigate:** do the following — Hb, WCC, urea, electrolytes, glucose, calcium, liver enzymes, and arterial gases. Also do blood cultures if the patient is febrile, a malarial film if the patient is from an area endemic for malaria, a toxicology screen if it is an overdose or poisoning case, or a CSF examination if there is meningism (beware rising intracranial pressure). Do ECG, EEG; X-ray the skull and chest; CT/MRI the head if indicated and available.
5. **Determine the cause and treat:**
   - *Coma with focal signs* — e.g. subdural or extradural haematoma or SOL may require definitive neurosurgical drainage and steroids, mannitol, etc., to lower intracranial pressure.
   - *Coma without focal signs* — e.g. hypoglycaemia (give 50 ml of 50% glucose IV); opiate poisoning (give IV naloxone); cerebral malaria (give artemisinin derivatives if available or quinine); overdose (give gastric lavage and/or appropriate antidote).
   - *Coma and meningism* — e.g. meningitis or subarachnoid haemorrhage, treat with antibiotics.
6. **Care:** nurse in the ITU or high-dependency ward.
   - Monitor the level of consciousness using the GCS.
   - Determine pupillary size, equality, and response to light.
   - Check vital signs.
     These should all be done at regular fixed intervals varying from every 15 mins to every 4 hrs depending on the clinical situation. Pay special attention to respiration, circulation, skin, bladder, and bowels.

Prognosis: depends mainly on the cause, depth, and duration of the coma. The combination of the absence of the pupillary light reflex and corneal and brainstem reflexes at 24 hrs indicates a grave prognosis. The persistence of deep coma for greater than 72 hrs also has a poor prognosis.

Glasgow coma score (GCS)

Assess on admission and then at regular intervals to follow progress and predict prognosis.

Best motor response
6 Carries out request (obeys a command)
5 Localizes pain
4 Withdraws limb in response to pain
3 Flexes limb in response to pain
2 Extends limb in response to pain
1 Does not respond to pain

Best verbal response
5 Orientated in time and place
4 Responds with confused but understandable speech
3 Spontaneous speech but inappropriate and not responsive
2 Speech but incomprehensible
1 No speech

Eye opening
4 Opens eyes spontaneously
3 Opens eyes in response to speech
2 Opens eyes in response to pain
1 Does not open eyes

Add together the best response in each group. Roughly:
GCS 1–8 = serious injury
GCS 9–12 = moderate injury
GCS 13–15 = minor injury

A simpler version can also be useful:
A Alert
V Responds to *vocal* stimuli
P Responds to *pain*
U Unresponsive

Headache

The brain parenchyma is insensitive to pain. Headaches result from distension, traction, or inflammation of the cerebral blood vessels and dura mater. Pain is referred from the anterior and middle cranial fossae to the forehead and eye via the trigeminal nerve, and from the posterior fossa and upper cervical spine to the occiput and neck via the upper three cervical nerves. Both infratentorial and supratentorial masses can lead to frontal headaches by causing hydrocephalus.

Causes of a headache

1. *Acute meningeal irritation:* due to subarachnoid haemorrhage or meningitis caused by bacteria, viruses, fungi, or metastases.
2. *Rising intracranial pressure:* see p. 400.
3. *Many infectious diseases:* cause a headache during the acute phase. Locally important infections need to be determined (e.g. malaria; meningitis — including TB; trypanosomiasis; typhoid, arboviral and typhus fevers; fungal infections).
4. *Giant-cell arteritis:* may rapidly result in blindness. Occurs in elderly people. There may be a tender engorged occipital or temple artery; ESR is markedly raised. Temporal artery biopsy may confirm the diagnosis, but do not delay giving steroids while awaiting biopsy.
5. *Migraine:* headaches which occur at intervals (not daily) and are associated with N&V, anorexia, photophobia, phonophobia, and in 20% of cases visual, mood, sensory, or motor disturbances. Most individuals have their first attack while young. Identify and avoid precipitating factors; give analgesia (paracetamol, NSAIDs, or codeine) together with metoclopramide 10 mg (not in children). Ergotamine is useful in 50% of patients. Chemoprophylaxis may work for regular migraines.
6. *Tension headache:* most common cause of headache. It is normally a benign symptom due to an identifiable cause (e.g. overwork, family stress, lack of sleep, emotional crisis). It is often a daily occurrence unlike migraine headache, getting worse as the day goes on. Visual disturbances, vomiting, and photophobia do not occur. Management involves thorough examination and reassurance of its benign course, analgesia (usually paracetamol 1 g qds), and rest. Ask about drugs, caffeine, and alcohol. Amitriptyline starting at 10 mg at night, increasing by 10 mg each week until side-effects occur, is also often of benefit. Tension headaches may be part of a **depressive illness**. Check for other signs or symptoms such as mood change, loss of appetite, weight or libido, or a disturbed sleep pattern.
7. *Analgesia-induced headache:* follows long-term and inappropriate use of analgesia for headaches. History reveals increasing and frequent use of often multiple forms of analgesia. Management involves reassurance followed by stopping all forms of analgesia. The headache initially gets worse before improving.
8. *Others:*
   - Trauma
   - Cluster headaches
   - Hypertension
   - Drugs
   - Indometacin-sensitive headaches

Pain may be referred to the forehead and temple from the orbits, paranasal sinuses, teeth, skull or spine pathology, and venous sinuses.

The major responsibility of a physician faced with a patient with a headache is to exclude a treatable, structural or dynamic cause. Specifically exclude either a SOL or meningitis. Check for:

- Localizing signs
- Papilloedema
- Neck stiffness
- Rash

Raised intracranial pressure (↑ICP)

Clinical features: include
- *Headache:* often worse in the morning due to CO_2 retention during sleep → cerebrovascular dilatation, possibly waking the patient from sleep; made worse by coughing, straining, standing up; relieved by paracetamol in the early stages.
- *Alteration in the level of consciousness* (drowsiness).
- *Vomiting* (may relieve the headache; sometimes the 1st sign of raised ICP).
- *Hypertension, bradycardia.*

Failing vision and decreasing consciousness are ominous signs. Papilloedema is frequently *not* present.

Pathophysiology: initially, mechanisms such as reducing CSF volume allow the CNS to compensate for rising ICP as may occur with a slow-growing tumour. However, if the ICP continues to rise or if the increase is acute and the compensatory mechanisms overwhelmed, the brain often becomes laterally displaced and pushed towards the foramen magnum at the base of the skull. The medial temporal lobe (or uncus) is then forced down through the tentorial hiatus, or a cerebellar tonsil is forced through the foramen magnum, causing the brainstem to become compressed (coning). This produces the following progressive changes:
- Level of consciousness decreases, drowsiness → coma
- Pupils become dilated and unresponsive, initially on the side of the mass, then bilaterally
- Posture becomes decorticate, then decerebrate
- Slow deep breaths → Cheyne–Stokes breathing → apnoea

Beware of ipsilateral hemiparesis and VI cranial nerve palsy as false localizing signs.

Causes: SOL; cerebral oedema; hydrocephalus. The cerebral oedema may surround a tumour or result from infection (cerebral malaria, encephalitis), trauma, or hypoxic cell death.

Management: if possible, establish the cause with a CT/MRI scan.
1. Sit the patient up at ~30–40° to increase venous drainage from the brain
2. Ensure adequate oxygenation — ventilate if necessary
3. Give mannitol 5 ml/kg of a 20% solution IV over 15–30 mins to reduce cerebral oedema
   - In severe oedema, dexamethasone 12–16 mg IV stat by slow IV injection may also be used
   - If less severe oedema, give dexamethasone 4 mg IM q6h
4. If the patient has a positive malaria blood film, see Chapter 2A for management of cerebral malaria
5. Control seizures if present
6. If a SOL is believed to be responsible, refer to a neurosurgeon. If the ICP progresses rapidly, urgent decompression with burr holes may be life-saving — see p. 426

Acute pyogenic (bacterial) meningitis

A multitude of microbes — bacteria, viruses, parasites, and fungi — can cause meningitis. However, bacterial meningitis is the most important since it has a high fatality rate and is readily treatable. All febrile patients with a history of headache should be examined for signs of meningism.

Aetiology

In children and adults, bacterial meningitis is frequently due to:
- *Neisseria meningitidis*   (Gram −ve intracellular diplococci)
- *Haemophilus influenzae* B (Hib)   (Gram −ve rods)
- *Streptococcus pneumoniae*   (Gram +ve capsulated diplococci)

Meningococcus causes epidemics (see p. 404), while previous head injury, sinusitis, otitis media, or pneumonia predispose to pneumococcal meningitis. Hib meningitis is most common in children <5yrs. Other bacteria are less common (e.g. *S. aureus*, *Pseudomonas* spp) or occur in particular groups or regions (e.g. *Streptococcus suis* in S.E. Asia; Group B streptococci and *E. coli* in neonates; *Listeria* in pregnant women, immunosuppressed, and neonates). **TB meningitis** is also an important cause of meningitis — see p. 406 and Chapter 2C.

Clinical features: there is sudden onset of intense headache, fever, N&V, photophobia, and stiff neck. Cardinal signs of meningism are:
- *Neck stiffness* — passively flex the head (chin towards chest); this results in pain and resistance in a patient with meningism.
- *Kernig's sign* — passively straighten the leg with hip flexed (>90°); this causes pain and resistance by stretching inflamed nerve roots.

Neurological signs are not normally focal in pyogenic meningitis and include: lethargy, delirium, coma, convulsions. Lower cranial nerve palsies and retention of urine is common in TB meningitis. Acute complications include raised ICP, seizures, sepsis, paralysis, SIADH.

Check the skin (particularly on the back, buttocks, and soles of the feet) and conjunctivae carefully for purpura. This is associated with meningococcal septicaemia which can be rapidly fatal. If present, treat for meningococcal infection immediately.

Diagnosis: blood cultures (1. insert cannula; 2. take out blood for culture; 3. immediately administer antibiotics through cannula if there is clinical suspicion of meningococcal septicaemia); lumbar puncture (if there is no evidence of SOL or raised ICP) for CSF examination. Take blood for FBC, U&E, (and malarial parasites).

Prognosis: mortality varies with age and organism. Perinatal, neonatal, and childhood mortality varies from 50–80%. Similarly, mortality is increased in old age. In adults, mortality with pneumococcus is 30–40%, *Haemophilus* 20–30%, meningococcus 10–15% (much higher with septicaemia). The main long-term complications include paralysis, deafness, visual loss, epilepsy, and mental retardation.

Management
1. On suspicion, give immediate antibiotics — see below.
2. Give supportive measures: fluids, oxygen, maintain normal electrolytes, generous pain relief, and tepid sponging to reduce temperature.
3. IV dexamethasone 0.4 mg/kg 12 hrly × 2 days is generally recommended for adults and children with acute bacterial meningitis in developed countries. But a very large recent study from Malawi suggests steroids confer no benefit in the treatment of bacterial meningitis in childhood.

Initial empiric antibiotic regimens for presumed bacterial meningitis in adults
Choose one of:
1. Benzylpenicillin 2.4 g (4 mega units) IV q4h for 10–14 days *and/or* Chloramphenicol 12.5–25 mg/kg or 1 g IV q6h for 10 days
2. Ceftriaxone 1–2 g IV q2h for 7–10 days
3. Ampicillin 2 g IV q6h for 10 days

Local recommendations based on antibiotic sensitivity:
1.
2.
3.

Chloramphenicol

The WHO reaffirms the value of chloramphenicol in infections such as meningitis and severe bacterial infections due to bacteria resistance to other antibiotics.

Chloramphenicol has one serious toxicity — aplastic anaemia. Estimates of frequency are 1 in 10,000 to 1 in 70,000 courses of therapy (which are similar to estimates of death due to penicillin anaphylaxis: 1 in 40,000 courses). The WHO's Expert Committee on the Use of Essential Drugs, after due consideration of the risks and benefits of chloramphenicol, concluded that it is essential for modern medical practice in all countries.

Epidemic meningococcal disease

There are at least 9 different serogroups of Meningococci, of which three — groups A, B, and C — cause outbreaks of meningitis. Serogroup A meningococcus is the most important. It is responsible for the explosive epidemics that continue to devastate sub-Saharan Africa on an almost annual basis. It is also the main cause of endemic meningitis in this area of Africa with rates that are higher than the epidemic rates in other parts of the world. Types A and C have both been responsible for large outbreaks in the rest of the world.

Some strains of meningococci appear to be more virulent than others. Large epidemics occur when such strains encounter populations of non-immune individuals in areas of poverty during particular climatic conditions (e.g. dry season, dust storm). In between epidemics, the bacteria survive in the community in the nasopharynx of carriers.

Vaccination: is essential for stopping an epidemic once it has begun. Kits for such campaigns are available from the WHO. Advice on organizing a campaign is also given in a WHO book — see below.

Chemoprophylaxis: only for household contacts of cases: rifampicin 600 mg (10 mg/kg for a child, 5 mg/kg for children <1 yr) PO bd for 2 days. (Alternatives: spiramycin 1 g PO bd (child: 25 mg/kg) PO bd for 5 days or ciprofloxacin 500 mg PO as a single dose.)

Viral meningitis

Enteroviruses, such as echo and coxsackie viruses, are important causes of epidemic viral meningitis worldwide, while arboviruses cause sporadic disease in endemic regions. Other causes of sporadic viral meningitis include polio, mumps virus, EB virus, HIV, varicella-zoster virus, CMV, and HSV.

Clinical features are similar to bacterial meningitis but the headache is less severe and the neck less stiff. It is diagnosed by examination of CSF. The identity of the causative virus during epidemics may already be clear. In sporadic cases, peripheral signs may suggest the aetiology such as genital or rectal lesions (HSV), skin blisters (herpes zoster), orchitis (mumps, lymphocytic choriomeningitis virus), rashes (enterovirus), parotid swelling (mumps). The prognosis is usually good, with complete resolution.

Other causes of meningitis
- Mycobacteria — *M. tuberculosis* (see Chapter 2C and below)
- Fungi — *Cryptococcus neoformans*, *Candida albicans*
- Parasites — *Naegleria*

For details on setting up a surveillance system and organizing the logistics of a mass vaccination campaign, see the following book: *Control of epidemic meningococcal disease: WHO practical guidelines* (Edition Fondation Marcel Merieux, 1995). Available from the WHO.

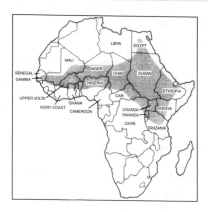

Fig. 8.1

Chronic meningitis

TB meningitis or *Cryptococcus neoformans* (also: disseminated fungal infections; cysticercosis in children) typically present with a longer history (>7 days), headache, and low-grade fever. Confusion and drowsiness are common and may be due to hydrocephalus. Papilloedema, visual symptoms, and cranial nerve lesions (particularly VI, VII, and urinary retention) may occur. Signs of infection at other sites (e.g. lungs) may also be found.

Diagnosis: the cause can be determined by examination of CSF; subsequently treat for the relevant infection. Both cryptococcal and TB meningitis occur commonly in immunosuppressed patients, particularly AIDS, but they also occur in previously healthy individuals. See Chapters 2B and 2C.

Eosinophilic meningoencephalitis

Follows CNS infection with the nematodes *Angiostrongylus cantonensis*, *Gnathostoma spinigerum*, or *T solium* (causing cysticercosis, see p. 434)

Angiostrongyliasis — results from the ingestion of infected snails or contaminated shrimps, fish, and vegetables. The larvae migrate to the brain where they induce an immune response to dead parasites and then to the eyes and lungs. Initial presentation is of acute, intermittent intense headache without fever; malaise; N&V; cranial nerve palsies; in some, meningism. If severe, there may be fever, decreasing GCS, and spinal cord involvement. The eyes are commonly involved.

Management: do not give antihelminthics since dying parasites elicit a strong immune reaction that can be fatal. It is normally a self-resolving condition — give sedatives, analgesia; the headache responds well to LP every 3–7 days. Eye involvement requires surgery to remove the nematode. Corticosteroids may help in severe disease.

Spinocerebral gnathostomiasis — frequently presents with intensely painful radiculitis followed by **rapidly advancing** myelitis → paraplegia with urinary retention or quadriplegia, or as a cerebral haemorrhage in a previously healthy person.

Primary amoebic meningoencephalitis (PAM)

PAM is a rare but frequently fatal infection that follows intranasal infection with *Naegleria fowleri* while swimming in warm fresh water. The amoebae invade the CNS through the cribriform plate and cause extensive tissue necrosis. Headache occurs first, then fever, meningism, coma, convulsions. The patients are seriously ill. The CSF shows neutrophils, red cells, and amoebae on **wet microscopy**. The prognosis is poor. *Acanthamoeba* cause a similar syndrome, granulomatous amoebic encephalitis (GAE), in immunosuppressed individuals.

Management: amphotericin B 1 mg/kg IV. Also give amphotericin intrathecally (via a reservoir) – start with 0.025 mg, then increase to 0.25–1 mg (TOTAL, not per kg) on alternate days.

Table 8.1

Cause	Normal CSF	Pyogenic Bacteria	TB	PAM	Virus	Cryptococcus
Appearance	Clear and colourless	Cloudy or purulent	Clear, yellowish, slightly cloudy	Clear or slightly cloudy	Clear	Clear or slightly cloudy
White cells (majority)	<5/mm³	>200/mm³ (neutrophils)	>10/mm³ (mononuclear)	>200/mm³ (neutrophils)	>10/mm³ (mononuclear)	>10/mm³ (mononuclear)
Glucose	2.5–4 mmol/l (45–72 mg%)	Markedly ↓ or absent	Low	Normal or slightly ↓	Normal	Low
Total protein	0.15–0.4 g/l	Raised	Raised	Normal or slightly ↓	Raised	Raised
Microscopy	None	Gram: pus	Ziehl–Neelsen: AFB present	Wet: motile amoebae	None	India ink+

Encephalitis

Virus infection of the brain parenchyma is termed encephalitis. It is characterized by impairment of cerebral function, in contrast to meningeal infection that does not involve actual brain tissue.

Epidemics of encephalitis occur seasonally in many parts of the world and are important causes of death and disability in the young and elderly. The equine encephalitides have recently caused widespread epidemics in South America. Herpes simplex virus encephalitis (HSV) is the most important cause of sporadic encephalitis worldwide since it is treatable and therefore should be considered in all cases. However, Japanese encephalitis far outstrips HSV in actual numbers.

Clinical features: high fever, headache, N&V, followed by convulsions, confusion, and changes in level of consciousness. Some patients also present with meningism, focal neurological signs, abnormal behaviour, and/or raised ICP. Severe cases result in prolonged coma, hemiparesis, dystonia, decorticate or decerebrate posturing, and respiratory failure. Neurological sequelae such as mental retardation, hemiparesis, and behavioural abnormalities are particularly common after Japanese encephalitis, untreated HSV encephalitis, and post-infectious/vaccination encephalomyelitis.

Diagnosis: is via lumbar puncture. LP is contraindicated if there is evidence of raised ICP or focal signs.

Management: except for HSV encephalitis (see below), management is supportive with careful control of seizures (using phenytoin) and pyrexia. Beware respiratory failure and raised ICP (p. 400). The effectiveness of corticosteroids in preventing cerebral oedema is unclear.

Post-infectious or post-vaccination encephalomyelitis

On rare occasions, infection or vaccination elicits an antiviral immune response that results in CNS immunopathology and an encephalitic picture. It usually occurs after infection with measles, rubella, herpes zoster, mumps, and influenza and after vaccination with the Semple form of the rabies vaccine, but the relative risk is very small compared with the benefits of vaccination.

Herpes simplex virus (HSV) encephalitis

HSV encephalitis should be considered in the differential diagnosis of any patient presenting with an encephalitic picture. Focal signs relate to the frontal and temporal cortices and limbic system. It is particularly important since it is the only encephalitis for which there is effective treatment.

Management: aciclovir 10 mg/kg q8h by slow IV infusion for 10–14 days. Untreated HSV encephalitis has a mortality rate of 40–70% and many survivors have neurological sequelae. Aciclovir markedly decreases mortality and the incidence of sequelae.

Japanese encephalitis

A common arboviral encephalitis of E., S., and S.E. Asia. Historically, it has been an infection of young children in wet season epidemics coincident with abundance of its mosquito vector. Widespread childhood vaccination campaigns in some countries have reduced the incidence of clinical disease. West Nile is a very closely related virus that causes encephalitis in parts of Africa and C. Europe and has recently spread to the USA.

Transmission: is via the bite of the *Culex tritaeniorhynchus* mosquito. The virus's primary hosts are birds such as herons, from which it is passed to domestic pigs by mosquitoes. It is amplified in these pigs before transmission to humans (a dead-end host). Most infections are subclinical — ~1 in 300 infections results in encephalitis.

Clinical features: after an incubation period of 6–16 days and a non-specific prodrome illness lasting a couple of days, the sudden onset of fever is accompanied by severe headache, meningism, N&V, and hyperexcitability, or decreased consciousness. Seizures are common in children. Neurological signs such as cranial nerve palsies, tremor and ataxia, parkinsonism, and upper limb paralysis develop. Together with a lowered consciousness level, they follow a variable course. Around 25% of patients die; many survivors have serious long-term neuropsychiatric disabilities (e.g. parkinsonism, paralysis, mental retardation). Spontaneous abortion and fetal death may occur in pregnant women. Japanese encephalitis virus is now a recognized cause of acute flaccid paralysis.

Equine encephalitides

Three alphaviruses — Western, Eastern, and Venezuelan equine encephalitis viruses (EEVs) — cause widespread epizootics of encephalitis in horses in the USA, C. America, and the northern regions of S. America. The EEVs are not common causes of human encephalitis, but VEEV has recently caused large epidemics in both horses and humans in Colombia and Venezuela. The virus is amplified during horse infections and may subsequently cause human encephalitis.

Transmission: rodents and birds are the primary hosts of these viruses; transmission to humans is via *Culex, Culiseta,* and *Aedes* mosquitoes.

Clinical features: most infections are subclinical. Some may manifest as a short febrile illness with rigors (in VEEV also: sore throat, features of URTI, and diarrhoea). In a few cases, the illness is biphasic: recovery from the febrile illness is followed by encephalitis. Adults do not normally have sequelae; in contrast, many young children and infants are left with permanent neurological effects after encephalitis. Mortality is high (~10%) in this group.

Rabies

A uniformly fatal infection, still common in many parts of the tropics, that is caused by the rabies virus (or, very rarely, a related lyssavirus). Once clinical symptoms have appeared, the patient will die. However, if the infection is caught soon after transmission and before the onset of clinical symptoms, rabies can be prevented by post-exposure vaccination. Increasing availability and affordability of vaccines and increasing their uptake by rural populations is pivotal in controlling rabies.

Transmission: is by the bite of an infected mammal, most commonly stray dogs (but also wild dogs, wolves, foxes, cats, and skunks) in endemic regions. The virus does not pass though intact skin; however, infected saliva can infect already damaged skin (e.g. by dogs' claws) and mucosae. Bites by vampire bats and inhalation of virus in bat-filled caves are methods of transmission in central and south America.

Clinical features: after an incubation period that normally lasts 20–90 days, prodromal symptoms develop: itching, pain, or paraesthesia at the site of the bite; followed by fever, chills, malaise, weakness, headache, and neuropsychiatric symptoms. Furious or paralytic rabies develops depending on the major locus of infection.

- *Furious (brain) rabies:* the pathognomic feature is hydrophobia — inspiratory muscle spasm (arched, extended back with arms thrown up) +/− laryngeal spasm, associated with terror. While initially stimulated by attempts to drink water or wash, it soon becomes provoked by many stimuli. It may end in convulsions with cardiorespiratory arrest. Other features include: hyperaesthesia; generalized arousal (lucid periods alternating with wild, hallucinating, or aggressive periods); cranial nerve defects; meningism; involuntary movements; ANS/hypothalamic changes — hypersalivation, lachriymation, ↑ or ↓ BP and temperature, SIADH, diabetes insipidus.
- *Paralytic (spine) rabies:* prodromal symptoms are followed by flaccid paralysis that ascends symmetrically or asymmetrically from the bitten area, pain, fasciculation, sensory disturbances; paraplegia and loss of sphincter control; ultimately, paralysis of muscles of respiration and swallowing.

Complications include: aspiration and bronchopneumonia; pneumonitis and myocarditis; pneumothorax after inspiratory spasms; cardiac arrhythmias; haematemesis; rarely, ↑ICP.

Diagnosis: history of dog or bat bite plus neurological features; immunofluorescence of viral antigen in base of hair roots in skin biopsy; isolation of virus from body fluids during 1st week.

Prevention: controlling the mammalian reservoir through vaccination; decreasing human exposure to infected mammals; vaccination of persons at high risk and those bitten by mammals post-exposure vaccination. See p. 412

Nipah virus encephalitis

Nipah virus has recently caused an outbreak of encephalitis in Malaysia and Singapore. The causative agent was a new paramyxovirus named *Nipah*, closely related to the *Hendra* virus described in Australia, and potentially a new genus. The Nipah virus is a zoonosis infecting pigs and almost all patients infected in this outbreak had direct contact with pigs. There is no specific treatment

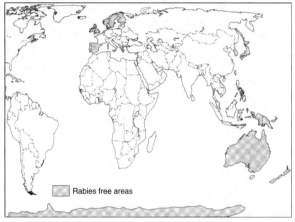

Rabies free areas

Fig. 8.2 Worldwide distribution of rabies.

Management of rabies infection

There is currently no effective treatment for a person who is showing signs and symptoms of rabies infection. In this situation, management is symptomatic with sufficient sedation and analgesia to relieve pain and terror. ITU care will prolong life by preventing or controlling complications.

Post-exposure prophylaxis

Vaccination within days of exposure is 100% effective in preventing the progression of the infection to encephalitis. However, the cheap Semple vaccine that is used most widely in the developing world is itself capable of initiating encephalitis. It is made by isolating virus from infected sheep's brains. Unfortunately, an immune response to sheep CNS components left in the vaccine can produce severe CNS disease with a 3% mortality.

Recent efforts to make the safer, tissue culture-grown, vaccine more affordable have involved using small doses intradermally (ID). Studies with such regimens have shown that they induce an immune response extremely quickly and that patients require fewer clinic visits. The regimens have been found to be 100% effective and without major side-effects.

Procedure: see box
- *Clean the wound* — this kills virus in superficial wounds. Scrub wound with soap/detergent and wash under running water for >5 mins. Liberally apply virucidal agent: 40–70% alcohol, 0.01% aqueous iodine. Debride as required.
- *Give anti-tetanus toxoid;* consider antibiotic cover.
- *Give vaccine.* The various regimens are below.
- *Give immunoglobulin* if possible, either human RIG 20 IU/kg or equine RIG 40 IU/kg. In the latter case, have drugs already drawn up to treat an anaphylactic reaction.

Vaccine regimens

Sheep brain vaccine (Semple) Give 2–5 mls of vaccine SC into the abdominal wall daily for 14–21 days. Boosters should be given after the course is finished.

Tissue culture vaccines
1. *2-site intradermal method (2–2–2–0–1–1)*
Days 0, 3, and 7:   0.1 or 0.2 ml ID at each of 2 sites (deltoids)
Days 28 and 90:   0.1 or 0.2 ml ID at 1 site (deltoid)
2. *8-site intradermal method (8–0–4–0–1–1)*
Day 0:   0.1 ml ID into 8 sites (2× deltoids, suprascapulum, lower quadrant abdominal wall, thighs)
Day 7:   0.1 ml ID into 4 sites (2× deltoids, thighs)
Day 28:   0.1 ml ID into 1 site
Day 91:   0.1 ml ID into 1 site
ID regimens require the use of Mantoux-like syringes and must cause a raised macule to appear immediately (like BCG vaccination).

Minor exposure
(including licks of broken skin, scratches, or abrasions without bleeding)
- Start vaccine immediately.
- Stop treatment if the dog remains healthy for 10 days.
- Stop treatment if dog's brain proves negative for rabies by appropriate Ix.

Major exposure
(including licks of mucosa and minor or major bites)
- Immediate rabies IG and vaccine.
- Stop treatment if dog remains healthy for 10 days.
- Stop treatment if dog's brain proves negative for rabies by appropriate Ix.

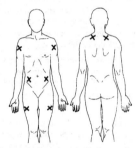

Fig. 8.3 Sites for the 8-site intradermal method of post-exposure vaccination. The use of multiple sites ensures that as many groups of lymph nodes are activated as possible, enhancing the immune response

Tetanus

Contamination of a wound with the bacterium *Clostridium tetani* can result in the production of a powerful exotoxin. This toxin tracks back up the nerves innervating local muscles, entering the CNS. The toxin also enters the blood and passes to other muscles where it is again transported back up peripheral nerves to the CNS. There it blocks the release of inhibitory neurotransmitters, resulting in widespread activation of both motor and autonomic nervous systems. Muscles of the jaw, face, and head are involved first because of the shorter axonal paths, but all muscle groups become involved in most cases. Activation of opposing groups results in rigidity. Protracted uncontrolled muscular spasms of the chest result in ineffective breathing and hypoxia. Death is due to respiratory complications, circulatory failure, or cardiac arrest.

Tetanus is easily prevented by vaccination: its incidence worldwide is directly related to the prevalence of immunization — where immunization rates are high, tetanus is a rare disease; where immunization rates are low, it is a common condition, particularly of neonates who become infected at birth. Immunization of pregnant women prevents neonatal tetanus. Currently ~800,000 people die each yr.

Transmission: *C. tetani* spores are ubiquitous in the environment and can infect even the most trivial cuts, typically on feet, legs, hands, and feet. Neonatal infection occurs via the cut umbilicus from the use of a dirty knife or the practice of applying dung to the stump.

Clinical features

There is an incubation period of 7–10 days, but this is variable and many patients cannot recall the injury. The ***period of onset*** is between the first symptom and the onset of spasms; it varies between 1 to 7 days and is a good prognostic indicator — the shorter the interval, the more severe the disease.

The first symptom is often stiffness of the masseters producing difficulty in opening the mouth — trismus. As the condition progresses, other muscle groups become rigid, including muscles of the face (producing characteristic look — risus sardonicus), skeleton (→ difficulty in breathing; opisthotonos; rigid limbs), and swallowing (→ aspiration).

Spasms are an exaggeration of the underlying rigidity and occur in more severe disease either as a reflex response to stimuli (touch, sounds, sights, emotions) or spontaneously. They may be mild and brief, or prolonged and very painful. Prolonged thoracic spasms may result in respiratory failure; laryngeal spasms in death from anoxia. In severe disease, the patient has a fever, tachycardia, and an unstable CVS, mostly due to involvement of the autonomic nervous system — see box.

Neonatal cases present with inability to suckle; they go on to develop characteristic opisthotonos.

Diagnosis: can be made on clinical features alone.

Prevention: by active vaccination of children and pregnant women (see Chapter 00); good wound toilet and passive vaccination following injuries; and provision of clean facilities for childbirth.

Grading of tetanus severity

- **Grade I (mild):** mild to moderate trismus; general spasticity; no respiratory problems; no spasms; little or no dysphagia.
- **Grade II (moderate):** moderate trismus; well-marked rigidity; mild to moderate but short-lasting spasms; moderate respiratory failure with tachypnoea >30–35/min; mild dysphagia.
- **Grade III (severe):** severe trismus; generalized spasticity; reflex and often spontaneous prolonged spasms; respiratory failure with tachypnoea >40/min; apnoeic spells; severe dysphagia; tachycardia >120/min.
- **Grade IV (very severe):** features of grade III plus violent autonomic disturbances involving the CVS. These include: episodes of severe hypertension and tachycardia alternating with relative hypotension and bradycardia; severe persistent hypertension (diastolic >110 mmHg); severe persistent hypotension (systolic <90).

Complications

- **Respiratory** collapse; aspiration, lobar, or bronchopneumonia (often due to Gram −ve organisms); anoxia due to prolonged laryngeal spasm; severe hypoxia and respiratory failure in severe tetanus if patient is not paralysed and ventilated; unexplained tachypnoea and respiratory distress; ARDS. Complications also include those of tracheostomy and prolonged ventilation.
- **CVS** (mostly mediated by ANS): persistent tachycardia, hypotension or hypertension; labile hypertension; severe peripheral vasoconstriction → shock-like state. Autonomic storms are characterized by sudden sinus tachycardia + severe hypertension followed by sudden bradycardia and hypotension; they may precede cardiac arrest. Increased vagal tone is shown by sudden bradycardia — sucking out of the trachea may lead to an arrest. Dysrhythmias include: SVT; junctional rhythms; atrial and ventricular ectopics; short bursts of self-resolving VT. Hyperthermia (hypothermia is very rare).
- **Sudden death** caused by many of the above complications, massive PE, or unidentified event.
- **Sepsis** most commonly iatrogenic.
- **Renal insufficiency.**
- **Mid-thoracic vertebral fracture** occurs during severe spasms; there are usually few sequelae and healing occurs without incident.

Management of tetanus

Management of severe tetanus can be extremely difficult, particularly in the open ward where conservative management has an appalling mortality rate. Ideally, ALL patients should be treated in an ITU setting.

However, careful management of the patient with particular attention to critical care and ventilatory support can markedly improve the prognosis where an ITU is not available.

If ventilators are limited, they should be kept for patients with:
- Grade IV disease
- Grade III disease uncontrolled by sedatives
- Serious respiratory complications

Give immediate care on admission (see box). Subsequent management depends on the severity of the condition.

Grade I — beware complications of septic wound. *Observe carefully* since grade I tetanus can progress to more severe disease. For sedation/muscle relaxation, give diazepam 5 mg PO tds (neonatal dose 2 mg PO tds). Alternative: chlorpromazine 50 mg (adult), 25 mg (child), or 12.5 mg (neonate) IM qds (phenobarbital can be added if essential).

Grade II — as for grade I but increase sedation/muscle relaxation. Increase dose of diazepam up to 4-fold in adults (do not exceed 80–100 mg/day because of respiratory depression). Give by slow IV infusion over 24 hrs.

The ideal sedative/muscle-relaxant schedule ensures continuous sedation such that the patient can sleep but can be woken up to obey commands. An objective guide is relaxation of abdominal muscles.

Perform a tracheostomy (may prevent death due to prolonged laryngeal spasm and anoxia). If laryngeal spasm occurs, promptly give chlorpromazine 50 mg IV (alternative: diazepam 10–20 mg IV).

Grade III — treat as for grade II but also paralyse and ventilate. Reduce diazepam dose to 30–40 mg over 24 hrs. Give pancuronium 2–4 mg (poorer alternative: gallamine 20–40 mg) IV, titrated for each patient to give sufficient neuromuscular blockade for efficient ventilation. Initially, give every 0.5–1 h (1st 1–2 wks), then extend interval as the patient improves. Check with periodic arterial blood analysis, if available. Spasms still occur under paralysis but they need not affect ventilation; pancuronium can be stopped when spasms cease. Continue ventilation until patient can be weaned off.

Grade IV — as above, with addition of drugs that act on the CVS if deemed *essential* for grossly deranged haemodynamics.
- Hypotension — give volume load; if ineffective or CI, use dopamine to keep systolic BP >100 mmHg.
- Hypertension (systolic >200, diastolic >100 mmHg) — propranolol 5–10 mg PO or nifedipine 5 mg sublingual.
- Bradyarrhythmia or persistent tachyarrhythmias.

Management on admission

All patients should receive:
- **Antiserum (antitoxin)** — preferably human tetanus immunoglobulin 150 units kg IM; otherwise equine antiserum 10,000 units by slow IV injection, but **beware anaphylactic reactions**. Some believe that a sensitivity test should be done first, but anaphylactic reactions can occur after a negative sensitivity test. Therefore it may be better to expect anaphylactic reactions in all patients receiving equine antiserum and have treatment ready drawn up in syringes.
- **Antibiotics** — metronidazole 500 mg IV q8h for 7–10 days (poorer alternative: benzylpenicillin 1.2 g IM or IV q8h for 8 days).
- **Local infiltration of antiserum** — is of uncertain efficacy but is recommended in some parts of the world.
- **Wound toilet** — performed after other steps, to remove necrotic tissue. Delay suturing.
- **Vaccination** — before discharge.

Critical care and nursing is essential

- Reduce external stimuli — physical examination must be gentle.
- Keep airway patent — use **gentle** suction to remove saliva and secretions at the back of the throat.
- Take exquisite care of the tracheostomy.
- Gently and frequently change the patient's posture.
- Use physiotherapy to keep lungs patent — give a small IV bolus of diazepam before physiotherapy. In the paralysed patient, perform physiotherapy when the action of pancuronium (gallamine) is at its maximum.
- Keep up patient's nutrition: 3500–4000 calories (including >100 g protein) by NG tube is required each day.

Overall aims of care

- Maintain adequate arterial PaO_2 and O_2 saturation.
- Maintain fluid, electrolyte, and acid-base balance.
- Maintain circulatory support in grade IV hypotensive patient. A central venous line is very useful if available.
- Prevent, detect, and promptly treat any infection.
- Detect early hyperpyrexia — treat with paracetamol and wet cloths.

Stroke

A rapidly developing episode of focal loss of cerebral function which lasts more than 24 hrs in a person with no history of recent head injury. In the industrialized world, most are due to cerebral infarction after a thrombotic or embolic event (~80%). The situation may differ in the developing world — see box. Around 20% of stroke patients die within the first month; strokes due to intracranial haemorrhages have a higher fatality rate than those following cerebral infarction.

Transient ischaemic attacks (TIAs) — are defined as an acute loss of focal cerebral or monocular function that lasts less than 24 hours. They are believed to be embolic events that are transient such that they produce ischaemia rather than infarction. They indicate that the person is at increased risk of a stroke (~5%/yr) and death due to thromboembolic events such as stroke or MI (~10%/yr).

Risk factors: include hypertension, ischaemic heart disease, atrial fibrillation, TIAs, peripheral vascular disease, DM, and smoking.

Clinical features: the neurological deficits are varied but commonly come on rapidly. It may be possible to relate the clinical features to the known anatomy of particular cerebral blood vessels but collateral blood supply makes this difficult. Infarcts affecting the cerebral hemisphere may cause contralateral hemiparesis (→ upper motor neurone paralysis after initial spinal shock), sensory loss, homonymous hemianopia, and/or dysphasia. Infarcts affecting subcortical structures such as thalamus and basal ganglia can cause mixed or isolated motor and/or sensory defects or ataxia. Brainstem infarcts can have profound affects: quadriplegia, visual and/or respiratory problems, locked-in syndrome. There is often a transient hypertension that settles.

Management: it is essential to ***think about rehabilitation*** early in the patient's illness. Do not ignore this issue until the patient has developed joint contractures that will prevent physical recovery.
- Give aspirin 150 mg daily if cerebral haemorrhage can be excluded.
- Take great care of the airway in the unconscious patient. Turn the patient often to avoid bedsores.
- Ensure adequate nutrition and hydration.
- Slowly and carefully lower very high BP (>130 diastolic; >240 systolic).
- If there is an identified source of thromboemboli (other than endocarditis), anticoagulate as for a DVT.
- Check for treatable causes such as giant-cell arteritis.
- Watch out for causes of neurological deterioration — see box.
- If there is evidence of cerebral oedema, consider giving mannitol.

Prevention: recovery for most patients is rarely complete and primary prevention is important. Reduce the risk of strokes by controlling risk factors, particularly hypertension and smoking, in individuals and populations. In patients who have had TIAs or previous strokes, it is important to control hypertension and reduce the chance of further thrombotic events by giving aspirin 75 mg PO od. Assuming no contraindications, anticoagulation is required for patients with AF, clotting disorders, or recurrent DVT.

Main causes of stroke in sub-Saharan Africa

- Hypertension (haemorrhagic stroke)
- Atherosclerosis (thrombotic stroke)
- Rheumatic heart disease (embolic)
- Others: Haemoglobinopathies
          HIV
          Subarachnoid haemorrhage
          Unexplained (mainly young persons)

Causes of neurological deterioration after stroke

- *Local* — extension of thrombus; recurrent embolism or haemorrhage; haemorrhagic transformation of the infarct; post-haemorrhage vasoconstriction; further ischaemia; cerebral oedema; brain shift and herniation; hydrocephalus; epileptic seizures.
- *General* — hypoxia (pneumonia, PE, cardiac failure); hypotension; infection; dehydration; hyponatraemia; hypoglycaemia or hyperglycaemia; drugs; depression.

Stroke rehabilitation

Without rehabilitation and physiotherapy, the patient risks spending the rest of her/his days in a wheelchair or bedbound. It is essential to start physiotherapy as soon as the patient is medically stable, to give the best chance of regaining hand and arm function and of walking. Aim to regain independence.

- Rehabilitation is a 24-hr process. Good work during the day can be ruined by a night spent sleeping in a bad position. It may be useful to teach the patient's relatives the basics of physiotherapy so that they can both look out for bad positioning and help the patient perform exercises.
- Initially, encourage the patient to participate in therapy for about 20 mins., 3 times a day. This can be increased with time.
- The patient needs regular turning to prevent bed sores (q4h).
- Physiotherapy should NEVER be painful. The expression 'no pain, no gain' has no place in rehabilitation.

General guidelines

- The stroke patient initially has decreased tone. At the beginning, therefore, rehabilitation attempts to increase power in the limbs. However, over time the tone may increase so much that the patient's limbs become spastic with fixed deformities. A hand left bunched up and curled under the arm is useless. Gentle repetitive exercises should be able to reduce the tone. Work on the opposite movements to those that cause the hand to bunch up: extension at the shoulder, elbow, wrist, and fingers.
- Normal movement is easier if the person is completely relaxed. This is accomplished by supporting the whole body as in Fig. 8.4.
- The aim of stroke rehabilitation is for normal movement. Some patients will neglect one side — ensure that the patient is able to see both arms and hands at all times. Reinforce the message that they are symmetrical. The patient can practise doing actions with weak limbs (e.g. picking up a cup, stepping from one foot to the other while sitting) by carefully noting the action with the normal limb, and then copying this with the weak limb.

Repetition of a movement over a period reinforces plastic adaptation. After a stroke, the brain has to relearn how to do things. It needs to practise. However, repetition can strengthen both bad and good habits, so it is essential to get the practised movements right.

Early stage

- It is important to support and position the patient carefully, paying particular attention to the hemiplegic shoulder to reduce the risk of injury. Nos. 1–3 in Fig. 8.4 show how to cushion the patient.
- The relatives or nurses should roll the patient carefully (no. 4 in Fig. 8.4). As the patient becomes stronger, teach rolling from side to side, and then how to get up from lying (nos. 5 and 6 in Fig. 8.4). The patient will often need help.
- Frequent changes in position are good.
- Aim to maintain muscle length (prevent contractures) with GENTLE passive/active movements into extension, taking particular care over the Achilles tendon, and the flexors of elbow, wrist, and fingers.

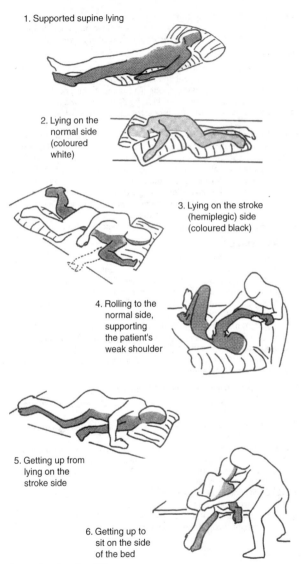

1. Supported supine lying

2. Lying on the normal side (coloured white)

3. Lying on the stroke (hemiplegic) side (coloured black)

4. Rolling to the normal side, supporting the patient's weak shoulder

5. Getting up from lying on the stroke side

6. Getting up to sit on the side of the bed

Fig. 8.4 (continued, p. 423)

- Encourage selective and controlled movements. It is better to work slowly to get good control of arm and hand movements than to be able rapidly to regain function with gross abnormal limb movements.

Basic principles for this early stage

- *Aim for symmetry* — sit the patient in a good position with adequate support (no. 7 in Fig. 8.4). Set the arms forward. Sit the patient out for short periods if trunk control is poor. This is important; practise transferring weight from side to side (no. 11 in Fig. 8.4) — this will make it easier for him/her to shift weight from one leg to the other while learning to walk again.
- *Aim for good control of movement* — in particular, the patient needs to be able to control the transference of body weight in sitting and in standing. The patient needs to lean forward to get up. This is best learnt with a high seat initially (and something in front to help build confidence; no. 9 in Fig. 8.4). With progress, the seat can be lowered and the front support shifted to the side, before trying a chair (no. 12 in Fig. 8.4).
- *Aim for trunk control* — in sitting before trying to stand and, in particular, during the act of moving from sitting to standing.
- *Aim for balance* — in standing and stepping before walking.

Walking stage

1. Aim for normal gait — equal stride length and equal time on both sides.
2. The patient may require support on one or both sides.
3. Start walking with the UNAFFECTED leg. This means that the patient must have already learnt to shift weight from leg to leg.
4. Walking aids — use a wheeled frame/rollator or a normal walking stick (a quadruped stick should be a last resort).
5. The patient may require help with a 'drop foot' (no. 13 in Fig. 8.4).
6. Use mime, gestures, repeating and rephrasing movements, and physical prompts to help the patient. Allow time for slow synapsing.
7. Little and often is a better way to build stamina and sustain carry over from one session to another.

Some 'don'ts' for stroke rehabilitation

1. **Do not ask the patient to try harder** — AVOID effort as it increases tone and gross patterns of movement.
2. **Do not ask the patient to squeeze a ball** — this encourages the arm flexors that are already too strong.
3. **Avoid a painful shoulder** — do not make any arm movements unless the whole shoulder, including the scapula, is relaxed and supple. Support for a weak arm (no. 8 in Fig. 8.4) may be useful temporarily (e.g. while concentrating on walking).
4. **NEVER lift under the stroke arm or pull it** — the muscles that hold the shoulder are weak and the joint easily dislocated.
5. **Prevent dislocation** — support the forearm and hand forwards with natural weight through the elbow (no. 7 in Fig. 8.4).

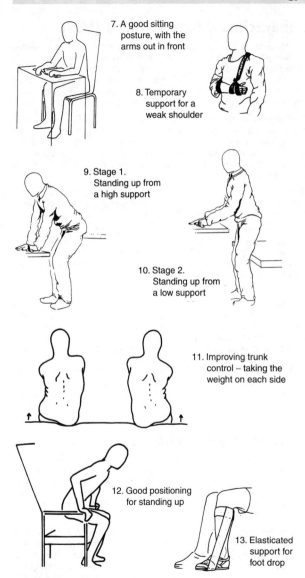

7. A good sitting posture, with the arms out in front

8. Temporary support for a weak shoulder

9. Stage 1. Standing up from a high support

10. Stage 2. Standing up from a low support

11. Improving trunk control – taking the weight on each side

12. Good positioning for standing up

13. Elasticated support for foot drop

Fig. 8.4 (*contd.*)

Subarachnoid haemorrhage (SAH)

An acute bleed into the subarachnoid space that produces a sudden intense headache, sometimes accompanied by nausea and vomiting. This is classically described as 'like being hit on the back of the head'. Most cases are caused by ruptured aneurysms. Other causes are rare mycotic aneurysms (due to endocarditis) and arteriovenous malformations (more frequent in young patients). 15% have no identified cause.

Clinical features: the conscious level may be impaired. The more severe the bleed, the lower the conscious level, and the worse the prognosis. Other features include: headache with meningism; vomiting; fits. Focal signs are rare. The patient is often irritable and drowsy; the headache may last for weeks. Complications include vascular spasm that contributes to cerebral ischaemia.

Beware: worsening conscious level, the appearance or worsening of a neurological deficit (e.g. development of hemiparesis, dilatation of a pupil), or systemic changes such as ↑BP that may indicate ↑ICP.

Diagnosis: is by clinical findings with LP (and early CT scan if available). The CSF is uniformly blood-stained in the first few days. Xanthochromia (straw-coloured supernatant) may be present if at least 6 hrs have elapsed since the onset of the bleed. It may be present for up to 14 days. However, if meningitis forms part of the differential diagnosis, the LP should not be delayed.

Management: involves neurosurgery in many cases to evacuate an intra-cerebral haematoma or clip the aneurysm. Medical treatment involves extended bed rest, analgesia, sedation (beware masking of deterioration in conscious level), and cautious control of hypertension. IV hydration (3 L/day) is strongly advised. Nimodipine (60 mg PO q4h for 2–3 weeks) decreases the incidence of vascular spasm.

Some SAH are preceded by minor herald bleeds that also elicit an intense headache +/− meningism or back pain. If suspected, refer for evaluation since surgical treatment at this time may prevent a later severe bleed. Rebleeding occurs in ~30% of cases; it is a common cause of death.

Subdural haemorrhage

A slow venous bleed that follows damage to veins crossing from the cortex to venous sinuses. It may even occur after a minor accident, such as stepping awkwardly off a bus, in those predisposed: elderly, alcoholics, people with clotting disorders, epileptics. Presentation can occur months after the forgotten accident as chronic bleeding slowly increases the size of the haematoma.

Clinical features: typically there is a lucid interval between the injury and the onset of neurological symptoms. Common acute symptoms include headache, vomiting, fluctuating levels of consciousness; less often, mood changes, irritability, incontinence, drowsiness. Signs may include changes in pupil size, distal limb weakness, and increased reflexes; less commonly, fits and dysphasia.

ubarachnoid haemorrhage (SAH)

.n acute bleed into the subarachnoid space that produces a sudden
ntense headache, sometimes accompanied by nausea and vomiting. This is
classically described as 'like being hit on the back of the head'. Most cases
are caused by ruptured aneurysms. Other causes are rare mycotic
aneurysms (due to endocarditis) and arteriovenous malformations (more
frequent in young patients). 15% have no identified cause.

Clinical features: the conscious level may be impaired. The more severe
the bleed, the lower the conscious level, and the worse the prognosis.
Other features include: headache with meningism; vomiting; fits. Focal
signs are rare. The patient is often irritable and drowsy; the headache may
last for weeks. Complications include vascular spasm that contributes to
cerebral ischaemia.

Beware: worsening conscious level, the appearance or worsening of a
neurological deficit (e.g. development of hemiparesis, dilatation of a pupil),
or systemic changes such as ↑BP that may indicate ↑ICP.

Diagnosis: is by clinical findings with LP (and early CT scan if available).
The CSF is uniformly blood-stained in the first few days. Xanthochromia
(straw-coloured supernatant) may be present if at least 6 hrs have elapsed
since the onset of the bleed. It may be present for up to 14 days. However,
if meningitis forms part of the differential diagnosis, the LP should not be
delayed.

Management: involves neurosurgery in many cases to evacuate an intra-
cerebral haematoma or clip the aneurysm. Medical treatment involves
extended bed rest, analgesia, sedation (beware masking of deterioration in
conscious level), and cautious control of hypertension. IV hydration
(3 L/day) is strongly advised. Nimodipine (60 mg PO q4h for 2–3 weeks)
decreases the incidence of vascular spasm.

Some SAH are preceded by minor herald bleeds that also elicit an
intense headache +/– meningism or back pain. If suspected, refer for evaluation since surgical treatment at this time may prevent a later severe
bleed. Rebleeding occurs in ~30% of cases; it is a common cause of death.

Subdural haemorrhage

A slow venous bleed that follows damage to veins crossing from the
cortex to venous sinuses. It may even occur after a minor accident, such as
stepping awkwardly off a bus, in those predisposed: elderly, alcoholics,
people with clotting disorders, epileptics. Presentation can occur months
after the forgotten accident as chronic bleeding slowly increases the size
of the haematoma.

Clinical features: typically there is a lucid interval between the injury and
the onset of neurological symptoms. Common acute symptoms include
headache, vomiting, fluctuating levels of consciousness; less often, mood
changes, irritability, incontinence, drowsiness. Signs may include changes in
pupil size, distal limb weakness, and increased reflexes; less commonly, fits
and dysphasia.

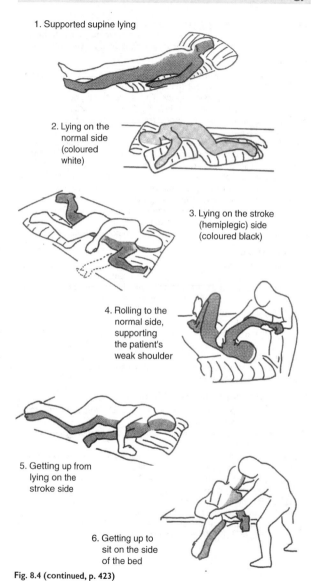

1. Supported supine lying

2. Lying on the normal side (coloured white)

3. Lying on the stroke (hemiplegic) side (coloured black)

4. Rolling to the normal side, supporting the patient's weak shoulder

5. Getting up from lying on the stroke side

6. Getting up to sit on the side of the bed

Fig. 8.4 (continued, p. 423)

- Encourage selective and controlled movements. It is better to work slowly to get good control of arm and hand movements than to be able rapidly to regain function with gross abnormal limb movements.

Basic principles for this early stage

- *Aim for symmetry* — sit the patient in a good position with adequate support (no. 7 in Fig. 8.4). Set the arms forward. Sit the patient out for short periods if trunk control is poor. This is important; practise transferring weight from side to side (no. 11 in Fig. 8.4) — this will make it easier for him/her to shift weight from one leg to the other while learning to walk again.
- *Aim for good control of movement* — in particular, the patient needs to be able to control the transference of body weight in sitting and in standing. The patient needs to lean forward to get up. This is best learnt with a high seat initially (and something in front to help build confidence; no. 9 in Fig. 8.4). With progress, the seat can be lowered and the front support shifted to the side, before trying a chair (no. 12 in Fig. 8.4).
- *Aim for trunk control* — in sitting before trying to stand and, in particular, during the act of moving from sitting to standing.
- *Aim for balance* — in standing and stepping before walking.

Walking stage

1. Aim for normal gait — equal stride length and equal time on both sides.
2. The patient may require support on one or both sides.
3. Start walking with the UNAFFECTED leg. This means that the patient must have already learnt to shift weight from leg to leg.
4. Walking aids — use a wheeled frame/rollator or a normal walking stick (a quadruped stick should be a last resort).
5. The patient may require help with a 'drop foot' (no. 13 in Fig. 8.4).
6. Use mime, gestures, repeating and rephrasing movements, and physical prompts to help the patient. Allow time for slow synapsing.
7. Little and often is a better way to build stamina and sustain carry over from one session to another.

Some 'don'ts' for stroke rehabilitation

1. *Do not ask the patient to try harder* — AVOID effort as it increases tone and gross patterns of movement.
2. *Do not ask the patient to squeeze a ball* — this encourages the arm flexors that are already too strong.
3. *Avoid a painful shoulder* — do not make any arm movements unless the whole shoulder, including the scapula, is relaxed and supple. Support for a weak arm (no. 8 in Fig. 8.4) may be useful temporarily (e.g. while concentrating on walking).
4. *NEVER lift under the stroke arm or pull it* — the muscles that hold the shoulder are weak and the joint easily dislocated.
5. *Prevent dislocation* — support the forearm and hand forwards with natural weight through the elbow (no. 7 in Fig. 8.4).

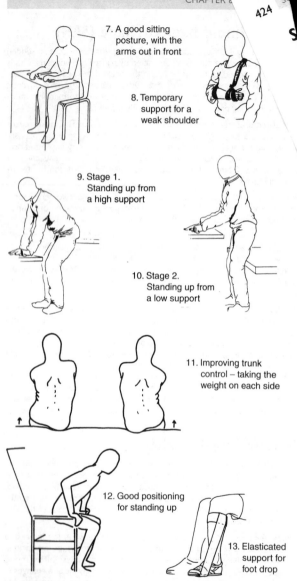

7. A good sitting posture, with the arms out in front

8. Temporary support for a weak shoulder

9. Stage 1. Standing up from a high support

10. Stage 2. Standing up from a low support

11. Improving trunk control – taking the weight on each side

12. Good positioning for standing up

13. Elasticated support for foot drop

Fig. 8.4 *(contd.)*

Management
This requires a neurosurgical opinion and if possible, a CT scan — evacuation through burr holes is recommended for most cases (see p. 426). Possibly, minor haematomas will resolve by themselves. The outcome is good in all ages — ~90% return to normal. Therefore, consider the diagnosis in a confused elderly person.

Extradural haematoma[1]

An arterial bleed that normally results from a skull fracture after head injury (e.g. assault, RTC). The haematoma enlarges rapidly and unless evacuated equally rapidly there is a high risk of brain herniation and the patient's death. Suspect when the conscious level declines in a patient with head injury. Unilateral dilation of a pupil, which is sluggish or unresponsive to light, is ipsilateral to the side of the haemorrhage.

Management: do a CT scan if possible to localize the expanding lesion. Further management depends on the distance to a neurosurgeon. If close, give mannitol before transferring the patient. If the neurosurgeon is remote, a burr hole will be required to prevent brain herniation.

In this situation, unless a burr hole is done rapidly, the patient will die or suffer brain damage. You and the patient have nothing to lose and everything to gain. An inelegant burr hole now will do much more good than an elegant operation one hour or more later.

How to do a burr hole

1. *Incision*
   - Shave the scalp if there is time.
   - Local anaesthetic is not usually necessary.
   - Make a 4 cm incision over the site of fracture or injury. This is usually in the temporal region — just above the zygomatic arch — curved as shown in Fig. 8.5 (no. 1) so that it can be enlarged.
2. *Incise right down to the bone.* Do not stop to control bleeding.
3. *Scrape back the pericranium* (periosteum) using a periosteal elevator (or similar instrument) to expose the skull.
   - Insert a mastoid retractor (no. 2 in Fig. 8.5) — this will stop all the bleeding.
   - Leave the retractor in.
4. *Perforate the bone using a perforator* (no. 3 in Fig.8.5)
   - Dark blood will ooze out.
   - The dura will not be seen as it is stripped away by the blood clot.
   - Do no more than **JUST** perforate the skull.
   - This will create a conical hole.
5. *Enlarge the perforation using a burr (no. 4 in Fig. 8.5)*
   - The burr will enlarge the hole so that it is nearly cylindrical.
6. *The blood clot will immediately ooze out.*
   - Suck the blood away by applying a sucker to the burr hole but **DO NOT INSERT SUCKER INTO THE CAVITY**. This will cause more bleeding and might damage the brain.
7. *It is now safe to transfer the patient* to a neurosurgical unit.
   - Leave the scalp retractor in. Organize for its return.
   - Leave in the endotracheal tube and leave a drip up.

[1] With many thanks to Mr C.B.T. Adams, Radcliffe Infirmary, Oxford.

1

2

3

4

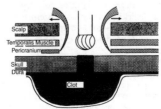

Fig. 8.5 How to do a burr hole.

Blackouts

The most common causes of blackouts are epilepsy and syncope. Causes of blackouts are given in the box. A reliable eyewitness account is helpful.

Syncope is the brief loss of consciousness due to an acute reduction in cerebral blood flow. It is the most common cause of recurrent episodes of disturbed consciousness and may be precipitated by anxiety or pain. It is due to reduced venous return to the heart and cardiac output or an inadequate response of the heart when ↑demand requires ↑cardiac output. Causes include hypotension, vagal slowing of the heart, neuropathy, dysrhythmias, aortic stenosis, vertebrobasilar ischaemia (TIAs), carotid-sinus syndrome.

Space-occupying lesions (SOL)

Classically present with focal neurological signs, ↑ICP, or seizures. Focal neurological signs can be used to localize the mass but beware the false localizing sign that can arise from the VI cranial nerve's long intracranial path.

Causes
* *Infection* — tuberculoma, cysticercosis, echinococcosis, bacterial or amoebic brain abscess, paragonimiasis, schistosomiasis, toxoplasmosis, fungal granulomata.
* *Tumour* — glioma, meningioma, metastases, lymphoma, pituitary adenoma, cysts.
* *Others* — aneurysm, haematoma.

Hydrocephalus

In older children and adults, the skull will not expand if the intracranial pressure rises. Blockage of CSF flow through the ventricles or a failure to reabsorb CSF results in a build up of pressure or hydrocephalus. While producing an increasing head circumference in young children, it results in rising intracranial pressure in older persons that will need urgent management. It exists in two forms:
* **Non-communicating hydrocephalus** — is due to blockage of CSF flow through the ventricles, normally at the foramina or aqueduct between ventricles and/or basal cistern. It is caused by any SOL, such as tumour or cyst, or stenosis of the aqueduct. The location of the blockage must be identified and the blockage removed surgically, or a shunt placed.
* **Communicating hydrocephalus** — is due to CSF obstruction in basal cisterns or subarachnoid space (the CSF still flows out of the ventricular system but it cannot be reabsorbed in the arachnoid villi). It may result from intracranial haemorrhage or meningitis (acute pyogenic or chronic); the cause is often unknown. Presents with a triad of dementia, incontinence, and gait disturbance (this condition is also called normal pressure hydrocephalus). Repeated lumbar taps with treatment of any underlying cause may be sufficient.

Causes of blackouts

- Vasovagal
- Hyperventilation
- Hypoglycaemia
- Epilepsy
- Hysteria
- Postural hypotension
- Cardiac arrhythmia
- Vertebro-basilar TIAs
- Hypoxia

It is important to measure blood levels of:
- Glucose
- K^+
- Mg^{2+}
- Na^+
- Ca^{2+}

Epilepsy

Epilepsy is the continuing tendency to have epileptic seizures — spontaneous paroxysmal discharges of neurons that result in clinical symptoms.

It is a common disease with ~40 million people affected worldwide. Its incidence is higher in the developing world than the industrialized world. Approximately 1% of the population has epilepsy due to higher incidence of infection and head injury. Unfortunately, at present, only ~15% of cases are treated adequately and many people suffer unnecessarily. As a result, a global campaign is being set up to increase public awareness of both the diseases and its causes. There is also a great need to both reduce its incidence in the developing world (by decreasing the number of head injuries and infections) and find ways of providing adequate supplies of affordable effective antiepileptic drugs to poorer countries.

Causes — 70% unknown, 30% known.

- *Infection* — cysticercosis, tuberculoma, schistosomiasis, paragonimiasis, sparganosis, hydatid disease, toxoplasmosis, toxocariasis, cerebral malaria, cerebral amoebiasis, syphilitic gumma, and HIV.
  Epilepsy can also be a late consequence of almost any meningeal or brain parenchyma infection.
- *Brain injury* — due to either head injury (such as assault or RTA) or antenatal head injury (may also be due to post-natal injury but this is now believed to be less important).
- *Unknown* — many may actually be due to very small areas of focal dys-genesis (hamartomas).
- *Eclampsia* — urgent delivery is required.
- Inherited diseases
- Alcohol
- Brain tumour or metastasis
- Metabolic causes
- Degenerative disorders (in elderly)
- Vascular disease
- Drugs

Clinical features: will depend on the class of seizure — see below.

- There may be an aura or warning before the attack.
- In grand mal attacks, the person has generalized convulsions usually with tonic-clonic movements of all four limbs. The patient loses consciousness and may bite his/her tongue and be incontinent of urine or, rarely, faeces.
- Post-ictally, there may be a period of confusion, drowsiness, a failure to remember the onset, and a headache with a tendency to sleep.

Seizure classification — important for choice of drug therapy

1. *Origin and spread of the seizure:*
   - A seizure that remains localized to its area of origin is a **partial seizure**.
   - A seizure that subsequently spreads from this region to involve the whole brain is termed a **secondarily generalized seizure**.
   - A seizure that originates in centrally positioned cells and activates all parts of the brain simultaneously is a **generalized seizure**.

Principles of antiepileptic drug therapy

1. Establish a clear clinical diagnosis
2. Get EEG supporting evidence if possible
3. Choose a drug, considering the:
   - Seizure type(s)
   - Patient's age
   - Price
   - Interaction with other drugs
   - Possibility of pregnancy
4. Give one drug only
5. Begin with modest dosage building up slowly over 2–3 months
6. Give full information to the patient concerning
   - Names and alternative names of the drug supplied
   - The main side-effects of the drug
   - The need for compliance with instructions
   - Possible interactions with other medications
7. Monitor progress, seizure frequency, and side-effects
8. Ensure adequate supplies

2. **Clinical features of the seizure**
   - *Partial seizures:* have signs and symptoms referable to a part of one hemisphere.

        Simple (consciousness is not impaired) (e.g. in focal motor seizures which may start in a toe, finger, or the angle of mouth).
        Complex (consciousness is impaired with signs of temporal lobe activity) (e.g. olfactory aura followed by automatism of facial expression, behaviour, hallucinations).
        Secondarily generalized.

   - *Generalized seizures:* do not have any features that are referable to only one hemisphere.

        Absences (petit mal) brief ~10sec pauses (e.g. stops talking mid-sentence, carries on where left off). Classically, has pathognomic 3Hz activity on EEG.
        Tonic-clonic (grand mal) sudden onset with loss of consciousness, body stiffens for up to 1 min. before jerking, post-ictal drowsiness.
        Myoclonic and **akinetic** seizures.

Management: if the seizure appears to have a focal onset, look for a treatable underlying cause, particularly infectious (if available, use CT or, better, MRI). Patients should be warned not to drive.

First-line drugs: see a formulary for details of use and side-effects.
- *Phenobarbital* — start at 1.5 mg/kg PO od, building up to 3.0 mg/kg (max 180 mg) od. First choice for partial and generalized tonic-clonic seizures. Should not be used to treat the seizures associated with cerebral malaria. Its side-effects in children appear to be acceptable.
- *Carbamazepine* — start at 100 mg PO bd, building up to 600 mg bd if tolerated. First choice for tonic-clonic seizures in association with partial seizures; reserve drug for partial seizures alone.
- *Sodium valproate* — start at 300mg PO bd, building up to 750mg bd (max = 2.5 g/day). First choice for typical absences, myoclonic and akinetic seizures, and tonic-clonic seizures in association with typical absences.
- *Phenytoin* — start at 2.5 mg/kg PO od, building up to 5.0 (max ~8.0) mg/kg PO od. Reserve drug for tonic-clonic and partial seizures (not for absences). It is a toxic drug and plasma levels should ideally be monitored.
- *Other drugs* — include clonazepam, ethosuximide, and the newer expensive drugs: vigabatrin, lamotrigine, gabapentin.

Changing drugs: persist with an old drug until it has been used at its maximum dose before considering a change. Introduce the new drug at its starting dose and slowly increase to its mid-range; then start to slowly decrease the dose of the old drug.

Stopping drugs: it is not clear how long any person needs to stay on antiepileptic drugs once the seizures have been controlled. An MRC trial of stopping medication in people who had not had a seizure for 2yrs showed that 59% of those who stopped medication were seizure-free at 2yrs compared to 78% who remained on medication. Discuss with the patient what they want: risk of recurrence vs. gravity of the side-effects.

Status epilepticus

Status epilepticus has recently been redefined: 'generalized, convulsive status epilepticus in adults and older children (>5 years old) refers to at least 5 min of (a) continuous seizures or (b) two or more discrete seizures'. This definition reflects the current uncertainty about the relationship between the duration of convulsions and CNS damage. Status epilepticus can result in death, permanent neurological damage, or the onset of chronic epilepsy — risk factors for such sequelae include aetiology, duration of attack, and systemic complications.

Aetiology: ~40% occur in known epileptics; other causes include fever or acute CNS infection (particularly in children), head injury, pesticide poisoning, stroke, eclampsia.

Management
- Stop seizures quickly.
- Prevent complications.
- Find and control the underlying causes.
1. Remove patient from potential danger.
2. Secure the airway, preferably with a Guedal airway, and give oxygen.
3. Do not attempt to intubate if the jaw is clenched. Wait for sedation to have its effect.
4. Give 50 ml 50% dextrose as IV bolus unless hypoglycaemia is excluded.
5. Give thiamine 250 mg by slow IV infusion over 20 mins if the patient is an alcoholic — ensure facilities for managing anaphylaxis are available.
6. Give diazepam 10–20 mg in 2–4 ml IV or PR at a rate of 1 ml/min. (For children, give 1mg per year of age.) This should control ~80% of patients. Second (and rarely third) doses may be needed.
7. Beware respiratory depression following bolus diazepam.

If convulsions continue after giving diazepam —
manage the patient in ICU if possible.

1. Give phenytoin 20 mg/kg as an IV infusion, at <50 mg/min, through a separate giving set. Once seizures are controlled, maintain with phenytoin 100 mg IV q6–8h.
2. (Alternatively, give phenobarbital 10 mg/kg as an IV infusion, at <100 mg/min. Do not give more diazepam. Beware respiratory depression and hypotension. Chlormethiazole is an alternative. Phenobarbital is preferred for fits associated with poisoning.)
3. Check for and treat raised ICP.

If convulsions continue after phenytoin

1. Exclude pseudostatus.
2. Check drugs have been given correctly.
3. Then give general anaesthetic and ventilate, whilst treating causative condition. Give thiopental 75–125 mg (3–5 ml of a 2.5% solution) IV over 10–15 secs. Give further doses according to response. Beware hypotension. If large amounts of thiopentone are infused over a long period, it will accumulate and delay recovery.

Cysticercosis

This condition, caused by the pork tapeworm, *Taenia solium*, is a common cause of epilepsy worldwide. Humans are the definitive host for this species and normally become infected by eating cysts in undercooked pork meat — see Fig. 8.6 for life cycle.

Accidental human ingestion of eggs in faecally contaminated food results in disease with marked morbidity of the CNS, muscles, skin, and eye. The symptoms are caused by the inflammatory reaction to the living and dying parasites (active disease) and long-term effects of the inflammatory reaction to the cysts — fibrosis, calcification, and granulation (inactive disease).

Transmission: by ingestion of food or water contaminated with pig faeces. Poor personal hygiene, particularly amongst food handlers, and faecal pollution of water and irrigated vegetables predispose to infection.

Clinical features: CNS involvement (neurocysticercosis) normally manifests as epilepsy. However, since the number and localization of cysts varies greatly, neurocysticercosis can manifest in a variety of ways including hydrocephalus, dementia (frontal lobe involvement; often in children); infarcts (due to vasculitis); basal meningitis; cranial nerve defects; spinal symptoms.

Subcutaneous and muscular cysts occur in 25% of cases with CNS involvement, but may also occur in isolation — the calcified cysts appear as small, round, painless, firm nodules. The rare involvement of cardiac muscle can result in conduction defects.

Ocular cysticercosis often presents with blurring of vision and the sensation of something moving in the eye. If untreated, it may progress to blindness and eye atrophy.

Diagnosis: active CNS lesions can be identified by CT or MRI; calcified inactive lesions can be seen on CT (and sometimes on X-ray). Serology.

Management
Drugs should not be given to patients with severe active neurocysticercosis because they may elicit a potentially fatal inflammatory reaction. In this situation, manage symptomatically until the disease has settled.

1. Treat inactive or mild CNS disease with praziquantel 10–20 mg/kg PO tds for 2–3 weeks or albendazole 7.5–15 mg/kg PO bd for 30 days. Albendazole may be more effective but may have more SEs.
2. Patients presenting with seizures and a single cyst can be managed with anticonvulsants alone.
3. Surgery is usually reserved for subarachnoid and intraventricular cysts causing compression and resulting in hydrocephalus or cord compression
4. Ocular infection should **not** be treated with drugs. Ocular cysts may need to be treated surgically.

Prevention: health education and public health measures to improve personal hygiene, meat inspection, sanitation on farms, and sewage disposal. Mass treatments in hyperendemic regions and interruption of the parasite's life cycles.

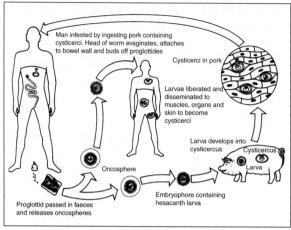

Fig. 8.6 Life cycle of *Taenia solium*.

Weak legs/paraplegia, non-traumatic

Ask the following questions:

- Was the onset gradual or sudden?
- Is the tone spastic or flaccid?
- Is there sensory loss, in particular a sensory level? — a strong clue to spinal cord disease.
- Is there any loss of sphincter control (bowels or bladder)?
- Is there normal sensation around the sacrum and good anal tone?

1. *Sudden weak legs with spasticity*
   - **Cord compression** — spinal or paraspinal infection or abscess due to TB, *Brucella*, pyogenic bacteria; tumours (metastases, Hodgkin's or Burkitt's lymphoma, myeloma); disc prolapse; Paget's disease. **Cord compression** is an emergency. It must be considered when there is a rapid progression of leg weakness and/or sphincter failure. Check the perineal area for loss of sensation (saddle anaesthesia).
   - **Other causes** — infectious or post-infectious myelitis; cord infarction (due to vasculitis, thrombosis of anterior spinal artery, trauma or compression, dissection of aortic aneurysm, surgery); tetanus; carcinomatous meningitis.

2. *Sudden weak legs with flaccidity/acute flaccid paralysis*
   - **Cauda equina compression** — a neurosurgical emergency. Causes: tumour; prolapsed disc; canal stenosis; TB; cysticercosis; schistosomiasis.
   - **Poliomyelitis** — see p. 438.
   - **Other causes** — acute cord trauma/infarction; myelitis (in early stages with back pain, fever, double incontinence, sensory loss at defined level surmounted by a zone of hyperaesthesia); Guillain–Barré syndrome; rabies; lumbosacral nerve lesion; hypokalaemic periodic paralysis.

3. *Chronic spastic paraparesis*
   - **Causes** — cord compression (e.g. cervical spondylosis); syringomyelia; tropical spastic paraparesis (TSP, due to HTLV-1); MND; subacute combined degeneration of the cord (vitamin B_{12} deficiency); konzo; and lathyrism.

4. *Chronic flaccid paraparesis*
   - **Causes** — peripheral neuropathies; myopathies; nerve trauma; and tabes dorsalis.

5. *Weak legs + no sensory loss: motor neurone disease (MND)*

6. *Absent knee jerks with extensor plantar responses*
   - **Causes** — Friederich's ataxia; taboparesis; MND; subacute combined degeneration of the cord; DM.

7. *Unilateral foot drop*
   - **Causes** — DM; stroke; prolapsed disc; MND; organophosphorous poisoning; common peroneal nerve palsy.

Principles of management of paraplegia

1. Prevention of pressure sores by turning every 2 hrs.
2. Attention to bladder and bowels (urinary catheter if incontinent).
3. Adequate hydration and nutrition.
4. Prevent complications: aspiration and pneumonia (ensure adequate swallowing), DVT (support stockings/heparin), contractures (physiotherapy), malaria (mosquito net).
5. Treat the underlying cause.

Poliomyelitis

This disease — usually of young children — is caused by the poliovirus, an enterovirus. The virus selectively infects and destroys anterior horn cells in the spinal cord, resulting in the cardinal sign of polio — acute flaccid paralysis (AFP). The clinical disease is relatively uncommon, however ~99% of infected people show no paralytic manifestations.

A worldwide vaccination effort is under way to eradicate it. Whilst polio has been a major cause of disability worldwide, it may soon be just a disturbing memory, unlike the other major causes — RTA and landmines.

Transmission: via ingestion of faecally contaminated food or water, or via droplet spread from the respiratory tract.

Clinical features: the prodromal symptoms are common to many infections and practically indistinguishable: fever, malaise, headache, drowsiness, sore throat.

In a minority, CNS disease (preparalytic disease) follows with abrupt onset of fever, headache, body pains, sensory disturbances, and neck stiffness — due to poliovirus meningitis. Flaccid paralysis then occurs in ~65%, developing asymmetrically over a variable time, particularly affecting the lower limbs. The paralysis rarely progresses after 3 days or after the temperature falls. There is some recovery of function over the following weeks or months, as some damaged anterior horn cells recover. Death is relatively uncommon but results from aspiration or airway obstruction (bulbar paralysis) or respiratory failure (respiratory paralysis). A rare complication is slow deterioration of limb or bulbar function after many years — the post-polio syndrome.

Diagnosis: is clinical, with retrospective serological analysis.

Management: is supportive. Bed rest is essential; give analgesia, sedation. Do not give any injections.

Prevention: vaccination and improved public health.

Guillain–Barré syndrome (GBS)

A post-infectious demyelinating peripheral polyneuropathy. Some form of infection, mainly respiratory or diarrhoea, precedes the onset of GBS by 1–2 weeks in ~60% of cases. It develops over a few hours (rarely), to several weeks, and is a medical emergency.

Respiratory arrest may occur without notice in severe cases; sudden death may also be caused by ANS disturbance of CVS function. These patients need constant observation, in an ITU setting if possible.

Clinical features: include progressive muscle weakness in the limbs of less than 4 wks' duration; distal paraesthesia (less often sensory loss). Back and limb pain may be occasionally present. Also cranial nerve palsies (particularly VII); ANS disturbances; ileus. Monitor respiratory function and heart rhythm; plasma exchange or high-dose immunoglobulin if available shortens the hospital stay. Recovery occurs over several weeks or months with remyelination of peripheral nerves.

Warnings

- Paralytic poliomyelitis is made worse by IM injections during the preparalytic phase (e.g. injections of antibiotics) or by the muscles becoming fatigued (e.g. after exercise), so a high index of suspicion in endemic regions is important to prevent polio being made worse.
- Patients must be carefully observed during the onset of paralysis for signs of life-threatening bulbar and respiratory paralysis. Nurse patients with weak swallowing on their side. Good nursing care, including frequent suction and observations, may delay the need for a tracheostomy — however, perform a tracheostomy early in serious cases.

Polio rehabilitation

Acute stage

1. Treatment at this stage is based on: (i) rest (ii) positioning.
2. Support the wrist and hands in a functional position with a splint or other support (e.g. pillow).
3. Support the ankle — maintain the ankle at 90° and avoid excessive inversion or eversion.

Subacute stage

1. Progress from passive movements, to active assisted movements, to active movements within the normal range. The movements will depend on the muscle groups affected
2. Progress to standing and walking with assistance — use walking aids if necessary (e.g. stick, crutches). Aim for the best possible function.

Avoid

1. Muscle shortening.
2. Malformation due to muscle imbalance.

Mono/polyneuropathies

The mononeuropathies are lesions of single nerves; polyneuropathies are lesions of multiple nerves normally due to systemic disease. In some conditions such as leprosy, multiple peripheral nerves may be involved simultaneously — this is termed mononeuritis multiplex. Polyneuropathies are symmetrical conditions and often affect the peripheries initially, producing a symmetrical glove and stocking distribution.

In the tropics, environmental toxins and nutritional deficiencies are important causes of peripheral neuropathies. They may be seen in epidemic form after toxins are released into the environment by industry or in an endemic form in particular regions. Some toxins are used in local forms of medicine or they may contaminate food, liquor, etc. They frequently produce an individually recognizable syndrome — as always, there is no replacement for local clinical experience. In these situations, treatment involves removal of the toxin and/or supplementation with the deficient nutrient. The effects of many neuropathies are permanent.

Causes

Single nerves can be damaged by:
- Trauma
- Compression
- DM
- Leprosy.

The latter two conditions will often develop into neuropathies affecting multiple nerves, causing a mononeuritis multiplex or widespread peripheral neuropathy.

Polyneuropathies can be caused by:

1. *Deficiencies:* vitamin B_1, B_6, and B_{12}; plus a variety of multiple nutrient deficiencies.
2. *Toxins*
   - Heavy metals: including lead (motor involvement), thallium (found in rodenticides → alopecia), arsenic (Mee's nail lines, changes in skin pigmentation, skin cancers)
   - Drugs: many but particularly isoniazid, ethambutol (affects optic nerve), sulfonamides, chloroquine, clioquinol, metronidazole, phenytoin, didanosine
   - Industrial chemicals/solvents (e.g. trio-ortho-cresyl phosphate)
   - Pesticides, particularly organophosphorous (OP) compounds
   - Excessive consumption of certain foods (e.g. cassava which contains a cyanogenic glycoside) can cause tropical ataxic neuropathy.
3. *Metabolic diseases:* DM, renal or liver failure, alcohol, hypothyroidism
4. *Infections:* leprosy, TB, HIV
5. *Other causes:* genetic diseases, malignancy, connective tissue disease

Table 8.2 WHO differential diagnosis of acute flaccid paralysis (WHO[ND])

	Polio	Guillain–Barré syndrome	Traumatic neuritis	Transverse myelitis
Onset of paralysis	24–48 hrs, from onset to full paralysis	From hrs to 10 days	From hrs to 4 days	From hrs to 4 days
Flaccid paralysis	Usually acute, asymmetrical, principally proximal	Usually acute, symmetrical, and distal	Asymmetrical, acute, affecting one limb only	Acute, affecting lower limbs, symmetrical
Muscle tone	Reduced or absent in the affected limb	Global hypotonia	Reduced or absent in the affected limb	Hypotonia in lower limbs
Deep tendon reflexes	Decreased to absent	Globally absent	Decreased to absent	Absent in lower limbs early, increased late
Sensation	Severe myalgia, backache, no sensory changes	Cramps, tingling, hypoanaesthesia of palms/soles	Pain in gluteus muscles, hypothermia	Anaesthesia of lower limbs, sensory level
Cranial nerve	Only when bulbar involvement is present	Often present, affecting nerves VII, IX, X, XI, XII	Absent	Absent
Respiratory insufficiency	Only when bulbar involvement is present	In severe cases; worsened by bacterial pneumonia	Absent	Sometimes
CSF findings	Inflammatory	Albumin–cells dissociation	Normal	Normal or a few cells
Bladder dysfunction	Absent	Transient	Never	Present

Leprosy (Hansen's disease)

Leprosy is a disease that still elicits immense stigma in many communities. It is a chronic inflammatory disease caused by *Mycobacterium leprae* infecting macrophages and peripheral nerve Schwann cells.

Its presentation and progress are determined by the patient's cell-mediated immune response to the mycobacterium. Most people (~95%) develop an effective immune response and clear *M. leprae*. A minority are unable to do so and develop clinical leprosy. The clinical features form a spectrum determined by the immune response (see Table 8.3). The two poles of the spectrum are tuberculoid (TT; paucibacillary) and lepromatous leprosy (LL; multibacillary). At the TT pole there is a strong (but ineffective) immune response to the bacteria which damages peripheral nerves and skin. At the LL pole, there is cellular anergy towards *M. leprae* with abundant bacillary multiplication. Between these two poles are the borderline patients — borderline tuberculoid (BT), borderline (BB), borderline lepromatous (BL) — with varying immunity and bacterial loads. The polar groups (TT, LL) are stable, but the borderline groups are unstable and experience tissue damaging reactions.

Transmission: untreated lepromatous patients discharge bacilli from the nose. Infection occurs when *M. leprae* invades via the nasal mucosa with haematogenous spread to skin and nerve. Leprosy bacilli can survive for several days in the environment. People in close contact with infected people have a greater, but still small, chance of becoming infected. The incubation period is 2–5 yrs for TT cases and 8–12 yrs for LL cases. HIV infection is not a risk factor for the development of leprosy.

Clinical features

- *Skin:* the most common lesions are macules or plaques; more rarely papules and nodules or diffuse infiltration. Indeterminate leprosy is an early form of disease often found in screening programmes; lesions can last for months before resolving or progressing to established leprosy.
- *Nerve damage:* occurs in peripheral nerve trunks — great auricular nerve (neck), ulnar nerve (elbow), radial-cutaneous nerve (wrist), median nerve (wrist), lateral popliteal nerve (neck of the fibula), and posterior tibial nerve (medial malleolus) — producing typical patterns of regional sensory and motor loss. Small dermal nerves are also involved producing patches of anaesthesia in TT/BT lesions and glove and stocking sensory loss in LL patients.
- *Other organs:* may be involved: eyes (can → blindness); bones (dactylitis, resorption); testes (orchititis, sterility); nasopharynx (nasal collapse).

Presentation of leprosy

Patients commonly present with skin lesions, weakness, or numbness due to peripheral nerve lesion or a burn/ulcer in an anaesthetic hand or foot.

Borderline patients may present in reaction with nerve pain, sudden palsy, multiple new skin lesions, pain in the eye, or systemic febrile illness.

The ulceration and digit loss seen in leprosy is due to secondary damage in neuropathic hands and feet and is not an intrinsic disease feature.

Table 8.3 Clinical features of leprosy

Classification	Skin lesions	Nerve involvement
Indeterminate	Solitary hypopigmented 2–5 cm lesion. Centre may show sensory loss although both doctor and patient are often uncertain about this loss. May become TT-like.	None clinically detectable.
Tuberculoid (TT)	Lesions with well-defined borders and sensory loss. The patch is dry (loss of sweating) and hairless.	May have 1 peripheral nerve affected. Occasionally presents as a mono-neuropathy.
Borderline tuberculoid (BT)	Irregular plaques with raised edges and sensory loss. Satellite lesions at the edges.	Asymmetrical peripheral nerve involvement.
Borderline (BB)	Many lesions with punched out edges. Satellites are common.	Widespread nerve enlargement. Sensory and motor loss.
Borderline lepromatous (BL)	Many lesions with diffuse borders and variable anesthesia	As above.
Lepromatous (LL)	Numerous nodular skin lesions in a symmetrical distribution. Lesions are not dry or anaesthetic. There are often thickened shiny earlobes, loss of eyebrows, and skin thickening.	As above.

Diagnosis is based on:
- A typical skin lesion (loss of sensation in TT/BT patients)
- Thickened peripheral nerves
- Skin smear from lesion edge/ear lobe positive for mycobacteria

Test skin lesions for sensation. Palpate peripheral nerves to assess enlargement/ tenderness. Assess nerve function by testing the small muscles' power and sensation in hands/feet. Many patients are unaware of their anaesthesia. Eye function should be checked (visual acuity, corneal sensation, and eyelid closure). Serology is not helpful.

Management

1. *Chemotherapy to treat the infection*

The WHO regimens are given in Table 8.4. More than 11 million people have been treated with such multi-drug regimens. Relapse rates are 0.1%/yr. Clinical improvement is rapid and adverse reactions are rare. These drugs are considered safe during pregnancy and breastfeeding. Patients are classified for treatment by the number of skin lesions present, paucibacillary have 2–5; multibacillary >5.

Table 8.4 WHO recommended multi-drug therapy regimens

Leprosy type	Drug treatment		Treatment duration
	Monthly supervised	Daily self-administered	
Paucibacillary (2–5 skin lesions)	Rifampicin 600 mg	Dapsone 100 mg	6 mths
Multibacillary (>5 skin lesions)	Rifampicin 600 mg	Clofazimine 50 mg	12 mths
	Clofazimine 300 mg	Dapsone 100 mg	

2. *Educate the patient about leprosy* Within 72 hours of starting chemotherapy, they are non-infectious. They can lead a normal social life. There are no limitations on touching, sex, sharing utensils. Leprosy is not a curse from God or a punishment. Gross deformities are not the inevitable end point of disease. Care and awareness of their limbs is as important as chemotherapy.

3. *Prevent disability* Monitor sensation and muscle power in patient's hands, feet, and eyes as part of routine follow-up so that new nerve damage is detected early. Treat any new damage with prednisolone 40 mg daily, reducing by 5 mg/day each month.

Patient self-awareness is crucial in minimizing damage. Patients with anaesthetic hands or feet need to inspect hands and feet (using a mirror) daily for injuries or infection and dress wounds immediately. Protect hands and feet from trauma ('trainers' are excellent for anaesthetic feet). Identify the cause of any injury so that it can be avoided. Soak dry hands and feet in water and then rub with oil to keep skin moist.

4. *Support the patient socially and psychologically*

Reactions

These are immune-mediated tissue-damaging phenomena and may occur before, during, or after treatment. They should be treated promptly to prevent serious nerve damage. Do not stop chemotherapy during a reaction.

1. **Reversal reaction (type 1 reaction)** — is due to delayed type hypersensitivity and occurs in patients with borderline leprosy, affecting up to 30% of BL patients. Skin lesions become erythematous; peripheral nerves become tender and painful. Loss of nerve function can be sudden, with foot-drop occurring overnight. Neuritis may occur without skin lesions or in a clinically silent form without nerve tenderness.

   Management: for severe reactions, prednisolone 40–60 mg PO od reduced every 2–4 wks over 20 wks. A few patients may require 15–20 mg prednisolone daily for many months. Response rates vary depending on the severity of initial damage but even promptly treated nerve damage will only improve in 60% cases.

2. **Erythema nodosum leprosum (ENL) (type 2 reaction)** — is due to immune complex deposition and occurs in 20% LL and 5% BL patients. It manifests with malaise, fever, and crops of painful, red nodules, which become purple and then resolve. If severe, plaques may form with necrosis and ulceration. Iritis is common; other signs are bone pain and swollen joints, painful neuritis, lymphadenopathy, iridocyclitis, orchitis, nephritis (rarely).

   Management: in moderate and severe cases (systemic features or painful nerves), treat in hospital with one of:

   • Prednisolone 60–80 mg PO od, reduced after 2 wks by 5–10 mg every 2 wks (best for short episodes).

   • Thalidomide 400 mg nightly for 4 wks. Once a satisfactory response occurs, reduce by 50 mg every 2–4 weeks (best drug but contraindicated in women of childbearing age and frequently not available). Causes drowsiness.

   • Clofazimine 300 mg daily, reduced after 3 months (preferred drug for premenopausal women; takes 3–4 wks to have its full effect so should be combined with prednisolone initially). It causes brown staining of the skin.

   • Treat iridocyclitis with steroid and homatropine eye drops.

   ENL is a difficult condition to treat and some patients develop a chronic relapsing form which may last for up to five yrs, but will then resolve. Mild symptoms can be controlled with paracetamol.

Ulcers

Ulcers in anaesthetic feet are the most common cause of hospitalization. Ulceration is treated by rest and cleaning. Ulcers should be carefully probed to detect osteomyelitis and sinuses that require surgical debridement. Unlike ulcers in diabetic or ischaemic feet, ulcers in leprosy heal if they are protected from weight-bearing. No weight-bearing is permitted until the ulcer has healed. Appropriate footwear should be provided to prevent recurrence.

Mental health

Section editor   **Oliver Howes**

Mental illnesses are a major public health problem. They account for 12.7% of the global burden of disease according to WHO estimates, and projections indicate this will increase. International surveys have shown that they are common throughout the tropics, and frequently not recognized or treated.

Lack of knowledge about mental illness is one explanation for under treatment: patients may not present, and when they do, their problems may be misdiagnosed or dismissed. Negative attitudes towards the mentally ill persist amongst the general population and health care professionals. The approach to mental illness should be fundamentally the same as that to physical ill health.

Mental illnesses are more common in people with physical illnesses, particularly chronic conditions, and may complicate the treatment of physical disorders. Conversely, in a patient with mental illness, beware ascribing physical symptoms as psychogenic — always rule out organic causes first.

Suicide and deliberate self-harm

Deliberate self-harm includes a wide range of behaviours that are characterized by an individual inflicting acute harm on themselves. It may take many forms, such as deliberate overdosing with medication, self-poisoning, self-cutting, strangulation, or burning. The motivations can vary widely and several may play a role simultaneously.

There are large variations between countries in the rates and methods used depending on socio-cultural, economic, and political conditions. The WHO multi-centre study found the lifetime risk for self-harm was 3% for women and 2% for men. In ~90% of cases the patient was suffering from a mental illness.

Consider the suicide risk in all patients with mental illnesses. Patients are rarely embarrassed and generally relieved to be tactfully asked about suicide. Build up to direct questions such as:

- 'Feeling as you've described recently, have you felt that life was a struggle?'
- 'Patients with similar difficulties to you sometimes tell me they feel suicidal?'
- 'Have you felt like that?'

Management

- *Treat physical problems* (e.g. injuries/poisoning). Be prepared for refusal of treatment and know local laws for dealing with this.
- *Assess future suicide risk:* see below.
- *Assess mental state and start appropriate treatment.* Consider affective disorders, alcohol or drug dependency, personality disorders, and chronic psychotic disorders.
- *Help the patient address the main problems.* These may be psychological, social (e.g. financial problems, relationship difficulties), or physical (e.g. chronic illness).
- *Enlist the help of others* (social workers, financial advisors, counsellors) where appropriate.

Assessment of future suicide risk

Be sympathetic and use a collateral history if necessary. You may need to wait until the patient is no longer under the influence of drugs/alcohol. See box for issues to be assessed.

Summarize risk and protective factors and use this to identify areas which can be improved. If risk is high and cannot be adequately reduced, the patient may need to be admitted, often against their will. If the patient goes home, agree a 'contract' with the patient specifying the steps that each side will take if their situation changes (e.g. techniques to alleviate acute distress, asking for help, seeking medical advice). It may be necessary to agree to remove dangerous/sharp objects from the patient's home, to lock windows, and even to ensure constant supervision. Agree times to meet again and discuss progress/problems.

Assessment of future suicide risk

Assess:

- *Intention of act*: what was their motivation? Ask about associated actions and thoughts, go through what led up to the act and afterwards. Was there planning/preparation? Why did they choose this method, and did they consider alternatives? Did they make any 'final acts' (e.g. writing a suicide note). Did they take precautions to avoid discovery? Did they take alcohol or other substances in addition? What did the act represent: a wish to die/for help/something else? Did they seek help/tell anyone? Was medical attention willingly sought or were they coerced?
- *Present feelings and intentions*: do they regret or feel guilty about the act or being discovered? Have they changed how they feel? If they go home, will they cope? What do they want now: to die/get help? Will they accept treatment?
- *Precipitation*: what problems led to the act? What can be done about them?
- *Resources*: what resources are available (self/friends/family/community/health services/etc.)?
- *Protective factors*: do they have hope for future improvement? Do they have supportive children/partner/family/friends or strong convictions or religious beliefs that would prevent them from committing suicide?
- *Personal history*: previous attempts, chronic pain or illness, social isolation, unemployment, and older age (all increase risk of eventual suicide).

Mood/affective disorders

Depression and bipolar affective disorder are the greatest cause of disability worldwide.

Depression

Major depression is common and globally the fourth leading cause of disease burden. Life expectancy is reduced.

Clinical features: persistent (>2 weeks) low mood (sadness/tearfulness), anhedonia (loss of interest or pleasure), and unexplained fatigue. Symptoms can be considered as cognitive, somatic, and affective — see box. Increasing severity is reflected by both more symptoms and increased level of impairment.

Differential diagnosis: consider drug-induced low mood (e.g. alcohol or other psychoactive substance dependency, or an adverse effect of steroids or beta-blockers), bipolar disorder, eating disorder, schizophrenia, or low mood 2° to chronic infection, anaemia, metabolic, or endocrine disturbance (e.g. hypothyroidism, renal failure, Cushing's syndrome).

Management

- Assess suicide risk (see previous page) — there is no evidence that asking about suicide 'puts ideas into their head'.
- Offer treatment addressing social, psychological, and medical issues.
- Engender hope in the patient and carers and encourage the patient to stop concentrating on negative ideas, or acting on them (e.g. leaving work).
- Avoid the 'pull yourself together' approach — the patients are caught up in guilt and feelings of failure and do not need outside blame.
- A problem-solving approach may be useful, focusing on small, defined steps.

Medication is useful for moderate and severe depressive episodes (>3 symptoms or marked severity), with 70–80% patients showing an improvement. See box.

Choice of antidepressant is influenced by:
- Toxicity (if the risk of overdose is high, avoid tricyclic antidepressants)
- Side-effect profile (avoid amitryptiline and imipramine in patients with heart disease)
- Symptoms: consider more sedative medication (e.g. amitryptiline, imipramine) in anxious or sleep-deprived patients

If patient does not respond: review diagnosis, psychological, and social issues and consider changing medication (ideally to an alternative class). Initially overlap the new treatment with the old, gradually building up the new whilst the old is reduced and withdrawn (except MAOIs, such as phenelzine, where two weeks washout is necessary to avoid interactions).

Recurrent depression

Repeated episodes of depression without mania. Consider long-term social support, psychological therapy directed at relapse prevention, and/or periodic 'top-up' sessions, or long-term prophylactic medication (antidepressant and possibly the addition of a mood stabilizer e.g. lithium).

ICD-10 definition of depression

Symptoms should last 2 weeks or more.
1. **2 of 3 core features:**
   - Low mood
   - Anhedonia
   - Fatigue

2. **Plus 1 or more of:**
   - Sleep disturbance (reduced sleep duration/quality, difficulty getting to sleep, waking during the night, and early morning waking)
   - Guilt, blaming self (out of proportion, or for events out of control such as natural disasters)
   - Appetite disturbance (decreased interest in food and appetite, but can be increased appetite, bingeing)
   - Poor concentration
   - Anxiety and nervousness
   - Low self-esteem
   - Negative thoughts about the future (hopelessness)
   - Reduced libido, menstrual disturbance
   - Suicidal thoughts or acts

Examples of drugs for treatment of depression

- Imipramine, initially 25 mg PO tds, max daily dose 200–300 mg
- Amitryptilline, initially 75 mg PO at night, max daily dose 200 mg
- Fluoxetine, initially 20 mg PO od, max daily dose 60 mg
- Citalopram, initially 20 mg PO od, max daily dose 60 mg

Start at a low dose and increase gradually over a few weeks, with regular reviews to assess side-effects, compliance, and suicidal ideation. Explain that side-effects generally fade after 2–3 weeks, and that maximum benefit builds up over 3–6 weeks, but only if medication is taken every day. They should seek medical advice before stopping medication, unless they have a severe adverse reaction. Once improved, discuss ways to maintain improvement and recommend they continue the antidepressant for 3–6 months, withdrawing gradually after this to avoid discontinuation syndromes (e.g. GI symptoms, chills, headaches, anxiety, and restlessness).

Bipolar affective disorder (BPAD)

A chronic affective disorder characterized by periods of mania and depression. The lifetime prevalence is about 0.5%, with peak onset in the mid-twenties.

Clinical features

Episodes of depression and mania or hypomania. Mania and hypomania are syndromes characterized by a triad of *affective*, *psychomotor*, and *cognitive* features — see box for list of symptoms.

Manic episode: is defined by the presence of 2 or more of these symptoms for at least 1 week.

Hypomanic episode: is defined by the presence of 2 or more of these symptoms for less than 1 week but not more than 2 days.
Manic episodes may not be recognized by the patient, so obtain a collateral Hx if possible. Enquire about high-risk behaviours (e.g. alcohol and drug taking, sexual activity, gambling, spending), work, and legal problems.

A *mixed affective state* is characterized by features of both depression and mania (e.g. concurrent increased psychomotor activity and decreased affect). It is more common in the elderly and may be a sign that the affective state is swinging towards the opposite pole.

Diagnosis: BPAD is diagnosed if there has been at least one clear manic or hypomanic episode and at least one clear depressive episode. Rapid cycling is defined as 4 or more episodes in one year. Rarely, individuals may experience only manic or hypomanic episodes: these episodes are termed BPAD manic type since they respond to treatment in a similar way to BPAD.

Differential diagnosis of manic episodes includes alcohol or drug misuse (particularly stimulants e.g. amphetamines, cocaine, khat), BPAD, medication (e.g. steroids, antidepressants, interferon, anti-TB drugs), schizoaffective disorder, CNS infection (HIV, neurosyphillis), stroke, or SOL.

Management: manic patients may need to be closely supervised, usually in a secure hospital environment with skilled nursing. Avoid confrontation (unless to prevent danger) and establish clear boundaries.

Manic episode
- Agitation and/or psychotic symptoms should be treated with an antipsychotic medication (e.g. haloperidol, chlorpromazine) which is discontinued once the episode has resolved.
- Sedative medication may be required for severe behavioural disturbance.
- Mood stabilizers are indicated for patients with chronic affective disorders (BPAD, recurrent depression, schizoaffective disorder). They are only effective if patient complies for at least 6 months — intermittent compliance may increase affective disturbance.

Depressive episode: see p. 453 for management.

Features of mania/hypomania

* Increased physical and mental energy, and activity levels (patients are talkative, restless)
* Decreased sleep (patients feel they need less sleep)
* Elevated mood (inappropriate)
* Irritability
* Impulsivity
* Disinhibition
* Increased perceptual acuity (e.g. colours, smells seem stronger)
* Grandiosity (feelings that they have special abilities or powers — these may be of delusional intensity)

Drug therapies for BPAD

Agitation and/or psychotic symptoms:

* Haloperidol 1.5–3 mg PO bd or tds (up to 15 mg/day in severe disturbance). 2–10 mg may be used either IM or IV for emergencies.
* Clozapine 12.5 mg PO od initially, gradually titrated up to 300 mg od (max 900 mg) over weeks. It is an atypical antipsychotic and, where available, can be effective when other drugs are ineffective. Monitor FBC weekly for 4 mths initially, and monthly thereafter (causes agranulocytosis).

Sedation:

* Diazepam 2 mg PO tds is a useful starting dose though up to 30 mg in divided doses may be needed. 10 mg by slow IV injection may be used in emergencies, but beware respiratory depression. Avoid IM if possible.

Mood stabilizers:

* Lithium carbonate — the dose required depends on the preparation used. Adjust dose to achieve a serum lithium concentration of 0.4–1 mmol/L 12 hrs after a dose on days 4–7 of treatment. Repeat every week until the dose is constant for 4 weeks; then check every 3 months. A common starting dose is 300 mg PO bd (less in elderly, renal failure, dehydration). Warn patients about signs of toxicity: coarse tremor, nausea, diarrhoea, confusion, fits. Blood levels should be measured weekly until stable, and then at least 6 monthly.
* (Alternatives: carbamazepine and sodium valproate are second-line options used by specialists.)

Acute psychotic disorders

Recent (days to few weeks) history of hallucinations, delusions, fear and suspiciousness, unusual behaviour, emotional lability, and/or speech abnormalities.

Differential diagnosis: a large number of conditions can cause acute psychotic conditions. Consider acute confusional state (delirium), epilepsy, intoxication or withdrawal from drugs or alcohol, chronic psychotic disorders, affective disorders and transient psychotic episodes (sudden onset related to significant stress), hypo- and hyperthyroidism, steroid psychosis.

Management

- Investigate and treat potential causes of acute confusional state (see Chapter 8), including drug or alcohol withdrawal. Use an antipsychotic to treat psychotic symptoms (see below), and continue for 3 months once the psychosis has resolved (beware lowered seizure threshold — haloperidol is less likely to cause seizures).
- Minimize the risk of harm to the patient with behavioural disturbance and others. Ideally treat in a safe, secure environment. Family help may be needed; don't place their safety at risk. Promote a calm, relaxed atmosphere and minimize stress. Avoid confrontation/argument and where it is necessary to intervene, do it calmly and firmly.
- Sedatives can be a useful short-term adjunct: use diazepam 5 mg 2–3 times daily or clonazepam 1 mg 2–4 times daily (long half lives), or a sedative antihistamine (such as chlorphenamine).

Chronic psychotic disorders

These conditions are characterized by persistent psychotic symptoms lasting greater than one month. Schizophrenia is most common, but others include paraphrenia ('late-onset schizophrenia'), schizoaffective disorder, affective disorders, delusional disorders, and drug-related psychoses (e.g. alcoholic hallucinosis). Patients may present via their family, via the police, or with physical illness because of self-neglect via a variety of routes.

Schizoaffective disorder: is characterized by the simultaneous occurrence of affective and schizophrenic symptoms with no clear predominance.

Management: is as for schizophrenia. However, these patients may benefit from a mood stabilizer and treatment of depression, in addition to antipsychotic therapy.

Delusional disorders: are characterized by predominance of stable and well-defined delusions (e.g. jealousy, sexual interest) without prominent hallucinations and abnormalities of affect or personality.

Alcoholic hallucinosis: shows prominent auditory hallucinations and occurs usually after chronic alcohol dependency. Symptoms persist into abstinence.

Management: both generally respond to management for schizophrenia (and continued abstinence from alcohol in the case of hallucinosis).

Schizophrenia

Clinical features and diagnosis

1. One-month history of one or more of the following (two symptoms if not clear cut):
   * *Delusions:* that the body, mind, or feelings are under external control, or that thoughts are being inserted, withdrawn, or broadcast from their mind, or other very bizarre beliefs.
   * *Hallucinations:* the experience of their thoughts being spoken aloud, or other persistent auditory, visual, olfactory, or somatic hallucinations.

Or

2. Two or more of the following:
   * Formal thought disorder (e.g. neologisms, incoherent speech)
   * Catatonic behaviour (e.g. stupor, mutism, posturing, waxy flexibility)
   * Negative symptoms (e.g. unexplained apathy, alogia, incongruous affect)
   * Social withdrawal

3. These symptoms occur in **clear consciousness**. There should not be a marked affective component. Where affective symptoms are present, they should not predominate or should develop after the main features.

Assessment

Consider the differential list for acute psychosis. Was there a precipitating factor? Exposure to high levels ($\rightarrow$ 35 hours per week) of expressed emotion (e.g. critical/hostile comments) is associated with increased risk of relapse.

Management

* This should be started as soon as possible since untreated psychosis is linked with increased disability.
* Acutely disturbed patients will need to be admitted to hospital and require intensive nursing. If this is not available, try to arrange a safe environment and engage the patient's family, as with management of acute psychosis.
* Treat with antipsychotic medication — see box.

If there is no or incomplete response:
* Assess compliance
* Discuss reasons for non-compliance (e.g. poor insight, intolerable side-effects).
* Address these reasons (e.g. give compliance therapy, switch antipsychotic drug to an alternative with fewer side-effects).

Depot (intramuscular) injections can aid compliance.

Psychological and social interventions: have been shown to be effective.
* Reduce levels of stress and 'expressed emotion'.
* Offer sheltered work or appropriate training, to help develop occupational and self-care skills.
* Encourage the patient to reach the highest level of functioning possible once the acute/severe symptoms have resolved.
* Activity or distraction may reduce the severity or burden of symptoms.

Education: is important for patient and family. Schizophrenia is a chronic illness, and treatment is often needed for life to prevent relapse.

Drug management of schizophrenia

1. **Treat with antipsychotic medication.** Drug-naïve patients should be started on a low dose (e.g. chlorpromazine 25 mg PO tds or haloperidol 1.5–3 mg PO bd or tds [3–5 mg bd or tds if severe]) and this dose increased gradually over several weeks. Benefit should become apparent after 2–3 weeks and continued improvement occurs for 3–6 months. The initial action of antipsychotics is largely sedative.

2. **Warn the patient about likely side-effects:** acute and chronic movement disorders, anticholinergic effects, increased appetite and weight gain, sedation, and hyperprolactinaemia (gynaecomastia, galactorrhoea, dysmennorrhea, and sexual dysfunction).

3. **Acute dystonia** (e.g. painful ocular deviation, neck twisting, or muscle spasms) may occur within hours and should be treated with an anticholinergic such as procyclidine 5 mg IM, which may need to be repeated.

4. **Chronic movement disorders**, such as Parkinsonism, will require dose reduction or drug change. If movement disorder persists, try an anticholinergic (e.g. procyclidine. 2.5mg PO tds, increasing gradually; daily max 30 mg). Akathisia (severe motor restlessness) can be very distressing — consider adding an anticholinergic or beta-blocker.

75% will respond to an antipsychotic. 85% will relapse within 2 yrs if they stop medication, compared to about 20% who continue. The 25% of patients who do not respond should be switched (gradual cross-tapering) to an alternative drug, ideally from a different class. Patients that remain psychotic despite adequate trials of antipsychotics are often termed 'treatment resistant'. The diagnosis should be reconsidered. Where the diagnosis remains schizophrenia, a trial of clozapine is warranted (~2/3 will respond to clozapine). Withdraw other antipsychotics and commence clozapine 12.5 mg PO od initially, gradually titrated up to 300 mg (max 900 mg) over 4 weeks. Monitor FBC weekly for 4 mths initially, and monthly thereafter (causes agranulocytosis).

Anxiety disorders

These are common and disabling conditions which include phobias, panic disorder, generalized anxiety disorder, and mixed anxiety and depression. Consider them in terms of cognitive, physical, and behavioural aspects (e.g. avoidance).

Clinical features

The anxiety is extreme, sometimes incapacitating, and out of proportion to the level of danger/threat. The anxiety may occur without trigger.

Physical:

- Palpitations
- Tachycardia
- Trembling
- Feeling of choking
- Dizziness
- Lightheadedness/faintness
- Chills or hot flushes
- Pounding heart
- Sweating
- Shortness of breath
- Chest pain/discomfort
- Unsteadiness
- Paraesthesia (perioral and peripheral)
- Nausea/abdominal discomfort (butter flies in stomach, diarrhoea, vomiting)

Psychological:

- Persistent excessive worry
- Fear of criticism or embarrassment
- Fear of losing control/going mad
- Tension
- Fear of being trapped
- Feelings of unreality (derealization or depersonalization)

Differential diagnosis: consider depression, drug and alcohol misuse (alcohol/drugs may be used to self-treat anxiety), thyrotoxicosis, Cushing's syndrome, anaemia, cardiac dysrhythmias, pulmonary disease, or seizures.

Common management principles

1. Describe the link between thoughts, feelings, and physical responses, which are part of the body's natural arousal system.
2. Identify and reduce chemical elements that predispose to anxiety (e.g. caffeine, cigarettes, theophylline, steroids, stimulants such as khat, or amphetamines).
3. Identify and reduce psychosocial stressors (e.g. work pressures).
4. Explain that withdrawing from/avoiding a situation only acts to strengthen the anxiety associated with it.

Medication is secondary

1. Anxiolytics (e.g. diazepam 2 mg PO tds, increased as necessary to 5–10 mg tds) are effective for short term (<2 weeks) use. Dependence and reinforcement of anxiety may occur with longer use.
2. Antidepressants (e.g. Imipramine, see before) are useful if depressive symptoms are present. SSRIs may be effective for panic disorder.
3. Beta-blockers (propranolol 40 mg od) are effective in reducing autonomic symptoms (e.g. palpitations and tremor).

Phobic disorder

Fear of a specific item or situation that is out of proportion to objective risks, beyond voluntary control, and not responsive to reasoning. It results in avoidance of situations in which this item or situation (the trigger) is expected (e.g. crowds, open spaces, travelling, social events). Patients may become confined to their house.

Management: anxiety reduction techniques (see box). Use graded exposure (e.g. to feared situation such as crowds) to reduce avoidance and escape the cycle of reinforcement:

- Start by thinking about or discussing the feared item/situation.
- Gradually increase exposure, with support, until it is experienced in full.
- Each step should be carried out regularly until it is no longer anxiety provoking.

Discuss alternative ways of viewing and challenging the fears.

Panic disorder

Recurrent, frequent, unexpected panic attacks characterized by >4 symptoms.

Management: practice anxiety reduction techniques regularly. Identify exaggerated fears (e.g. 'palpitations mean I'm having a heart attack') and restructure them by helping the patient to come up with alternative explanations that reflect the evidence.

Obsessive-compulsive disorder

Recurrent obsessional thoughts or compulsive acts, present most days for 2 weeks. They may be thoughts, images, impulses, or ideas that repeatedly take the same characteristic form. Obsessional thoughts are recognized as the patient's own (cf. schizophrenia), and the patient usually makes an (often unsuccessful) effort to resist such thoughts/acts.

Differential diagnosis: includes depression, psychotic disorders, tic disorders, and physical brain disorders.

Management: cognitive behavioural techniques and antidepressants (e.g. clomipramine).

Anxiety reduction techniques

These techniques need to be practised, ideally daily, to develop the ability to relax before and during stressful situations. Generally, the more they are practised, the more effective they are. They can be used prior to or during anxiety provoking situations to reduce anxiety levels.

1. ***Progressive muscle relaxation:*** in a quiet, comfortable environment, work through the body's muscle groups, tensing then relaxing each in turn: feet, then legs, then thighs, etc. Concentrate on the relaxed feelings.
2. ***Controlled breathing:*** practise breathing in and out to a slow count of 4 each. Continue this for 5 mins to reduce hyperventilation (causing paraesthesiae, carpopedal spasms, etc.).
3. ***Imagery:*** visualize a scene that is calm, safe, and relaxing. Concentrate on the details, smells, sounds, and feel of the place.
4. ***Distraction:*** focus attention away from anxious thoughts and sensations and on to something relaxing and absorbing.

Mental retardation (learning disability)

A condition of arrested or incomplete development of the mind leading to functional disability. Impairment is global (i.e. manifest in cognitive, social, language, and motor development), apparent during the developmental period (onset before age 18), and results in reduced ability to meet the daily demands of life. The prevalence of moderate to severe retardation varies from 1–20/1000 worldwide.

Differential diagnosis: consider specific learning difficulties (e.g. language acquisition), motor disorders (e.g. cerebral palsy), sensory problems (e.g. in the past, deaf people were often inappropriately considered as mentally retarded), hyperkinetic disorder, and autistic spectrum disorders.

Assessment

An informant such as a parent is essential.

1. *Record nature and extent of mental retardation* — take a developmental history and consider delay in communication and social interaction; motor function and self-care; and functional academic skills.
2. *Identify additional problems* — such as self-harm or harm to others; impulsive or dangerous behaviour.
3. *Determine aetiology* — see box.
4. *Identify coexisting psychiatric diagnoses* — prevalence is 2–4-fold higher in people with mental retardation than the general population.

Classification

The WHO has subclassified mental retardation into mild, moderate, and severe.

- *Mild:* development is slow, but most people achieve full independence.
- *Moderate:* achieve some language and self-care skills but require on-going assistance and supervision. Independent living is uncommon.
- *Severe:* is usually apparent in the first few years of life. The person is rarely capable of more than simple speech and needs assistance with daily tasks of living.

Management

- *Consider and investigate treatable causes:* this can be difficult due to limited resources, cultural practices, and a lack of interest from health professionals.
- *Aim to maximize functioning:* provide the optimal environment for development. Treat sensory impairment.
- *Encourage carers to reward desirable behaviours* and to reduce the 'attentional reward' of disruptive behaviours. Consistency and perseverance with this approach usually works to reduce disruptive behaviour.
- *Support the family:* offer encouragement, periodic 'respite' admission, support groups, literature. Specialist educational provision may be appropriate if available.
- *Medication:* is indicated for specific comorbid conditions (e.g. epilepsy, hyperkinetic disorder, depression).

Aetiologies of moderate to severe mental retardation

1. **Prenatal (50–70%)**
   Genetic
   - Fragile X
   - Down's syndrome
   External factors
   - Congenital infections with herpes simplex 2, rubella, HIV, toxoplasmosis, syphilis, cytomegalovirus.
   - Exposure to toxic substances such as medications, alcohol, cocaine.
   - Maternal disorder such as diabetes and pre-eclampsia.

2. **Perinatal (10–20%)**
   - ***Delivery problems*** resulting in asphyxia, neonatal sepsis, encephalitis.

3. **Postnatal (5–10%)**
   - ***Brain damage*** due to trauma, toxic agents (e.g. lead poisoning), iodine deficiency, malnutrition.

Disorders due to psychoactive substances

The diagnosis of a dependence syndrome (ICD-10 criteria) should be made if three or more of the following is present:

- **Strong desire/compulsion** to take the substance
- **Difficulties controlling** substance-taking behaviour in terms of onset, termination, or levels of use
- **Withdrawal**: a physiological state when use of the substance has been stopped or reduced. The patient may use the substance to relieve or avoid withdrawal symptoms
- **Tolerance**: increased doses are required to achieve a given effect
- **Neglect of alternative interests**: obtaining and taking the substance gradually grows to dominate the individual's life
- **Continued use despite evidence of harmful consequences**: the user must be aware of these consequences

Harmful use is substance abuse not fulfilling the above criteria but causing significant damage to mental or physical health. There are often major social consequences.

Clinical features: acute withdrawal state, low mood, anxiety symptoms, sleep difficulties, physical complications (e.g. trauma, GI disease in alcohol dependence), cognitive impairment, unexplained change in behaviour (e.g. irritability, reduced personal care or functioning), and legal or social problems (e.g. missed work).

Withdrawal states

Many states show these general effects: anxiety, tremor, fever, sleep disturbance, tachycardia, gastro-intestinal disturbance.

- *Opiate withdrawal:* muscle aches, dysphoria, agitation, insomnia, diarrhoea, shivering, yawning, fatigue, hypertension, lacrimation, rhinorrhoea, dilated pupils, and piloerection ('gooseflesh').
- *Alcohol withdrawal:* fits, confusional states including delirium tremens (severe confusional state with visual and auditory hallucinations and paranoid ideation); risk of Wernicke's encephalopathy (ophthalmoplegia, nystagmus, and ataxia with confusion due to thiamine deficiency).
- *Benzodiazepines/barbiturates:* weight loss, vivid dreams (REM sleep rebound), tinitus, irritability, impaired memory and concentration, perceptual disturbance (hypersensitivity to sound, light and touch, derealization and depersonalization), confusional states and fits.

Withdrawal states usually begin 4–12 hours after the last dose, peak at 48–72 hours, and last 7–10 days. However, the onset of benzodiazepine withdrawal occurs usually 1–14 days after the last dose and may last many months. The confusional states and fits associated with alcohol, benzodiazepine, and barbiturate withdrawal are potentially life-threatening. Withdrawal states should be avoided as much as possible by using a gradual reducing regime and being treated rapidly when identified (see p. 466).

Questions to assess alcohol and/or substance use

- Are you concerned by your use of alcohol/the substance?
- Can you control your use of it?
- Have you thought you should cut down?
- Have friends commented on your use of it?
- Has your use of it led you to neglect your friends/family/work?
- Has your use of it led you to be in trouble with the police?
- Do you take it as soon as you can after you wake up?

Management of dependence

There is increasing evidence that patients are in a state in which ability to control substance use is reduced — it is not just 'a lack of willpower'. Ask 'open' questions and use 'reflective listening', clarify concerns, convey empathy and collaboration, and help the patient to reach their own conclusions about the effects of substance misuse. Educate the patient that dependence is an illness with serious health consequences, and stopping or reducing use will bring mental and physical benefits, and explain the symptoms of withdrawal. Abstinence should be the goal in the majority of cases, although controlled, reduced levels of use are sometimes appropriate. Relapses are common, and it may take several attempts to control or stop substance use.

For patients willing to stop now or control their use, help them:

- Set a definite day to quit/begin controlled use.
- If reducing use, agree a clear and highly specific goal for reduction (e.g. no more than 4 units of alcohol per day and two alcohol-free days per week).
- Agree strategies to control use (e.g. slow down drinking to no more than one unit/hour, introduce alternative behaviour to substance use such as drinking fruit juice, chewing gum, exercise).
- Identify high-risk situations (social or stressful occasions) and form a menu of strategies to avoid or cope with these.
- Make specific plans to avoid substances (e.g. develop assertiveness skills to respond to friends who are using substances).
- Identify family members/friends who will support them.
- Discuss symptoms and management of withdrawal.

If the attempt is unsuccessful:

- Identify areas of success (e.g. cut down use for a period).
- Discuss situations and triggers for relapse and identify whether these can be altered.
- Try again.

Alcohol withdrawal

Admission may be advisable, particularly if there is a Hx of previous severe withdrawals (e.g. confusion, fits) or poor physical health (e.g. liver failure) or mental health (e.g. suicidal ideation). A reducing dose of a substitute benzodiazepine is given over 5 days — see box.

- Higher doses may be required. As an in-patient this judgement can be based on symptoms of withdrawal, with more frequent dosing.
- A short-acting drug (e.g. lorazepam 1 mg) may be used instead for patients with significant liver failure.
- B-complex vitamins should be given parenterally to avoid or treat Wernicke's encephalopathy.

Benzodiazepine withdrawal

Change to an equivalent dose of a long-acting benzodiazepine such as diazepam (e.g. lorazepam 0.5 mg is equivalent to diazepam 5 mg). Then gradually reduce the dose to nothing. If dependency is chronic, this may take many weeks or months.

Benzodiazepine regimen for alcohol withdrawal

Chlordiazepoxide:

Day 1	30 mg tds
Day 2	20 mg qds
Day 3	30 mg bd
Day 4	10 mg bd and 20 mg od
Day 5	10 mg bd

Reactions to severe stress

Adjustment disorders and bereavement

An adjustment disorder is a state of emotional disturbance and impaired social functioning that develops shortly after (<3 months) or during a stressor. There may be affective, cognitive, and behavioural symptoms. Stressors may take many forms (e.g. bereavement, diagnosis of a major illness, migration). Adjustment disorders are common in people with physical disorders, and should be considered if rehabilitation is slower or poorer than expected.

Bereavement: may be abnormal in form and/or severity compared to cultural norms. Four stages have been described:
1. Shock and numbness
2. Preoccupation (yearning or anger, etc.)
3. Disorganization (loss is reluctantly accepted)
4. Resolution

These may not necessarily occur in this order. It is abnormal when symptoms are not related to the loss — such as feelings of worthlessness or inappropriate guilt. Abnormal perceptions involving the lost person (e.g. hearing them whispering) can be a feature of normal bereavement, but hallucinatory phenomena not involving the lost person are indications of a bereavement disorder.

Differential diagnosis: depressive disorders, obsessive-compulsive disorder, physical causes of weight loss and anorexia (e.g. intestinal parasites, malaria, Crohn's syndrome).

Management
- Allow the individual to talk about the loss and its circumstances, and to discuss the feelings that are provoked, particularly guilt and anger.
- Involve the carers and family, and aim to increase social support.
- Identify steps that can be taken to modify causes of stress.
- Medication should be avoided unless there is depression or pychosis. If there is severe insomnia, hypnotics may be used — but only for <2 weeks.

Post-traumatic stress disorder

A delayed/protracted response within 6 months of a stressful event. There may be repetitive, intrusive re-experiencing of the event ('flashbacks' or dreams), autonomic disturbance, affective symptoms, suicidal ideation, and alcohol/drug abuse.

Management: give gradual, supported exposure to the stressful event (either through imagination or in person where safe) — as for anxiety/phobias — leading to lessening of arousal and habituation. Cognitive behavioural techniques may also be used. Antidepressants (e.g. SSRIs) are useful but benzodiazepines are not indicated.

Further Reading

Hawton K et al. (1999) *Cognitive behaviour therapy for psychiatric problems: a practical guide*. Oxford University Press.

Patel V (2003) *Where there is no psychiatrist; a mental health care manual*. Gaskell Press (Royal College of Psychiatrists).

WHO (1996) *Diagnostic and management guidelines for mental disorders in primary care. ICD-10*. Hogrefe & Huber, Gottingen, Chapter V.

http://www.nimh.gov

http://www.mentalhealth.com/main.htm

Ophthalmology

Section editor   **Allen Foster**

Sources:
J Sandford-Smith. *Eye diseases in hot climates*. Butterworth-Heinemann, Oxford 1990.
E.Sutter. *Hanyane – A Village Struggles for Eye Health*. MacMillan, London 1989
Int. Resource Centre. *Journal of Community Eye Health*. ICEH, 11 Bath St., London.

Global blindness

The WHO estimates that 45 million people worldwide are blind (corrected visual acuity of less than 3/60 in the best eye). This figure is increasing by 1–2 million per year because of an increasing ageing population. By far the majority live in the developing world. A further 135 million people have low vision (corrected acuity of less than 6/18 to 3/60).

Cataract is the commonest cause of blindness worldwide, with an estimated 20 million blind people and over 100 million eyes justifying cataract surgery because of severe visual impairment. In 1999 an estimated 10 million cataract operations were performed worldwide. It is calculated that as many as 30 million cataract operations need to be performed annually if cataract blindness is to be controlled in the next 10 years.

Trachoma and onchocerciasis are blinding ocular infections responsible for approximately 15% of all blindness. Both occur in poor communities. Blindness can be prevented through relatively simple, low cost interventions including the use of anti-microbials. Vitamin A deficiency is a major cause of blindness in children and again occurs in poor communities.

Visual loss due to Refractive Errors, particularly myopia, is an increasing problem especially in Asia. Refraction followed by the appropriate spectacle correction will restore sight but for people living in isolated communities the 'refractionist' and spectacles are often not available or affordable.

These five diseases (cataract, trachoma, onchocerciasis, vitamin A deficiency, and refractive errors) are all avoidable (preventable or curable) and constitute at least 70% of all cases of blindness worldwide.

Introduction

People attending with an eye complaint are usefully considered according to the main symptom, namely:

1. Visual loss, so that they cannot see in the distance with one or both eyes
2. Red painful eye(s), with or without a history of trauma
3. Inability to read print, or see near objects, due to presbyopia after 40 years of age
4. A variety of other specific symptoms – e.g. watering eyes, flashing lights, etc.

In this section, emphasis is placed on the causes, diagnosis, and management of patients presenting with 'visual loss' or 'red eye'. The final paragraphs describe some eye diseases that are seen in the tropics.

Visual loss

Examination

1. measure the visual acuity without and with a pinhole
2. examine the cornea and pupil with a torchlight
3. after dilating the pupil, examine the optic disc and retina with an ophthalmoscope

Refractive errors

There are five different types of refractive errors:

- Myopia – short-sightedness, causing poor distance vision
- Hypermetropia – long-sightedness, giving difficulty with near vision in young people
- Astigmatism – due to a different refraction in two axes of the eye
- Aphakia – the refractive error due to absence of the lens
- Presbyopia – poor accommodation giving difficulty in reading after the age of 40 years, which is treated with reading spectacles that usually have a number between +1.00 and +3.00 dioptres

Most people with poor distance vision due to refractive errors have myopia. The visual acuity usually improves with a pinhole. Myopia can be corrected with minus lenses.

Cataract

Cataracts are the commonest cause of bilateral blindness worldwide. They cause gradual and progressive decrease in visual acuity.

Diagnosis: when complete, they can be seen as a white opacity in the pupil, while earlier cataracts give a grey-white appearance to the pupil. Examination of the fundus of the eye with an ophthalmoscope, after dilation of the pupil, shows an opacity in the red reflex with obscuration of fundal detail due to the lens opacity. The pupil reaction to light is normal in an uncomplicated cataract.

Management: cataracts are treated by surgery to remove the lens and replace it with an artificial intro-ocular lens (IOL). Surgery is usually performed under local anaesthesia. The results in experienced hands are very good. The patient may need corrective spectacles post-operatively to obtain optimal vision.

Corneal opacity

Diagnosis: there is a white opacity on the cornea, which usually obscures a clear view of the pupil. This may follow a corneal ulcer, injury, or be due to a specific eye disease such as trachoma, vitamin A deficiency, or leprosy.

Management: if both eyes have severe visual loss, then a corneal graft or optical iridectomy may be considered to try and improve the vision. Specialist care and very good follow up are essential to obtain reasonable results.

Glaucoma

The glaucomas are responsible for 10–20% of all cases of blindness. Glaucoma may be acute with a red painful eye, or chronic with gradual progressive loss of vision due to optic nerve damage.

Diagnosis: of chronic glaucoma is difficult until most vision has been lost when a raised intra-ocular pressure (IOP), with 'pathological cupping' of the optic disc, and poor pupil reaction to light are evident.

Management: of glaucoma consists of lowering the IOP with life-long eye drops or (hopefully) one time filtration surgery. Treatment does not restore sight, but is given in an effort to preserve the remaining vision.

Table 10.1 Common causes of poor distance vision

	Refractive error	Corneal Opacity	Cataract	Diseases of Optic Nerve and Retina
Causes	Myopia Astigmatism Aphakia (Hypermetropia)	Corneal ulcer Trachoma Vitamin A deficiency Leprosy	Usually age related. Also:- Eye injuries Diabetes Iritis	The glaucomas Optic atrophy Macula degeneration Diabetic retinopathy hypertensive retinopathy Retinal detachment Hypertensive retina
Signs and symptoms	Vision improves with a pinhole.	White scarring of the cornea in a quiet white eye Pupil difficult to see. Absent or poor red reflex.	White or grey pupil. Pupil reacts to light. Absent or poor red reflex.	Cornea and lens should be clear. Pupil may not react normally to light. Specific signs seen with an ophthalmoscope in the retina or optic nerve.
Management	Spectacles	Often no treatment. Surgery may be considered when both eyes are affected.	Cataract removal if the visual acuity is less than 6/60, or if the person's lifestyle is affected.	That of the cause.

Red eye

History and Examination
1. ask about any known cause, particularly any injury
2. measure the visual acuity
3. carefully examine the eyelids, conjunctiva, cornea, and pupil with a torch

Injuries to the eye

First ask about any injury to or foreign body into the eye.

Corneal or conjunctival foreign bodies (FB).
The history is usually straightforward. The FB may be obvious or you may need to evert the upper eyelid to check the conjunctiva for objects scratching the cornea each time the patient blinks.
To remove the FB:
- Lie the patient flat
- Local anaesthetic drops are applied to the conjunctiva
- Light the eye, so that the FB is easily visible
- Loupe magnification is useful
- Lift off the FB with the corner of a thick piece of paper, or carefully with a needle.

Give an antibiotic eye ointment and eye pad for 1 day.

Corneal abrasion
This occurs when something scratches the cornea, removing some of the epithelial cells. There is sudden severe pain and photophobia. To confirm the diagnosis, one can apply fluorescein to stain the cornea where there is no epithelium. Treat with an antibiotic eye ointment and eye pad until the pain has gone and epithelium completely healed.

Hyphaema
If there is a severe blunt injury then bleeding may occur inside the eye. A level of blood (hyphaema) may be visible between the cornea and iris. This will usually resolve over a few days with rest. Avoid using aspirin; if the eye is painful give acetazolamide 250 mgs qds for 3–7 days to lower the IOP. If the hyphaema has not resolved by 5 days, an eye specialist should be consulted.

Perforating eye injury
If the eye has been perforated, then this is serious. Be very careful examining the eye as pressure may aggravate the injury. Gently apply an antibiotic eye drop (not ointment), put an eye pad over the eye, and refer the patient to a specialist immediately. If this is not possible then conservative treatment with antibiotic eye drops every 3 hours and an eye pad is probably better than a non eye surgeon 'having a go'.

Red eye with no injury

If there is no history of eye injury, then there are 4 conditions that should be considered in the differential diagnosis of an acute red eye:

* Conjunctivitis
* Corneal ulcer
* Iritis
* Acute glaucoma

Conjunctivitis

Infective conjunctivitis

Infection or inflammation of the conjunctiva is common in the tropics. The important causes and a method for differentiating them are given on the following page.

Diagnosis: there is irritation of the eye with discomfort but normal vision. The eye is red with increased discharge (see Table 10.2). Severe disease may produce swelling of the eyelids (chemosis).

Management: give an antibiotic eye ointment (or drops) 4 times per day for 5–7 days. Do not pad the eye.

Ophthalmia neonatorum

This is a specific conjunctivitis occurring within the first 4 weeks of life. It is usually due to *Neisseria gonococcus* or genital *Chlamydia*. The lids are very swollen and covered with pus.

Management: is with an appropriate systemic and topical antibiotic to which *Neisseria* is sensitive – see Chapter 2B.

Chlamydial conjunctivitis (trachoma)

This is discussed later in the section on specific eye diseases.

Epidemic haemorrhagic conjunctivitis

This is a highly contagious viral conjunctivitis usually due to an enterovirus. After a 1–2 day incubation period, multiple petechial haemorrhages occur. Most patients recover quickly.

Management: if possible, prescribe an anti-microbial agent such as povidone iodine 1% eye drops to help reduce transmission and reassure the patient.

Allergic conjunctivitis

Children may develop an allergic conjunctivitis called vernal conjunctivitis. There is severe itching and irritation with a mucus discharge, sometimes with swelling and pigmentation around the cornea.

Management: with anti-inflammatory agents is difficult and not without serious side effects. If at all possible, children with severe disease should be seen and treated by an eye specialist.

Table 10.2 Common causes of non-traumatic acute red eye

	Conjunctivitis	Corneal ulcer	Iritis	Acute glaucoma
Pain	Irritation	Moderate to severe	Moderate	Severe
Vision	Normal	Variable loss	Variable loss	Severe loss
Redness	Especially in the fornices	Around the cornea	Around the cornea	Around the corneal limbus
Cornea	Normal	Opacity on cornea	Keratic precipitates seen with magnification	Oedematous and hazy
Pupil	Normal	Normal	Constricted and irregular	Half dilated and fixed
Special features	Discharge, often bilateral	Stains with fluorescein	Irregular pupil may be more obvious as the pupil is dilated	Raised IOP
Treatment	Topical antibiotics	Topical antibiotics or antimicrobials.	Dilate pupil and give topical steroids if certain of diagnosis	Acetazolamide 250 mg qds Drops to lower IOP Surgery is usually needed

Table 10.3 Common causes of conjunctivitis

	Age and state of patient	Secretions	Special features	Treatment
Bacterial	Any	Purulent	Red and swollen Purulent discharge	Topical antibiotics for 5 days
Ophthalmia neonatorum	First 4 weeks of life	Purulent	Very red and swollen Purulent discharge	Systemic and topical antibiotics for 10 days
Viral	Any	Watery	May have corneal lesions	Symptomatic only
Chlamydial (Trachoma)	Usually young children	Mucopurulent	Follicles and papillae on upper lid	Azithromycin tablets or tetracycline ointment for 6 weeks
Allergic (Vernal)	Children	Stringy mucus	Very itchy Large papillae Infiltrate and pigmentation around cornea	Chromoglicate and possibly steroid eye drops for symptoms.

Corneal ulcers

A corneal ulcer may occur spontaneously or follow minor trauma. There are many causes – the main ones are summarized opposite.

Diagnosis: there is usually severe pain and blurred vision. On examination, there is redness around and an opacity on the cornea, which usually stains with fluorescein. In severe cases, there may be a fluid level of pus inside the eye called a hypopyon. If infective the causative organism may be identified by gram stain and culture of a scraping from the edge of the corneal ulcer.

Management: depends on the cause, and is summarized opposite.

Uveitis

Inflammation of the uvea may involve both anterior uvea (iris and ciliary body) and posterior uvea (choroid). Anterior uveitis is termed iritis or iridocyclitis; posterior uveitis choroiditis. There are many causes including: leprosy; onchocerciasis; toxoplasmosis; TB; and syphilis, but most cases have no known cause.

Iritis

Clinical features: the pain of iritis varies from mild to severe, and is usually associated with blurring of vision and photophobia. Blood vessels around the margin of the cornea (the limbus) are dilated. The iris constricts and adheres to the front of the lens, making the pupil irregular. With iris dilatation, adhesions may be seen before they break, leaving iris pigment on the front of the lens. WBC and protein exudate collect in the anterior chamber in acute diseases, and can be seen with a slit lamp microscope.

Management: involves dilating the pupil to break any posterior synechiae (cyclopentolate 1% or atropine 1%), and anti-inflammatory agents (prednisolone 0.5 to 1.0% drops) to reduce the inflammation.

Choroiditis

Clinical features: presents with visual loss because of involvement of the overlying retina. It is not usually painful but a severe attack may cause some discomfort. A white inflammatory lesion may be seen in the retina. Once the inflammation has settled, characteristic scars occur with pigment atrophy and hypertrophy.

Management: requires treatment of the cause, often with systemic anti-inflammatory agents.

Acute glaucoma

If the IOP increases suddenly over hours or days then the eye becomes red and very painful with severe loss of vision. The condition, acute glaucoma, is unusual in people under 50 years of age. It may occur spontaneously or as a complication of a complete white cataract. The cornea appears hazy and the pupil is semi-dilated and fixed to light. The IOP is very high.

Management: give acetazolamide 500 mgs stat and then 250 qds. The patient should be seen by an eye specialist and laser treatment or surgery is often required.

Table 10.4 Common causes of corneal ulceration

Cause	Predisposing factors	Clinical features	Treatment
Herpes simplex	Fever	Irregular branch-like ulcer.	Aciclovir ointment
Bacteria	Trauma	Often severe, hypopyon may be present	Intensive topical, or sub-conjunctival antibiotics
Fungus	Humid areas	Often severe, hypopyon may be present	Antifungal agents
Vit A Deficiency	Malnutrition Measles Malabsorption	Dry cornea. Central 'punched out' oval ulcer, often in a quiet eye	Vitamin A 200,000 i.u. stat immediately, then after 1 day, and 2 weeks
Exposure ulcer	Leprosy Eyelids open	Eyelids do not close Lower third oval ulcer	Antibiotics Tape eye closed ? Tarsorrhaphy

Trachoma

Trachoma is a chronic conjunctivitis due to repeated infection with *Chlamydia trachomatis*, serotypes A, B, and C. Inflammation from active trachoma infection leads to conjunctival and tarsal plate scarring which causes the eyelashes to turn in. The lashes rub on the cornea, producing ulceration, scarring, and blindness.

Transmission: the disease occurs particularly in poor dry areas of the world in which there is inadequate water supply and poor community sanitation. The classic trachoma environment can be described as:
- Dry: lack of water
- Dirty: lack of sanitation
- Discharge: lack of personal hygiene

Transmission of trachoma from child to child and child to mother occurs through:
- Flies: flies go from individual to individual
- Fingers: direct contact with ocular discharge
- Family: within the family, child to child

Clinical features and diagnosis: see the 5-point WHO grading system opposite. TF and TI are found mainly in pre-school children; TS, TT, and CO occur more commonly in women than men, starting at around the age of 15 and gradually increasing in prevalence.

How to examine the eye for trachoma: requires good light (sunlight or strong torch) and x2–2.5 magnification. Examine each eye separately.
1. Look for trichiasis (either inturned lashes or previously removed eyelashes). Push upper lid upwards slightly to expose lid margins.
2. Check cornea for opacities.
3. Check inside of upper eyelid by everting it. Ask the patient to look down; gently take hold of eyelashes between thumb and first finger of left hand, and evert the upper eyelid using a glass rod or similar instrument in the right hand. Steady the everted lid with left thumb and examine the conjunctiva for follicles, intense inflammation, and scarring.

Management: either
- azithromycin 20 mg/kg PO as a single dose, *or*
- for pregnant women, erythromycin 500 mg PO bd for 7 days, *or*
- tetracycline 1% topical ointment both eyes bd for 6 weeks.

Studies are still evaluating the merits of mass community treatment vs. targeted treatment of affected individuals. Entropion and trichiasis will require surgery (the bilamellar tarsal rotation procedure).

Prevention: of trachoma is considered under the acronym SAFE (see box opposite). Control requires first identifying a community with blinding disease. This can be done using the grading scheme and a survey of 1–10 yr old children for TF and TI, and women over the age of 15 yrs for TT. A prevalence of TF in excess of 20%, or TT in excess of 1%, would identify a community with severe disease.

Trachoma grading - see colour plates

Signs must be clearly seen in order to be considered present. Grading is important for community prevalence surveys to decide whether mass treatment is warranted.

Normal: the normal conjunctiva is pink, smooth, thin, and transparent. Over the whole area of the tarsal conjunctiva, there are normally large deep-lying blood vessels that run vertically. The dotted line shows the area to be examined.

Trachomatous inflammation – follicular (TF): *the presence of five or more follicles in the upper tarsal conjunctiva.* Follicles are round swellings that are paler than the surrounding conjunctiva, appearing white, grey, or yellow. Follicles must be at least 0.5 mm in diameter.

Trachomatous inflammation – intense (TI): *pronounced inflammatory thickening of the tarsal conjunctiva that obscures more than half of the normal deep tarsal vessels.* The conjunctiva appears red, rough, and thickened. There are numerous follicles, which may be partially or totally covered by the thickened conjunctiva.

Trachomatous scarring (TS): *the presence of scarring in the tarsal conjunctiva.* Scars are easily visible as white lines, bands, or sheets in the tarsal conjunctiva. They are glistening and fibrous in appearance. Scarring, especially diffuse fibrosis, may obscure the tarsal blood vessels.

Trachomatous trichiasis (TT): *at least one eyelash rubs on the eyeball.* Evidence of recent removal of inturned eyelashes should also be graded as trichiasis.

Corneal opacity (CO): *easily visible corneal opacity over the pupil.* The pupil margin is blurred viewed through the opacity. Such corneal opacities cause significant visual impairment (worse than 6/18 vision), and therefore visual acuity should be measured.

WHO's SAFE strategy for the global elimination of trachoma

S Surgery for entropion and trichiasis
A Antibiotics for infectious trachoma
F Facial cleanliness to reduce transmission
E Environmental improvements such as control of disease-spreading flies and access to clean water

Specific eye conditions

Vitamin A Deficiency and xerophthalmia

Xerophthalmia is dry eyes due to vitamin A deficiency, which may lead to corneal ulceration and blindness, particularly during the presence of measles infection.

See Chapter 15. Patients with acute corneal lesions should be referred, whenever this is possible, to a hospital for treatment of their general condition as well as of their eye disease.

Ocular leprosy

Leprosy (Chapter 8) can affect the eyelids, cornea, or pupils by damaging the nerves to the eye or by causing iritis.

Eyelids: nerve damage causes an inability to close the eye (lagophthalmos), with resulting corneal exposure, ulceration, scarring, and blindness.

Management: requires protection of the cornea when the patient is asleep by applying ointment and strapping the upper eyelid to the cheek. If severe and permanent, or if there is evidence of corneal ulceration, then a lateral tarsorrhaphy will be required to protect the cornea. This consists of sewing the upper and lower eyelids together over the lateral third of the eyelid margins.

Cornea: ophthalmic nerve damage results in anaesthesia of the cornea. The patient does not blink as much as usual and may also be unaware of minor trauma to the cornea, causing corneal ulceration, scarring, and blindness.

Management: prevent by early recognition of the problem, and educating the patient to protect her cornea during the day by blinking, and at night with ointment and strapping of the eyelid to the cheek. If these measures fail, then a permanent lateral tarsorrhaphy is required.

Pupil: there may be acute iritis with a red painful eye, and small irregular pupil. This may occur as part of an erythema nodosum leprosum reaction (Chapter 8). Leprosy also causes a chronic low-grade iritis in which the pupil is very small and irregular, and will not dilate. The eye is usually white in chronic iritis.

Management: in acute iritis, the pupil should be dilated immediately and the patient kept on atropine and topical steroids. In chronic iritis, it is important to keep the pupil dilated and to maintain the patient on mydriatics for life.

Onchocerciasis

Onchocerciasis is an infection of the skin and eye due to the filarial worm *Onchocerca volvulus* (Chapter 11). Inflammation can affect the:

- cornea, causing acute punctate keratitis which may lead on to sclerosing keratitis and corneal scar;
- iris, causing iritis and posterior synechiae;
- choroid and retina, causing chorioretinitis, night blindness, and chorioretinal atrophy most marked temporal to the macula; *and*
- optic nerve, causing optic neuritis and secondary optic atrophy.

HIV infection and the eye

The ocular manifestations of HIV infection include:
- Herpes zoster ophthalmicus
- Squamous cell carcinoma of the conjunctiva
- CMV retinopathy

Herpes zoster presents initially with pain over one side of the head and face followed by a vesicular rash. The eyelids are always involved and there may be a keratitis and iritis, which can cause raised intra-ocular pressure. The disease tends to be severe in HIV positive patients with corneal involvement. Treatment is with oral aciclovir 800 mg 5x/day.

Squamous cell carcinoma of the conjunctiva appears as a raised irregular lesion, usually on the temporal conjunctiva, that grows to invade the fornices, lids and cornea. Treatment is by wide surgical excision where possible.

Cytomegalovirus (CMV) infection of the retina is the most common opportunistic infection of the eye and the major cause of blindness in AIDS patients. It is bilateral in 50% of cases. The appearance is one of red haemorrhages and yellow necrotic tissue. It is progressive and can destroy the whole retina. Treatment if available, is with
- ganciclovir 60 mg/kg IV q8h for 2–3 weeks, then 5 mg/kg/day, *or*
- foscarnet 5 mg/kg q12h IV for 2–3 weeks, then 90–120 mg/kg/day.

However, both have severe side effects and are expensive.

Dermatology

Section editor **Diana Lockwood**

Rashes

Basis of rashes

- The skin varies in thickness and quantity of hair or sebaceous glands. Rashes affecting only one component of the skin will have a distribution which reflects this component (e.g. hair follicles in folliculitis or dermatomes in shingles).
- The lesions differ according to the depth of the inflammation. Near the surface it causes vesiculation and scaling, while deep dermal or subcutaneous inflammation results in nodule formation.
- The rate of development is determined by the type of inflammatory response. Erythema, wheals, and blisters are more acute; white cell infiltration, purpura, and pustules take longer; while ischaemic necrosis and exfoliation are more chronic responses.
- The distribution of the lesion may be typical — see Figs. 11.1 and 11.2.
- Endogenous rashes tend to be symmetrical; in contrast, a biting insect produces asymmetric lesions. Unlike the rashes of 2° syphilis, the site of the 1° chancre is not influenced by host symmetry. Fungus infections tend to be more obvious on one side of the body, whereas psoriasis is usually exactly symmetrical.

Common rashes

Maculopapular rashes

Extensive:

- Scabies
- Rubella
- Measles
- Body lice
- Chickenpox
- 2° syphilis

Sparse:

- Gonococcaemia
- Lichen planus
- Typhoid rose spots
- Flea bites

Hypopigmentation

- Post-inflammation
- Pityriasis alba
- Pinta
- Tinea versicolor
- Vitiligo
- Post-kala azar dermal leishmaniasis
- Leprosy
- Yaws

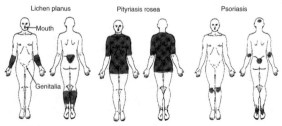

Fig. 11.1 Some characteristic rash distribution.

Nodules
- Onchocerciasis
- Fungal infections
- Erythema nodosum
- Leprosy
- Kaposi's sarcoma
- Gout
- Cutaneous leishmaniasis

Plaques/crusts
- Fungal infections
- Kaposi's sarcoma an eschar (rickettsia) or chancre (trypanosomiasis)
- Leprosy
- Cutaneous leishmaniasis
- Psoriasis
- Impetigo
- Pinta

Urticaria
- Drugs
- Schistosomiasis
- Strongyloidiasis
- Gnasthostomiasis
- Loiasis

Petechiae
- Meningococcaemia
- Typhus
- Viral haemorrhagic fevers
- Causes of DIC

Vesicles
- Herpes zoster
- Papular urticaria
- Herpes simplex
- Vasculitis
- Orf
- Monkeypox

Pustules
- Bacterial infection
- Irritant folliculitis
- Psoriasis

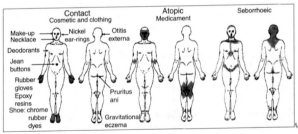

Fig. 11.2 Common patterns of dermatitis/eczema.

Urticaria

Transient swelling and/or flushing of the skin due to release of inflammatory mediators in the skin. This release is stimulated by allergens (e.g. food, drugs) binding to IgE, immune complex disease and complement activation (due e.g. to antivenom, penicillins, infections), or molecules that release histamine directly (e.g. drugs such as morphine, shellfish). The reaction may be accompanied by joint pains, stomach aches, and fever.

Urticaria is life-threatening when:
• It is part of an anaphylactic reaction
• Angioedema involves the upper respiratory tract
• It is part of a severe systemic disease (e.g. septicaemia, SLE).

Papular urticaria: itchy and persistent papules following damage to epidermis, often by an insect bite. They are intensely pruritic and commonly blister.

Chronic urticaria: urticaria lasting >2–3 months. Most commonly due to parasite infection in the tropics. Check for worm infection (hookworm, tapeworm, roundworm), trichinosis, onchocerciasis, dracunculosis, lymphatic filariasis, strongyloidiasis. Other causes: drugs, food additives.

Management: Remove the stimulus, treat any infection. Give oral antihistamines (e.g. chlorphenamine 4 mg q4–6h or promethazine 10–20 mg tds).

Drug eruptions

Adverse drug reactions commonly follow both western and altenative therapies. Drug rashes tend to occur in a symmetrical pattern; the rashes are commonly erythematous, urticarial, purpuric, or ischaemic. Exfoliation or vesiculation are rare.

Ask the patient about previous reactions to drugs. Without this priming, it is unlikely that drugs given for just a few days could have caused the rash. The exception is when an infection primes the body to a medicine (e.g. cough mixture or antibiotics). In general, most drugs take >5–10 days to initiate a reaction.

Erythema multiforme (Stevens–Johnson syndrome): a reaction to virus infection (e.g. HSV, Orf), drugs (e.g. thiacetazone in HIV +ve patients, sulfonamides), neoplasms, or certain systemic diseases. There are coin-shaped or target lesions on the hands, feet (to a lesser extent the trunk), and mucosae — mouth, genitalia, eyes. If the mucosal blistering is severe, it is termed Stevens–Johnson syndrome and is often accompanied by fever (sometimes with anterior uveitis, pneumonia, renal failure, polyarthritis, diarrhoea).

Management of drug eruptions
• Stop the use of all drugs likely to have caused the reaction; give prednisolone 1mg/kg if the reaction is acute and severe. Nurse patients with Stevens-Johnson syndrome as if they had extensive burns.
It is possible to restart the drugs one by one to identify the causative drug (unless the drug causes anaphylaxis), but there is a high risk of morbidity. Only essential drugs should be restarted.

Cutaneous larva migrans

Infection with filariform larvae of canine hookworms (*Ancylostoma caninum* or *A. braziliense*) for whom humans are not true hosts. Larvae migrate ~1–2 cm per day in the skin, leaving a red irregular track, most often on the feet. They cannot complete their life cycle and die eventually after some months.

Management: albendazole 400 mg PO od for 3 days *or* ivermectin 150–200 mcg/kg PO stat. Tiabendazole cream or 10–15% suspension can also be applied topically.

Larva currens

A cutaneous eruption resulting from autoinfection into the skin (often of the buttocks/perianal area) by *Strongyloides stercoralis*. The urticarial wheals are linear and move ~1–2 cm per hour; the abdomen and buttocks are most affected. See Chapter 2D.

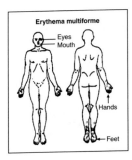

Fig. 11.3

Skin ulcers

- **Leprosy** should be considered in any patient with a painless burn, injury, or ulcer of a limb.
- **Diabetes** with neuropathy often leads to ulcers on the feet, with reduced sensation.
- **Trauma** is a very common cause of ulceration, particularly in children. Bites, wounds, and cuts often become 2° infected leading to ulceration.

Management of leg ulceration

1. Identify and, if possible, eliminate the cause of the ulcer.
2. Check for arterial disease (absent peripheral pulses).
3. Prevent venous stasis by elevating the legs above the heart (do this during the day by raising the mattress with e.g. a chair). Elevation should be 45° for most people; if peripheral pulses are absent, do not raise the feet >23cm above the heart. Use compression bandages if difficult to raise legs.
4. Apply clean dressing using short pieces of bandage that do not completely encircle the leg. Dressings wet with saline will encourage healing and soften crusts.

Tropical ulcer

Ulcers due to mixed bacterial infection which predominantly occur on the foot, ankle, or lower leg following minor trauma. A small round painful ulcer forms which then spreads rapidly, exposing the underlying muscles and tendons. The patient is febrile. After a few weeks, the ulcer stops spreading and the pain diminishes. Good treatment in the early stages encourages the ulcer to heal. Neglected ulcers become fibrosed and may be the site of a future squamous cell CA.

Management: if noted early, the ulcers respond well to antibiotics and daily dressing. Large ulcers may need antibiotics followed by skin grafting. Chronic ulcers should be excised and grafted.

Buruli ulcer

A chronic necrotizing skin disease of tropical forest areas caused by infection with *Mycobacterium ulcerans*. The method of transmission is not known but is presumed to occur through broken skin. The infection starts as a painless nodule which breaks down to form an ulcer that is relatively painless and has edges that may be undermined for 5–15 cm. Necrosis is caused by a bacterial exotoxin. There are few systemic signs (although lymphadenopathy occurs). The ulcer may spread rapidly, or become 2° infected. Without treatment, healing is slow and may lead to scarring, contractures, and deformities. Diagnosis is on typical clinical picture or AFB in the ulcer's base.

Management: completely excise nodule if recognized early. At the ulcer stage: treat any 2° infection, irrigate ulcer with saline, excise all diseased tissue, and cover the wound by skin grafting. Antibiotics (streptomycin, rifampicin) have weak activity.

Infective causes of skin ulcers include: bacteria (streptococci, staphylococci); non-venereal treponematoses; anthrax; mycobacteria; fungal infections; leishmaniasis.

Some causes of skin ulcers

Ulcers on penis or vagina	See Chapter 2B
Ulcers on breast	Infection or cancer
Ulcers on foot or leg	Diabetes
	Leprosy
	Venous disease
	Arterial disease
	Tropical ulcer
	Sickle cell disease
	Chronic osteomyelitis
	Dracunculiasis
Ulcers anywhere	Cutaneous leishmaniasis
	Bacterial infection
	Typhus eschar
	Trypanosomal chancre
	Anthrax
	Buruli ulcer

80% of skin diseases in tropical rural areas are fungal, bacterial, viral or parasitic infections. These are relatively easy to treat.

Key conditions that need to be recognized:

- Staphylococcoal and streptococcal impetigo and pyoderma
- Tinea infections
- Scabies
- Eczema / dermatitis (commoner in urban settings).

Essential laboratory procedures for diagnosing skin diseases:

- Mycology: skin scapings and hair examination in KOH preparations
- Serology for syphilis
- Slit skin smear - for leishmaniasis and leprosy
- Skin snips for onchocerciasis

Dermatitis (eczema)

An inflammatory reaction of the skin that may occur as a (usually asymmetrical) response to an external irritant or as a symmetrical endogenous response to a stimulus (atopic eczema).

- **Irritant dermatitis:** the most common form of dermatitis, generally affecting the hands following contact with industrial irritants at work. The skin is dry and unsupple with deep cracks which may become infected. Previously damaged skin is more susceptible to irritants.
- **Contact allergic dermatitis:** sensitization to an allergen, normally over months or years, results in the onset of dermatitis within hours of subsequent exposure to the allergen (e.g. cosmetics, nickel in zips, buttons, stainless steel watches, or jewellery, food, plants, medicines, metals). Irritant dermatitis is a risk factor for contact dermatitis. Patch testing identifies the specific allergen.
- **Atopic eczema:** is due to an IgE response to foods or environmental agents. The skin is very itchy and dry; it becomes damaged by repeated scratching. 2° infection produces lymphadenopathy.

Psoriasis

Clinical features: the classic lesion is a sharply demarcated silvery plaque, often more active at the edge with a clear centre. Initially, or as plaques resolve, they may be atypical (e.g. scaleless, exudative, red). Plaques occur most commonly on knees, elbows, scalp; also navel, natal cleft, hairline. Lesions in flexures have decreased scale, and are red, shiny, and liable to crack and macerate. Distinct forms occur:

- *Guttate psoriasis:* small poorly defined lesions (often red with little silvery scale) that occur across the whole body; often in children after streptococcal sore throat or vaccination.
- *Palmar/plantar psoriasis:* the lesions develop deep cracks and sterile pustules and the nails become involved. Need to differentiate this from fungal infection.
- *Generalized pustular psoriasis:* fever, arthropathy, bright red erythema followed by the development of multiple pustules. Can occur after stopping steroid therapy. It is self-resolving.
- *Polyarthritic psoriasis*

Management of eczema

1. Eliminate or avoid known irritants or allergens.
2. Avoid soaps (these dry the skin) and wash with emollients to keep the skin moist.
3. Apply steroid creams to affected areas 1–2 times daily. Use the least potent steroid that works for short periods of time only. Avoid strong steroids in children.
4. Severe chronic allergy can be relieved by prednisolone and other immunosuppressive drugs (e.g. azathioprine). Rebound often occurs when steroids are stopped.
5. Treat 2° *Staph. aureus* infection vigorously with flucloxacillin or erythromycin.

Breastfeeding may reduce the risk of atopic eczema. This is worth emphasizing for infants with a family history of eczema.

Management of psoriasis

This is a chronic condition — many treatments have been suggested. Options include:
1. Emollients and reassurance for mild cases.
2. Coal tar applied twice daily to the lesions. Build up from a low concentration initially.
3. Dithranol ointments and creams.
4. Systemic therapy may be required occasionally for generalized illness, particularly in the elderly. Use methotrexate or cyclosporine.
5. Corticosteroids: potent topical steroids should be avoided because they may lead to relapse or vigorous rebound on withdrawal. A weak steroid (e.g. hydrocortisone 1%) can be used for short periods on the face or in flexures. Systemic steroids should usually be avoided.

Skin cancers

Long-term exposure of pale skin to strong sunlight is a risk factor for all these tumours. Pale-skinned people should be encouraged always to use sunscreen on sun-exposed parts of their body, and wear a hat outdoors. Dark-skinned people with depigmenting disease or albinism are at high risk of developing skin cancer.

Actinic keratoses

The lesions are caused by chronic exposure of pale skin to intense sunlight. Dry, wrinkled areas of skin that become pale scaly crusts with a red base — they are pre-malignant — while they may disappear in some individuals, in others they develop into one of the malignancies described below. They should be treated before this change takes place.

Management: freeze lesions with liquid nitrogen, or apply topical fluorouracil daily.

Squamous cell carcinoma

Initially a fleshy dry nodule that breaks down to form an ulcerating lesion with hard raised edges. They occur in actinic keratoses, on the lips, or inside the mouth of long-term smokers, or at the edges of chronic ulcers and areas of inflammation. They are locally very invasive but do not metastasize systemically.

Management: early wide local excision is essential; the tumour often infiltrates further into neighbouring tissue than is apparent. If the tumour is removed only at its obvious margins, infiltrations will be left behind and the tumour will recur.

Basal cell carcinoma

Initially a slow-growing papule that breaks down in the centre, becoming an ulcer with a rolled 'pearl-coloured' edge. Occurs on the face above a line drawn between the chin and ears. Untreated, they infiltrate slowly causing extensive damage, but do not metastasize.

Management: involves curettage and cauterization of the ulcer's base, or cryotherapy. Fluorouracil cream may be used after surgery.

Melanoma

Any pigmented lesion that is variably coloured, changes shape or colour, starts to bleed, or ulcerates, should be considered a potential melanoma. Pigmented satellite lesions around a mole also suggest a melanoma. They frequently originate in moles; therefore people with many moles should be encouraged to examine them regularly and report changes to a doctor. Melanoma is extremely invasive and may only be recognized when metastasized to the CNS or other sites. The original lesion may be quite innocuous.

Management: is immediate, wide local excision.

The non-venereal treponematoses

These disfiguring conditions primarily affect children in communities with poor hygiene. Like syphilis, they have three stages, with a long period of latency before the manifestation of 3° disease. Unlike syphilis, the 3° lesions are infective, which causes problems for their eradication since it is difficult to identify latent carriers.

Transmission: direct person–person through skin contact. Spirochetes cannot penetrate intact skin, so abrasions are probably required.

Clinical features

1. *Yaws:* the 1° lesion is a papule which develops into a round/oval 2–5 cm painless, itchy papilloma. It normally heals in 3–6 months. Weeks to years after this lesion resolves, multiple 2° lesions occur in crops on any part of the body and last up to 6 months. They are papules or papillomas of various shape; they may ulcerate and form yellow-brown scabs. Other lesions include dermatitis or hyperkeratosis of palms and soles, local lymphadenopathy, dactylitis, long bone swelling, rarely, osteitis of nasal bones. After a latent period, the disease reappears with necrotic destruction of skin and bones (gummas). Other clinical features include hyperkeratosis, palatal destruction and 2° infection, sabre tibia, bursitis.

2. *Endemic syphilis (bejel):* a 1° lesion is rarely seen — the first lesions are usually painless ulcers of lips and oropharynx. In addition, there is osteoperiostitis of long bones, condylamata lata, angular stomatitis, rarely, a 2° syphilis-like rash, and generalized lymphadenopathy. Late lesions include bone destruction (as in yaws), skin ulcers, and palmar and plantar keratosis.

3. *Pinta:* primarily affects the skin. Satellite lesions surround the 1° papule; there is regional painless lymphadenopathy. 2° stage plaques appear within a few months; these plaques change their colour and occur anywhere on the body. The 3° disease involves depigmentation and atrophy of the skin.

Diagnosis: motile spirochaetes can be seen on dark-field microscopy of lesion exudates. There are no serological or morphological features that differentiate syphilis-causing *T. pallidum* from the other treponemes. The precise diagnosis is clinical.

Management: a single dose of benzathine penicillin G 0.9 g IM (alternatives: erythromycin 250–500 mg PO qds or amoxicillin 500 mg tds for 15 days).

Prevention: identification of active cases, followed by treatment of all contacts. If >10% in a community are actively infected, all should receive penicillin.

	Yaws	Bejel	Pinta
Organism	T. pertenue	T. pallidum	T. carateum
Age group	15–40	2–10	10–30
Occurrence	Africa S. America Oceania	Africa Middle East Asia	Latin America
Climate	Warm, humid	Dry, arid	Warm

Varicella-zoster infection

This herpesvirus causes two conditions: *chickenpox* (or varicella) following $1°$ infection and *shingles* (or zoster) following reactivation of latent virus. Transmission is by inhalation of nasopharyngeal droplets or contact with vesicular fluid. After viraemic spread and $1°$ disease, latency occurs in sensory ganglia and motor neurones. Reactivation normally occurs only once. It affects just one sensory ganglion, leading to vesicles and pain involving that dermatome only.

Chickenpox

May be severe in the 1st week of life and adults; generally it is a mild infection of children. There is prodromal fever, headache, and malaise followed by itchy papules or vesicles looking like drops of water on the face/trunk. Lesions 'crop' daily, moving distally with lesions progressing from papules to vesicle, pustule, and scab in about 8 days. After a few days, all stages are present at once (cf. poxviruses). The scabs fall off on the 10th day without scarring, unless lesions become $2°$ infected.

Complications: $2°$ bacterial infection (streptococci, staphylococci) is common in children; pneumonitis (mainly seen in adults, especially smokers); mild encephalitis (ataxia); thrombocytopenia

Zoster (shingles)

Paraesthesia and shooting pains can occur in the affected dermatome for several days before the appearance of a rash and mild fever. The vesicles scab after 3–7 days; they may become $2°$ infected. Zoster typically involves one dermatome; scanty distant blood-borne vesicles occur.
- Complications of ophthalmic zoster are conjunctivitis, keratitis, periorbital swelling.
- Postherpetic neuralgia is very painful and difficult to treat; it can be reduced by early use of amitriptyline 10–25 mg nocte.
- Zoster (or a zoster scar) in a patient <40 years old suggests HIV infection. Zoster in HIV patients can be more severe, deeper, more prolonged, and affect >1 dermatome. Chickenpox is not a feature of HIV.

Management: if within 2 days of onset, give aciclovir 800 mg PO 5 times daily for 5 days; in severe infections, give aciclovir 5mg/kg IV q8h (10 mg/kg in immunocompromised patients).

Poxvirus infections

Although smallpox was eradicated in 1976, it might become an agent of bio-terrorism and re-emerge. It carries ~50% mortality; there is no effective treatment, and smallpox control relies upon isolation of all cases and vaccination of all contacts. Two closely related poxviruses — monkeypox and tanapox — still cause occasional infections. The rash (1–2 lesions in tanapox; many covering the whole body in monkeypox) is preceded by a 2–3 day prodromal period with fever and other systemic signs.

Lymphadenopathy occurs in monkeypox, characteristically involving both femoral and inguinal nodes. Unlike chickenpox, the lesions are always at the same stage, and the peripheries are involved early. Both infections tend to resolve without treatment. Human–human transmission has been reported within households with monkeypox.

Cutaneous leishmaniasis (CL)

A widespread disease, caused by *Leishmania* parasites, that manifests in different ways depending on the infecting species. After the bite of a sandfly, *Leishmania* multiply in skin macrophages, killing cells and producing the characteristic ulcer. The balance between infection and immune response determines whether the infection remains focused in the skin, healing over months, or becomes disseminated across skin and mucosae

Transmission: occurs via the bite of *Phlebotomus* and *Lutzomyia* sandflies. For zoonotic CL, reservoirs are rodents or dogs; *L. tropica* is anthroponotic.

Clinical features: weeks to months after a bite, a nodule develops at the bite site. This grows slowly (up to 5 cm) and is covered by a crust. This may drop off to expose a painless ulcer which is dry or exudative, depending on the species. It heals over months or years, leaving a 'tissue paper' scar. Satellite lesions occur; 2° infection is uncommon. *L. mexicana* may cause lesions of the pinna — chiclero ulcer — that takes years to heal, often destroying the pinna.

Certain forms do not resolve spontaneously, but are uncommon compared to the vast numbers of classical CL:

- **Mucocutaneous leishmaniasis (MCL):** 2° lesions occur months to years after 1° lesion has healed. Starting on the upper lip or nostril edge, MCL eventually destroys the mucosa and cartilage of the nasopharynx, larynx, or lips. *L. braziliensis* is the most important cause (others: *L. guyanensis*, *L. panamensis*).
- **Disseminated cutaneous leishmaniasis (DCL):** 1° nodule spreads slowly without ulceration while 2° lesions appear symmetrically on limbs and face. Some individuals are not able to mount an immune response to *Leishmania*; their infection (anergic DCL) continues to spread and responds only transiently to chemotherapy. Usually DCL is caused by *L. mexicana* or *L. aethiopica*.
- **Recidivans leishmaniasis:** usually caused by *L. tropica*; often on the cheek; the lesion heals in the centre but nodules with scanty parasites persist at the edges for years.

Diagnosis: identification of Giemsa-stained parasites in skin smears taken from the edge of active ulcers.

Management: *Leishmania* are killed at 40–42°C, so heating the wound by radiofrequency or heat pads improves healing. The most common drug treatment is local infiltration of sodium stibogluconate or meglumine antimoniate into lesions: 1–3ml of undiluted antimonials is injected into the base and edges of the lesion. This is repeated 2–3 times weekly for 2–3 weeks. If the injections are very painful, lignocaine 2% can be mixed in the syringe. **See box for systemic therapy**.

pentavalent antimony

• Amphoteracin B if ø resp. to pentavalent antimony after 1 month

• Aldara cream + pentavalent antimony = faster healing

Systemic therapy – Old World CL

L. tropica and *L. major* cause CL in the Old World, do not cause MCL, and usually self-heal without problems in most patients. Only needs systemic treatment if

- Sores too large or badly sited for local therapy
- Ulcerated or severely inflamed sores, or overlying a joint
- Disease with lymphatic spread
- Lesions with involvement of cartilage

Treatments

Oral fluconazole 200 mg od for 6 weeks is effective in *L. major* CL
Injections of antimonials or amphotericin B– see below.

Systemic therapy – New World CL

CL from Central or South America could be caused by *L. braziliensis*. If in doubt, consider all New World CL to be *L. braziliensis*, because differentiation from *L. mexicana* is usually impossible geographically, clinically, or parasitologically- unless PCR available. Treating *L. braziliensis* CL should prevent subsequent MCL.

Treatments Note: Once healing has begun, complete epithelialisation is likely to occur after treatment.

- 10–20mg/kg/day sodium stibogluconate by IM or slow IV route, or meglumine antimoniate by deep IM for 20 days.   4 mins
- Pentamidine isothionate 4mg/kg/day on alternate days x 3 injections
- MCL responds better to amphotericin B 1mg/kg alternate days to total dose 30 mg/kg

Diffuse CL

DCL is almost impossible to cure: give sodium stibogluconate or meglumine antimoniate 20 mg/kg IM od for several months after clinical improvement; relapse is common

Local treatments for CL – suitable for Old World CL and *L. mexicana*

- Intra-lesional infiltration of sodium stibogluconate or meglumine antimoniate
  Is widely used: 1 ml of undiluted antimonial is injected into the base and edges of the lesion. This is repeated 2–3 times weekly for 2–3 weeks. If the injections are very painful, lignocaine 2% can be mixed in the syringe.
- *Leishmania* are killed at 40–42°C, so heating the wound by radiofrequency or heat pads improves healing.
- Cryotherapy is used successfully used in Old World CL, either alone or combined with intra-lesional antimonial
- Topical treatment with paromomycin 15% ointment is effective in *L. major* and *L. mexicana*

Filariasis

The filariases are caused by filarial worms which live in lymphatics, blood vessels, skin, or connective tissue. The larval stages are inoculated by biting mosquitoes or flies, each specific to a particular filaria. The adult worms produce millions of microfilariae. Disease is due to the host immune response to the worms, particularly dying worms, and its pattern and severity vary with the site and stage of each species. The worms are long-lived; microfilariae survive 2–3 years and adult worms 10–15 years. The infections are chronic and worst in individuals constantly exposed to reinfection. Serology for anti-filaria antibodies is usually positive. Symbiotic *Wolbachia* (rickettsia) are found within all filariae pathogenic to humans, and may contribute to pathology. Multiple infections with different filariae are possible; therefore check for multiple infection and bear this in mind when deciding therapy.

Onchocerciasis ('river blindness')

Onchocerca volvulus occurs in areas with fast-flowing rivers and biting *Simlium* blackflies, the parasite's vector. In the west African savannah, it was a common cause of blindness until the onchocerciasis control programme reduced its prevalence. It still causes blindness in other savannah regions, while skin manifestations are more prominent in other areas.

Clinical features: there is considerable variation, possibly due to differences in the infecting strain of *O. volvulus*.

- *Subcutaneous nodules* containing adult worms are conspicuous over bony prominences (e.g. iliac crests, ribs, knees, trochanters).
- *Microfilariae* migrate from nodules into the skin and ocular tissues. Host inflammatory reactions occur to dead or dying microfilariae — see box.
- *Ocular lesions:* include transient punctate keratitis and potentially blinding conditions such as sclerosing keratitis, iridocyclitis, optic atrophy.

Diagnosis: confirmed by finding microfiliariae in skin snips or the eye. Ask the patient to put their head between their knees for >2 mins before examining the anterior chamber with a slit-lamp. If skin snip and eye examinations are both negative but onchocerciasis is still strongly suspected, perform the Mazzotti test. Give DEC 50 mg PO; increased pruritis within 24–48 hrs indicates that the patient is infected.

Management

- Ivermectin 150 mcg/kg PO stat clears microfilariae from the skin for about 6–9 months. Repeat the dose when the patient is symptomatic (typically each 6–12 months) throughout the lifespan of the adult worms (15–20 yrs).
- Doxycycline 100 mg PO bd, which acts on the *Wolbachia* rickettsiae within the filariae, can reduce microfilariae in skin for 12–18 months.

Prevention: long-term ivermectin mass distribution programmes; vector control programmes.

Forms of dermal onchocerciasis

- *Acute papular onchodermatitis:* small scattered itchy papules, +/– vesicles and pustules, +/– skin oedema, often on the trunk and upper limbs.
- *Chronic papular onchodermatitis:* larger itchy, hyperpigmented, often flattopped, papules +/– areas of hyperpigmentation.
- *Lichenified onchodermatitis:* itchy, hyperpigmented papulo-nodules or plaques which become confluent. The itching is intense initially; the rash is asymmetrical, often affecting one or both legs.
- *Atrophy:* loss of elasticity with excessive wrinkles particularly on the buttocks; inelastic folds of inguinal skin form hanging groins, often filled with enlarged lymph nodes.
- *Depigmentation (leopard skin):* patches of decreased pigment or loss contrasted with normally pigmented skin around hair follicles.

Dracunculiasis (Guinea worm)

The Guinea Worm eradication programme has reduced the prevalence of this disease to scattered foci in semi-desert areas south of the Sahara (see map). A disease of people without a clean water supply caused by *Dracunculus medinensis*, which infects people after they drink water containing its vector — small copepod crustaceans. Released larvae migrate into body cavities where they mature and mate. Months later, adult females (50–100 cm long) migrate in the subcutaneous layers of the skin to the extremities where an ulcer forms and the tip of the worm protrudes. On contact with water, large numbers of larvae are released from a loop of the worm's uterus which prolapses to the skin surface.

Clinical features: include a systemic hypersensitivity reaction to infection. Most are identified later when the female worm is seen migrating under the skin or the blister forms or bursts. The tissue around the worm becomes extremely painful and almost always 2° infected with bacteria. Some worms migrate to sites such as brain, joints, or eyes, resulting in cerebral/subdural abscesses, arthritis, or blindness.

Diagnosis is clinical.

Management: female worms can be removed before they form a blister by making a small incision in the skin at their midpoint and pulling the worm out with careful traction and massage along its track. Metronidazole for 1 week reduces inflammation and eases the removal. After a blister has burst, analgesics will be needed before the worm can be pulled out. Keep the blister clean and covered.

Prevention: involves improving the water supply or filtering drinking water through cloth to remove the crustaceans.

Loiasis

Loa loa is transmitted in the central African rainforests by bites of *Chrysops* horse flies.

Clinical features: as the injected larvae mature, they migrate away from the site in the subcutaneous layers (producing itching, prickly sensations) or deeper fascial layers (pain, paraesthesia). Transient Calabar swellings occur at intervals, lasting between a few hours and days. These odematous lumps occur on the limbs and are an immune response to migrating adult worms — the overlying skin is slightly inflamed. Worms migrating beneath the conjunctiva produce acute eye irritation; the worm is clearly visible for some minutes to hours.

Diagnosis: clinical or serological; microfilariae can also be found in filtered blood samples collected around mid-day.

Management: DEC 1 mg/kg on day 1; 1 mg/kg bd on day 2; 2 mg/kg bd on day 3, and 2–3 mg/kg tds from day 4–21, all PO. Start persons with heavy microfilaraemia at a low dose and give steroid cover for first 2–3 days (risk of meningoencephalitis with dying microfiaria). Check for mixed infection with *O. volvulus* before using DEC — if present, use ivermectin as there is risk of mazzotti reaction. Doxycycline 100 mg bd PO for 6 wks will produce a more gradual reduction of microfilaraemia by acting on *Wolbachia* rickettsiae.

Prevention: a weekly dose of DEC 300 mg PO may be an effective prophylactic; otherwise, reducing vector contact is important.

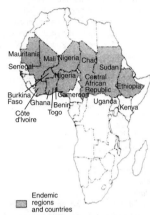

Fig. 11.4 Worldwide distribution of dracunculiasis (2000). Foci of transmission occur in remote areas in these countries.

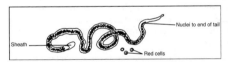

Fig. 11.5 Appearance of *Loa loa* microfilaria on a blood film.

Lymphatic filariasis

A highly variable disease that is caused by infection of the lymphatic system with one of three species of nematode: *Wuchereria bancrofti*, *Brugia malayi*, and *B. timori*. Variation is due to differences in parasite strain, the host's immune response, and the intensity of infection. For example, growing up in an endemic region produces immunological tolerance and high rates of infection but low rates of severe immunologically-mediated disease. Immigrants to endemic areas have higher rates of severe disease. Pathology is caused by direct effects of the adults in the lymphatics plus the effects of the host's immune response. Microfilariae do not cause lymphatic pathology but do cause tropical pulmonary eosinophilia (TPE).

Transmission: via the bite of mosquitoes. Mosquito species differs according to region and particular filiariae.

Clinical features: fall into following categories:

1. *Seropositive, asymptomatic patients without microfilaraemia.* Common in endemic regions.
2. *Asymptomatic microfilaraemia.* Many people have parasites but there is no apparent disease.
3. *Acute lymphatic filariasis*
   - Filarial fever — (chills, rigors, headache, bone & joint pains, malaise, +/− delirium) may be due to 2° infection in some cases. Fever lasts 3–7 days and may recur over many years.
   - Limb lymphadenitis and lymphangitis — may produce severe pain; attacks occur at the same time as fever. Nodes may form abscesses.
   - Epididymo-orchitis (painful swelling of spermatic cord) +/− scrotal oedema +/− hydrocoele — most common form of acute lymphatic filariasis. Often recurs, sometimes repeatedly, causing chronic disease.
4. *Chronic lymphatic filiariasis.* A progressive and cumulative disease, probably requiring 10–20 yrs of exposure. It may overlap with acute disease. Features include:
   - Hydrocoele — normally contains clear, straw-coloured liquid but may become blood- or lymph-stained. Repeated tapping of fluid causes fibrosis and abscess formation; fluid may contain microfilariae.
   - Lymphoedema (elephantiasis) of the legs — is common, and usually asymmetrical. Normally starts at the ankle, spreading onto the foot and up the leg. Grade I lymphoedema is transient and pitting, responding well to rest and elevation. Later, grade II oedema develops; it is non-pitting, and becomes brawny.
   - Gross swelling — occurs in grade III, with skin thickening, hyperkeratosis, and papillomatous changes.
   - Chyluria and lymphuria — rupture into the renal pelvis or bladder of damaged lymphatics draining (i) intestines → fat in urine (chyluria) or (ii) other organs → lymph in urine. Blood is often present. Chronic chyluris can result in malabsorption. Clotting can occur in both cases, producing urine retention.

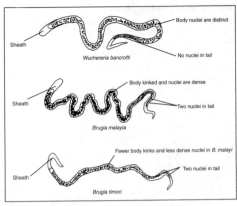

Fig. 11.6 Blood film appearances of the microfilariae lymphatic filariasis.

Tropical pulmonary eosinophilia

An allergic alveolitis caused by microfilaria being destroyed in the lungs. TPE presents with persistent dry cough (often nocturnal); dyspnoea and wheeze (resembling asthma); occasionally crepitations; fever; mild haemoptysis. TPE is more common in south India and Sri Lanka than other geographical areas. If untreated, irreversible lung damage occurs. Peripheral eosinophilia is high, and filarial serology usually strongly positive. Treatment with DEC produces rapid clinical, CXR, and lung function test improvement.

Other complications of filariasis: arthritis of the knee joint, endomyocardial fibrosis, skin rashes, thrombophlebitis, and nerve palsies have all been attributed to filarial disease with negative blood films (the microfilaraemia having been destroyed by the immune response).

Diagnosis: examination of stained films of blood, or by collecting 20 ml of anticoagulated blood and syringing through a polycarbonate filter (pore size 20 mm). The filter is then examined under a coverslip. Microfliariae can be found in the blood around midnight unless the patient is from the South Pacific, when day and night bloods are needed. Serological tests are useful.

Management

- DEC 2 mg/kg PO tds for 12 days for *W. bancrofti* infection. Lower doses may be adequate for *Brugia* infections: 1–2 mg/kg PO tds for 6–12 days.
- Mass chemotherapy for *W. bancrofti* requires 6 mg/kg PO in 3 divided doses during 24 hrs, on 12 occasions, at weekly or monthly intervals. Again lower doses may suffice for *Brugia*: 1–2mg/kg PO tds, on 6 occasions.
- Ivermectin, albendazole, and coumarin have all shown promising results in clinical trials.
- Doxycycline 100 mg PO bd for 6 weeks, active against symbiotic *Wolbachia*, may also be effective.
- Surgical management is required for severe hydroceles and lymphoedema; radical surgery may have long-lasting benefits.
- Conservative treatment can prevent deterioration in lymphoedema and elephantiasis: nocturnal leg elevation, firm pressure bandaging and elastic stockings, careful foot care, control of infections, careful use of diuretics. Also see box.

Prevention: education to reduce vector–human contact; systematic chemotherapy of individuals and mass chemotherapy of communities with >5% prevalence of infection. Routine addition of DEC to table salt has been used with success in China.

The realization that elephantiasis can be profoundly reduced by simple hygiene and early treatment of infections has stimulated a new approach. Patients are now encouraged to:
• Wash the affected part twice daily with soap and water
• Raise the affected limb at night
• Exercise, to promote lymph flow
• Keep nails clean
• Wear shoes
• Use antiseptic or antibiotic creams to treat small wounds or abrasions, or in severe cases systematic antibiotics.

Such measures help to halt disease progression in those with slight lymphatic damage. People with advanced lymphoedema or elephantiasis can also be helped by these simple methods, as collateral lymphatic channels re-establish lymph flow if kept free from 2° infection. Examples of simple patient information leaflets are available from; *http://www.filariasis.org* the WHO filariasis programme and from *http://www.who.int/ctd/filariasis/ Specific_information/WHO_docs.html*

Infestations

Lice

There are three species of medical importance:

- The head louse (*Pediculus capitis*)
- The body louse (*P. humanus*)
- The pubic or crab louse (*Phthirus pubis*)

The body louse is also important as the vector of epidemic typhus (*Richettsia prowazeki*), relapsing fever (*Borrelia recurrentis*), and trench fever (*Bartonella quintana*). Transmission is by close personal contact, increased by poverty, overcrowding, and poor hygiene. The lice pierce the skin to take a blood meal, injecting saliva and defecating at the same time. A rash occurs due to a hypersensitivity reaction to the saliva. Blue macules <1 cm in diameter occur during pubic louse infection possibly due to injection of an anticoagulant. The body louse lives in the person's clothes, passing onto the skin only to take a blood meal. The other two lice infect the skin directly. Eggs are laid and firmly glued to hairs where they can be seen — the 'nits'.

Management: for body lice, the patient does not need treatment, but clean clothes by a very hot wash, then ironing the seams; or by dusting clothes with 1% malathion powder. For head and pubic lice, apply 0.5% malathion liquid on the affected parts for 0–2 hrs. (Alternatives to malathion in case of resistance: carbaryl 0.5–1%; permethrin 1–5%; phenothrin 0.2–0.5%.) Treat 2° infection for *S. aureus*.

Scabies

Sarcoptes scabiei is transmitted by close personal contact. It is not a disease of poverty. During the first few weeks following 1° transmission, sensitization to mite faeces and saliva occurs. Reinfestation results in almost immediate irritation and, in some cases, a generalized urticaria.

Scabies is extremely irritating to young children. Infection causes small itchy papules and linear burrows, particularly in the finger webs and on the flexor wrist surface. Other sites commonly include elbows; axillae; genitalia (particularly scrotum); peri-umbilicus; breasts. Head infestation is common in infants. The itching is worse at night. Macules and pustules occur; scratching results in 2° bacterial infection. The female burrows into the dermis to lay eggs — burrows can be seen as 0.5–1.5 cm long irregular tracks.

Diagnosis: is either clinical or by finding a female in one of the burrows with a needle.

Management: treat the whole group at the same time since some members may be asymptomatic. Malathion 0.5%, permethrin 5% cream, or benzylbenzoate 25% can be used: apply to the body and leave on for 24 hrs before washing off. Malathion and permethrin are applied twice, 1 week apart; benzyl benzoate is applied on 3 consecutive days. Itching may persist for some days, but does not usually indicate treatment failure. Severe, hyperkeratotic ('Norwegian') scabies is seen in HIV +ve patients, and may require repeated applications to penetrate the crusts; addition of a single dose of ivermectin 200 mcg/kg PO stat improves cure rates.

Female *Pediculosis capitis*

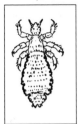

0.3 mm length

Female *Pediculosis humanus*

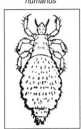

0.4 mm length

Female *Phthirus pubis* with ovum within

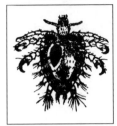

0.3 mm length

Female *Sarcoptes scabiei*

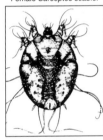

0.4 mm length

Fig. 11.7

Bone, joint, and soft tissue infections

Section editor **Tony Berendt**

Infections of skin

Skin infections can be divided into:

- **Pyodermas:** pus is formed within the skin; a localized infection
- **Spreading infections:** diffuse infection spreading along tissue planes

Pyodermas

1. Impetigo

Superficial infection of the epidermis, often at sites of skin damage (e.g. cuts, eczema, chickenpox blisters, scabies, insect bites). A golden-yellow vesicle quickly bursts to become an area of epidermal loss, which crusts over and enlarges. There may be a little pus under the edges of the lesion. Impetigo is highly contagious: 1° lesion → satellite lesions elsewhere on the skin (spread by patient's own fingers) → infection of contacts. *Staph aureus* and *Strep pyogenes* are most commonly found, often together.

Management

- Give systemic antibiotics (see table 12.1)
- Apply topical antiseptics (e.g. Gentian violet or chlorhexidine)
- Soak off crusts in saline or weak antiseptic

2. Furuncles (boils), carbuncles, and abscesses

Staph aureus causes abscesses in the dermis or subcutaneous fat. A furuncle (boil, pimple) is a collection of pus in a hair follicle or a sebaceous/sweat gland in the skin. Carbuncles are furuncles which have spread deeper (often 2° to patient squeezing or sitting on the furuncle) so multiple points of pus are seen. An abscess is a collection of pus at a deeper level — indicated by swelling, erythema, warmth, and fluctuance. Tenderness is common in all skin infections, but pressure on an abscess is very painful.

Management

- Drain pus and remove necrotic tissue and debris. The abscess cavity should be packed and left to heal by 2° intention — do not suture or allow the opening to close until the interior has healed.
- If the infection spreads in the surrounding soft tissues, give 1–2 wks of antibiotics (see Table 12.1). If antibiotics are unavailable or in short supply, drainage and good wound care alone may suffice.

Spreading infections

These are more commonly caused by beta-haemolytic streptococci (BHS) (e.g. Group A BHS, also known as *Strep pyogenes*) than by *Staph aureus*, except when surrounding a staphylococcal abscess.

1. Erysipelas

Spreading infection in the epidermis, producing a large area of red, shiny, tender skin. The patient is unwell and febrile. The involved area is sharply demarcated from normal skin because the dermo-epidermal junction limits the spread of the inflammatory response in a lateral direction. Erysipelas is common on the face. Severe infection produces skin blistering; necrotic tissue encourages toxin production so the infection becomes worse if the infection is not treated.

Management: antibiotics (see Table 12.1).

Soft tissue infections

Insect bites, reduced access to antibiotics, poverty, and malnutrition contribute to a high incidence of soft tissue infections in the tropics. Some conditions, such as pyomyositis (infection of muscle), are particularly common in the tropics compared to temperate zones.

Table 12.1 Causative organisms and antibiotic choice for soft tissue, bone, and joint infections in the tropics

Condition	Microbiology	Treatment choices	Duration
Superficial infections			
Impetigo **Furuncles** **Carbuncles** **Abscesses** **Erysipelas** **Cellulitis** **Bursitis**	Group A beta-haemolytic streptococci *Staph aureus*	1st flucloxacillin or co-amoxiclav 2nd cephalosporin 3rd erythromycin or clindamycin 4th co-trimoxazole If associated chronic ulcer, wound, water contact, or trauma, add ciprofloxacin + metronidazole	Until clinical resolution, usually 5–14 days
Deep infections			
Acute septic arthritis **Osteomyelitis** **Pyomyositis** **Necrotizing fasciitis**	*Staph aureus* Group A beta-haemolytic streptococci; Mixed flora	1st penicillin or cephalosporin + clindamycin 2nd co-amoxiclav If associated wound, diabetes, ulcer, or water contact, add ciprofloxacin + metronidazole	>6 weeks **or** until clinically cured for >1 week or until ESR normal for >1 week

Usual adult doses

Intravenous route:

Benzylpenicillin 1.2–2.4 g IV q6h

Flucloxacillin 1–2 g IV q6h

Cefuroxime 750 mg – 1.5 g IV or IM q6h to q8h

Co-amoxiclav 1.2 g IV q8h

Erythromycin 500 mg – 1 g IV q6h

Clindamycin, ciprofloxacin, erythromycin, and metronidazole are all very well absorbed PO and seldom require IV administration

Oral route:

Oral flucloxacillin and cefuroxamine have incomplete bioavailability; not advised for severe infection. Penicillin is incompletely absorbed, so choose amoxicillin 0.5–1 g PO tds or ampicillin 0.5–1 g PO qds

Flucloxacillin 500 mg – 1 g PO qds

Cefuroxime 250 mg PO bd

Co-amoxiclav 625 mg PO tds

Erythromycin 500 mg PO q6h

Clindamycin 300 mg PO q6h

Ciprofloxacin 500 mg PO bd

Metronidazole 800 mg PO initially, then 4–500 mg PO tds; or 1g tds PR (reduced to bd after 3 days)

2. Cellulitis

Infection involves the dermis and usually subcutaneous fat as well. There is obvious diffuse swelling and the erythematous area is not so clearly demarcated from uninvolved skin as it is in erysipelas. It commonly involves the lower leg, spreading from breaks in the skin: minor injuries, fungal infection (e.g. athletes foot), scabies, or insect bites which have been scratched. Always bear in mind an underlying abscess, which may form within cellulitis, especially in the hand. When cellulitis is near the knee or elbow but spares the extremity, consider an underlying prepatellar, pretibial, or olecranon bursitis.

Management: see Table 12.1

Scaling and desquamation are normal after some days of infection; blisters may require aspiration; and subcutaneous abscesses can develop despite antibiotics. Recurrence is relatively common: if multiple recurrences occur, prolonged courses of treatment, long-term prophylaxis, or standby antibiotics to take at the onset of symptoms can be helpful.

3. Bursitis

Bursitis most commonly involves the elbow or the knee, and presents as cellulitis over the joint, or as a red painful swelling. The pathogens are usually BHS or *Staph. aureus*. Although bursitis often restricts the movement of the joint, this is related to the mechanical effects of the swelling and the associated tenderness of the soft tissues, and careful examination can usually distinguish bursitis from the much more serious condition of septic arthritis.

Management: see box

In chronic bursitis, suspect TB, underlying osteomyelitis (erosion of bone detectable on X-ray), or chronic septic arthritis.

4. Necrotizing fasciitis

Necrotizing fasciitis is a medical and surgical emergency with high mortality. The most common cause is Group A BHS, but other organisms (e.g. *Vibrio vulnificus* acquired from contact with water, or mixed aerobe/anaerobe infections following abdominal or perineal wounds) can also cause necrotizing fasciitis.

Infection spreads very rapidly in the loose connective tissue adjacent to the fascial plane, leading to necrosis of fascia and thrombosis of blood vessels that supply the skin or muscle. The pace of spread and severity of the underlying process are greater than the time it takes devascularized skin to necrose. As a result, necrotizing fasciitis typically causes severe systemic upset (often with high fever and shock) and pain that seem disproportionate to the local physical signs.

Management: see Table 12.1

Development of fixed tissue staining, echymoses, superficial blistering (early in disease, not late as in cellulitis, and on obviously unhealthy skin) makes the diagnosis probable.

Management of cellulitis

- Antibiotics (see Table 12.1).
- If cellulitis is 2° to a chronic ulcer, in a diabetic, or follows water contact, broaden the antibiotic cover to include Gram –ve rods and anaerobes.
- Consider wound debridement and cleaning.
- Drain underlying abscesses (esp. in the hand).
- Rest and elevate the limb.

Management of bursitis

- Antibiotics for 2–3 weeks (see Table 12.1)
- Needle aspiration to remove some pus without surgery — this is useful for diagnosis and symptom relief.
- Avoid incision and drainage where possible: the synovial fluid produced in the bursa produces a high volume wound drainage, can delay healing, and sometimes produces a synovial fistula.

Management of necrotizing fasciitis

- Early surgery is mandatory: explore the fascial plane and excise the affected area back to bleeding tissue.
- Broad-spectrum antibiotics (see Table 12.1): high-dose penicillin *plus* gentamicin *plus* metronidazole is a good 1st choice. Where available, add clindamycin (beneficial in animal models of necrotizing fasciitis). Adjust antibiotics when cultures are available from surgical samples.
- Intensive care support and reconstructive surgery — without these, prognosis is poor.

Infections of muscle

Pyomyositis

Also called tropical pyomyositis, it is a 1° bacterial infection of striated muscle that is common throughout the tropics and subtropics, particularly in young men.

Clinical features: there are three characteristic phases

1. *Woody phase:* the affected muscle is painful and is hard and woody on palpation. The patient may have little systemic illness; this phase may last for days–months. The condition is difficult to diagnose, and can sometimes be mistaken for a tumour.
2. *The muscle liquefies → intramuscular abscess,* with a very tender swollen muscle. Ultrasound shows intramuscular collections; for psoas abscess, CT or MRI scanning may be necessary (**note**: psoas abscess is also a complication of lumbar spinal infections and does not always represent 'pure' pyomyositis). Gram stain and culture of pus usually reveals *Staph. aureus* (rarely *Strep. pyogenes*).
3. *A bacteraemic illness +/– multiple abscesses* in different muscles.

Management
- Antibiotics for >3 weeks (see Table 12.1).
- Drain abscesses surgically or percutaneously, depending on circumstances.

The overall prognosis is generally good.

Gas gangrene

A spreading and necrotizing infection within muscle, characterized by severe systemic illness, muscle pain, and crepitus due to gas formation. Gas gangrene is generally caused by *Clostridium perfringens*, which produces toxins that cause muscle necrosis. The infection is acquired through environmental (particularly soil) contamination of deep wounds involving muscle.

Management
- For established gas gangrene, extensive surgical removal of dead tissue is needed, often with excision of massive areas of muscle (for trunk wounds) and early amputation (for limb infection).
- The effect of the toxin on the whole body means that without successful treatment, the infection is fatal.
- High-dose penicillin is important, but unlikely to be effective without surgery.

Prevention: through good wound care/wound debridement

Septic tenosynovitis

Infections of the tendon sheath occur predominantly in the hand and the traumatized foot (including the chronically ulcerated).

Aetiology: as well as common bacteria, tenosynovitis in the non-traumatized hand can be caused by atypical mycobacteria such as *M. marinum, M. cheloniae,* and *M. kansasii,* and environmental fungi such as *Sporothrix schenkii.* If related to trauma or ulceration, a wide range of organisms may be involved. It can also occur 2° to disseminated gonococcal infection, sepsis with other bacteria, or *M. tuberculosis.*

Clinical features: swelling of one or more fingers, palm, or dorsum of the hand. Swelling in the foot can be minimal if fluid drains via an ulcer.

Diagnosis: can be clinical, confirmed by surgery, or made with ultrasound or MRI.

Management
- Generally requires drainage of the involved tendon sheath — to control the infection and to prevent adhesions and long-term stiffness.
- Tendons heal slowly if exposed — soft tissue or skin cover is important.
- See Table 12.1 for antibiotics: for pyogenic infections, treat for 2–4 weeks; for mycobacterial or fungal infections, use standard courses for the pathogen.

Septic arthritis

Bacteria infect the joint by blood spread or by direct inoculation (trauma, ulceration, or iatrogenic). Bacterial multiplication in the joint leads to acute inflammation — this causes destruction of articular cartilage and resorption of exposed bone, resulting in deformity, chronic osteomyelitis, and even joint fusion. Bacteraemia and septicaemia may occur. If pus tracks and discharges externally, a sinus is formed.

Clinical features

Although most cases of acute or chronic infection involve a single joint, multiple joint involvement occurs in 5–10% of cases.

- *Acute septic arthritis:* fever, pain, and loss of function. The joint is highly irritable; the patient resists both active and passive movement. Usually the joint is obviously swollen, warm, and tender to touch, with little or no erythema unless accompanied by bursitis or cellulitis.
- *Chronic septic arthritis:* swollen and painful joint, but little systemic illness. There may be obvious deformity or crepitus from gross joint destruction.

Complications: without timely and effective treatment, joint destruction ensues. There may be osteomyelitis, septicaemia, and — in the young child — growth plate disturbances leading to deformity or limb length discrepancy. Complications are much more likely if treatment is delayed.

Diagnosis: FBC, CRP, ESR, and biochemistry assess patient's general state, but lack specificity. Plain X-rays determine extent of joint damage. MRI reveals the extent of bone and soft tissue infection, and aids surgical planning. Blood cultures are positive in <50%. Microscopy of aspirated synovial fluid shows neutrophils; bacteria may be seen on Gram stain; cultures often positive if antibiotics have not been previously given.

Management

- Systemic antibiotics (see Table 12.1) penetrate inflamed joints well. For uncomplicated infections of normal joints, treat for 2 wks for streptococci and 3 wks for staphylococci and Gram –ve bacteria. Even shorter durations of therapy can be used for gonococcal arthritis. In joints with extensive pre-existing arthritis and exposed bone, or in compromised hosts (rheumatoid arthritis is a good example of both), treat for longer.
- Infections of the hip and shoulder joints require arthrotomy or arthroscopic washout.
- Infections in other joints can often be managed by a diagnostic tap before antibiotic therapy, followed by daily aspirates. Proceed to surgery if it fails to settle within 5 days. There is no place for continuous irrigation of the joint: this carries the risk of introducing antibiotic-resistant bacteria (e.g. *Pseudomonas*).
- Chronic septic arthritis generally requires surgery.

Causes of bone and joint infections

- Skin infections can seed via the bloodstream to give septic arthritis and acute osteomyelitis.
- If ineffectively treated, these acute conditions become chronic (e.g. when surgery is unavailable and prolonged courses of antibiotics are unaffordable).
- Major cause is injuries on roads and in factories, armed conflict, and landmine injuries.
- Some 1° infections of bone and joint are more common in the tropics: TB, brucellosis, melioidosis, histoplasmosis, and blastomycosis.

Organisms causing acute septic arthritis

- *Staph. aureus* — most common in all age groups and all countries
- *Haemophilus influenzae* — in populations without access to HIB vaccine
- Beta-haemolytic streptococci of all groups (including Group B in pregnancy, neonates, and diabetics)
- Enterobacteriaciae (e.g. *E. coli*) — in neonates and elderly
- *N. gonorrhoeae* — in sexually active individuals

Organisms causing chronic septic arthritis

- The same organisms as acute septic arthritis
- *M. tuberculosis*
- *Brucella*
- Occasionally fungi (e.g. *Sporothrix schenkii*)

Osteomyelitis

Acute 1° haematogenous bone infection presents in a similar fashion to acute septic arthritis. Chronic osteomyelitis may follow septic arthritis, but is also seen in spinal infections (discitis and vertebral osteomyelitis), fracture-fixation infections, and the diabetic foot. Organisms causing acute osteomyelitis are largely the same as those causing acute septic arthritis.

Clinical features

- *Acute osteomyelitis:* fever, localized bone pain, and loss of limb function. Osteomyelitis can cause septic arthritis, especially in young children.
- *Chronic osteomyelitis:* chronic drainage from wound or sinus tract, pain, flares of intercurrent acute infection, impaired function, and/or chronic ill health. Visible or palpable bone in a wound makes osteomyelitis highly likely. An orthopaedic implant or an open fracture with a chronically draining wound is almost certainly infected.

Diagnosis: anaemia, ↑WBC, ↑CRP, ↑ESR indicate the ill health of acute or chronic infection.

X-rays: become abnormal after 7–10 days, as involved bone is demineralized (lytic areas), attempts to heal (periosteal reaction), and in parts dies (sclerotic areas). Changes evolve over a few weeks; the process is aggressive. There may be evidence of loosening of metalware.

Other imaging: US can show abscesses adjacent to bone and delineate sinus tracts. CT is useful for assessing bony union, bone destruction, and sequestrum formation, and soft tissue collections. MRI detects marrow oedema, cortical breaches, sinus tracts, and soft tissue collections, but is less useful in patients with extensive metalware or recent surgery.

Treatment

- *For acute osteomyelitis:* give antibiotics (see Table 12.1) for >4 weeks. Use IV, then perhaps oral route. Evaluate need for surgery.
- *For chronic osteomyelitis:* evaluate surgery, patient's general fitness, and goals of treatment.

1. *Control of intermittent flares* — esp. if flares infrequent and respond to antibiotics. Monitor for progression of bone involvement.
2. *Suppression with long-term antibiotics* — if surgery impossible for technical reasons, unaffordable, or worse than disease. Long-term antibiotics can lead to drying of sinuses, improvements in general health, and reductions in pain.
3. *Surgical exploration, debridement, and excision* — with subsequent antibiotics. Aim to remove all dead bone, ensuring the skeleton is stable and soft tissue covers the bone at the end of surgery. Dead space inside debrided bone can be filled with muscle, cancellous bone graft (usually delayed until infection is arrested), or antibiotic-laden carriers. Antibiotics added to acrylic bone cement will generate very high local levels. With expert surgery >90% of cases can be arrested. However, even without surgery or antibiotics, spontaneous long-term arrest can occur if sequestra discharge spontaneously. Many patients can live with their bone infection for long periods; in some situations, this may be the best that can be achieved.

Spinal infections

Common causes are *Staph. Aureus*, *Brucella* spp, and TB. Initial blood-borne seeding to disc space is followed by involvement of adjacent vertebral bodies. Paraspinal muscles may also become involved, with collections (e.g. psoas abscesses). Retropulsion of disc and inflammatory tissue, or spinal epidural abscess, may compress the spinal cord, resulting in paralysis.

Clinical features: unusually severe backache, especially night pain; sudden paraparesis on a background of back pain and/or fever.

Diagnosis: plain X-rays may show irregularity and destruction of end-plates adjoining the infected disc space (which becomes reduced in height). MRI is best investigation. CXR or sputum examination may provide evidence of TB; the organism may be cultured from blood, aspirate of paraspinal or disc space abscesses, or guided biopsy of the disc.

Management
- Antibiotics (see Table 12.1). Treat pyogenic infections of the spine for 6–12 weeks.
- Surgery is reserved for cases with acute spinal epidural abscess, persistent pain, mechanical instability, recurrent infection with abscess formation, or cord compression.
- Patients with spinal TB infection can recover completely on anti-TB medication, even if presentation is with paralysis.

The diabetic foot

The dramatic worldwide increase in type II diabetes has brought an increase in patients with foot complications. These arise from diabetic peripheral neuropathy, with or without ischaemia, plus impaired systemic resistance to infection. A foot ulcer precedes most amputations in diabetics; most patients undergoing amputation for non-traumatic causes are diabetic. Good long-term glycaemic control is important.

- Motor neuropathy leads to increased curvature and height of the arch of the foot, resulting in hyperextension and subluxation at MP joints, and clawing at the IP joints. This produces pressure on metatarsal heads, heel and clawed toes, the tips of toes, and over the PIP joints.
- These deformities coexist with a sensory neuropathy which means that the patient does not perceive pain until too late (or not at all).
- The patient may also sustain penetrating injuries or burns without knowing.
- The autonomic neuropathy results in its dry, fissured skin which is more susceptible to injury and infection.
- There is also impaired white cell function.
- Peripheral vascular disease, if present, further impairs healing of ulcers.

Clinical features: soft tissue infection and loss, draining sinuses with exposed bone, sometimes necrotizing fasciitis or septicaemia. Purulent drainage suggests infection, as does erythema, swelling, pain (which often occurs to some extent, despite neuropathy), and systemic symptoms.

Diagnosis: blood tests may show ↑WBC, ↑CRP, ↑ESR, ↑glucose, and ↑creatinine. Plain foot X-rays may show gas in the soft tissues, bone destruction, and/or changes consistent with infection or diabetic osteopathy. Serial X-rays may show progressive changes over weeks. MRI is best imaging.

Management

- Assess fever, cardiovascular stability, hydration, and diabetic control.
- Examine sensation, peripheral perfusion (Buerger's test, palpation of pulses, and Doppler assessment including ankle-brachial pressure indices), and presence of cellulitis, necrosis, swelling, or crepitus.
- Debride the ulcer to determine its extent. If possible, probe with a sterile metal probe: palpable bone suggests underlying osteomyelitis.
- See Table 12.1 for antibiotics. Durations: (a) 72 hrs for amputation through healthy tissue; (b) 1–2 wks for amputation through infected soft tissue, without residual infected bone; (c) 4 wks for amputation or surgery through ischaemic or severely infected soft tissues, including deep tissue involvement (e.g. tendon sheaths); (d) 4–6 wks for osteomyelitis, fully resected, with restoration of soft tissue cover; (e) 6–12 wks for osteomyelitis with residual infected or dead bone.
- Surgery for significant soft tissue necrosis, abscess drainage, or bone death.
- Vascular surgical input if ischaemic; may be able to avoid amputation.

Diabetic foot ulcers often recur without special attention to foot care and footwear. Appropriate long-term care, with offloading of pressure points, is also essential to obtain 1° healing of ulcers, even if not infected. Improve glycaemic control, stop smoking, and control blood pressure.

Fungal skin infections

Cutaneous infections

Dermatophytoses (tinea): common skin infections caused by fungi, particularly *Trichophyton* and *Microsporum spp.* They cause scaling or maceration between the toes (tinea pedis); itchy, scaly, red rash with definite edges in the groin area (tinea cruris); annular lesions with raised edges (often itchy) anywhere on the body (tinea corporis); scaling and itching of the scalp with loss of hair (tinea capitis). Treat with local application of Whitfield's ointment (benzoic acid compound) or clotrimazole for 2–4 weeks; for severe cases and nail involvement, use 4–6 weeks of griseofulvin 10 mg/kg PO (alternatives: terbinafine or itraconazole).

Pityriasis versicolor: a superficial, hypopigmented, macular rash normally of the upper body. If extensive, can indicate a chronic infection with sweating (e.g. TB or AIDS). Treat with 2% selenium sulfide shampoo, Whitfield's ointment, or itraconazole 200 mg PO od for 5 days

Superficial candidosis: in addition to vaginal and oral infection, *C. albicans* can infect moist folds of skin (groin, under breasts, nappy area of baby) producing a very red rash and skin damage. Treat with topical nystatin or clotrimazole and keep dry.

Subcutaneous infections

Mycetoma (Madura foot): chronic infection of subcutaneous tissue, bone, and skin that is due to environmental organisms, either fungi (eumycetes, producing eumycetomas) or bacteria (actinomycetes or Nocardia spp. producing actinomycetomas), probably introduced into deep tissue by a thorn. The infecting organisms grow very slowly, typically forming 'grains' that are macroscopic colonies of fungi or bacteria. Mycetomas commonly occur on the foot or leg, but may occur anywhere. They start as an area of hard swelling; infection eventually spreads from subcutaneous tissues to invade and destroy bone. There is considerable swelling and usually multiple sinus tract formation, through which grains may discharge, but pain is rarely severe.

Diagnosis: on X-ray, underlying bone is expanded, eroded, and ultimately destroyed. There is some local lymphatic involvement. The cause needs to be determined by microscopy of the sinus discharge.

Management: fungal mycetomas rarely respond to systemic antifungals and frequently require amputation. Actinomycetomas may respond to streptomycin or rifampicin for 2–3 months plus cotrimoxazole for many months until there is clinical improvement.

Sporotrichosis: Sporothrix schenckii probably enters the subcutaneous tissue through an abrasion. It may present as a single ulcer or nodule. In the lymphangitic form, the fungus spreads down the lymphatics, forming nodules at intervals which may then ulcerate through to the skin. Chronic lesions may look like psoriasis or a granuloma.

Treatment: saturated aqueous solution of potassium iodide mixed with milk, 0.5–1 ml PO tds, increased in small increments to 3–6 ml tds, until 1 month after clinical resolution. (Alternative: itraconazole 100 – 200 mg od.)

Skin signs of systemic fungal infection

- Systemic mycoses such as histoplasmosis, blastomycosis, coccidioidomycosis, paracoccidioidomycosis, and other fungal infections in immunocompromised individuals, often show skin signs.
- Such signs include purpura, ulcers, slow spreading verrucose plaques, nodules, papules, pustules, and abscesses.

Endocrinology

Section editor **Theresa Allain**

Diabetes mellitus

Diabetes mellitus (DM) is a syndrome caused by the lack, or diminished effectiveness, of endogenous insulin. DM is characterized by hyperglycaemia and deranged metabolism. Several forms of the disease exist and their prevalence throughout the world varies greatly.

Type I DM: is essentially an autoimmune disease of Caucasians, with highest prevalence occurring in northern Europe. In India there are 6–70 cases per 100,000; estimates from tropical Africa suggest 3 per 100,000. It is usually of juvenile onset and is the most common form of childhood DM; however, the increasing prevalence of type II diabetes in children and adolescents may reverse this order within a few decades. Type I DM may be associated with other autoimmune diseases in the patient or family. Environmental factors may be important, since a seasonal variation in onset has been noted and migrants tend to assume the risk of the country to which they have migrated. Patients always need insulin and are prone to ketoacidosis.

Type II DM: accounts for more than 90% of global cases of DM. Its prevalence is increasing massively worldwide due to the changes in diet and lifestyle accompanying globalization and is directly associated with increases in obesity. The number of cases of DM is expected to double by 2025, this increase being most marked in non-Europid populations. 50% of the Pima Indians of the USA and Micronesians of Nauru, 10% of Mauritians, and 6% of Indian Asians have type II DM. Asians in S. Africa have a prevalence of 20%. Although, historically, black Africans and Chinese have had a low rate, this is changing with 7% of urban black South Africans and 5% of Hong Kong Chinese affected. The worldwide diabetes epidemic is associated with an early age of onset of type II DM, some even presenting in childhood.

Maturity onset diabetes of the young (MODY) presents similarly to type II DM. 20% of type II diabetics eventually need insulin treatment.

Malnutrition-related DM (MRDM): accounts for 1% of diabetes presenting in a tropical setting. The WHO subdivides this disease into two classes:
• Protein deficient pancreatic diabetes (PDPD)
• Fibrocalculous pancreatic diabetes (FCPD)
Both occur in young patients of low body weight. High doses of insulin are required, but ketoacidosis does not occur. Tropical calcific pancreatitis (see Chapter 7) may be a cause of FCPD. Another theory is that consumption of cyanide-containing foods (e.g. cassava/manioc/tapioca, ragi in India, and kaffir beers in Africa) on a background of protein-calorie malnutrition leads to build-up of toxic hydrocyanic acid, resulting in direct damage to the pancreas. Conversely, some believe that the malnutrition is a result and not a cause of the diabetes.

Other types of DM
• *Gestational*
• *Secondary* — due to drugs (steroids, thiazide diuretics); pancreatic disease (chronic pancreatitis, TCP, post-surgery); endocrine disease (Cushing's, acromegaly, phaeochromocytoma, thyrotoxicosis).

Presentation
- **Acute:** ketoacidosis, weight loss, polyuria, polydipsia.
- **Subacute:** as above, but occurring over a longer time, plus lethargy, infection (pruritis vulvae, boils).
- **Chronic:** may present with complications — infection, cataract, microangiopathy (retinopathy, neuropathy, nephropathy) and macroangiopathy (MI, claudication), foot ulcers.

Diagnosis
Diagnosis requires:
- One abnormal blood glucose concentration if symptomatic.
- Two separate abnormal measurements if asymptomatic.

Abnormal values are:
- A fasting venous plasma glucose levels = 7.0 mmol/l, *or*
- Random glucoses = 11.1 mmol/l.

Always check urine ketones on diagnosis, if moderate or heavy the DM is likely to be type I.

PDPD — as above plus: onset <30 yrs of age, BMI <19, a history of childhood malnutrition, and no ketoacidosis. Such patients will require >60 units of insulin per day.

FCPD — needs the additional criteria of recurrent abdominal pain and evidence of pancreatic calculi in the absence of alcoholism, gallstones, or hyperthyroidism.

The glucose tolerance test (GTT)

This should only be used for epidemiological research and diagnosing gestational DM. The patient must be on a normal carbohydrate intake prior to the test. Fast the patient overnight, then take a plasma glucose (fasting sample).

Give 75 g oral glucose in 300 ml water (1.75 g/kg in children) and measure plasma glucose 2 hrs afterwards. DM is diagnosed if the fasting venous plasma glucose is = 7.0 mmol/l and/or the 2 hr sample is = 11.1mmol/l.

Screening for glycosuria is not a cost-effective way of diagnosis in the general population. However, this is an appropriate method of screening for gestational DM. If glycosuria is present, proceed to GTT.

Type I or type II diabetes?

The following features favour type I DM — *ignore age and glucose level:*
- Non-fasting ketonuria *(test everyone)*
- Short history
- Marked weight loss *(from any weight)*
- Family history of type I DM
- Personal/family history of autoimmune disease

Management of diabetes mellitus

Patient education and motivation is the key to success. The aim of treatment is to restore normoglycaemia and avoid complications. If home monitoring of control is not feasible, the aim is for the absence of symptoms of hyper- or hypoglycaemia.

Children are more likely to develop serious ketoacidosis, so the advice of a paediatrician should always be sought on admission. Glycaemic control is especially important during pregnancy, as hyperglycaemia in the first trimester carries a 3-fold increased risk for fetal abnormality and birth complications.

Education

Emphasize the importance of diet and adhereing to treatment. If possible, teach monitoring of blood and urine glucose levels. If on insulin or sulfonylureas, advise the patient to have access to sweets at all times; alert the patient/family/colleagues about symptoms of hypoglycaemia. The diet should avoid large amounts of rapidly absorbed carbohydrates (eg. sugar, sweets, fizzy drinks), but include regular meals of complex carbohydrate. Long periods of physical activity without food should be avoided. Explain the importance of foot care and the need to avoid walking barefoot. Where possible, arrange for appointments with a dietician and chiropodist or a nurse skilled in these areas. Stress the need for regular follow-up.

Conservative management

Treatment should always begin with a healthy diet: low in fat, sugar, and salt; high in starchy carbohydrate and fibre; with moderate protein; eaten at regular times. Note that fruit and fruit juice contain a lot of natural sugar. In urban areas, processed foods may be favoured but should be avoided because of high fat, sugar, and salt content. Obese patients should lose weight. CVS risk factors should be minimized (e.g. stop smoking, control hypertension, lower high cholesterol, advise regular exercise).

Oral drug therapy

Rx will depend upon the type of DM and drug availability. In uncomplicated, newly diagnosed, type II DM try a 3-month trial of diet and exercise. If conservative treatment has not achieved glycaemic control after 3 months, patients should be started on metformin if they are overweight or a sulfonylurea if they are slim. Sulfonylureas stimulate insulin secretion and insulin sensitivity and cause hypoglycaemia; tolbutamide (0.5–1.0 g bd) is short-acting and the preferred treatment. Gliclazide (40–160 mg od) and glibenclamide (2.5–15 mg od) are longer-acting and, particularly in elderly patients, cause hypoglycaemia. Metformin (500 mg–1 g tds with food) does not cause hypoglycaemia but may cause anorexia, diarrhoea, and, rarely, lactic acidosis. It should not be used in patients with renal, heart, or liver failure. If these drugs alone do not work, they may be combined. Should this still be insufficient, one of the drugs can be replaced with a single, once-daily injection of long-acting insulin. Patients who are still hyperglycaemic despite maximal oral therapy require changing entirely to insulin treatment. This is most likely if they are losing weight. In obese patients who require insulin, co-treatment with metformin reduces weight gain.

Insulin

Comes in one strength (100 units/ml). Soluble insulin is short-acting, peaking at 2–4 hrs and lasting up to 8 hrs. Medium-acting insulins are suspensions, peaking at 4–6 hrs, and lasting up to 16 hrs. Long-acting insulins may last up to 32 hrs.

Treatment regimes are varied, and ultimately will depend upon the availability of different insulins, access to home monitoring, and lifestyle of the patient. Most will require 20–60 units per day.

- Start with 0.5 units/kg/day, 2/3 given in the morning and 1/3 in the evening. Make 1/3 short-acting and 2/3 long-acting. With this twice-daily regime, the insulin injections should be given 20 mins before breakfast and evening meal. Avoidance of hypoglycaemia relies on the patient being able to take 3 meals a day at predictable times and 2 snacks, one mid morning and one before bed.
- An alternative regime, that gives more flexibility but also requires more injections, is to take a single injection of long-acting at bedtime and 3 injections of soluble during the day, shortly before each meal.
  Test glucose before each mealtime initially and adjust the previous insulin dose up or down by 2 units at a time.

Diabetic treatment with intercurrent illness

The stress of illness increases basal insulin requirements. If calorie intake is reduced, then reduce long-acting insulin by ~20% and short-acting in proportion to size of meal reduction. Check blood sugar regularly. In some cases a sliding scale or GKI regime may be needed.

Sliding scale

Infuse 1 litre of 5% dextrose with 20 mmol K^+ at 100 ml/hr. Add 50 units of soluble insulin to 49.5 ml of normal saline in a 50 ml syringe (i.e. 1 unit/ml) and infuse this into a separate vein (or IV line) at a rate according to the blood glucose as follows:

Blood glucose	Units/hour
<4.5	0.5–1
4.5–6.4	2
6.5–11	3
11.1–17.1	4
>17	5

GKI regime

Add 15 units of soluble insulin to 500 ml 10% dextrose with 10 mmol K^+. Infuse at 100 ml/hr and check the blood glucose hourly. Make up new bottles with altered insulin units according to;

Glucose	Insulin in bottle
<5	6
5–15	15
>15	25

N.B. Unless the blood glucose is quite stable, the GKI regime tends to be more wasteful as new bottles need to be made up frequently.

Diabetic follow-up

Diabetes is an increasingly common problem, even in tropical, rural areas. The complications of diabetes can be devastating but simple measures, such as good blood pressure control, are effective at reducing the risk of complications. Some complications, such as cataract, can be easily identified and addressed. It is therefore essential, even in resource poor areas, to establish locally accessible diabetic clinics in which patients can be regularly reviewed. Follow-up is necessary with all diabetic patients, in order to:

- Identify and resolve problems with treatment
- Encourage adherence with treatment and maintain education
- Monitor foot care
- Prevent and monitor for the development of long-term complications

Frequent follow-up and tight control are essential during pregnancy.

Prevention of complications

1. ***Good glycaemic control:*** assess glycaemic control via
   - Symptoms
   - Home urine testing (aim for 0–0.25%),
   - Home glucose records (aim for 3.5–6.5 mmol/l)
   - History of hypoglycaemic attacks
   - Glycosylated Hb (HbA$_1$c; indicates mean glucose level over the last 8 weeks — aim for <8%)
2. ***Control of hypertension:*** is more effective at preventing complications than good glycaemic control. Target BP is 130/80 mmHg. ACE inhibitors are the drug of first choice but all antihypertensive drugs are probably effective
3. ***Stopping smoking***
4. ***Control of hyperlipidaemia***
5. ***Aspirin for those with vascular disease***

Clinic checklist

Ideally every 6 months check:

1. Treatment and glucose control
2. Injection sites
3. Feet: pulses, numbness, sores, nail care
4. Eyes:
   - Check acuities (with glasses if worn, otherwise use pin hole)
   - If acuity drops, check for cataracts
   - If no cataracts, maculopathy is likely (more common in type II DM)
   - Check fundus for retinopathy — if cotton wool spots or new vessels are present, refer for laser treatment
5. Urine dipstick for albumin — albuminuria or a rise in BP may indicate nephropathy. Exclude UTI; check serum creatinine. Albuminuria warrants aggressive treatment of BP
6. BP
7. If macrovascular disease or nephropathy is present, check lipids

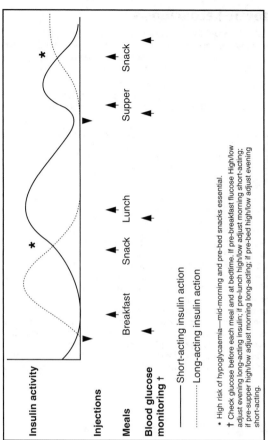

Insulin activity

Injections

Meals
Breakfast   Snack   Lunch   Supper   Snack

Blood glucose monitoring †

— Short-acting insulin action
······· Long-acting insulin action

* High risk of hypoglycaemia—mid-morning and pre-bed snacks essential.

† Check glucose before each meal and at bedtime. If pre-breakfast flucose High/low adjust evening long-acting insulin; if pre-lunch high/low adjust morning short-acting; if pre-supper high/low adjust morning (long-acting); if pre-bed high/low adjust evening short-acting.

Fig. 13.1 Balancing insulin action and meals. How to monitor and adjust insulin doses with a typical twice-daily regime of short- and long-acting insulin.

Risk of morbidity in patients with DM

Condition	Relative risk
Limb amputation	40
Renal failure	25
Blindness	20
Myocardial infarction	2–5
Stroke	2–3

Diabetic ketoacidosis

Without insulin, glucose is unable to enter cells. The body is therefore forced to make alternative substrates for metabolism, in the form of ketones produced in the liver. Lack of insulin eventually leads to hyperglycaemia and a build-up of acidic ketones. This may be precipitated by infection.

Clinical features: there is often a gradual deterioration over several days — ask a relative if the patient cannot give a proper history. There may be hyperventilation (with sweet, ketotic breath), vomiting, hyperglycaemia, and coma.

Investigations: FBC, U&Es, bicarbonate, blood gases, infection screen (urine and blood cultures, CXR). Test the urine for ketones. Blood glucose may not be very high. The seriousness of the condition is governed by pH, HCO_3 levels, and the level of ketones.

Management

1. Correct dehydration first (may be life-threatening) with 1.5–2 litres/hr of normal saline for 2 hrs.
2. Give soluble insulin 1.5 units/hr IV (or 6 units/hr IM) until the blood glucose is <14 mmol/l. Then either switch to a GKI regime, a sliding scale, or (if neither are available) halve the rate of infusion to 0.75 units/hr IV.
3. Measure K^+ hourly, since hypokalaemia can result as hyperglycaemia is corrected and glucose enters cells, taking K^+ with it. Give 20–60 mmol K^+ IV depending upon the measured levels (unless there is oliguria, when K^+ should be withheld).
4. Monitor vital signs, blood glucose, and K^+ every hour.
5. Prevent complications, including aspiration, DVT. Pass an NG tube to decompress stomach. Be alert to shock, cerebral oedema, and DIC.
6. If unconsciousness is prolonged, give 5000 IU heparin sc bd.

Giving bicarbonate is unnecessary — insulin and fluid will correct the pH provided the underlying cause (e.g. infection) is treated. If there is gross acidosis without ketosis, consider aspirin overdose or lactic acidosis in elderly diabetics.

Hyperglycaemic hyperosmolar non-ketotic coma (HONK)

Affects older, type II diabetics. There is usually a more gradual history with intense dehydration and severe hyperglycaemia (>35 mmol/l). There is no acidosis or ketosis and the plasma osmolality may be >340 mmol/kg. (Work out approximate plasma osmolality by: 2[Na^++ K^+] + [urea] + [glucose] mmol/l.) Treat as for ketoacidosis, but correct the osmolality slowly (over ~3 days) using half normal or normal saline to avoid cerebral oedema after large fluid shifts. DVT is more likely, so use heparin prophylaxis from the outset. Consider other precipitants such as silent MI.

Hypoglycaemia

This is usually due to administration of excess insulin or sulfonylureas. It presents with altered (often aggressive) behaviour, sweating, tachycardia, and, rarely, fits and coma of rapid onset. If the patient is unable to take sugar orally, treat with 50ml of 50% dextrose followed by a saline flush to avoid damaging the vein. Improvement should be rapid. Then feed them quickly with complex carbohydrate. If IV access fails, try 0.5–1 mg glucagon IM to attempt to promote conversion of hepatic glycogen to glucose (repeated doses of glucagon become less effective as glycogen stores become depleted). If a long-acting insulin or sulfonylurea has been taken, the patient will need monitoring and may require further IV dextrose for 48 hrs. In prolonged resistant hypoglycaemia, give dexamethasone 10 mg IV stat then 4 mg IM 6h to combat cerebral oedema.

Diabetic nephropathy

Early disease is manifested by microalbuminuria; this may progress to frank proteinuria (detected by dipstix) and a gradual decline in renal function, leading over 10–15 yrs to end-stage renal failure. In type I DM, nephropathy develops ~7–10 yrs after onset; in type II it may be present at diagnosis. Retinopathy is usually present in both type I and II diabetics with nephropathy.

Management

- *Good glycaemic control:* careful monitoring is essential, since requirements for insulin and oral hypoglycaemics tends to fall in CRF, due to reduced renal excretion and reduced insulin resistance. Avoid glibenclamide (risk of hypoglycaemia) and metformin (risk of lactic acidosis).
- *Control blood pressure* to prevent progression of renal damage. Target BP is 130/80. Patients are at high risk of hypertension since salt and fluid loads are less well handled. There may be a need for massive diuretic therapy, unless dialysis is possible.
- *ACE inhibitors* slow progression of nephropathy, even in normotensive diabetics with microalbuminuria.
- *Restrict dietary protein* to 0.6–0.8 g/kg body weight/day to slow progression. However, be careful to avoid malnutrition, particularly if there is intercurrent illness.
- *Control hyperlipidaemia*

Advanced nephropathy in the diabetic patient is also strongly correlated to the risk of coronary disease and cardiovascular death. Watch for the abrupt onset of pulmonary oedema or congestive heart failure, which may be the first signs of severe ischaemic heart disease.

Thyroid disease

The gland may become enlarged either diffusely (goitre) or in single or multiple nodules and in each case the patient may be euthyroid, hypothyroid, or hyperthyroid.

Hypothyroidism (myxoedema)

Clinical features: include weight gain, lethargy, constipation, dislike of cold, menorrhagia, hoarse voice, depression, dementia, cerebellar ataxia, myopathy, angina, infertility, dry skin, galactorrhea, and vitiligo. Examination reveals coarse features, bradycardia, goitre, CCF, non-pitting oedema, ascites, pleural effusion, delayed reflexes, loss of the outer third of the eyebrows.

Diagnosis: ↑TSH, ↓T_4 (and T_3). FBC may show macrocytic anaemia (check B_{12}/folate) or iron deficiency (menorrhagia); ECG may show bradycardia and ischaemia; cholesterol and triglycerides may be ↑. Positive antithyroid antibodies suggest an autoimmune cause.

Management: thyroxine 50–150 mcg od, adjusted according to clinical state (aim to keep TSH <5 mU/l). In the elderly/those with ischaemic heart disease, begin with 25 mcg/day and monitor for angina or tachycardia (propanolol may be needed e.g. 40 mg od). Usually required lifelong; if De Quervains is suspected, withdraw thyroxine after 6 months and monitor. If area is iodine deficient, use Schiller's iodine (1:30 diluted Lugol's iodine) 2 drops od for 6–12 months.

Myxoedema coma

A very rare condition with 50% mortality. Often precipitated by infection, MI, CVA, or trauma. Look for hypothermia, hyporeflexia, bradycardia, paralytic ileus, and fits.

Investigations: take blood for T_3 & T_4, TSH, FBC, U&Es (may have hyponatraemia), glucose (hypoglycaemia), cultures, and ABGs (hypoxia and hypercapnia).

Management: give O_2 and treat any precipitating cause.
- If available, give 12.5 mcg T_3 by slow IV injection, repeated 6–12h.
- Give hydrocortisone 100 mg q8h IV (especially if pituitary hypothyroidism suspected).
- Pass NG tube and, unless there is paralytic ileus, administer T_4 300 mcg od.
- Rehydrate with normal saline, avoiding CCF. Hyponatraemia is usually due to water retention so fluid restriction may be necessary.
- Correct hypothermia and hypoglycaemia.
- Monitor for pancreatitis and arrhythmias.
- After 3 days, start thyroxine PO od at the usual dose.

Compensated euthyroidism/subclinical hypothyroidism

Raised TSH, normal T3 and T4, clinically euthyroid. Usually follows treatment for thyrotoxicosis or at an early stage of autoimmune hypothyroidism. If possible, measure thyroid autoantibodies. Treat with thyroxine if antibody positive, hypercholesterolaemia, or subfertility. Otherwise monitor TFT 6 monthly.

Causes of goitre or thyroid nodules

- Physiological (either endemic or sporadic) colloid goitre
- Nodular goitre
- Hyperplasia (Graves')
- Goitrogens
- Dyshormonogenesis
- Thyroiditis
- Tumours (benign and malignant)

Causes of hypothyroidism

- *Iodine deficiency:* see Chapter 15. Previously widespread (e.g. >50% of countries in Africa). May be endemic, especially in mountain areas, or sporadic (pregnancy/puberty). Iodination programmes have improved the situation but endemic goitre is still seen in many adults.
- *Autoimmune hypothyroidism:* usually occurs in women. If a goitre is present, Dx is Hashimoto's thyroiditis; if none, Dx is atrophic hypothyroidism. Associated with previous Graves' disease, IDDM, Addison's disease, pernicious anaemia; rarely with thyroid lymphoma.
- *Post thyroidectomy or radioiodine treatment.*
- *Drug-induced:* anti-thyroid drugs, amiodarone, lithium, iodine.
- *Post-viral thyroiditis (De Quervains):* often follows 6 weeks after a viral prodrome. Goitre is tender. Inflammatory markers are raised. Can be hypo-, hyper-, or euthyroid. Self-limiting illness usually lasts 6 months but may require treatment in interim.
- *Dyshormonogenesis:* a number of defects, all autosomal recessive.

Abnormal TFTs in non-thyroidal illness: 'sick euthyroid syndrome'. Seen in severe illness, starvation, or fasting. TSH ↓ or normal, T3 ↓, T4 ↓ or normal. Patient may be clinically hypothyroid. Does not require treatment; abnormalities correct when the underlying problem is treated. If abnormalities persist, consider hypopituitism.

Amiodarone-associated thyroid abnormalities: abnormal TFTs are common on amiodarone as well as true thyroid dysfunction. The drug blocks conversion of T4 to T3, so may see raised T4, normal/↓T3 and normal/↑TSH. True thyroid dysfunction more likely if thyroid autoantibody positive. Only treat if clinical hypo-/hyperthyroidism supported by TFTs.

Hyperthyroidism (thyrotoxicosis)

Occurs more commonly in women

Clinical features: weight loss, diarrhoea, oligomenorrhoea, tremor, emotional lability, heat intolerance, sweating, itch, fatigue, polyuria/polydipsia, hair thinning, and eye protrusion. Examination may reveal tachycardia, AF, fine tremor, thyroid eye disease, goitre/nodule(s), thyroid bruit, myopathy. **Complications** include heart failure, AF, osteoporosis, gynaecomastia.

Diagnosis: suppressed TSH, ↑T3 & T4. Nuclear thyroid scanning is best way to differentiate toxic nodules and multinodular goitres from Graves' disease (diffuse increased uptake) and hyperthyroid thyroiditis (decreased uptake). Scan can be done while taking antithyroid drugs. USS, thyroid autoantibodies, ECG, FBC, U&Es also useful. Test the visual fields and acuity.

Management

1. Gain rapid symptom control with propranolol 40 mg qds.
2. Start carbimazole at 40 mg od for 4–6 weeks (may have to increase to 60 mg if not achieving control). Propylthiouracil is an alternative.
   - In Graves' disease, options are then to either reduce the dose according to TFTs and maintain on 5–10 mg od for 12–18 months before stopping, *or*
   - 'Block and replace' — leave on 40–60 mg carbimazole and once TSH starts to rise add 50–150 mcg/kg levothyroxine for 18 months. Block and replace is simpler as it does not require regular monitoring of TFTs and may be associated with lower relapse rates.
   - With both regimes ~50% will relapse, usually in the next 18 mths.
   - N.B. in the West 0.1% have **agranulocytosis on carbimazole**, therefore tell the patient to return if they have a sore throat shortly after starting treatment; check the FBC.
3. Radioiodine is best treatment for toxic nodule or multinodular goitre. A single treatment should lead to cure with minimal risk of hypothyroidism. Radioiodine can be used for Graves' (usually reserved for relapsed cases) but occasionally inadequate treatment requires a repeat dose and post-treatment hypothyroidism is common.
4. If carbimazole is used to treat toxic nodules/multinodular goitres the lowest effective dose should be used and treatment is usually lifelong.
5. Surgery is useful for large goitres but runs similar risks of over- and under-treatment as radioiodine in Graves' disease.
6. Patients should be made euthyroid with drugs before surgery or radioiodine to avoid thyroid storm.

In pregnancy the lowest dose of antithyroid drug should be used and, if possible, the fetus should be checked for goitre by US scanning before delivery

Subclinical hyperthyroidism

Suppressed TSH, normal T3 and T4. Found in multinodular goitre and after treatment for Grave's. Patients are usually clinically euthyroid. Not thought to require treatment but may be associated with increased cardiovascular morbidity and mortality.

Causes of hyperthyroidism

- **Toxic multi-nodular goitre:** common in areas of recently treated iodine deficiency.
- **Graves' disease:** genetic pre-disposition leads to antibodies to TSH receptors and a diffuse goitre. There may be ophthalmopathy, pre-tibial myxoedema (oedematous swellings above the lateral malleoli and shins), anaemia, $\uparrow$ESR, $\uparrow$Ca^{2+}, and abnormal LFTs. It is associated with IDDM and pernicious anaemia.
- **Toxic adenoma:** nodule producing T3 and T4.
- **Thyroiditis:** post-partum or triggered by viral illness (mumps, coxsackie). The goitre may be painful. Self-limiting condition.
- **Others:** medication, follicular carcinoma of the thyroid, choriocarcinoma, struma ovarii (ovarian tumour secreting T3 & T4).

Thyroid eye disease

This occurs in the presence of specific autoantibodies causing retro-orbital inflammation and lymphocyte infiltration. It occurs with autoimmune hyper- and hypothyroidism and may precede thyrotoxicosis.

Clinical features: gritty sore eyes, blurred vision, double vision, eye pain, and/or protrusion. Ophthalmopathy is worse in smokers and in those in whom hypothyroidism occurs during the course of treatment. Examination may reveal lid lag, lid retraction, proptosis, conjunctival oedema, corneal ulceration, papilloedema, optic atrophy, impaired colour vision (earliest sign of optic nerve compression), ophthalmoplegia.

The main risks to sight are exposure keratitis and optic nerve compression; ask the patient to shut his/her eyes and check eye closure is complete. Where available, a CT scan or US may be used to demonstrate thickening of rectus muscles and can demonstrate optic nerve compression.

Management: stop smoking. Pay close attention to maintaining the euthyroid state. Protect the cornea: wear sunglasses at all times to keep out dust/wind, tape eyelids shut with micropore in bed, consider tarsorraphy. Try hypromellose eye drops for lubrication. Use an eye patch for diplopia. Steroids (80mg od prednisolone) work but systemic side-effects of the doses required are unacceptable for long-term use. Orbital radiotherapy and surgical decompression are effective. These options should be reserved for situations where sight is threatened; seek expert advice.

Cushing's syndrome

Cushing's syndrome is due to chronic glucocorticoid (i.e. cortisol) excess. The most common cause is treatment with steroids/ACTH analogues. It is important to differentiate this cause from endogenous overproduction of cortisol. Cortisol is normally released after ACTH stimulus from the hypothalamo-pituitary axis and Cushing's syndrome is classified as either ACTH dependent (i.e. excess stimulus) or ACTH independent (i.e. ↑cortisol without ↑ACTH). Also consider alcoholic pseudo-Cushing's, depression, and ectopic ACTH from carcinoma.

Clinical features: moon face, obesity, impaired glucose tolerance, hypertension, hypogonadism, osteoporosis, purple striae, limb wasting and myopathy, hirsutism, thin skin, bruising, peripheral oedema, ↑ infection, poor wound healing, hypokalaemia, psychological change (depression/mania/psychosis). Increased pigmentation if ACTH high.

Diagnosis

Do an overnight dexamethasone suppression test (screening test); give dexamethasone 1–2 mg PO at 11 p.m. Take blood for plasma cortisol at 9 a.m. (normal <170 nmol/l: higher in Cushing's syndrome; N.B. the OCP gives false high values).
If this tests abnormal proceed to 2 or more of (including Liddle test):
- 24-hr urinary free cortisol (normally <700 nmol/24 hrs).
- 9 a.m. and midnight cortisols — loss of diurnal variation.
- Insulin-induced hypoglycaemia — see no rise in serum cortisol
- The Liddle Test: give dexamethasone 0.5 mg 6h for 2 days then check 9 a.m. serum cortisol and urinary 17 OHCS on the second day. If they are not suppressed, a diagnosis of Cushing's can be made.

Expert help is required for investigation and management.

Addison's disease

Adreno-cortical insufficiency, leading to ↓ gluco- and mineralocorticoids.

Clinical features: weakness, apathy, anorexia, weight loss, abdominal pain, oligomenorrhoea. There may be hyperpigmentation, vitiligo, hypotension, and sexual dysfunction. Dehydration in crises.

Investigations: synacthen tests. Check for hyperkalaemia, hyponatraemia (may be SIADH), uraemia, acidosis, hypercalcaemia, and eosinophilia. Get a CXR (looking for signs of TB) and AXR.

Causes: idiopathic (probably auto-immune, associated with other such diseases), adrenal TB, adrenal metastases, HIV, fungal infection.

Management: treat cause. Replace steroids with hydrocortisone, 20 mg in morning, 10 mg at night, and adjust the dose according to plasma cortisol (aim for 700–850 nmol/l) and clinical symptoms (↑ if postural hypotension, ↓ if patient becomes Cushingoid). Warn the patient about not stopping steroid treatment abruptly and if possible give syringes to give the hydrocortisone IM if vomiting prevents oral therapy. Explain that they need to take more hydrocortisone during intercurrent illnesses. There should be 6m follow-up.

Management of Cushing's syndrome

ACTH-dependent:

- Iatrogenic (ACTH or synacthen treatment) — treat by ↓ dose.
- Cushing's disease; ACTH-producing pituitary adenoma — treat either surgically or medically with metyrapone.
- Ectopic ACTH (or, rarely CRH) production from tumours, especially small-cell bronchial Ca — treat the cause.

ACTH-independent:

- Iatrogenic (prednisolone or dexamethasone treatment) — ↓ dose.
- Alcohol excess — reduce alcohol intake.
- Cortisol-producing tumours (adrenal adenoma or Ca) — remove tumour.

Addisonian crisis

Hypotension and shock in a known Addisonian patient or someone on long-term steroids who has omitted their tablets. Often there is preceding infection, trauma, or surgery.

Management:

- Take bloods for urgent ACTH and cortisol.
- Resuscitate with colloid then crystalloids.
- Give 100 mg hydrocortisone IV stat, then q6–8h
- Culture blood, urine, and sputum.
- Give a broad-spectrum antibiotic.
- Monitor for hypoglycaemia.
- Change to oral hydrocortisone after 72 h if stable.

Hyperaldosteronism

Excessive aldosterone production independent of the renin angiotensin system. Typically there is hypertension, hypokalaemia, alkalosis, and mild hypernatraemia. May be present in 1–5% of patients with 'essential' hypertension. Suspect if K^+ low before treatment of BP or persistent hypokalaemia on thiazides. Check plasma K^+, aldosterone ($\uparrow$), and renin ($\downarrow$). Most cases are due to adrenocortical adenoma (Conn's syndrome); rarely, adrenal hyperplasia and Ca. In 2° hyperaldosteronism (e.g. heart or liver failure, diuretic therapy) aldosterone and renin are both raised. Also consider elevated non-aldosterone mineralocorticoids in congenital adrenal hyperplasia — in which case both aldosterone and renin are low.

Management: can be medical with glucocorticoids (e.g. dexamethasone 0.75 mg in morning, 0.25 mg at night, or spironolactone 100–400 mg daily) or surgical. Treat 2° disease by treating the cause. Give K^+ replacements.

Hypopituitarism

The pituitary produces ACTH, GH, FSH, LH, TSH, and prolactin. $\downarrow$ production of one or more of these is termed hypopituitarism and may be due to: infarction (post-partum haemorrhage), cysts, granulomatous disease, abscesses, congenital defects, stroke, basal skull fracture, pituitary adenoma, hypophysectomy, and irradiation. There may be atrophy of the breasts, small testes, hair loss, thin skin, hypotension, visual field defects (bilateral hemianopia, initially of upper quadrants). Investigate with: lateral skull XR, assessment of visual fields, U&Es, FBC, TFT, testosterone/oestrogen, cortisol, CT head. Endocrine testing requires stimulation tests. A specialist centre is needed for treatment, which involves replacement of hydrocortisone, thyroxine, and oestrogen/testosterone.

Hyperprolactinaemia

Presents with amenorrhoea, infertility, galactorrhoea in women, and impotence in men. There may be visual field loss due to pressure effects. Causes may be physiological (pregnancy, stress), drugs (metaclopramide, haloperidol, methyldopa, oestrogens, TRH) or disease — pituitary disease (adenoma or stalk compression), CRF, hypothyroidism, sarcoid. Treat the underlying cause. If cause is pituitary adenoma, give bromocriptine (first line, often the only treatment required), surgery, and radiotherapy.

Acromegaly

Caused by ↑ secretion of GH from a pituitary tumour (in children, in whom epiphyseal plates have not yet fused, it results in gigantism). Adults have coarse features, prominent mandibles and hands and feet, large tongues, arthralgia, muscle weakness, and paraesthesiae (carpal tunnel syndrome). There is an increased risk of Ca colon, DM, HT, and cardiomyopathy. Diagnose by ↑IGF1 levels or failure of GH to suppress during an oral glucose tolerance test. Treatment is usually a combined approach between medicine (bromocriptine or, preferably, somatostatin if available), surgery, and radiotherapy.

Diabetes insipidus (DI)

Results from a failure of ADH action either due to lack of production (cranial DI) or renal insensitivity (nephrogenic DI). There is reduced water resorption by the kidney, polyuria, and polydipsia.

- *Cranial causes:* head injury, metastases, sarcoid, meningitis, and surgery.
- *Nephrogenic causes:* ↓K^+, ↑Ca^{2+}, drugs (e.g. lithium), sickle cell disease, renal failure, pyelonephritis, and hydronephrosis.

Diagnosis: by early morning urine osmolality (if >800 mosmol/l DI is excluded), U&Es, water deprivation test.

Treatment: for cranial DI is DDAVP replacement. For nephrogenic, remove underlying cause. May take weeks to recover; thiazides and indometacin 100 mg/day reduce urine output during this time.

Phaeochromocytoma

A tumour, usually in the renal medulla producing catecholamines. May be inherited as part of the multiple endocrine neoplasia syndrome (MENIIa) and associated with neurofibromatosis and medullary thyroid cancer. There is hypertension, cardiomyopathy, weight loss, hyperglycaemia, and crises of fear, palpitations, tremor, and nausea. Test the urine for HMMA or VMA. Cautiously reduce the BP with phenoxybenzamine 10 mg od (increased each day by 10mg, up to 1–2 mg/kg in 2 divided doses) and propranolol 20 mg tds. Add phentolamine 2–5 mg IV repeated if necessary during crises. Surgery provides the only cure.

Haematology

Section editor   **Saad Abdalla**

Disorders of red blood cells: anaemia

Clinical features and approach to dealing with anaemia

Anaemia is the most common manifestation and clinical feature of disease in the tropics. Prevalence and morbidity are highest in pre-school children and pregnant women. Although less common amongst other groups, it is still a major health problem. Anaemia is present when there is a decreased level of haemoglobin (Hb) in the blood — below the reference level for the age, sex, and pregnancy state of the individual. This fall in Hb is often, but not always, accompanied by a fall in the PCV. Alterations in the total circulating plasma volume as well as of the total circulating Hb mass determines the Hb concentration, allowing for altitude effect.

Anaemia can result from:

- Increased red cell loss
  - Haemolysis
  - Haemorrhage or chronic blood loss
- Decreased red cell production

These groups are not mutually exclusive and frequently overlap.

Causes of importance in the tropics are:

- Nutritional deficiencies (iron, folate, and vitamin B_{12})
- Infections (malaria, hookworm, schistosomiasis, TB, HIV)
- Inherited disorders of red cells (G6PD deficiency, thalassaemias, sickle-cell disease)

Classification: is useful in terms of management. It is based on the size and haemoglobin content of red cells (the red cell indices), mean cell volume (MCV), and mean cell haemoglobin (MCH). These values indicate the type of anaemia whether microcytic and hypochromic, normocytic or macrocytic, and may suggest an underlying abnormality before there are any clinical features of anaemia.

The diagnosis of anaemia should always lead to investigation of the underlying cause. The history, examination, and blood film will help determine the aetiology.

Symptoms: depend on the acuteness and the severity of anaemia. Symptoms can occur when anaemia is chronic; however, many patients are asymptomatic. Symptoms which relate to the underlying cause include non-specific complaints such as fatigue, headache, faintness (common in the general population), dyspnoea, palpitations, intermittent claudication, tinnitus, anorexia, and bowel disturbance. Susceptibility to infections increases with chronic and severe anaemia, especially in megaloblastic anaemia.

Signs: may be divided into general and specific.

- *General:* pallor of mucous membranes; signs of hyperdynamic circulation (tachycardia, bounding pulse, cardiomegaly, and systolic flow murmurs); rarely, papilloedema and retinal haemorrhages after an acute bleed (can be accompanied by blindness); heart failure, especially in the elderly.
- *Specific:* koilonychia (ridging and spoon-shaped nails) in iron deficiency anaemia; jaundice (haemolytic anaemia); bone deformities (thalassaemia major); leg ulcers (sickle-cell disease); splenomegaly in a number of conditions such as hyperreactive malarial splenomegaly and thalassaemias.

Aetiology

1. *Blood loss*
  Acute
  Chronic
  - Hookworm
  - Menstruation
  - Childbirth

2. *Decreased red cell production*
  Nutritional deficiencies
  - Iron, folate, vitamin B12
  - Protein, vitamins A, C, & E, riboflavin, pyridoxine, copper
  Depressed bone marrow function
  - 2° anaemias   Infections (e.g TB), chronic liver or renal disease, carcinomatosis
  - HIV infection
  - Aplastic anaemia   Drugs/chemicals, infiltration, idiopathic, irradiation, congenital
  - Ineffective erythropoiesis   Thalassaemias α and β

3. *Increased red cell destruction*
  Abnormalities of red cell constituents
  - Hb   Sickle-cell disease
  - Enzymes   G6PD deficiency
  - Membrane   Elliptocytosis, ovalocytosis, spherocytosis
  Abnormal haemolysis
  Immune haemolysis   Autoimmune, transfusion, fetomaternal incompatibility

  Non-immune haemolysis   Infections (e.g. malaria), hypersplenism, drugs and chemicals, venoms, burns, and mechanical injury

Table 14.1 Classification of anaemia according to RBC size

Red cell appearance	Microcytic	Normocytic	Macrocytic
Indices	Low MCV	Normal MCV	High MCV
Bone marrow	Micronormoblastic or Normoblastic	Normoblastic	Megaloblastic or Macronormoblastic
Diagnosis	Iron deficiency Chronic disease	Acute blood loss Malignancy	Vit B$_{12}$ deficiency Folate deficiency

Laboratory findings in anaemia

Red cell values: these vary with age, sex, pregnancy state, genetic and environmental factors. The values given are ranges, adjust them according to your local area.

	Hb (g/dl)	PCV (%)	MCV (fl)	MCH (pg)
Birth	13.5–19.5	0.44–0.64	–	–
10–12 yrs	11.5–14.5	0.37–0.45	77–91	24–30
Men	13.0–18.0	0.40–0.54	76–96	27–32
Women	11.5–16.5	0.37–0.47	76–96	27–32

Leukocyte and platelet counts: distinguish isolated anaemia from pancytopenia. The white blood counts *increase* in haemolytic anaemia, infections, and leukaemias, and there may be abnormal leukocyte or neutrophil precursors. Platelets may be increased in chronic inflammation and post sickle cell crisis.

Reticulocyte count: *increases* with the severity of the anaemia, as in chronic haemolysis. A dampened reticulocyte level in the face of anaemia suggests: impaired marrow function (hypoplasia, carcinomatous infiltration, lymphoma, myeloma, acute leukaemia, tuberculosis); deficiency of iron, vit B_{12}, or folate; lack of erythropoietin (renal failure); reduced tissue oxygen consumption (myxoedema, protein deficiency); ineffective erythropoiesis (thalassaemia major, megaloblastic anaemia, myelodysplasia, myelofibrosis, congenital dyserythropoietic anaemia); chronic inflammatory or malignant disease.

Iron studies (see Table 14.2): help distinguish between the different types of microcytic anaemia.

Hb colour scale: a new WHO test gives a good approximation of Hb levels in areas without laboratory facilities.

Blood film: viewed under a simple light microscope, anisocytosis and poikilocytosis point towards specific causes of anaemia. The WCC and its differential, platelet number, and morphology, as well as the presence or absence of abnormal cells, can also be obtained from the film.

Bone marrow: examination when the diagnosis is in doubt can be invaluable. *Aspiration* enables assessment of the appearance of developing cells, the presence of abnormal cells, and the proportion of cell lineages. Fragments of marrow are needed on the slide in order to assess cellularity. Romanowsky technique and a stain for iron assesses the iron stores in the reticuloendothelial system (macrophages).

Trephine biopsy: may be indicated if the bone marrow aspirate is a dry tap due to fibrosis or increased cellularity (because of leukaemia) or infiltration (lymphoma, multiple myeloma and carcinoma). A core of bone marrow is taken from the posterior iliac crest with a trephine needle. The bone marrow trephine is fixed in formalin, decalcified, and sectioned, and then viewed under a microscope. It provides a structural view of the marrow. Although less valuable than an aspirate, since individual cell details cannot be seen, it nevertheless gives a reliable indication of cellularity of the presence of abnormal infiltrates in the marrow.

Anaemia in pregnancy

Defined by the WHO as a Hb level <11 g/dl in a pregnant woman. This means that >20% women will become anaemic. A small fall in Hb is a physiological response to the pregnant state. Those most prone to a drastic drop in their Hb are those who start pregnancy anaemic (e.g. those with menorrhagia, hookworm, malaria, haemoglobinopathies, poor diet, frequent pregnancies, and twin pregnancies).

Anaemia in pregnancy is associated with the increased risk of haemorrhage, puerperal infection, and thromboembolic problems. The mother takes longer to recover and there is the increased risk of infection postpartum.

Screening: includes looking for causes of anaemia, especially for haemoglobinopathies, sickle-cell disease, G6PD deficiency, and malaria.

Management includes:

1. *Fortification with oral iron* supplements (~750 mg extra iron is needed during pregnancy, of which 300 mg is required by the baby, mostly after 30 weeks of gestation). 100 mg of Fe and 350 mcg of folic acid are in 1 tablet of Pregaday.

2. *Parenteral iron* may be given to those with iron-deficiency anaemia unable to tolerate oral iron: give 5% iron dextran by slow IV infusion.

   $$\text{Dose (ml)} = [0.0476 \times \text{weight (kg)} \times [14.8 - \text{Hb level (g/dl)}]]$$
   $$+ \ 1 \text{ ml/5 kg body weight to a maximum of } 14$$

   Contraindications: asthma, renal/liver disease.

3. The rise in Hb takes place over 6 weeks, so ***blood transfusions*** may be needed for late, severe anaemia (Hb <9 g/dl). 1 unit should increase Hb by 0.7 g/dl.

4. *Treatment of infections* particularly malaria.

Microcytic anaemia

Four common types: iron-deficiency anaemia, thalassaemia, anaemia of chronic disease, and sideroblastic anaemia.

Iron-deficiency anaemia

The most common cause of anaemia worldwide, particularly in children and pregnant or breastfeeding women in whom it is a major cause of illness and death. It is the most important cause of microcytic, hypochromic anaemia in which MCV, MCH, and MCHC are all reduced.

Specific clinical features are brittle nails, koilonychia, atrophy of the papillae of the tongue, angular stomatitis, brittle hair, and a syndrome of dysphagia and glossitis (Plummer–Vinson syndrome).

Causes include:

- *Poor diets* — low in animal protein, foods high in factors which inhibit iron absorption. Most iron in food is non-haem iron and not readily absorbed.
- *Chronic blood loss* — hookworm, schistosome, and whipworm infection; GI losses (oesophageal varices; hiatus hernia; peptic ulcer; Ca of stomach, caecum, colon, or rectum; colitis; angiodysplasia; diverticulosis); haematuria; pulmonary haemosiderosis; menorrhagia.
- *Increased demands* — prematurity, growth, pregnancy.
- *Malabsorption* — coeliac disease, gastrectomy.

Diagnosis: take good dietary, menstrual, and medication history; do iron studies (see Table 14.2). Blood film shows microcytic (MCV <80 fl) and hypochromic (MCH <27 pg) red cells, poikilocytosis (pencil shapes), anisocytosis, and target cells. There is a low reticulocyte count relative to the degree of anaemia. Erythroid hyperplasia is seen along with ragged normoblasts in the bone marrow. Stool examination may show hookworm ova or other parasitic infestation. GI tract investigation may be warranted in some individuals, rectal examination and FOB is required in all.

Management

1. Find and treat the underlying cause.
2. Give iron *replacement* as ferrous sulfate 200 mg/8h PO, before food. It takes 6 months to replenish iron stores. Parenteral iron, given as dextran or iron sorbitol, may be indicated in severe malabsorption and in UC and Crohn's disease. Monitor the response to iron with Hb — expect a rise of 1 g/dl each week — and reticulocyte count. Reduce to once a day and, if necessary, after food in cases of intolerance.
3. Correct associated deficiencies.
4. In severe anaemia, blood transfusions may be necessary to prevent sudden death. It is very important not to overload the circulation and precipitate or worsen cardiac failure. The use of exchange transfusion, fast-acting diuretics, and intra-peritoneal transfusion may avoid overload.

Prevention:

- Prophylactic iron to high-risk groups: pregnant women, infants, and pre-school children
- Antihelminthics to children
- Fortify one or more staple foods

Table 14.2 Diagnostic tests in hypochromic anaemia

	Fe deficiency	Chronic disease	Thalassaemia trait	Sideroblastic anaemia
MCV	Reduced	Normal or reduced	Low	Acquired = high Congenital = low
MCH	Reduced	Normal	Low	As MCV
MCHC	Reduced	Normal	Low	As MCV
Serum Fe	Reduced	Reduced	Normal	Raised
TIBC	Raised	Reduced	Normal	Normal
Serum ferritin	Reduced	Normal/ increased	Normal	Raised
Bone marrow iron stores	Absent	Present or may be increased	Present	Increased
Erythroblast iron	Absent	Absent	Present and may be heavy	Ring sideroblasts present
Hb electro-phoresis	Normal	Normal	HbA2 raised in β+ form	Normal

Anaemia of chronic disease

Anaemia associated with chronic inflammatory or malignant disease.

Causes

1. *Chronic inflammatory disease*
   - **Infectious** TB, lung abscess, osteomyelitis, pneumonia, SBE.
   - **Non-infectious** RA, SLE, other connective tissue disorders, sarcoidosis, Crohn's disease.

2. *Malignancy*
Carcinoma, lymphoma, sarcoma.

Clinical features: of general anaemia plus specific features of non-progressive mild microcytic or normocytic and normochromic anaemia. Reduced serum iron and TIBC. Normal or raised serum ferritin levels.

Management: is to treat the underlying cause. There is no response to iron supplements. In many cases, it is complicated by the presence of another form of anaemia (such as iron, vitamin B$_{12}$ or folate deficiency), renal failure, bone marrow failure, hypersplenism, or endocrine abnormality.

Sideroblastic anaemia

A refractory anaemia with hypochromic cells in the blood and increased marrow iron. Defined by the presence of pathological ring sideroblasts in the bone marrow. Divided into hereditary and acquired anaemia.

- **Hereditary form** occurs in males; females are carriers and are rarely symptomatic.
- **Acquired forms** are either 1° (myelodysplasia FAB type 2 WHO RARS) or 2° (myeloproliferative disorders, drugs such as TB chemotherapy especially isoniazid, alcohol, lead, conditions such as haemolytic anaemia, megaloblastic anaemia, and malabsorption).

Management: in 2° disease, treat the underlying cause. The hereditary diseases often respond well to high-dose pyridoxine therapy. Give folic acid replacement, especially if megaloblastic anaemia supervenes. In severe cases, repeated blood transfusion is often the only option, bringing with it the dangers of transfusion such as iron overload and viral infections.

Normocytic anaemia

Normocytic, normochromic anaemia is seen in anaemia of chronic disease, in some endocrine disorders (hypopituitarism, hypothyroidism, and hypoadrenalism), and in some haematological disorders (aplastic anaemia and some haemolytic anaemias). It is also seen following acute blood loss before iron stores are reduced. If there is a reduced white cell or platelet count, consider bone marrow failure and perform a bone marrow biopsy.

Management: treat the underlying cause. If the blood loss is severe and shock a possibility, consider blood transfusion to replace and maintain the blood volume.

Hookworm

The soil-transmitted helminths *Ancylostoma duodenale* and *Necator americanus* probably infect more than 900 million people in the tropics and subtropics, flourishing in areas of poverty and malnutrition. They are the most common cause of anaemia worldwide.

Transmission: filariform larvae penetrate the skin (usually the feet) and migrate to the small intestinal lumen, maturing to adult worms as they do so. There they attach to the mucosal surface, resulting in chronic, low-grade blood loss. The adult female sheds eggs into the faeces.

Infection can result in a daily loss of 1 mg of iron per 10,000 ova per gm of faeces, irrespective of the species. Subacute hookworm anaemia has an element of haemorrhage in its aetiology; acute hookworm anaemia is rare and follows extremely heavy infections. Heavy infections may also lead to hypoproteinaemia and malabsorption.

Whipworm

Trichuris trichiura is one of the most prevalent helminths in the world. Heavy infestations (>800 worms, which = 16,000 ova per gm of faeces) can result in the loss of 4 ml blood or 1.5 mg iron per day. (See Chapter 2D for more information.)

Diagnosis and treatment: see p. 128 for details. Treatment consists of treatment of the anaemia and elimination of the parasites. Albendazole is the drug of choice; mebendazole and levamisole are alternatives.

Prevention: in most areas where hookworm and whipworm are prevalent, reinfection is almost certain. In many instances treatment follows one of two routes: routine drug treatment of a whole target population at set intervals (e.g. yearly) — especially of children; or drug treatment given only to those who are symptomatic. In either case, education about safe disposal of faeces and the wearing of footwear is vital if the cycle is to be broken.

Macrocytic anaemia

Occurs in two forms — megaloblastic and non-megaloblastic — which are distinguished by the bone marrow findings at biopsy.

Megaloblastic anaemia

Characterized by the presence of megaloblasts (large erythroid cells with delayed nuclear maturation) in the bone marrow. There may also be a white cell abnormality (giant metamyelocytes). The blood film characteristically shows oval macrocytes and hypersegmented neutrophils. These changes occur in:

- Vit B_{12} and folic acid deficiency
- Abnormalities of red blood cell metabolism, transport, and synthesis
- Congenital enzyme deficiencies (orotic aciduria)
- Acquired enzyme defects (some antimalarials, chemotherapy)

The aetiology is often multiple.

Clinical features: are general symptoms of anaemia and mild jaundice, glossitis, angular stomatitis, weight loss, purpura due to thrombocytopaenia, megaloblastosis of epithelial cell surfaces, neuropathy (subacute combined degeneration of the cord only with lack of vit. B_{12}), sterility, reversible melanin skin pigmentation, decreased osteoblastic activity, and increased susceptibility to infections. Many remain asymptomatic.

Investigations: show a raised MCV (>95 fl) and MCH, normal MCHC, oval macrocytes, low reticulocyte count, moderately reduced WCC and platelets in severe cases, and hypersegmented nuclei in neutrophils. Bone marrow is hypercellular with erythroblasts. Giant metamyelocytes are present. Serum unconjugated bilirubin, hydroxybutyrate, and LDH are raised. Serum iron and ferritin are normal or raised.

Management: is with replacement, fortification, and dietary modification. Consider prophylactic treatment in patients after partial gastrectomy or ileal resection, pregnancy, severe haemolytic anaemia, on dialysis, and in the premature. Folic acid 5 mg PO od for 4 months; maintenance depends on underlying disease. Vit. B_{12} replacement is with hydroxycobalamin 1 mg IM 3× per week, for 2 weeks (6 injections), and maintenance with 1 mg every 3 months.

Non-megaloblastic macrocytic anaemia

Causes: include alcoholism (with or without associated liver disease), reticulocytosis (after recent bleed or in chronic haemolysis), hypothyroidism, myelodysplastic syndromes, sideroblastic and aplastic anaemia.

Investigations: reveal normoblastic, macrocytic anaemia, with round RBCs without hypersegmented neutrophils. Check ESR (malignancy), LFT (including γGT), T4. Exclude vit. B12 and folate deficiency — their levels should be normal. Bone marrow examination for myelodysplasia, aplasia, and myeloma.

Management: diagnose and treat the underlying disease.

Table 14.3 Causes of folate and vitamin B_{12} deficiencies

	Folate	Vitamin B_{12}
Inadequate intake	Seasonal shortage Boiling bottle feeds Prolonged storage of food Anorexia Famine Inappropriate weaning foods Prolonged cooking/reheating Feeding infants with goats milk Alcoholism	Breastfeeding by B_{12}- deficient mothers Veganism Alcoholism
Malabsorption	Diarrhoea in infancy Acute enteric infections *Giardia lamblia* Systemic infections (TB, pneumococcus) Strongyloides Coeliac disease Crohn's disease	Pernicious anaemia Gastrectomy Chronic *G. lamblia* HIV infection Ileocaecal TB Strongyloides Tropical sprue Crohn's disease
Increased physiological demands	Growth Pregnancy/lactation	
Increased pathological demands	Haemolysis Malignant disease	
Metabolic problems	Pyrexia	Nitrous oxide Chronic cyanide Intoxication (cassava)

Haemolytic anaemias

Anaemia due to a reduced red cell life span (normally 120 days) and therefore increased red cell turnover. The bone marrow is able to compensate up to 5 times the normal turnover rate given adequate hematinics and a healthy marrow (compensated haemolysis); if haemolysis exceeds this or there are deficiencies or associated disease, anaemia results.

Causes: the haemolysis is due to genetic or acquired causes. The aetiology is important since it influences therapy.

Genetic
- Membrane defects   Hereditary spherocytosis, elliptocytosis, S.E. Asian ovalocytosis
- Haemoglobin defects   Thalassaemias, sickle-cell disease, other haemoglobinopathies
- Enzyme defects   G6PD and pyruvate kinase deficiency

Acquired
- Immune   — isoimmune   — Haemolytic disease of the newborn, blood transfusion
-             — autoimmune   — Warm or cold antibody mediated, drug-induced
- Non-immune   — infections   — Malaria, septicaemia, parvovirus, hypersplenism
-             — membrane   — Paroxysmal nocturnal haemoglobinuria, liver disease
-             — physical damage   — Cardiac haemolysis (especially metal valves), microangiopathic anaemia, burns, venoms

Distinguishing between the different causes involves identifying clinical and laboratory features of increased Hb breakdown and compensatory increase in RBC production. The approach should therefore attempt to identify features of:
- *Increased red cell destruction:* jaundice, unconjugated hyperbilirubinaemia, increased urinary urobilinogen, increased faecal urobilinogen
- *Increased red cell production:* polychromasia, reticulocytosis, bone marrow erythroid hyperplasia
- *Intravascular haemolysis:* reduced/absent haptoglobins, reduced haemopexin, haem/methaemoglobin, positive Schumm's test (methaemalbumin), haemosiderinuria, haem/methaemoglobinuria

Clinical features: are of general anaemia with jaundice; hepatosplenomegaly; leg ulcers due to sickle-cell disease. In the history, check for family history, ethnic origin, drugs, previous anaemia, jaundice, dark urine.

Investigations: FBC, reticulocytes, bilirubin, LDH, screen for G6PD deficiency, haptoglobin, urinary urobilinogen. Blood films to look for malaria parasite, polychromasia, macrocytosis, spherocytes, elliptocytes, fragmented cells, and sickle-cells. Direct antiglobulin test (DAT) and urinary haemosiderin (stains Prussian Blue).

Genetic causes

Hereditary spherocytosis: AD inheritance. Blood films: spherocytes and RBCs show increased osmotic fragility. **Clinical features:** mild anaemia (8–12 g/dl) and splenomegaly and gall stones. **Diagnosis:** blood film and osmotic fragility tests. **Treatment:** splenectomy (delay if in early childhood) and give pneumococcal and haemophilus vaccines.

Hereditary elliptocytosis: AD inheritance. Usually asymptomatic +/− mild haemolysis in homozygotes. There may be episodes of jaundice and moderate splenomegaly following intercurrent infections (malaria may cause severe anaemia). Some elliptocyte variants are said to be resistant to invasion by *P. falciparum*. There is no evidence to confirm this. If **treatment** is required then splenectomy may help.

South-east Asian hereditary ovalocytosis: AD inheritance. Common in Malaysia, Indonesia, Philippines, PNG, and Solomon Islands. It is not associated with haemolytic anaemia. There appears to be a resistance to malarial parasites, probably due to reduced penetration of merozites.

Pyruvate kinase deficiency: AR inheritance. May present with neonatal jaundice. Later haemolytic anaemia with splenomegaly and jaundice may occur. **Diagnosis:** is by enzyme assay. **Treatment:** is non-specific; splenectomy may improve severe cases.

Acquired causes

Drug-induced immune haemolytic anaemia: occurs when antibodies to drugs bind to RBC membrane bound drug (e.g. high-dose penicillin), form immune complexes, or cause the development of autoantibodies (methyldopa, mefenamic acid, L-dopa).

Autoimmune haemolytic anaemia (AHA): can be caused by cold or warm antibodies. They may be 1° (idiopathic) or 2° (lymphoma or generalized autoimmune diseases like SLE).
- Warm AHA presents as chronic or acute anaemia. Remove underlying cause and treat with steroids (prednisolone 1mg/kg od, then gradually reduce) +/− splenectomy.
- Cold AHA presents as chronic anaemia made worse by a drop in temperature, Raynaud's phenomenon, or acrocyanosis. Treatment is to keep warm. Chlorambucil may help; splenectomy does not usually help especially if there is an underlying lymphoma.
- Paroxysmal cold haemoglobinuria is caused by Donnath–Landstiener antibody (mumps, measles, chickenpox, syphilis) sticking to RBCs in the cold, causing a complement-mediated lysis on rewarming.

Glucose-6-phosphate dehydrogenase (G6PD) deficiency

G6PD deficiency has a sex-linked inheritance. It affects over 2 million people in west Africa, Mediterranean, Middle East, and S.E. Asia. Where *P. falciparum* is or was endemic, G6PD deficiency confers a genetic advantage to female carriers.

Distribution: see Fig. 14.1 which shows the world distribution of G6PD deficiency. Superimposed are three zones where different G6PD variants reach polymorphic frequencies: zone I (Gd^{Mediterranean}), zone II (Gd^{Mediterranean}, Gd^{Canton}, Gd^{Union}, Gd^{Mahidol}), and zone III (GdA$^-$).

Clinical features

- Haemolytic anaemia in response to oxidative stress produced by drugs such as primaquine or sulfonamides and food such as fava beans.
- Haemolysis in response to infection (viral or bacterial).

Symptoms arise due to rapidly developing intravascular haemolysis with haemoglobinuria. Many patients remain asymptomatic. Possible precipitants are listed below.

Precipitants of haemolytic anaemia in G6PD deficiency

- Antimalarials   Primaquine, chloroquine, Fansidar, Maloprim
- Sulfonamides/   Co-trimoxazole, sulfanilamide, dapsone,
  sulfones   sulfasalazine
- Antibiotics   Nitrofuantion, chloramphenicol, quinolones
- Analgesics   Aspirin (in high doses), phenacetin
- Antihelminths   betanaphthol, stibophen, nicidazole
- Miscellaneous   Vitamin K analogues, naphthalene, probenecid,
                                 fava beans (possibly other vegetables),
                                 food additives

Diagnosis: is by detecting the enzyme deficiency through one of many screening tests. These tests rely on NADPH production in the presence of adequate amounts of G6PD and its detection by direct fluorescence or by reduction of a coloured dye (e.g. methylene blue) to its colourless form. These are sensitive, simple, and inexpensive for detecting hemizygous males and heterozygous females outside of a crisis.

Following a crisis, especially in the African A$^-$ type of deficiency, blood should be centrifuged and the older cells at the bottom of the column tested, or the dye tests should be delayed for 6 weeks. During a crisis, the blood film may show contracted and fragmented cells, called 'bite' cells and 'blister' cells, which have had Heinz bodies removed by the spleen. There are also features of intravascular haemolysis. In presence of hyposplenism, Heinz bodies may be seen in special preparations.

Management: withdraw any drug that could have precipitated the crisis and maintain a high urine output (in an attempt to prevent pre-renal failure). Give a blood transfusion if one is warranted. G6PD-deficient babies are prone to neonatal jaundice and in severe cases phototherapy and exchange transfusion are necessary. The jaundice is usually due to the deficiency affecting neonatal liver function.

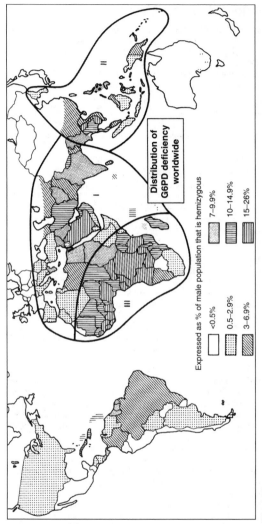

Distribution of G6PD deficiency worldwide

Expressed as % of male population that is hemizygous

- <0.5%
- 0.5–2.9%
- 3–6.9%
- 7–9.9%
- 10–14.9%
- 15–26%

Fig. 14.1

Sickle-cell anaemia

A severe haemolytic anaemia caused by inheritance of a point-mutated gene. The mutation results in a Glu-Val amino acid substitution in position 6 of the β-globin chain of haemoglobin molecule and the formation of HbS. When deoxygenated, the HbS molecules polymerize into long fibres and cause the RBCs to sickle. Sickled RBCs are rigid and block the microcirculation in various organs, causing infarcts. They also haemolyse easily.

Classification: sickle-cell *disease* arises from the homozygous form, HbSS, while the sickle-cell *trait* is due to heterozygous inheritance, HbAS. The trait is rarely symptomatic, unless crises are precipitated by severe anoxia or infection. The sickle gene is most common in Africa and the Indian subcontinent with a high rate of homozygous individuals, and less common in the Mediterranean and in the mixed populations of the Americas.

Clinical features: severe haemolytic anaemia punctuated by crises (see below). Typically, there is anaemia (Hb 6–8 g/dl; reticulocytes 10–20%) and jaundice early in life; often with painful swelling of hands and feet (dactylitis or the hand–foot syndrome leading to digits of varying length). Young sicklers alternate periods of good health with periods of acute crises. Later, chronic ill health supervenes because of damage to various organs from previous crises.

Complications: include renal failure (papillary necrosis of kidneys due to medullary infarction); failure to concentrate urine leads to dehydration and crisis; nocturnal enuresis is common; glomerulosclerosis is a rare, severe complication; bone necrosis; infections (salmonella osteomyelitis); leg ulcers; splenomegaly in infancy and early childhood which subsequently becomes reduced in size due to infarction (autosplenectomy); proliferative retinopathy; priapism. Micro-infarcts can result in chronic liver damage; bilirubin gallstones are common findings. Survival is strongly linked to socio-economic conditions.

Crises

- *Painful vascular-occlusive crises:* are frequent and precipitated by infections, acidosis, dehydration, or deoxygenation (altitude, operations, obstetric delivery, stasis of the circulation, exposure to cold, violent exercise). Infarcts may occur in bones (hips, shoulders, and vertebrae), the lungs, and spleen. The most serious crises can involve the CNS (in 7% of patients) and spinal cord.
- *Visceral sequestration crises:* are due to sickling within organs and pooling of blood, often with severe exacerbation of anaemia. A severe chest syndrome with pulmonary infiltrates is a common cause of death. Hepatic and girdle sequestration crises and splenic sequestration may lead to severe illness requiring exchange transfusions.
- *Aplastic crises:* may occur due to infection with parvovirus and/or folate deficiency, and are characterized by a sudden fall in Hb and reticulocytes, usually needing transfusion.
- *Haemolytic crises:* are characterized by an increased rate of haemolysis with a fall in Hb but a rise in reticulocytes. They usually accompany a painful crisis.

Sickle-cell disease and pregnancy

- Sickle-cell disease predisposes to abortion, pre-term labour, stillbirth, and sickle-cell crises. To prevent severe anaemia, treat with folate supplements. Exchange transfusions with top-up transfusions to maintain levels of HbS below 30% may be carried out in the more severe cases with repeated crises or life-threatening complications in pregnancy.
- Sickle-cell trait is not a problem, except that pyelonephritis is more common. are characterized by an increased rate of haemolysis with a fall in Hb but a rise in reticulocytes. They usually accompany a painful crisis.

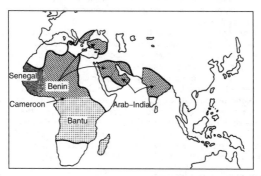

Fig. 14.2 Distribution of haemoglobin S gene and its haplotype to the Mediterranean and West Asia

Laboratory findings
- Hb 6–8 g/dl
- Sickle cells and target cells in the blood film; features of splenic atrophy (Howell–Jolly bodies) may also be seen
- Screening tests for sickling in deoxygenated blood (e.g. with dithionate and Na_2HPO_4)
- Hb electrophoresis

Management: see box, plus
- *Prophylaxis:* avoid precipitating factors, especially dehydration, hypoxia, infections, circulation stasis, and cooling of the skin surface.
- *Give folic acid and improve general nutrition and hygiene.*
- *Protect against infection:* vaccinate against pneumococcus and give regular oral penicillin.
- *Hydroxycarbamide:* useful for those who present with frequent crises.
- *Crises:* bed rest, rehydrate with oral fluids and/or IV infusions of normal saline. Give antibiotics if there is infection and bicarbonate if acidotic. Strong analgesics including opiates may be required. Transfuse blood only if there is severe, symptomatic anaemia. Exchange transfusion may be needed for either CNS involvement or a visceral sequestration crisis.
- *Pregnancy and anaesthesia:* particular care is needed. Routine transfusions may be considered throughout pregnancy to those with bad obstetric history or a history of frequent crises. Before delivery or major surgery, patients may require an exchange transfusion or be transfused repeatedly with normal blood to reduce the proportion of circulating HbS to less than 30%.

Other sickling syndromes

HbSC disease: occurs in west Africa. The pathophysiology is the same as that for HbSS but the severity is greatly reduced, with most patients being asymptomatic. HbSC is the most common form of sickle-cell disease to present with complications during pregnancy in west Africa. The Hb value is intermediate between that of HbSS and normal, the MCV is lower than in HbSS, while the reticulocytes are moderately raised. Electrophoresis shows two major fractions in the position of HbS and HbC.

HbSβ⁰ thalassaemia: occurs mostly in N. Africa, Sicily, and in mixed populations of the Americas. Clinically similar to HbSS; it can be very difficult to distinguish. The MCV is usually low The definitive diagnosis is made when one parent carries the $β^S$ gene and the other has β thalassaemia trait.

HbSβ⁺ thalassaemia: is the doubly heterozygous condition most commonly seen in Liberia and other parts of west Africa. Anaemia is mild and irreversibly sickled cells are rare. Definitive diagnosis with Hb electrophoresis shows HbA 5–30%; the balance is HbS.

HbSD^Punjab: HbD interacts with HbS leading to a disease similar to HbSS. It is seen amongst Sikh and mixed populations. There is moderately severe anaemia; the peripheral blood film resembles HbSS.

Sickle-cell trait: is the inheritance of HbAS and results in a benign condition. Complications occasionally arise due to microinfarcts in the renal medulla and spleen. There is strong evidence, more than with any other inherited abnormality of RBCs, that the trait confers partial protection against serious effects of *P. falciparum* malaria.

Maintenance of health in sickle-cell disease

Early diagnosis
- Good laboratory techniques — HbS solubility, Hb electrophoresis
- Screening — Pregnant women, newborn of mothers with S gene, anaemic children and siblings of patients
- Increased clinical awareness

Education
- Parents, patients, general public, and health professionals

Sickle-cell clinics
- Prevent Infection — Prophylactic antimalarials and penicillin immunization against pneumococcus, meningococcus *H. influenzae* B, and hepatitis B, where possible
- Nutrition — Folic acid supplements, general nutritional advice
- Advice — Avoid cold, fatigue, dehydration, alcohol; attend clinic regularly; report when ill and pregnant

Hydroxycarbamide
- Consider hydroxyurea in patients with repeated crises and severe crises after recovery.

Hospital
- Prompt treatment of crises — Rehydration, Analgesia, Antibiotics

Obstetrics
- Careful supervision of pregnancy, delivery, puerperium
- Encourage the woman to have less than 3 pregnancies

Thalassaemia

The thalassaemias are a heterogeneous group of genetic disorders which result from a reduced rate of synthesis of α or β chains of Hb (^{0} indicates total suppression, $^+$ partial suppression). Each individual has two genes for β-globin and four for α-globin. Changes in the normal ratio between these chains leads to globin precipitation; anaemia results from ineffective erythropoiesis and haemolysis. It is possible to correlate clinical severity with genetic deficit.

Distribution: is in a band stretching across the Mediterranean, Africa, and Asia, and in immigrant populations from these areas.

Thalassaemia minor

Is of heterozygous inheritance and the carrier is often asymptomatic. Few have palpable splenomegaly.

Diagnosis: Hb is 9–11 g/dl; the blood film shows moderate anisocytosis, microcytosis, and hypochromia with a few target cells, a few tear drop cells, and cells with punctate basophilia. Marrow biopsy shows mild–moderate erythroid hyperplasia. Electrophoresis shows that the HbA2 is raised to 4–6.5%; the HbF is also raised to about 3% in approximately half of patients.

Management: includes early diagnosis so as to avoid unnecessary treatment of the hypochromic anaemia with iron, offer reassurance that the condition is benign, and allow for genetic counselling.

Thalassaemia intermedia

Thalassaemia intermedia is less severe than major. HbE/β thalassaemia is the most common form: >40,000 born each year in S.E. Asia are affected. It may also result from the inheritance of homozygous β$^+$ thalassaemia in West Africa, various δβ thalassaemias, and Hb Lepore (crossover between δ and β genes) disorders.

Clinical features: there is a wide range of severity, ranging from mild haemolytic anaemia in HbC/β thalassaemia to severe β thalassaemia major-like disease in HbE/β thalassaemia. Morbidity and mortality are high in the latter condition, especially during childhood, with splenomegaly, recurrent infections, gallstones, skeletal deformities, and chronic leg ulcers.

Diagnosis: hypochromic, microcytic anaemia with target cells. Anaemia is worse in patients with hypersplenism, folate deficiency, intercurrent infection, and in pregnancy.

Management: involves continuous surveillance, folate therapy, active immunization, and antimalarial prophylaxis to prevent infections, and prompt treatment of any that do occur. Give blood only at times of severe anaemia or when there is a high risk of growth retardation and skeletal abnormality — a high transfusion regime with iron chelation is then indicated. Hypersplenism may increase transfusion requirements; splenectomy should be considered in this situation.

Clinical classification of thalassaemias

Hydrops fetalis	Fatal 4-gene deletion α^0 thalassaemia
Thalassaemia Major (see p. 570)	Transfusion-dependent, homozygous β^0 thalassaemia (β^0/β^0) or co-inheritance of thalassaemia traits (e.g. β^0/β^+) in some cases
Thalassaemia intermedia	Most double heterozygous (β^0/β^+) β thalassaemias
	W. African β^+/β^+ thalassaemias
	Co-inheritance of β thalassaemia with a β-chain variant (e.g. HbE/β^+)
	β thalassaemia with hereditary persistence of fetal Hb
	HbH disease
Thalassaemia Minor	β^0 thalassaemia trait
	β^+ thalassaemia trait
	Hereditary persistence of fetal Hb
	α^0 thalassaemia trait
	α^+ thalassaemia trait

α **thalassaemia:** has 4 varieties defined according to the number of defective α-globin genes on chromosome 16. Absence of 1 or 2 genes is very common in Africans and produces a mild anaemia with a low MCV. Epidemiological studies from Melanesia and Papua New Guinea suggest that α^+ thalassaemia has been selected for by malaria.

HbH disease — the child has β^4 Hb (HbH) due to a lack of α chains. HbH is present in 5–30% throughout life with moderate haemolytic anaemia (Hb 7–10 g/dl). Children may have growth retardation and skeletal abnormalities; there is a variable degree of splenomegaly.

Hb Bart's hydrops fetalis — a fatal condition in which the fetus lacks all α genes. The infant is stillborn or dies shortly after delivery.

β thalassaemia major

β thalassaemia major is an autosomal recessive disease of children of two heterozygotes or carriers of β thalassaemia trait. Either no β chains (β⁰) or reduced amounts (β⁺) are produced. Excess α chains are precipitated in RBCs and in erythroblasts resulting in ineffective erythropoiesis and haemolysis. The greater the α-chain excess, the more severe the anaemia. Over 100 different genetic defects have now been discovered. β thalassaemia major is often due to inheritance of two different mutations, each affecting β-globin synthesis (compound heterozygotes).

Clinical features

- *Failure to thrive:* at 3–6 months of age when the switch from γ to β-chain production should take place.
- *Hepatosplenomegaly:* due to excess haemolysis, extramedullary haemopoiesis, and, later in the disease, iron overload from transfusions. Splenomegaly increases blood requirements by increasing red cell destruction and pooling and by causing plasma volume expansion.
- *Bone expansion:* as a result of intense marrow hyperplasia leads to the characteristic thalassaemic faces: prominent frontal and parietal bones, maxillary enlargement, and flattening of the nasal bridge. There is cortical thinning of many bones (↑ tendency to fracture) and bossing of the skull with 'hair-on-end' appearance on X-ray.
- *Infections:* are common for a variety of reasons. Anaemic children are prone to bacterial infections. If splenectomy has been carried out without prophylactic penicillin afterwards, pneumococcal and meningococcal infections are likely. Severe gastroenteritis can be caused by *Yersinia enterocolitica* associated with desferrioxamine treatment of iron overload. Transmission of viral hepatitis is also increased.

Diagnosis: severe hypochromic microcytic anaemia with raised reticulocyte count, normoblasts, target cells, and basophilic stippling in the blood film. Electrophoresis shows absent HbA, raised HbF, and variable HbA2.

Management

- *Transfusion:* aim to keep Hb within 9–14 g/dl range, suppressing the patient's own abnormal erythropoiesis. This requires 2–3 units every 4–6 weeks. Fresh blood filtered to remove WBCs gives the best red cell survival with the fewest transfusion reactions.
- *Folic acid:* give regularly if there is suspicion of dietary insufficiency.
- *Chelate excess iron:* with desferrioxamine 1–2 g with each unit of blood that is transfused. Give by syringe pump driver, 20–60 mg/kg over 8–12 hrs, 4–7 days per week. Commence in infants after 10–15 units of transfusion. Excess desferrioxamine in high doses, especially in children, may lead to high tone deafness, retinal damage with night blindness and loss of visual acuity, and growth retardation.
- *Give vitamin C:* 200 mg od to increase iron excretion.
- *Splenectomy:* may be needed to reduce the amount of blood required. Delay until after 6 yrs because there is increased risk of life-threatening infections post-splenectomy before this age. Immunize, particularly against pneumococcus, prior to splenectomy.
- *Immunize:* against hepatitis B.
- *Beware endocrine disorders.*

Iron overload due to repeated transfusions: each 500 ml unit of blood contains 250 mg of iron. Iron accumulation leads to liver damage, endocrine damage (failure of growth, delayed or absent puberty, DM, hypothyroidism, hypoparathyroidism), and myocardial damage. In the absence of intensive iron chelation, death occurs in the second or third decade, usually from CCF or cardiac arrhythmias. Clinically apparent abnormalities usually appear after ~50 units (12 g of iron). However, organ damage and skin pigmentation occur before this.

Thalassaemia and pregnancy

In thalassaemia major, the duration of cell survival is reduced. Do not treat with iron as this will increase the already high levels of iron. Transfusions are the mainstay of management. Thalassaemia minor causes a moderate but persistent anaemia during pregnancy. This causes fetal hypoxia, compensatory placental hypertrophy, mild intrauterine growth retardation, an increased frequency of fetal distress during delivery, and a high frequency of low Apgar scores (3 or less at 1 minute), but no significant increase in perinatal mortality. HbF has α chains and the fetus may be anaemic or in severe cases stillborn if there is absence of α chain production. β thalassaemia does not affect the fetus.

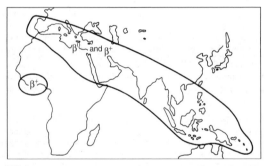

Fig. 14.3

Disorders of white blood cells

Leukopenia can result from failure of production, inhibition of release from the bone marrow, increased margination in the circulation, and pooling in an enlarged spleen. It is often due to a combination of these factors.

Lymphomas

Burkitt's lymphoma (BL)

A lymphoblastic lymphoma, which is the most common childhood cancer in tropical Africa. There is a peak incidence at 5–9 years, with a male predominance. There are three epidemiological patterns:

1. It is endemic in tropical Africa and PNG, in areas with high malaria endemicity, with a peak at 4–9 years.
2. It has intermediate incidence in north Africa, western Asia, and South America.
3. It occurs sporadically in the West.

Endemicity can be correlated with frequent childhood exposure to and infection with Epstein–Barr virus before the age of 1 year, with hyperendemic malaria, and with a chromosomal translocation t(8;14)(q24:q32). BL also occurs as a complication of HIV infection.

Clinical features: often presents with tumours of the jaw, but may involve other bones and also solid organs and GI involvement. Histology shows a 'starry sky' appearance (isolated histiocytes on a background of abnormal lymphocytes). Aspirates of tumour show large blasts with deeply basophilic cytoplasm and numerous vacuoles.

Management: a single dose of a cytotoxic drug (e.g. cyclophosphamide 30 mg/kg IV) produces a spectacular, but often short-term remission in some patients.

Non-Hodgkin's (non-Burkitt's) lymphoma (NHL)

Heterogeneous group of tumours of B and T cell origin. Low-grade lymphomas run an indolent course but are incurable, while the high-grade ones are more aggressive in nature but long-term cure is achievable. High-grade NHLs are more common in Asia and Africa and, in Africa, have a strong association with malarial endemicity.

Clinical features: NHL is rare before 40 years. Lymphadenopathy is common but extra nodal spread occurs early, so first presentation may be in the skin, gut, CNS, or lungs. Although often symptomless, systemic symptoms are as for HL. Marrow involvement may cause pancytopenia; infection is common.

Diagnosis: as for HL. Staging is less important in the low-grade NHL since 70% have spread at presentation, but may be more important in high-grade tumours. Consider LN biopsy, CXR, (CT), Ba meal.

Management: symptomless low-grade tumours may not need therapy and occasionally show remission. Chlorambucil or cyclophosphamide may control any symptoms which do occur. Splenectomy may help if splenomegaly is a major feature. Surgery may be used for local bulky disease. Optimum treatment for high-grade tumours is 6 weeks of doxorubicin, cyclophosphamide, vincristine, bleomycin, and prednisolone. If it is a lymphoblastic tumour, then treat as for ALL — see box.

Changes in the differential WCC

Neutrophilia >7.5 × 10⁹/l

Acute bacterial infections (eg *Staphylococcus* spp)
Some cases of severe malaria
Tissue damage, haemorrhage, haemolysis
Malignancies, stress states, DKA
Drugs, chemicals, steroids, renal failure, pregnancy

Basophilia >0.1 × 10⁹/l

Hypersensitivity, myxoedema, iron deficiency
Chronic haemolysis

Lymphocytosis >3.5 × 10⁹/l

Childhood infections, viral infections
Protozoan infections (malaria, toxoplasmosis)

Monocytosis >3.5 × 10⁹/l

Protozoan (malaria) and rickettsia infections
Chronic bacterial infection: TB, Brucella, SBE

Eosinophilia >0.44 × 10⁹/l

Parasitic infections (intra- or extra-GI tract)
Asthma, atopy, drugs, lymphoma
Connective tissue disease, malignancies
Convalescence from viral or other infections

(Values >30% are likely to be due to Katayama fever, infection with
Strongyloides or *Schistosoma mansoni/japonicum*, or lymphoma).

Neutropenia <2.0 × 10⁹/l

- Acute malaria
- Typhoid
- Hypersplenism
- Megaloblastosis

- Cytotoxic therapy

- Aplastic anaemia

- Felty's syndrome

- AIDS
- Brucellosis
- Viral infection in early stages
- Overwhelming bacterial infection
- Idiosyncratic reactions to drugs
- Bone marrow infiltration (e.g. leukaemia)
- Exposure to chemicals (e.g. benzene)

- Miscellaneous (ethnic, familial, cyclic, chronic, idiopathic)

Lymphopenia <1.5 × 10⁹/l

- Viral infections
- Corticosteroids
- Acute leukaemias

- AIDS
- Lymphoma

Hodgkin's Lymphoma (HL)

A malignant proliferation of the lymphoid cells that is characterized histologically by Reed–Sternberg cells. HL is not common, with an annual incidence of ~3/100,000 in the West. In the developing world, there are high incidences during childhood in central and south America, north Africa, W. Asia, and sub-Saharan Africa. There is a predominance of MC and LD forms — see box. EBV exposure and infection has been linked to its aetiology, especially in the under 15 and over 50 age ranges.

Clinical features: presentation is with enlarged, painless lymph nodes, usually in the neck or axillae. 25% have general symptoms of malaise, fever, weight loss, night sweats, pruritus, and lethargy. Signs include lymphadenopathy, weight loss, anaemia, hepatosplenomegaly.

Diagnosis: FBC, blood film, ESR, LFTs, uric acid, Ca^{2+}, LN biopsy for definitive diagnosis, CXR, bone marrow biopsy. Staging laparotomy involves splenectomy with liver and LN biopsy, superseded by CT scanning where available.

Management: for stages Ia and IIa is radiotherapy, and for stage IIa–IVb chemotherapy: 'MOPP' (Mustine, (chlormethine), Oncovin (vincristine), Procarbazine, Prednisolone). SEs: radiation lung fibrosis, hypothyroidism, nausea, alopecia, infertility (men), infection and second malignancies (AML and NHL), and myelosuppression.

Adult T-cell leukaemia/lymphoma (ATL)

The type C retrovirus, human T-cell lymphotropic virus type 1 (HTLV-1), is associated with both ATL and, in a few infected individuals, tropical spastic paresis/HTLV-1 associated myelopathy (TSP/HAM). The virus is endemic in much of the tropics, and becoming more widespread amongst IV drug abusers and homosexuals in N. and S. America and western Europe. HTLV-2 is a similar virus which is endemic amongst aboriginal groups in central America. It is now spreading in the USA and Europe via blood transfusions and IV drug abuse.

Transmission: is by sexual intercourse, breastfeeding, and exchange of blood. Male-to-female transmission is more effective than female-to-male, and enhanced by other STIs. Seroprevalence rises slowly with age, compatible with the slow rate of transmission in endemic areas.

Clinical features: five phases are recognized:
1. Asymptomatic
2. Acute ATL (two-thirds have lymphadenopathy, hepatosplenomegaly, and skin lesions: papules, nodules, plaques, tumours, ulcers)
3. Chronic ATL (with skin lesions, mild lymphocytosis, protracted course)
4. Smouldering ATL (skin rashes and low count of ATL cells; remains stable for many years)
5. Lymphoma type (clinically like NHL, poor prognosis)

Diagnosis: include LN biopsy, FBC, WCC ($30–130 \times 10^9$/l), bone marrow biopsy, CXR (pulmonary infiltration and osteolytic lesions).

Management: is supportive; most patients die within 12 months.

Classification of Hodgkin's lymphoma

Classification (in order of incidence)	**Prognosis**
Nodular sclerosing (NS)	Good
Mixed cellularity (MC)	Good
Lymphocyte predominant (LP)	Good
Lymphocyte depleted (LD)	Poor

Staging

I	Single LN area
II	>2 areas on same side of the diaphragm
III	LN on both sides of the diaphragm
IV	Spread beyond LNs
A	no systemic symptoms
B	presence of weight loss >10% in last 6 months, unexplained fever >38°C, night sweats

5-year survival overall 80%; depends on stage and grade.

Leukaemias

The crude incidence of leukaemias is probably the same in tropical and non-tropical areas, but there are distinct differences in the age and gender distribution of the four main types. There are relatively few diagnostic problems which are peculiar to the tropics, but there are severe limitations in their management, especially of acute leukaemias.

Acute lymphoblastic leukaemia (ALL)

This is a neoplastic proliferation of lymphoblasts.

Clinical features: are due to malignant infiltration (lymphadenopathy, hepatosplenomegaly, bone pain), anaemia, haemorrhage or thrombosis, and infections following immune depression.

Diagnosis: is by blood film (blast cells) and bone marrow biopsy, which shows infiltration by blast cells. The WCC is raised in two-thirds of patients.

Management: involves
1. Supportive care — transfusion for anaemia; platelet transfusion for haemorrhage due to thrombocytopenia; allopurinol for hyperuricaemia
2. Prevention of infection with antibiotics and antimalarials
3. Chemotherapy consists of:
- Remission induction with vincristine, prednisolone, L-asparaginase, and daunorubicin, followed by
- CNS prophylaxis with intrathecal methotrexate and cranial irradiation
- Maintenance chemotherapy — mercaptopurine (daily), methotrexate (weekly), and vincristine and prednisolone (monthly) — required for 2–3 yrs. Relapse is common in the blood, CNS, and testes.

Acute myeloblastic leukaemia (AML)

This is a neoplastic proliferation of blast cells derived from myeloid elements within the bone marrow.

Clinical features: as for ALL, except that in tropical Africa between 10–25% of all patients and about one-third of boys may present with a chloroma — a solid tumour arising from the orbit (may occur at other sites). Gum hypertrophy is seen particularly in M4, M5. DIC is common in M3.

Diagnosis: can be made with the non-specific esterase reaction which is strongly positive with M5 and M4. The myeloperoxidase and Sudan black reaction help distinguish between ALL L2 and AML M1.

Treatment
- *Supportive* — as for ALL (transfusions, platelets, allopurinol). Survival without treatment is about 2 months.
- *Chemotherapy* — requires specialist centres. A cure rate of 30–50% is achievable in patients optimally treated, according to WHO/FAB subtypes. Bone marrow transplantation is reserved for those with a sibling matched donor or in those who relapse, but it is expensive and needs sophisticated facilities. In AML M3, all-trans-retinoic acid (ATRA) therapy is beneficial.

Classification of acute leukaemias

Common ALL	75%; defined with a specific CD10 antibody; phenotypically pre-B; commonly 2–4 yr olds; M = F
T-cell ALL	Any age; peak in adolescent males; may present with mediastinal mass and high WCC
B-cell ALL	Rare; very poor prognosis; surface Igs are present on blast cells
Null-cell ALL	Undifferentiated; lacking any markers

Morphological classification of AML

FAB method	**WHO definition**
M0	AML minimally differentiated
M1	AML without maturation
M2	AML with maturation
M3 Acute promyelocytic leukaemia	AML with t(15; 17) (q22; q12)
M4	Acute myelomonocytic leukaemia
M5	Acute monoblastic and monocytic leukaemia
M6	Acute erythroid leukaemia
M7	Acute megakaryoblastic leukaemia

Chronic lymphocytic leukaemia (CLL)

Monoclonal proliferation of well-differentiated lymphocytes. 90–95% are B cells; variants include: hairy-cell leukaemia (5–10%; usually of B-cell origin); T-CLL (1%); and B- or T-prolymphocytic leukaemias (<1%).

Clinical features: onset can be insidious with bleeding, weight loss, infection, anorexia. It is asymptomatic in 25%. Signs include hepatosplenomegaly and enlarged rubbery non-tender lymph nodes. The spleen can be enormous in areas of malarial endemicity.

Diagnosis: blood film shows marked lymphocytosis, often with normochromic normocytic anaemia and thrombocytopaenia. Bone marrow biopsy will show infiltration by the malignant clone.

Management
- *Curative antimalarial therapy* followed by long-term prophylaxis results in partial reduction of spleen size and peripheral WCC.
- *Chemotherapy* is not always needed, but may postpone marrow failure. Give chlorambucil 150 mcg/kg PO od until lymphocyte count is reduced. Start a maintenance dose of 100 mcg/kg 4 weeks after ending the first course. Prednisolone will help autoimmune haemolysis.
- *Radiotherapy* is used for relief of lymphadenopathy or splenomegaly.
- *Supportive care* involves transfusions and prophylactic antibiotics.

Prognosis: some remain stable for years or even regress. Usually the nodes enlarge. Death is commonly due to infection. Median survival is about 8 years, but it is stage-dependent and shorter in tropical countries.

Chronic myeloid leukaemia (CML)

Uncontrolled proliferation of myeloid cells. 90% of cases have the Philadelphia chromosome t(9;22)(q34;q11), resulting in a BCR/ABL gene fusion. Those without it have a poorer prognosis.

Clinical features: presentation is chronic and insidious with weight loss, lethargy, sweats, fever, haemorrhage, anaemia, bruising, gout, abdominal pain, gross hepatosplenomegaly, generalized lymphadenopathy.

Diagnosis: WCC grossly elevated (up to >500×10⁹/l); reduced Hb; reduced leucocyte ALP (on stained film); plasma uric acid and ALP are increased.

Management
- *Chemotherapy:* hydroxycarbamide 1–2 g PO od reduced to a maintenance dose of 20–30 mg/kg od to keep WCC near normal. This has now superseded busulfan 2–4 mg/24 h PO until WCC is 20×10^9/l as treatment in the chronic phase. Monitor FBC to avoid pancytopenia. Transformation may be signalled by lack of response to previously effective therapy. Treatment of transformed CML is poor.
- *Autologous bone marrow transplant* is another option, starting with chemotherapy and whole body radiotherapy followed by autografting of patient's previously stored haemopoietic stem cells.
- *Allogenic transplantation* from an HLA matched donor should be considered where facilities are available during the chronic phase if <55 years.

Epidemiology of CLL and CML

Most CLL patients are >40 yrs; the M:F ratio is 2:1. The lowest incidence rates are in C. and S. America; the highest in Scandinavia and Canada. In tropical Africa, CLL occurs from 17 years with equal sex distribution. It is rare in India, S.E. and Far-East Asia. B-CLL has been associated with HTLV-1 infection in Jamaica and Nigeria.

CML accounts for 15% of leukaemias. In the West, it occurs most often during middle age, but in developing countries with younger populations CML can occur in patients <40 yrs. There is a slight male predominance.

Staging of CLL

Stage	**0**	Absolute lymphocytosis >15 × 10^9/l
	I	Stage 0 + enlarged lymph nodes
	II	Stage I + enlarged liver or spleen
	III	Stage II + anaemia (Hb <11 g/dl)
	IV	Stage III + platelets <100 × 10^9/l

Prognosis of CML: is variable. Typically there are 3 phases: a chronic symptomatic phase (which lasts months or a few years), an accelerated phase (where there is failure of adequate response to therapy, with increasing splenomegaly and impaired BM function), and then rapid blast transformation (with features of acute leukaemia and usually rapid death).

Myeloproliferative disorders

A group of disorders characterized by proliferation of haemopoietic stem cells, usually manifesting predominantly in proliferation of one cell series. The proliferating cells retain their ability to differentiate. The disorders share several features such as malaise, itch, and varying degrees of splenomegy. Night sweats, fever, and weight loss are more common in CML and myelofibrosis. Each may undergo transformation to acute leukaemia.

Polycythaemia: is an inaccurate term often used to denote a high haematocrit. The causes of a raised PCV may be relative (from dehydration due to alcohol, diuretics) or absolute (1° – polycythaemia rubra vera — or 2° due to chronic hypoxia (smoking, chronic lung disease, cyanotic heart disease, or altitude) or to increased secretion of erythropoietin (renal disease/tumours, other tumours secreting EPO).

Polycythaemia rubra vera (PRV): also called primary polycythaemia, is characterized by a high PCV (up to 70%), variably raised WBC and platelets, and splenomegaly (60%). Presentation varies but includes sludging (TIAs) and thromboembolic events (CNS disturbances, angina), haemorrhagic tendency, and gout. An absolute increase in red cell mass makes the diagnosis; the marrow shows active erythropoiesis. WBC, platelets, uric acid, leukocyte ALP are raised (decreased in CML). Treatment is to keep PCV <50% by venesection. Hydroxyurea or busulfan can be used especially when platelets are markedly raised. Prognosis is variable.

Essential thrombocythaemia: is characterized by persistently raised platelet counts of above >500×10^9/l without an underlying reactive cause. Platelet morphology and function may be abnormal; presentation may be bleeding or thrombosis. Symptomatic treatment is with hydoxyurea. Prognosis is good. Busulfan has also been used in the past for treatment of ET and other myeloproliferative disorders, but because of its leukaemaogenic potential, its use should be limited to older patients above the age of 60 years.

Multiple myeloma (MM)

MM is a plasma cell neoplasm (IgG: 55%, IgA: 25%, light chain: 20%) which produces diffuse bone marrow infiltration and focal osteolytic deposits. The incidence in the West is 5–10/100,000, with a peak age of 70 yrs and an equal sex distribution. The incidence is higher in the Black population in the Caribbean and Africa and secondary immigrants to the West. Young patients are common in Africa: ~65% of patients are 40–60 yrs old; patients in their late 30s are not uncommon.

Clinical features: bone pain and tenderness is common, particularly in spine, ribs, long bones, and shoulders. Pathological fractures may occur due to lytic bone lesions. Ca^{2+} increases in 30%. Renal failure results from light chain precipitation, hyperuricaemia, and high Ca^{2+}. Also: anaemia, infection, neuropathy, blurred vision, haemorrhages, and exudates in retina, bleeding, and amyloidosis (macroglossia, nephrotic syndrome, cardiac failure, and organomegaly).

Diagnosis: increased plasma cells on bone marrow biopsy more than 30% with atypical or primitive features; distribution may be patchy; M band or urinary light chains (Bence–Jones protein); osteolytic bone lesions ('pepper-pot' skull). Beware rise in Ca^{2+}, urea, creatinine, and uric acid.

Differential diagnosis of thrombocytosis

- Chronic bleeding, especially when associated with iron deficiency
- Inflammation (including collagen diseases)
- Malignancy
- Post-splenectomy
- Kawasaki disease
- Essential thrombocythaemia

Management of multiple myeloma

Supportive analgesia for pain and transfusions for anaemia. Solitary lesions may benefit from radiotherapy. Intermittent melphalan chemotherapy (150 mcg/kg daily od for 4 days, repeated every 6 weeks) is standard. Therapy must be monitored with a FBC after each course as melphalan can cause marrow suppression. Consider multiple therapy if there is no response or relapse. An alternative approach especially in younger patients, where facilities permit, is to treat with VAD followed by high-dose melphalan with autologous stem cell rescue of preharvested stem cells. This may lead to a better prognosis in responders, with a median survival of 4–5 yrs. Thalidomide 100–400 mg at night can be used in relapsed or resistant disease and can lead to good responses in 30–40% of cases. Side-effects include somnolence, fatigue (dose related), rashes (discontinue treatment), constipation; long-term usage leads to peripheral neuropathy. Dexamethasone 20 mg/mL for 4 days every month can be added to treatment or used as a single agent. Death is commonly due to renal failure, infection, or haemorrhage.

Prognosis: 50% alive at 2 yrs. Survival is worse if urea is >10 mmol/l or Hb <7.5 g/dl.

Splenomegaly

The spleen has two major immunological functions: phagocytosis and antibody production. The large number of parasitic, bacterial, and viral agents in the tropical world ensures that these functions are stretched to their capacity and induce splenomegaly of varying magnitude. Splenomegaly is therefore a common physical sign in the tropics.

Clinical features: splenomegaly can cause abdominal distension and discomfort. It may also lead to hypersplenism — pancytopenia then occurs as cells become trapped and destroyed in the spleen's reticuloendothelial system, resulting in symptoms of anaemia, infection, and bleeding. The spleen is recognized clinically by its movement with respiration, enlargement towards RIF, +/− presence of a notch, and the fact that one cannot get above it. AXR may help. Check for lymphadenopathy and liver disease.

Investigations: FBC, ESR, LFTs; liver, marrow, or LN biopsy.

Mild splenomegaly (<5 cm below the costal margin):
- *Acute infections* — malaria, septicaemia, viraemias, hepatitis, trypanosomiasis, brucellosis, toxoplasmosis, typhus.
- *Subacute, chronic infections* — TB, brucellosis, syphilis, hydatid disease, meningococcal septicaemia, histoplasmosis, bacterial endocarditis.
- *Miscellaneous* — megaloblastic anaemia, iron deficiency anaemia, immune thrombocytopenia, RA, hyperthyroidism, multiple myeloma, SLE, sarcoidosis, amyloidosis.

Moderate splenomegaly (5–10 cm below the costal margin):
- *Chronic haemolysis* — recurrent malaria, haemoglobinopathies, hereditary spherocytosis.
- *Portal hypertension* — hepatic cirrhosis.
- *Haematological malignancies* — CLL, lymphomas, acute leukaemias, PRV.

Massive splenomegaly (>10 cm below the costal margin):
Infections — hyperreactive malarial splenomegaly (HMS; formerly called tropical splenomegaly syndrome), schistosomiasis, leishmaniasis.
Blood disorders — thalassaemia major, CML, myelofibrosis.
Miscellaneous — splenic cysts, tumours.

Splenectomies

Indications for splenectomies include trauma, haemolytic anaemias, ITP, and, occasionally, for purposes of diagnosis.

Post-operatively there may be a prompt, transient rise in the platelet count. All patients, particularly children, are at increased risk of septicaemia (post-splenectomy sepsis), especially with encapsulated bacteria such as pneumococcus. Prophylactic antibiotics for children are recommended in the form of penicillin V until age 20 yrs. Pneumococcal, meningococcal, and *H. influenzae* B vaccines are recommended. Prophylaxis against malaria should also be given.

Disorders of haemostasis

Abnormal bleeding results from disorders of:

1. **Initiation of haemostasis:** involving the vascular endothelium and platelets. Manifests as purpura and haemorrhage from or into skin and mucous membranes.

2. **Consolidation of haemostasis:** involving the coagulation and fibrinolytic pathways. Manifests clinically as uncontrolled haemorrhages from or into deeper tissues.

Purpura

Disorders of the initiation of haemostasis result from abnormalities of the endothelium (vascular purpura), abnormalities of platelet function, or thrombocytopenia.

Vascular purpura: damage to vascular endothelium is a common cause of purpura and haemorrhage in the tropics. Infections are important, causing haemorrhage through either direct toxicity to the endothelium (the haemorrhagic fevers — see Chapter 3), or immune damage. In immunocompromised patients, herpesviruses (HSV, VZV) and arboviruses (O'nyong–nyong, African chikungunya) can also cause fatal haemorrhage.

Defective platelet function: thrombocytopathy can complicate the course of some of the haemorrhagic fevers (Lassa, dengue, Marburg, Ebola), alcoholism, hepatic cirrhosis, uraemia, paraproteinaemias, leukaemias, and myeloproliferative disorders. It can also result from ingestion of drugs such as NSAIDS.

Thrombocytopenia: an abnormally low platelet count may result from defective production, increased destruction or consumption in the peripheral blood, splenic pooling, or a combination of these. Conditions such as immune thrombocytopenic purpura (ITP) have no epidemiological or clinical features particular to the tropics, except that patients tend to develop splenomegaly and anaemia.

Onyalai

A profound acquired immune thrombocytopenia of young people in southern Africa which differs from ITP. Clinical features include haemorrhagic bullae on mucous membranes and less frequently the skin (including the soles of the feet), epistaxis, and cerebral haemorrhage. The bleeding normally lasts for ~8 days, but can persist for months and often recurs. Acutely, there is ~3% mortality due to haemorrhagic shock and cerebral haemorrhage. Transfusion is required; splenectomy may be necessary to control bleeding — this is followed by a return to normal platelet counts, but there may be a fatal recurrence post-splenectomy.

Causes of haemorrhage due to vascular endothelial damage

Infections

• Direct toxicity	Viruses (dengue, yellow fever, Lassa fever, other haemorrhagic fevers), bacteria (typhoid, Gram-negative sepsis, meningococcal septicaemia)
• Early immune damage	Measles, scarlet fever, chickenpox, rubella, TB
• Late immune damage	Henoch–Schonlein purpura, purpura fulminans

Drugs

• Idiosyncratic reactions	Streptomycin, isoniazid, penicillin, aspirin, sulfonamides, quinine, etc.

Others
• Uraemia, scurvy, dysproteinaemias (multiple myeloma), fat embolism
• Congenital conditions (e.g. Ehlers–Danlos, Osler–Weber–Rendu)
• Senile purpura

Causes of thrombocytopenia

Reduced production	• Infections (eg typhoid, brucellosis) • Megaloblastic anaemia • Alcoholism • Marrow infiltration (e.g. leukaemia) • Aplastic anaemia • Drugs/chemicals: cytotoxic drugs, idiosyncratic reactions, overdose, occupational exposure (e.g. benzene)
Increased consumption or destruction	• Infections (eg malaria, trypanosomiasis, dengue) • Hypersplenism • Chronic hepatic disease • DIC • Immune mechanisms: ITP, Onyalai, acute viral infection, AIDS, drugs (quinine, penicillin), lymphomas, CLL, autoimmune diseases

Coagulation disorders

These conditions occur in two forms:

1. **Congenital:** haemophilia A (factor VIII deficiency); haemophilia B (Christmas disease, factor IX deficiency), and von Willebrand's disease (deficiency or abnormality of von Willebrand's factor, previously known as factor VIII-associated protein).
2. **Acquired:** malabsorption (vit K deficiency), liver disease, disseminated intravascular coagulation (DIC), and snake envenomation.

Congenital forms

Clinical features: bleeding into joints and muscles is common; it can lead to crippling arthropathy and haematomas with nerve palsies. Boys may also present with haemorrhage post-circumcision. Cerebral haemorrhages may result from the increased ICP of persistent coughing.

Diagnosis: is by history, FHx, increased APTT, and factor VIII or IX assay.

Management: seek expert advice.

- *Haemophilia A:* avoid NSAIDS and IM injections. With minor bleeding, apply pressure and elevate the limb. Desmopressin (0.3–0.4 mcg/kg every 12–24 hrs IV in 50 ml 0.9% saline over 20 mins) raises factor VIII and may be sufficient. Major bleeding requires either factor VIII infusion or cryoprecipitate (rich in factor VIII and can be prepared easily — see box). There is a high risk of HIV transmission with cryoprecipitate. Recombinant factor VIII is also available.
- *Haemophilia B:* is best treated with virus-inactivated factor IX concentrate; cryosupernatant or FFP can be given in its absence but there is increased risk of HIV transmission.
- *Von Willebrand's disease:* should be managed with desmopressin although cryoprecipitate may also be required.

Blood products and HIV/hepatitis viruses: HIV, hepatitis B and C, and other micro-organisms can be transmitted in blood products that have not been heat inactivated. Such products should only be used when the advantages are judged to outweigh the risks of infection.

Acquired hypoprothrombinaemias

Vitamin K deficiency

- Haemorrhagic disease of the newborn is the result of vitamin K deficiency in premature infants and infants of mothers on anti-TB therapy, anticonvulsants, or warfarin. Infants may also present later, between 1–3 months of age, with intracranial haemorrhage. It is prevented by prophylactic vitamin K 1 mg IM. On the first day of life vitamin K should be given IV. Be aware of anaphylaxis.
- Malabsorption — see Chapter 7. Diagnosis is via a prolonged PT, which reverts rapidly to normal following treatment with vitamin K 10 mg IV; the response will be partial if there is liver disease.

Vitamin K antagonism: is seen with the competitive inhibitor warfarin. Inadvertent overdose, simultaneous administration of other potentiating drugs, and accidental ingestion may all cause haemorrhage. Warfarin's anticoagulant effect remains for a few days after withdrawal; if the bleeding does not resolve, give vitamin K 5–10 mg carefully by slow IV injection.

Liver disease: see box.

Haemostatic measurements (for children >2 yrs and adults)

Blood platelets	$150–400 \times 10^9/l$
Prothrombin time (PT)	11–14 seconds
Partial thromboplastin time (APTT)	23–35 seconds
Blood fibrinogen levels	2–4 g/l
Fibrinogen degradation products (FDP)	<10 mg/l

PT is used for measuring the extrinsic coagulation pathway. Since factor VII has the shortest half-life of the coagulation factors, it is the first factor to become reduced after giving warfarin. Therefore the PT is used to measure anticoagulation due to warfarin.

APTT is used for measuring the intrinsic coagulation pathway. It is therefore used to measure anticoagulation due to heparin.

To prepare a cryoprecipitate and cryosupernatant

Collect donor blood into a multipack plastic blood-collection set. Centrifuge the unit or allow it to sediment; separate the plasma into a second pack and freeze this at −20°C or colder for 24 hrs. Thaw the plasma at 4°C and centrifuge; the cryoprecipitate remains in the bag while the cryosupernatant is separated into a third bag. Both should be stored at −20°C until used.

Liver disease and coagulation disorders

Bleeding in liver disease is multifactorial:

1. During acute infectious hepatitis, a mild disorder of haemostasis consisting of reduced levels of factors V, VII, and X and a prolonged PT is not unusual.
2. In liver failure, there is severe coagulation factor deficiency, hypofibrinogenaemia, and DIC.
3. Patients with chronic hepatic disease or cirrhosis show impairment of synthesis of all vitamin K-dependent factors and fibrinogen and reduced platelet function. The PT is prolonged and vitamin K has little or no effect.

Bleeding with liver disease should be treated by transfusion of cryosupernatant, FFP, or factor concentrates.

Disseminated intravascular coagulation (DIC)

DIC is the widespread or uncontrolled deposition of fibrin in the circulation, followed by increased activation of fibrinolysis. It may be accompanied by a microangiopathic picture and is triggered by a large number of conditions.

Mechanisms

1. Damage to the endothelium with activation of the intrinsic pathway of the coagulation cascade.
2. Release of thromboplastin-like materials from tissues with the activation of the extrinsic pathway.
3. Injection of procoagulants in snake venom.
4. During pregnancy, there is normally a potential hypercoagulable and hyperfibrinolytic state. A wide range of obstetric disorders can trigger severe DIC — see box.

The dominant feature is haemorrhage, which is multifactorial. The end state is one of depleted platelets, coagulation factors, and fibrinogen. DIC is therefore known as 'consumption coagulopathy'. Fibrinogen degradation products (FDPs) are released into the circulation where they have an antithrombin activity. Their incorporation into clots makes the clots friable.

Clinical features: presentation is usually with the underlying condition. DIC can range from a minor derangement of coagulation without bleeding to a severe haemorrhagic state. It is a dynamic condition which can progress rapidly. The common manifestations of bleeding include haemorrhage in mucous membranes, skin, venepuncture sites, or from the uterus.

Microangiopathic haemolytic anaemia: results from subacute and chronic DIC. Fibrin deposition in small blood vessels may cause ischaemia, tissue necrosis, and renal failure; pituitary failure and adrenal failure are rare complications.

Diagnosis: the platelet count is reduced; APTT, PT, and thrombin times are prolonged; and plasma FDPs raised. In severe DIC, the simple clotting time is prolonged. Microangiopathic haemolytic anaemia shows features of intravascular haemolysis: there are many small, fragmented RBCs with bizarre shapes (schizocytes) in the peripheral blood.

Management

1. Treat the underlying condition; if this has a rapid response, the DIC will correct spontaneously.
2. Restore and maintain blood volume via transfusion of whole blood (if unavailable, use concentrated RBCs plus saline, or saline and colloids).
3. If haemorrhage cannot be controlled, give platelets, FFP, and/or cryoprecipitate to restore the missing coagulation factors.

Main causes of DIC in the tropics

Acute
- Infections   Viraemia, liver disease, sepsis, renal disease, protozoan infections
- Obstetric   Septic abortions, abruptio placentae, ruptured uterus, amniotic fluid embolus
- Shock   Accidental trauma — birth anoxia, head injury, fractured femur; surgical trauma, burns, heat stroke
- Envenoming   Snake bites, *Lonomia achelous* caterpillars
- Others   Acute hepatic necrosis, cytotoxic therapy, incompatible blood transfusion

Subacute
- Obstetric   Pre-eclampsia, eclampsia, retention of dead fetus; hydatidiform mole
- Malignancy   AML M3
- Others   Purpura fulminans

Chronic
- Metabolic
- Malignacy   e.g. prostatic carcinoma

Nutrition

Section editor **Saskia van der Kam**

Causes of weight loss and malnutrition

Around 100 million children worldwide suffer from moderate malnutrition and ~10 million are severely malnourished and at risk of death. The syndrome of malnutrition can be a 1° complaint or 2° to another illness. The 1° cause of malnutrition is a negative balance between dietary intake and physical needs. There are three major underlying factors: lack of food/decline in food security; infectious diseases; and caring practices for dependents. These elements seldom occur in isolation and they often reinforce each other.

Food security

The economic base (e.g. harvests, labour), accessibility to markets and fields, safe movement, and terms of trade all determine food security. Internal conflicts and war are the greatest threats.

Infections

Malnutrition is both a cause and a consequence of infection, with a vicious circle of malnutrition and infections. The malnourished become immuno-suppressed, so infections last longer and are more severe. Infections reduce appetite, leading to reduced food intake. Infections often lead to malabsorption to some degree (e.g. diarrhoea may be directly caused by *Giardia lamblia* or *Strongyloides stercoralis* or 2° to measles). Infections deplete specific body stores, which are often marginal in health: vitamin A during measles; antioxidant vitamins like A, C, E; iron deficiency (in hookworm infection). Finally, some chronic diseases have catabolic effects (e.g. HIV, TB, and kala azar).

The combination of lack of appetite and increased requirements leads to malnutrition that in turn worsens the infection. To decrease the burden of infections, interventions improving health are essential to ensure a good nutritional status: preventive health services (e.g. vaccinations, MCH) and curative medical care (e.g. clinics) as well as safe water and waste disposal.

Caring practices

These are determined not only culturally but also by the financial resources and time available to families for their children, disabled, orphans, and elderly. Sometimes malnutrition is linked to chronic emotional deprivation by caretakers who, because of ignorance, poverty, or family disintegration, are unable to provide the child with the nutrition and care he/she requires. The time available to care givers is important, and can decrease considerably in times of economic recession and migration of men. Deep-rooted gender inequalities can be important underlying factors like the workload on women who have to be carers as well. The resulting lack of care and mental well-being for the dependent results in a lack of appetite and a lack of thriving in general.

Successful prevention and treatment of malnutrition should address the three underlying causes of malnutrition — a combination of medical, nutritional, and social care and help to improve the economy.

Vulnerability

- The people who are physically dependent in a community are vulnerable: children, the elderly, and the disabled.
- Those with special or increased nutritional needs are vulnerable (e.g. pregnant and lactating women, and AIDS patients).
- Socially marginalized minorities or disempowered groups have often limited access to economic resources and markets.
- Also vulnerable are people in unhealthy environments (e.g. refugee camps and shanty towns).
- Vulnerability often affects the entire family or community.

Defining and assessing malnutrition

Severe malnutrition is a medical syndrome in two major forms — kwashiorkor and marasmus. They are often mixed: marasmic–kwashiorkor.

Clinical features of marasmus (see Fig. 15.1)

- Emaciated: thin, flaccid skin (the 'little old man' appearance), fat and muscle tissue grossly reduced, prominence spine and ribs
- Behaviour: alert and irritable
- Electrolyte imbalance, dehydration, possibly associated with diarrhoea and vomiting
- Infection, often with minimal signs: urinary, ear, respiratory, diarrhoea
- Normal hair
- There are no biochemical or haematological changes diagnostic of the condition

Clinical features of kwashiorkor (see Fig. 15.2)

- Oedema: pitting, bilateral including lower extremities. May be localized or extensive, including the eyelids. It may mislead an observer into thinking that the child is plump and well.
- Thin: subcutaneous fat may be present, but emaciation may occur as well.
- Skin lesions: atrophy, patches of erythema and/or hyperpigmentation, desquamation, hypopigmentation, usually beginning around the perineum. Skin breakdown leads to ulceration.
- Hair: becomes dry, thin. It may also become depigmented (achromotrichia), appearing brown, yellowy-red, or white.
- Diarrhoea and vomiting is non-specific: in chronic malnutrition it may be 2° to malabsorption owing to GI damage. Hepatomegaly is common. There may be hypovolaemia, even in an oedematous child.
- Behaviour: the child is lethargic, apathic, and miserable, with reduced expression and comprehension.
- Infections: especially URTIs which may progress rapidly to pneumonia and death.

Aetiology

Although marasmus and kwashiorkor are clinically different, the aetiology is quite similar with a lack of several nutrients (energy, protein, vitamins, and minerals) and variable immunosuppression. Deficiencies exist in various combinations; depletion of body stores of the various elements occurs at different speeds.

Marasmus most often results from inadequate energy provision in the diet of growing children combined with chronic or repeated diarrhoea. When stores are depleted, the body catabolizes tissues to provide essential elements; the result is cessation of growth, emaciation, and marasmus. The patient utilizes subcutaneous fat, then muscular tissue, as alternative energy sources. The disease develops in infants on prolonged breast-feeding with inadequate supplementation, or inadequate artificial feeding with overdiluted cow or powdered milk. The latter may also expose the child to infective agents resulting in diarrhoea, compounding the situation.

Kwashiorkor develops due to another reaction to a lack of nutrients: alternative, less effective metabolic pathways develop that have detrimental results. For example, lack of some essential nutrients means the growth or repair of cell membranes is less effective. Leaking cell membranes result in an excess of sodium in the interstitial space, causing oedema. The condition is

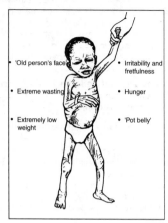

Fig. 15.1 Typical signs and symptoms in marasmus

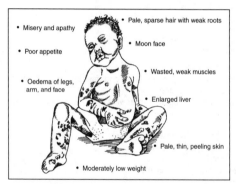

Fig. 15.2 Typical signs and symptoms in Kwashiorkor

Other key points in physical examination

- Spleen enlargements and tenderness
- Ascites
- Sunken fontanel, sunken eyes
- Neck suppleness
- Breath sounds
- Lymph nodes enlargement and tenderness
- Corneal lesions suggestive of vitamin A deficiency
- Evidence of ear, mouth, or throat infection
- Infection or purpura of skin

worsened by acute infections because free radicals are produced to kill the infective agents. However, if not controlled by antioxidants, these free radicals cause tissue damage; a lack of such antioxidants in kwashiorkor means the cell membranes are not protected and oedema is made worse. Thus kwashiorkor is often accompanied by a history of illness and infection.

Zinc and selenium deficiencies are thought to contribute to kwashiorkor. Although a lack of protein is an important element in the aetiology of kwashiorkor, the syndrome can also be caused by a lack of micronutrients in foods that are rich in proteins.

Other causes of nutritional oedema are the consumption of badly prepared cassava (Konzo), containing cyanide, and the consumption of infected beans and peanuts (aflatoxin).

Points in the history and physical examination

History

- Behaviour and activity changes (crying, irritable, apathy)
- Usual diet before current illness, complaints about lack of food or the quality of food, recent change in diet
- Breastfeeding history — is child suckling? Is mother healthy?
- Food and fluids taken in past few days; thirst?
- Recent illness (measles, diarrhoea, malaria, cough, infections) and treatments
- Recent sinking of eyes
- Duration, frequency, and nature of any vomiting or diarrhoea
- Time when urine was last passed
- Contact with measles or TB
- Deaths of siblings
- Birth weight
- Milestones reached (e.g. sitting, standing)
- Immunizations

Physical examination

- General appearance, behaviour, mood (apathy, irritable), level of consciousness, facial appearance
- Signs of shock: cold hands or feet, weak pulse, decreased consciousness, thirst
- Pulse
- Temperature — hypothermia/fever?
- Respiratory rate and type
- Pallor, jaundice
- Weight and length or height
- Oedema
- Enlarged or tender liver, jaundice
- Abdominal distension, bowel sounds, tenderness

Classification of malnutrition[1]

	Well-nourished	Malnutrition		
		Mild	Moderate	Severe
Symmetrical oedema?	NO	NO	NO	YES = oedematous malnutrition[2]
Weight for height	90–120%[3] (+2 to −1SD)	80–89% (−1 to −2SD)	70–79% (−2 to −3SD)	<70% = severe wasting[4]
Height for age	95–110% (+2 to −1SD)	90–94% (−1 to −2SD)	85–89% (−2 to −3SD)	<85% = severe stunting

(continued)

Notes:

1. The diagnoses are not mutually exclusive. A child can have severe wasting and oedematous malnutrition, or severe wasting and severe stunting, etc.

2. Corresponds to the definitions of 'kwashiorkor' and 'marasmic kwashiorkor' in other classifications. To avoid confusion with the clinical syndrome of kwashiorkor (which includes other features), the term 'oedematous malnutrition' is preferred here.

3. % of the median WHO standard and standard deviation (SD). For 'weight for age' and 'weight for height', one SD unit is about 10% of the median, except in children less than 6 months old. For 'height for age', one SD unit is about 5% of the median.

4. This corresponds to 'marasmus' (without oedema) or 'grade III malnutrition'. To avoid confusion, the term 'severe wasting' is preferred.

Table 15.1 Simplified WHO reference chart: weight-for-length and weight- for-height by sex

Boys' weight (kg)						Girls' weight (kg)				
-4SD 60%	-3SD 70%	-2SD 80%	-1SD 90%	Median	Length or Height (cm)	Median	-1SD 90%	-2SD 80%	-3SD 70%	-4SD 60%
1.8	2.2	2.5	2.9	3.3	50	3.4	3	2.6	2.3	1.9
1.9	2.3	2.8	3.2	3.7	52	3.7	3.3	2.8	2.4	2
2	2.6	3.1	3.6	4.1	54	4.1	3.6	3.1	2.7	2.2
2.3	2.9	3.5	4	4.6	56	4.5	4	3.5	3	2.4
2.7	3.3	3.9	4.5	5.1	58	5	4.4	3.9	3.3	2.7
3.1	3.7	4.4	5	5.7	60	5.5	4.9	4.3	3.7	3.1
3.5	4.2	4.9	5.6	6.2	62	6.1	5.4	4.8	4.1	3.5
4	4.7	5.4	6.1	6.8	64	6.7	6	5.3	4.6	3.9
4.5	5.3	6	6.7	7.4	66	7.3	6.5	5.8	5.1	4.3
5.1	5.8	6.5	7.3	8	68	7.8	7.1	6.3	5.5	4.8
5.5	6.3	7	7.8	8.5	70	8.4	7.6	6.8	6	5.2
6	6.8	7.5	8.3	9.1	72	8.9	8.1	7.2	6.4	5.6
6.4	7.2	8	8.8	9.6	74	9.4	8.5	7.7	6.8	6
6.8	7.6	8.4	9.2	10	76	9.8	8.9	8.1	7.2	6.4
7.1	8	8.8	9.7	10.5	78	10.2	9.3	8.5	7.6	6.7
7.5	8.3	9.2	10.1	10.9	80	10.6	9.7	8.8	8	7.1
7.8	8.7	9.6	10.4	11.3	82	11	10.1	9.2	8.3	7.4
8.1	9	9.9	10.8	11.7	84	11.4	10.5	9.6	8.7	7.7
7.9	9	10.1	11.2	12.3	86	12	11	9.9	8.8	7.7
8.3	9.4	10.5	11.7	12.8	88	12.5	11.4	10.3	9.2	8.1
8.6	9.8	10.9	12.1	13.3	90	12.9	11.8	10.7	9.5	8.4
8.9	10.1	11.3	12.5	13.7	92	13.4	12.2	11	9.9	8.7
9.2	10.5	11.7	13	14.2	94	13.9	12.6	11.4	10.2	9
9.6	10.9	12.1	13.4	14.7	96	14.3	13.1	11.8	10.6	9.3
9.9	11.2	12.6	13.9	15.2	98	14.9	13.5	12.2	10.9	9.6
10.3	11.6	13	14.4	15.7	100	15.4	14	12.7	11.3	9.9
10.6	12	13.4	14.9	16.3	102	15.9	14.5	13.1	11.7	10.3
11	12.4	13.9	15.4	16.9	104	16.5	15	13.5	12.1	10.6
11.4	12.9	14.4	15.9	17.4	106	17	15.5	14	12.5	11
11.8	13.4	14.9	16.5	18	108	17.6	16.1	14.5	13	11.4
12.2	13.8	15.4	17.1	18.7	110	18.2	16.6	15	13.4	11.9

SD = standard deviation or Z-score. Length is measured < 85 cm.

Measuring malnutrition

Malnutrition is assessed by a combination of clinical features (described above) and athropometry (body measurements). The indicators used are:

- *Wasting:* weight for height, mid upper arm circumference (MUAC), body mass index (BMI)
- *Stunting:* height for age
- *Wasting and stunting combined:* weight for age
- *Kwashiorkor:* bilateral oedema

Weight for height, height for age, weight for age

These are all indicators that compare the patient with a reference population: the weight of the patient with a certain height, is compared to the weight of the similar height in the reference population. The comparison is expressed as a simple % of the median (e.g. if the patient weighs 8 kg and the reference value for the same height is 10 kg, the patients has 80% weight for height). Alternatively, the comparison can be expressed as a number of standard deviations from the median (See Table 15.1, previous page). All reference values are derived from tables. These indicators are used up to a height of 163.5 cm for female and 174.5 cm for male adolescents.

Using growth charts

A commonly used monitoring tool is the weight for age or growth chart (see Fig. 15.3). This chart has three solid reference curves on it:

- The upper one is 97th centile curve, below which 97% of a healthy population of children will lie.
- The middle one is the median curve, or 50th centile, below which 50% of a healthy population of children will lie.
- The lower one is the 3rd centile curve, below which only 3% of a healthy population will lie.

The dotted curve represents 60% of the median curve; no healthy child's weight is below this line.

Although there is some variation between boys and girls (separate charts for each sex exist), healthy children of either sex have weights between the 97th and 3rd centile curves. The slope of the curve shows the rate at which the child gains (or loses) weight and should be roughly the same as that of the reference curve.

Weighing a child once will only give an estimate of the child's growth and nutritional status since children vary greatly in weight. If a single measurement falls below the 3rd centile, the child is probably malnourished. If it falls below the 60% line, it is almost certainly malnourished.

Weighing a child at regular intervals and recording the results on a growth chart gives much more information. For example, a child's weight may fall just below the 3rd centile, but remain parallel to it as the child grows and eats a healthy diet — indicating that the child is simply one of the 3% of small, well-nourished children. The clinician should be alerted when weight plots cross the reference lines or deviate abnormally. This indicates a child is becoming malnourished, not growing normally, or even losing weight.

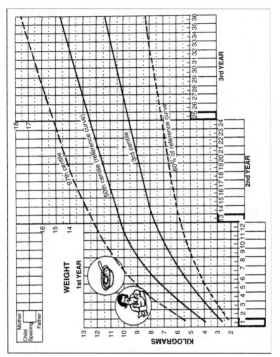

Fig. 15.3 Standard growth chart showing centiles

Common mistakes with growth charts

- Writing January in the first box instead of the child's birth month
- Writing the month in which the child was first weighed instead of his/her birth month in the first box
- Missing out months
- Writing the months as numbers and confusing them with ages
- Forgetting to miss out blank boxes if the child has not been weighed for several months
- Not using the calendar and estimating the child's age each time
- Recording a child's weight in the wrong year
- Putting the weight dot the wrong side of the kilogram line

Mid upper arm circumference (MUAC)

Fig. 15.4 shows an arm circumference for age chart. The reference line on the chart rises very steeply in the first year. MUAC is thus not very useful for children <1 yr of age. From the age of 1 yr, however, it rises only slowly and may be used to assess nutritional status, since there is little variation between ages. The MUAC is less sensitive than weight for height assessments, and regularly gives false positives and false negatives, caused by less precise measuring and by interpopulation differences. Therefore, the MUAC is most often used as a rapid assessment tool, to pre-select for a more thorough examination.

Above 5 yrs there are is agreed MUAC cut-off, although MUAC is a useful anthropometric tool for adults. MUAC assessment must always be combined with clinical examination for signs of malnutrition (e.g. extreme weakness, inability to walk, extreme pallor) and social indicators (e.g. lack of care giver for elderly/disabled). The most widely used cut-off points are listed in the box — these should be adapted according to context.

Body mass index (BMI)

The BMI takes into account the size (height) of the patient when assessing weight and is found by: weight (kg) ÷ height (m)^2. The BMI is used for assessment of adults. The inter- and intra- population variability of BMI is great, so it is not possible to establish general cut-off points useful in all populations. Any cut-off points should be adapted according to the local context and combined with clinical examination. The BMI is no better than MUAC as an anthropometric tool for adults.

Oedema

Oedema should always be checked. In children, bilateral oedema is considered to be kwashiorkor unless proven otherwise. Assessment of oedema is not always easy (firm pressure of the thumb for 3 seconds on both feet). Sometimes fat feet are confused with oedematous feet, especially if the child has discoloured hair.

Oedema in adults: bilateral oedema can be a symptom of severe adult malnutrition. Oedema > grade 3 carries a poor prognosis and represents severe malnutrition in adults. However, oedema in adults can also be a sign of many other pathologies (renal, cardiac, hepatic).

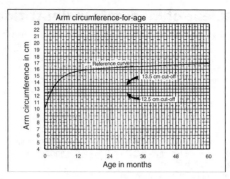

Fig. 15.4

MUAC cut-off points for malnutrition in children, adults, pregnant women, and the elderly

	Severe	Moderate	At risk
Children 1–5 yrs	<110 mm	110–125 mm	125–125 mm
Adults	<160 mm	160–185 mm	
Pregnant/lactating women	<170 mm	170–185 mm	185–210 mm
Elderly*	<160 mm	160–175 mm	

*MUAC is generally low among the elderly due to loss of muscle

Classification of oedema in children

Feet	+
Feet + legs	++
Feet + legs + other parts of the body	+++

Classification of oedema in adults

Grade	Extent of oedema
0	Absent
1	Minimal oedema on the foot or ankle
2	Obvious oedema on the foot or ankle
3	Oedema up to the knee (tibial)
4	Oedema up to the groin (inguinal area)
5	Total body oedema (anasarca)

Treatment of moderate malnutrition

In developing countries, 50% of child mortality is associated with malnutrition, in particular moderate malnutrition. Even this level of malnutrition reduces immune competence, so infections last longer and are more severe. Children may unnecessarily die from a infection (e.g. URTI). Thus moderately malnourished children (weight for height <80%) should receive nutritional suplementation of at least 500 kCal per kg per day (14 grams of protein) with fortified foods.

Discharge: the child after several weeks on 85% weight for -height (adolescents: 80% weight for height).

- Moderately malnourished adolescents and adults are normally not treated. They are less vulnerable and diagnosing moderate malnutrition among adults is difficult.
- Pregnant and lactating women require nutritional support: their nutrition determines the quality of the breast milk (micronutrients) and the health of the baby. If a woman is thin, the quantity of breast milk is usually not affected; but when her food intake drops to <1700 kCal/day the baby will suffer.

It is essential to treat infections at an early stage.

Treatment of severe malnutrition

The principles of treatment of severe malnutrition are similar for all age groups combining therapeutic nutritional treatment with intensive medical care. All people who are severely malnourished (oedema, weight for height <70% or MUAC as above or BMI <16) should be treated regardless of age.

Discharge: when moderate malnutrition is reached, there is no oedema, and patients are in a good clinical condition and gaining weight. Adults should not be discharged on an increase in MUAC or BMI, but on a weight gain of 10–15% .

For treatment, nutritional and medical components are combined. It is based on routine protocols applicable for all patients, and adapted for specific problems. Nutritional treatment is divided in three phases:

1. Initiation
2. Transition
3. Rehabilitation

Monitoring of:

- Weight
- Height
- Oedema
- Vomiting
- Diarrhoea
- Temperature
- Heart rate
- Respiratory rate

is essential in the initial and transition phases of the treatment in order to intervene quickly at the first signs of fluid overload and/or infection. In the rehabilitation phase, the monitoring can be less intensive.

Nutritional support for sick people

All severely ill patients need energy-dense food fortified with vitamins and minerals to promote recovery. Being sick often alters metabolism, resulting in increased needs for micro- and macro-nutrients, at the same time as a reduced food intake because of malabsorption, diarrhoea, and loss of appetite. Fever increases the energy needs by 5–10 kCal/kg/day. Losses by diarrhoea and vomiting should be replaced.

Food should be easily digestible, palatable, and soft without strong odours and spices, and fortified with micronutrients such as vitamin A, B, C, and zinc, magnesium, and selenium.

Patients with TB, kala azar, shigellosis, and measles in particular need supplementary feeding with energy, protein, and vitamin-rich food.

Nutrition in people with HIV/AIDS

Good nutrition is one of the pillars of successful HIV/AIDS management, in order to maintain immune competence and strength and minimize the nutritional impact of 2° infections. HIV/AIDS patients (even when asymptomatic) need an increased food intake:

- Up to an extra 400 kCal/day (10–15% increased energy intake), with a minimum of 2500 kCal/day
- The extra need for protein depends on the physical state
- At least the recommended daily intake (RDA) or more of vitamins A, B, C, E, and minerals (e.g. selenium, folic acid, zinc)

NB A high consumption of vitamin A, zinc, and iron can have a detrimental effect.

Nutritional education should start once a person is identified as HIV +ve. Focus on how to meet increased dietary needs and prevent opportunistic infections and improve hygiene. Support the entire family, look into food security, hygiene, and care of the patient.

To optimize dietary intake: eat small, frequent meals (smaller portions, snacking, softer food) and a variety of foods, including body-building food (legumes, cereal, animal products), protective foods (fruits and vegetables, fortified food), and energy foods (sugar, starch and fat, staple foods).

Problems

- **Nausea and vomiting:** eat frequent small meals and avoid fatty food and food with strong smells; drink enough.
- **Mouth sores:** avoid hot and spicy foods, eat soft, mashed, liquid food.
- **Lack of appetite:** eat frequent small meals that are easy to digest.
- **Drink:** enough to maintain fluid balance.
- **Time doses of drugs:** with side-effects such as nausea, in relation to meals.

Therapeutic nutritional treatment

Initiation phase

The aim of this phase is to stabilize and readjust the metabolism. Severely malnourished people are extremely fragile with disturbed metabolisms and electrolyte balances, and as a consequence cannot handle large amounts of food.

- The quantity given in the initial phase is delicate: if too little is given, malnutrition will continue. Overfeeding (too large quantities of food, too high osmotic value of the food) and overhydration (IV fluids, oral rehydration fluids) increases the risk of congestive heart failure. Early signs are increased respiratory rate, increased heart rate, and lung sounds.
- Give the food frequently and in small amounts (e.g. 8 times over 24 hrs) throughout the day and night — this avoids overloading.
- Patience is required: nearly all malnourished patients have poor appetites when first admitted. If the patient fails to take at least 80 kCal/kg/day, use a NG tube. At each feed the food should be offered by mouth, after which the remainder is given by NG tube. When the patient takes three-quarters of the daily diet orally, the tube can be removed.

Severely malnourished patients do not tolerate the usual amounts of dietary protein, fat, and sodium, and require a diet low in these ingredients and in osmolality, but high in carbohydrate. Special food items are therefore used.

- ***Frequency***: 8 meals over 24 hrs (night feeding is required to prevent hypoglycaemia)
- ***Quantity***: see box
- ***Food***: therapeutic milk. In order of suitability: F-75, SDTM, diluted HEM, undiluted F100, undiluted HEM
- ***Monitoring***: general appearance, appetite, vomiting, diarrhoea, oedema, heart rate, respiratory rate
- ***Duration:*** must be an inpatient (for close monitoring); lasts 2–7 days. When the patient regains appetite, is lively and interested, recovering from medical complications, and oedema is absent (or greatly reduced), he/she can go to the transition phase.

Transition phase

The aim of this phase is to monitor closely the intake of larger amounts of food with a higher osmolality and sodium content, in order to intervene quickly if heart failure develops due to fluid overload. Monitoring of vital functions is essential.

- Frequency: 8 meals over 24 hrs
- Quantity: increased by 35–50% (see box)
- Food: therapeutic milk. In order of most suitable: F100, HEM
- Monitoring: general appearance, vomiting, oedema, heart rate, respiratory rate. If any of these signs occur, the patient must return to the initiation phase.
- Duration: after 1–3 days, when the patient is able to tolerate larger amounts of food without complications, he/she can go on to the rehabilitation phase.

Rehabilitation phase

The aim is to promote rapid growth and to regain strength.
- **Frequency**: 6 meals over 24 hrs (night feeding not required).
- **Quantity**: at least double the initiation phase (see box).
- **Food**: 3 meals of therapeutic milk (in order of most suitable: F100, HEM) plus one meal of porridge (fortified, energy dense) and a local meal. You have to add one RTUTF for home consumption.
- **Monitoring**: general appearance, weight, height, oedema. If deterioration in any of these signs occurs, then place the patient back in initiation phase.
- **Duration**: about 20 days.

Types of therapeutic milk

- **F75** — designed for the initial phase: 75 kCal/100 ml, isotonic, low sodium, 5 kCal % protein, 32 kCal % fat
- **F100** — designed for the transition and rehabilitation phases: 100 kCal/100 ml, low osmolality, medium sodium content, 10 kCal % protein, 50 kCal % fat
- **SDTM (specially diluted therapeutic milk)** — is 75% diluted F100; 1 litre of F100 plus 350 ml water supplies 75 kCal/100 ml, isotonic, medium sodium, 10 kCal % protein, 50 kCal % fat
- **Alternative SDTM** — 50 g DSM, 75 g sugar, 25 g oil, and 850 ml of clean water
- **HEM (high-energy milk)** — a home-made preparation of 80 g DSM, 60 g oil, 50 g sugar, 3 g mineral mix (when available) added to 1 litre of water: 100 kCal/100 ml, high osmolarity, high sodium, 10 kCal % protein, 50 kCal % fat
- **RTUTF (ready to eat therapeutic food)** — (e.g. BP100®, Plumpynut®) designed for the rehabilitation phase, doesn't require cooking nor heating but must be consumed with water and can be used at home

Don't give any therapeutic milk (F100, F75, SDTM, HEM) for use at home.

Quantity of food per phase for particular age groups (kCal/kg/day)

Age	Initiation phase	Transition phase	Rehabilitation phase
<7 yrs	100	135–150	200
7–10 yrs	75	135–150	200
11–18 yrs	55	70–90	100
19–75 yrs	40	50–60	80
>75 yrs	35	50–60	80

Medical treatment

Medical treatment aims to treat infections, restore deficiencies, and prevent complications. The majority of severely malnourished people have similar medical conditions, so all should receive the following routine medical treatments. Therapy should start on admission, and continue as needed through all phases of treatment.

- Rehydration
- Antibiotics
- Measles vaccination
- Malaria test and treatment
- Folic acid supplement
- Intestinal worm treatment
- Vitamin A supplement
- Iron supplements
  (starting only after 14 days)

These can be adapted if the patient has illness on admission or during treatment.

Bacterial infections

Nearly all severely malnourished patients have bacterial infections when first admitted. These may be multiple and signs of infection such as fever and inflammation may be absent. Early treatment with effective antimicrobials improves the nutritional response to feeding, prevents shock, and reduces mortality. Routinely all patients receive a broad-spectrum antibiotic (e.g. amoxicillin 500 mg PO tds for >5 days [250 mg tds for children under 10 yrs; if under 20 kg, then 20–40 mg/kg daily in divided doses; infants <3 months, max dose of 15 mg/kg od]). Treatment can be adapted if a specific infection is detected or if the treatment is not effective. A good second-line drug is IV/IM ceftriaxone.

Measles

All children aged 6 months–15 yrs should be vaccinated against measles, unless a vaccination card proves previous vaccination. Children immunized between 6–9 months should be re-vaccinated at 9 months, as their immune response may be limited.

Malaria

Test on admission by blood film or dipstick; if positive, treat with best available combination therapy including artesunate derivatives where available.

Intestinal worms

Give all patients (except women in 3rd trimester of pregnancy) albendazole 400 mg or mebendazole 500 mg, both PO stat.

Important principles of medical therapy

- The principal route of administration of food and medicines is oral, by mouth, or NG tube. IV infusions are given only in extreme situations (shock, unconsciousness).
- Transfusions for anaemia should only be given in extreme cases (Hb<4 mg/dL).
- IM injections, when required, should be given in the buttock using a small-gauge needle and the smallest possible volume.

Dehydration in malnourished patients

Many malnourished patients have acute or chronic diarrhoea, and dehydration is common. However, dehydration is easily over diagnosed, and treatment with salt solutions risks overloading the weak patient (especially kwashiorkor patients). (For signs of dehydration, see Chapter 2D.) In malnourished patients, dehydration is difficult to recognize and easily confused with septic shock. The box opposite may help differentiate septic shock from dehydration. With incipient septic shock, the patient is usually limp, apathetic, and profoundly anorexic, but is neither thirsty nor restless. With established septic shock, superficial veins can be dilated or constricted, and dyspnoea is common.

Choose 'oral rehydration solution for the severely malnourished' — called ReSoMal. Use the oral route whenever possible; IV infusion may lead to overhydration and heart failure. Full-strength normal ORS **should not be used** since total body sodium is high and potassium low in the malnourished. In the absence of pre-packaged sachets of ReSoMal, dilute one standard sachet of ORS in 2 litres of water (instead of 1 litre) and add: 50 g sucrose (25 g/l) and 2 packets of mineral mix powder or 40 ml (20 ml/l) of mineral mix solution.

Mildly dehydrated patients, or after vomiting and diarrhoea
1 dose of ReSoMal can be administered in the following quantities:
- <10 kg   50 ml
- 10–30 kg   100 ml
- Adolescents, adults, and elderly   200–300 ml

Antimicrobial treatment for infantile diarrhoea is discouraged and anti-diarrhoeal drugs should not be given.

Severely dehydrated, severely malnourished patients
- Should receive ReSoMal 70–100 ml/kg body weight over 12 hrs to restore normal hydration.
- Start at 10 ml/kg/hr for the first 2 hrs (checking the patient's condition every 15 mins).
- Reduce to 5ml/kg/hr for the remaining 10 hrs (checking the patient's condition hourly).
- Use an NG tube at first and switch to oral administration as the patient's condition improves.
- Assess the patient frequently, in particular note the presence of thirst, diarrhoea, urine output, and level of consciousness.
- If the respiratory or pulse rate increases, the jugular veins become distended, or there is increasing abdominal distension, stop giving ReSoMal immediately and restrict fluids.

IV fluids
Only give fluids IV if the patient is unable to swallow and an NG tube cannot be used (severely dehydration or septic shock). Use:
- Half-strength Darrow's solution with 5% dextrose, *or*
- Ringer's lactate with 5% dextrose, *or*
- 0.45% (half-strength) normal saline with 5% dextrose (+ 20 mmol/l of KCl if available)

Change to NG tube administration as soon as possible. After the patient's condition improves, start the F-75 diet, initially with an NG tube but changing to oral administration as soon as the patient can tolerate it.

Clinical features of dehydration and septic shock in severely malnourished patients

	Moderate dehydration	Severe dehydration	Septic shock
Diarrhoea	Yes	Yes	Yes/no
Mental state	Restless and irritable	Lethargic and/or coma	Lethargic
Recent sunken eyes	Yes	Yes	No
Thirst	Drinks eagerly	Drinks poorly	Drinks poorly
Cool hands or feet	No	Yes	Yes
Weak/absent radial pulse	No	Yes	Yes
Urine flow	Reduced	Poor	Poor
Hypothermia	No	No	Yes/no
Recent weight loss	Yes	Yes	No

Tachycardia and tachypnoea

Cut-off points for tachycardia and tachypnoea are different for severely malnourished children compared to healthy children:

Tachycardia for malnourished:
<12 yrs	>120 beats per min
Adults	>100 beats per min

Tachypnoea for malnourished:
<2 months	>55 breaths per min
2–11 months	>45 breaths per min
12–59 months	>35 breaths per min

Micronutrient deficiencies

- **Vitamin A deficiency**: severely malnourished patients are at risk of developing blindness owing to vitamin A deficiency. Give to all severely malnourished patients on admission, day 2, and on discharge.
- **Folic acid deficiency**: if the therapeutic food is not fortified (e.g. HEM without vitamin mix), the patients should receive oral folic acid 5 mg daily.
- **Other micronutrients**: many patients are also deficient in riboflavin, ascorbic acid, pyridoxine, thiamine, and the fat-soluble vitamins (D, E, K). These are replaced by the fortified therapeutic foods.

Anaemia

Most malnourished patients are anaemic, due to chronic dietary iron deficiency, infections (malaria, hookworm), nutrient deficiencies (folic acid, vitamin C). Iron metabolism is deranged and erythrocyte production impaired. During the treatment of malnutrition, anaemia may worsen because the growing tissues require nutrients and there is increased circulating volume (mobilizing oedema, rehydration). Iron metabolism is deranged in malnutrition — iron is in reactive forms (free radicals) which damage tissues. This can worsen the condition (e.g. increase oedema). Iron in the gut can increase bacterial proliferation, leading to diarrhoea.

- Only after metabolism becomes normal (usually 14 days) should patients receive supplementation with 1–2 mg/kg/day of elemental iron.
- Use ferrous sulfate as tablets or crushed and dissolved into food.
- Those with moderate anaemia should receive 3 mg/kg/day elemental iron for 3 months (start after 14 days).

Severe anaemia in severely malnourished patients

This is often due to lack of utilization of iron (will be resolved through nutritional treatment), or expansion of blood and plasma volume (dilution develops during treatment), but not iron deficiency. Therefore, even severe anaemia in the initial phase is left untreated unless the patient has signs of heart failure. Transfusion for aneamia is often only effective in the first 24 hours of admission when the Hb is 3–4 g/dL (haematocrit <12%), with signs of heart failure. Transfusion is not recommended with a Hb >5 g/dL.

- If there are signs of heart failure, do an exchange transfusion. Withdraw 2.5 ml/kg of blood before starting the transfusion and at hourly intervals during it, so that the volume transfused = that removed.
- Give 10 ml of packed cells (or whole blood) per kg body weight slowly over 3 hrs.
- If there are signs of liver failure (purpura, jaundice, tender hepatomegaly) give a single dose of vitamin K 1 mg IM.
- During the blood transfusion, closely monitor vital signs and symptoms for congestive heart failure every 15 mins.
- Steroids should not be used, and no other drugs given.
- After the transfusion, feed by NG tube as outlined.

Micronutrient deficiencies

Micronutrients are categorized as either Type I or Type II.

Type I nutrient deficiencies result in specific deficiency diseases, and do not always affect growth but will affect metabolism and immune competence before signs are apparent: vits A, B_1, B_2, B_6, B_{12}, C, D, E, iron, calcium, copper, manganese, iodine, folic acid, selenium deficiencies.

Type II nutrient deficiencies do not show specific clinical signs. They affect metabolic processes and result in growth failure, wasting, increased risk of oedema, and lowered immune response: sulfur, potassium, sodium, magnesium, zinc, phosphorus, water, essential amino acids, nitrogen deficiencies.

Specific problems

Hypoglycaemia: (blood glucose <3 mmol/l or <54 mg/dl) is often a result of infection, and leads to hypothermia, lethargy, and confusion. Often confusion is the only sign before death. Give 1 ml/kg of 50% glucose IV upon admission, followed by 50 ml of 10% glucose (or sucrose) by NG tube to prevent recurrence. Further glucose may be required; close monitoring is required. As consciousness recovers, begin feeding or give 60 g/l Sucrose (glucose) in sterile water. Give prophylactic antibiotics as outlined below. Hypoglycaemia is prevented by immediate feeding on admission, feeding frequently, night feeding, and immediate treatment of infections.

Hypothermia: (rectal temp <35.5°C) is often associated with infections and usually occurs in the early morning. The patient will need warming through staying and sleeping with the caretaker and a warm environment (lamps, heater, blankets). Adopt the 'kangaroo' technique: the mother lies supine with her child on her chest, covered by her clothes and blankets. Avoid hyperthermia by over-heating. All hypothermic patients with malnutrition should be treated for hypoglycaemia and infection.

Diarrhoea: is commonly seen on admission and during treatment. Severely malnourished patients often have soft green, red, or brown coloured stools during the first days of treatment. This is normal and transient.
Watery stools can be due to excess osmolarity of the food, premature transfer to the next phase, or poorly balanced food. Adjust the diet by giving F75 or SDTM or just dilute the food by a third with water.
Milk intolerance may develop in the first few days, although it is rare and should be diagnosed only if there is copious, watery diarrhoea that occurs promptly after milk feeds are begun and that improves when milk is reduced or stopped. In such cases, milk should be substituted (totally or partially) by another liquid, but milk feeding should be attempted again before discharge, to determine whether the intolerance has resolved.
Profuse, sudden watery diarrhoea with or without fever could be due to bacterial or viral infections in the gut or elsewhere (e.g. pneumonia, malaria, otitis media).
Bloody diarrhoea (check!) could be shigella.
Profuse whitish diarrhoea could indicate cholera. Always check for dehydration and treat accordingly.

Congestive heart failure: unexpected sudden death a few days after admission — when the patient is eating well and gaining weight — is often because of congestive heart failure due to fluid overload. This could be a result of overhydration (too much ReSoMal or ORS) or overfeeding (too much food or liquid during one meal, high-protein diet, high-sodium diet) or blood transfusions. The symptoms are tachypnoea, tachycardia, prominent jugular veins, pulmonary congestion, cold hands and feet, and oedema. Early signs are increased respiratory rate and/or increase in oedema. These signs of incipient heart failure are easily confused with pneumonia.

Table 15.2 Clinical features of pneumonia and congestive heart failure

Symptom	Pneumonia	Congestive heart failure
Fever	Yes (but not always in severely malnourished)	No (unless concomitant infection)
Respiration	Tachypnoea Lower chest wall indrawing, head nodding, grunting, nasal flaring	Tachypnoea Superficial, no chest indrawing
Pulmonary auscultation	Coarse crackles or silence	Basal fine crackles
Cardiac auscultation	Tachycardia	Gallop rhythm, heart murmur, apex beat displaced
Jugular vein*	Normal	Prominent (raised pressure)
Liver*	Normal	Enlarged, tenderness and pain
Extremities	Warm or cyanosed and cold	Cyanosed and cold
Oedema	No oedema or no increase (in case of kwashiorkor)	Sudden increase (puffy eyes)
History	Cough?	Signs of severe anaemia Occurs during transfusion or rehydration Occurs when increasing feeds

* Hepatomegaly and hepato-jugulo reflux (when compressing the liver) are early and specific signs of CHF, especially in small children.

Incipient heart failure: should be treated by stopping oral intake. If the patient's respiratory rate is back to normal (after 12–24 hrs) start feeding cautiously, initially with small amounts.

In heart failure with fluid overload:
- Stop all oral and IV fluids; the treatment of heart failure takes precedence over feeding, even if it takes 24 hrs.
- Give furosemide 0.5–1.5 mg/kg IV (max 20 mg/day in children).
- Never use diuretics to reduce oedema in oedematous malnutrition, so check the JVP to establish if the circulation is overloaded or not.
- Give digoxin 20–30 mcg/kg IV stat (PO if IV not possible) if the diagnosis of heart failure is definite, once the plasma potassium concentration has been corrected. Maintenance dose is 5–10 mcg/kg od
- Provide oxygen.
- Sit the patient upright with legs down if possible.

Specific infections

Severely malnourished patients may not show the typical signs and symptoms of infection. During the treatment both malaria and cross-infections from other patients become more common. The most common infections are:
- Pneumonia
- URTI
- UTI
- Otitis media
- TB

Others include: hepatitis B, malaria, HIV/AIDS, and dengue.

Keep in mind that oral dosages must be higher because of malabsorption and decreased immune response in severely malnourished.

Otitis media: occurs frequently — signs are non-specific (fever, restlessness), although the child may pull on his/her ears due to pain. If the tympanic membrane ruptures, there may be a purulent discharge. Examine the ear with an otoscope and treat with co-trimoxazole or amoxicillin for 5 days. A cotton wick will help to dry any discharge.

TB and HIV/AIDS: are important and interrelated causes of treatment failure. The tuberculin skin test may be negative in severe malnutrition, becoming positive as the nutritional status improves.

N.B. Malnutrition can result from unrecognized serious congenital abnormalities, inborn errors of metabolism, malignancies, immunological disease, and other diseases of major organs.

In general, whatever the identity and treatability of the underlying disease, malnutrition should be treated as above. The condition of the patient will improve, resulting in prolonged and improved quality of life.

Rashes

Skin changes (which include areas of hypo- and hyperpigmentation) are common in kwashiorkor and can easily become infected. They usually resolve as the child's nutritional status improves. However, in the intervening period they should be disinfected, and then left dry and exposed.

- If the skin is very painful or infected, apply zinc and castor oil ointment, petroleum jelly, or paraffin gauze dressings.
- Use nystatin cream/ointment and oral nystatin if the skin becomes infected with *Candida* spp.
- Disinfect bacterially infected skin with chlorhexidine-cetrimide or bathe in 0.01% potassium permanganate solution for 10–15 mins daily. Povidone-iodine 10% may also be used (sparingly for large lesions, since it is systemically absorbed). Children with this condition must receive systemic antibiotics (flucloxacillin or co-trimoxazole).

Scabies

Very common and can lead to serious skin infections. Give ivermectin 150–200 mcg PO stat on empty stomach or apply 25% benzyl benzoate to the skin (not recommended for children). Trim the patient's fingernails and treat the family.

Candidiasis

Common infection in severely malnourished patients. Lesions in the mouth are painful and impair feeding.

- Treat with nystatin: 100,000 IU as oral suspension or lozenges qds after food, usually for 7 days, but continuing for 48 hrs after lesions have resolved. Immunosuppressed patients may need higher doses.
- Use a NG tube to allow feeding in the presence of very painful oral lesions.

Breastfeeding as treatment of malnourished infants

In areas where malnutrition is prevalent, breastfeeding should be encouraged. Breast milk increases immunity, is hygienic, clean, and cheap, with a good supply. Artificial feeding in circumstances of poverty is associated with contamination (teats, bottles, milk left standing too long, unclean water) and with dilution (no money to buy more milk, sharing with siblings). This can result in malnutrition through a combination of inadequate intake of artificial milk and repeated episodes of diarrhoea.

In times of insecurity, anxiety, and migration, breast milk might be reduced. Mothers often think they produce less breast milk and are not able to produce more because they are themselves malnourished. However, breast milk production only suffers in quantity with an intake of less than about 1700 kCal/day. In contrast, quality (especially of micronutrients) is quickly affected by the mother's diet. Therefore a mother's complaint that she does not have enough milk should be properly investigated.

When the milk production is reduced or stopped, breastfeeding should be encouraged and the mother supported with, amongst other things, nutritious food. Only if there is no other option should a supply of artificial feeding be secured and the mother (or caretaker) trained in using the milk in a safe way.

Pregnant women who are HIV +ve have two choices: exclusive breastfeeding with abrupt weaning at 3–6 months or exclusive artificial feeding (no breast milk at all). Mixing methods of feeding, by prolonging breastfeeding, increases the risk of HIV transmission. In exclusively breastfed infants, the risk of HIV is <15%. The use of artificial milk can increase the risk of mortality, depending on the hygienic and economic circumstances of the mother. Exclusive artificial feeding may stigmatize the mother more than exclusive breastfeeding. The public health approach in areas where the prevalence of HIV is high is to promote exclusive breastfeeding and abrupt weaning, regardless of HIV status. Women in advanced HIV stages are recommended to adopt artificial feeding.

Talk to the mother about breastfeeding
- Why it helps her baby to breastfeed exclusively
- That it takes patience and perseverance
- That the baby should be allowed to suckle at least 10 times in 24 hrs, more if it wants (offer the breast every 2 hrs, suckle on demand, suckle longer, breastfeed at night)
- That she should have enough to eat and drink and enough time to rest
- That she should keep her baby near her, for plenty of skin to skin contact
- That she should avoid teats, feeding bottles (they are not hygienic and make the baby 'lazy'), and pacifiers

Signs that a baby is not getting enough milk

- Poor weight gain
- Small amounts of concentrated urine (strong smelling and yellow)
- Baby unsatisfied after a breast feed
- Baby refuses to breastfeed
- Baby takes long breast feeds
- No milk extracted when pressed
- Breast milk not produced after delivery
- Mother's breasts do not enlarge

Milk supplementation

The supplemental suckling method induces lactation by providing additional therapeutic milk to the infant while he/she is suckling. The infant's suckling should stimulate the production of milk by the mother. The infant's efforts are rewarded by milk flow, which in turn stimulates suckling. This method is useful if an infant is not interested or is too weak to suckle from a breast that does not yet produce milk.

For the first 1–2 days, give the full amount of artificial feed for a baby of his/her weight or the same amount that he/she has been having before. As soon as the mother's breast milk begins to flow, she can start to reduce the daily total by 30–60 ml each day. If a baby is still breastfeeding sometimes, the breast milk supply increases in a few days. If a baby has stopped breastfeeding, it may take 1–2 weeks or more before much breast milk comes.

Check the baby's weight gain and urine output to make sure that he/she is getting enough milk. If not the case, do not reduce the artificial feed for a few days — if necessary, increase the amount of artificial milk for a day or two.

Supplemental suckling technique

1. Use a fine NG tube.
2. Attach the tip of the NG tube to the mother's breast at the nipple (at the top or side — see Fig. 15.5).
3. Put the other end of the tube in the cup of diluted therapeutic milk.
4. The breast with tube is offered to the infant. Ensure that the tip of the NG tube is in the infant's mouth.
5. Keep the cup at least 20–30 cm below the level of the baby's mouth.
6. If the presence of the tube is discouraging the baby from attaching, slip the tube into the mouth once the infant has started to suckle.
7. Help the mother to regulate the flow of milk from the tube, so that the baby does not feed too fast, thereby stimulating the breast too little.
   The flow can be regulated by:
   • Closing the tube a bit with a paper clip, loose knot, or finger pinch
   • Lifting or lowering the container
   • Attaching the tube to a syringe and using the piston

Alternative: the supplement can also be put into the side of the infant's mouth using a syringe or dropper while the infant is suckling

• Remind the mother to let her infant suckle at any time she is willing — not only when she is using the supplementer.
• Keep the NG tube clean by rinsing with chlorinated water. The tube should be changed every day.

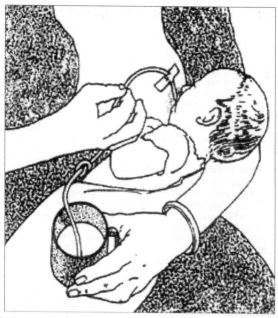

Fig. 15.5

Severe malnutrition in infants

Feeding problems — due to sickness or the absence of the infant's mother, insufficient breast milk (stress, war, drought), inappropriate alternative infant feeding (unsafe bottle feeding) — can be causes of severe malnutrition as well as illness in infants.

Diagnosis of severe malnutrition in young infants (<6 months of age or 65 cm in length) is not only based on low weight, because a low weight for height (W/H) index may result from low birth weight (<2.5 kg).
Criteria are:
- W/H below 70%, *and either*
- Weight loss or growth stagnation (for 1–2 weeks), *or*
- Poor clinical status (illness, apathy, etc.)

Three-phase nutritional treatment
- *Starting phase (1–15 days):* the total caloric intake (breast milk plus diluted therapeutic milk) should be 105 kCal/kg/day (140 ml/kg/day SDTM). The supplemental suckling technique should be used.
- *Mid phase (2 days):* when breast milk output increases after 10 to 15 days, SDTM can gradually be reduced to half the amount (52 kCal/kg/day = 70 ml/kg/day SDTM) for 2 days, and then stopped completely.
- *Final phase (minimum of 4 days):* the infant should be exclusively breastfed under close supervision.

Treatment for non-breastfed infants: increase the amount of SDTM from 105 kCal/kg/day to 120 kCal/kg/day. Once a non-breastfed infant has gained weight for 3 consecutive days (in the starting phase), SDTM can be gradually replaced by 'normal' breast milk substitutes, following the same principles. Make sure the calorie intake is gradually increased to 120–150 kCal/kg/day (120 kCal/kg/day is normal intake; 150 kCal/kg/day is for extra growth).

Monitoring: monitor weight gain on a daily basis. A special maternity type scale (10 g precision) is necessary. If an infant loses weight for 3 consecutive days, either the amount of food offered is not enough (breast milk plus therapeutic milk), or underlying medical or social problems must be addressed.

Medical treatment: severely malnourished infants require a medical check-up and treatment. The rationale is similar as that for the treatment of severe malnutrition in non-infants. (Mothers also require a medical check-up and treatment, including a malaria test.) Use syrup, suspensions, or drops when available. Give:
- Antibiotics — amoxicillin: infants <3 months, max dose of 15 mg/kg od; otherwise 20–40 mg/kg daily in divided doses for children less than 20 kg; for at least 5 days.
- Vitamin A — 50,000 IU days 1, 2, and at discharge; mothers should be given 200,000 IU.
- Folic acid — 5 mg on day 1

Principles of nutritional treatment of infants

- Stimulate breastfeeding.
- Supplement with specially diluted therapeutic milk (SDTM) through the supplemental suckling technique if breastfeeding is insufficient. F75 should not be used.
- Use a 3-phase treatment regimen to gradually decrease supplement and increase breast milk.

All of the following conditions should be met before discharge:

- Satisfactory clinical status and absence of infections.
- Minimum weight gain of 100–125 g/week without therapeutic milk supplementation for 7 days (minimum 5 g/kg/day, target 10 g/kg/day).
- For breastfed infants — active suckling and well-established breast milk production.
- For non-breastfed infants — a supply of breast milk substitutes must be ensured and the caretaker should be aware about safe hygienic methods for preparation and about the dangers associated with artificial feeding.

Neonatal tetanus

Difficulty in suckling starting 3–21 days after birth can be an early sign of neonatal tetanus. Obtain a detailed history of the mother's vaccination status and umbilical cord care.

Complications

Hypothermia: is a major cause of mortality in malnourished infants. It is therefore important to keep infants warm: skin to skin contact (kangaroo position); give mother hot beverages; provide blankets and hats.

Dehydration: use Re-So-Mal.

Malaria: test on admission and then on clinical basis. Sulfadoxine-pyrimethamine should not be given to children <2 mths old.

Anaemia: iron is given as treatment for anaemia not as routine therapy. Give 2 mg/kg tds (preferably as a syrup, e.g. Galfer or Fersamal) for >3 mths, but only after 14 days of nutritional treatment. When the Hb is <5 g/dl, consider blood transfusion after careful medical evaluation.

Candidiasis: is frequent in newborns — treat with nystatin.

Patient care and facilities

Treatment facility: the setting to treat severely malnourished patients depends on availability of hospital or health centre, number of patients, workload of mothers, distance from home, and culture — see box.

Psycho-social and educational considerations

Psycho-social support: during the treatment, create a positive and stimulating atmosphere by organizing entertainment — plays, toys, songs, dance. Organize professional, culturally appropriate care for patients and caretakers who have an apparent psycho-social problem (e.g. marriage/ relationship, alcoholism, domestic violence, sexual violence, trauma). Involvement of caretakers in organization of activities (kitchen, entertainment) increases the ownership of the treatment.

Treatment of adults and adolescents: follows the same principles as for children. However, the psycho-social context is different: adults may be depressed and anorexic; they often don't have caretakers; the physical tolerance for milk-based diets is low and on top of that they have their own opinions about foods (e.g. a diet based on milk is only accepted the first few days; porridge is often a problem too; adults like to add salt to their food).

Educate: patients and caretakers about proper feeding (with the resources available), feeding the sick (e.g. HIV/AIDS), breastfeeding, and hygienic food handling.

Check that

- Caretakers (or patients) know how to deal with anticipated problems before discharge.
- There is a caretaker and economic support for the family (e.g. by the community).
- Follow-up visits have been arranged for education and social support (e.g. 1 wk, 2 wks, 1 mth, and 6 mths after discharge).

It might be possible to form support groups in which people discuss with each other the problems they face and the possible solutions (eg. HIV/AIDS patients).

Monitoring

All patients should be weighed daily and the weight plotted on a graph. The expected weight gain for children is 10–15 g/kg/day. A child who does not gain at least 5 g/kg per day is failing to respond. Examine the patient carefully at least twice a day in the initial phase, measuring temperature, pulse rate, BP, and RR.

Accurate records should be kept of all patients who fail to respond and of all deaths due to malnutrition. Periodic review of these records can help to identify areas where management practices should be carefully examined and improved.

In a TFC, using these data, the coverage, success, and mortality rates should be regularly evaluated using the following criteria:

Coverage rate: the number of severely malnourished children admitted, divided by the total number of severely malnourished children in the population (i.e. refugee camp), based on the latest survey. Target TFC >80%

Success rate: the number of children reaching criteria for discharge, divided by the number of children admitted within a given period. Target TFC >80%

Mortality rate: the number of deaths in the centre, divided by the number of children admitted at the centre within a given period. Target TFC <5%

Therapeutic feeding centre (TFC) (or TFC ward in hospital): highly efficient facility specializing in treatment of severely malnourished. Ideally a 24-hr facility. An alternative set-up is to give phase 1 and transition phase care in 24-hr care units, and the rehabilitation phase in day care, or even as outpatient (every 3 days, or weekly). The TFC is only feasible with >20 patients.

In hospitals without a special TFC ward: malnutrition is dealt with as any other disease. Ensure the doctors and nurses are trained to avoid common mistakes (see p. 624). The feeding and monitoring of the treatment should be properly organized. In hospitals, the risk of cross infections is high, so discharge as soon as possible to a follow-up facility.

Health centre: if only a few cases are presenting with severe malnutrition, give treatment through the regular health staff. Health centres often only offer day care, but a night nurse can monitor an occasional critical patient. During the initial phase, patients come back daily; in the rehabilitation phase, the contact is less frequent.

Home based care: treatment meant for uncomplicated severely malnourished cases and alternative for phase 2. It is based on RTUTF (ready to eat therapeutic food), access to a health facility, and well-trained home visitors. Complicated cases based are sent to a hospital.

Failure to respond to treatment

A severely malnourished patient should show signs of improvement within a few days and continue to improve thereafter.

Criteria for failure to respond — see box.

Assessment of failure to respond

The patient should be examined, weighed, measured, and the results charted. Check the patient's recent health (oedema, temperature, vomiting, diarrhoea, medical problems, immunization e.g. measles), feeding practices (eating well, night feed), and play (sits, crawls, stands, or walks; mental state has improved — smiles, responds to stimuli, interested in surroundings).

Poor practices in treatment unit

- Incorrect food prescription
- Incorrect food preparation (too much energy and protein during phase 1; high-sodium diet)
- Improper preparation (kitchen)
- Poor organization of food distribution
- Lack of feeding at night
- Poor storage and hygienic handling (heating, cooling, hand washing, etc.)
- Failure to monitor food intake (patient disliking food, food eaten by siblings)
- Underlying infections (e.g. UTI, ARI, otitis, candidiasis, TB, AIDS, cross-infections)
- Malabsorption (improper management of diarrhoea, hurrying to intermediate or rehabilitation phase)
- Poor organization of facility (failure to distinguish between phase I and II)
- Lack of support and time for feeding (~15 mins is needed to feed one patient; 1 staff member is needed for 10 patients)
- Lack of blankets
- Poor medical treatment: e.g. diuretics for oedema; iron supplement at admission; IV fluids given unnecessarily; wrong use of oral rehydration solution; vitamin A and antibiotics not given.
- Lack of psychological and emotional support (e.g. unrecognized depression, anorexia)

Causes of poor practices

- Poor training of staff; inadequate skills; poor staff attitudes (especially in hospital setting)
- Poor motivation of staff — insufficient salary, insecurity
- Lack of funds for food items, drugs, proper measuring and weighing machines, etc.
- Incorrect focus on diseases instead of malnutrition (esp. on paediatric wards)

Criteria for failure to respond

1° *failure to respond*	*Time after admission*
• Fails to regain appetite	By day 4
• Fails to start to lose oedema	By day 4
• Oedema still present	By day 10
• Fails to gain weight at >5 g/kg/day	By day 10

2° *failure to respond*	
• Fails to gain >5 g/kg/day for 3 successive days	During rehabilitation

Vitamin A deficiency

Vitamin A is required for rhodopsin production in the retina and also for an effective immune response. Its deficiency causes increased susceptibility to systemic infections, in particular measles, and eye complications (xerophthalmia) which causes blindness in about 250,000 children each year.

Clinical features: eye signs approximate to severity and duration of vitamin A deficiency and are classified XN, X1, X2, X3, and XS:

Night blindness (XN): occurs due to rhodopsin deficiency in retinal cone cells. Difficult to assess in children — ask the mother whether the child bumps into objects in poor lighting.

Conjunctival xerosis (X1a): dryness of the conjunctiva results in increased susceptibility to infection and trauma.

Bitot's spots (X1b): are white foamy spots on the surface of the conjunctiva, commonly at the corneoscleral junction on the temporal side. As the cornea is not involved, vision is normal. Spots may be bilateral or pigmented and may persist beyond the period of vitamin A deficiency.

Corneal xerosis (X2): similar to X1a, but the cornea is now involved. Most common in children aged 2–4 yrs and may be the start of visual impairment.

Corneal ulceration (X3a): may be superficial or deep. If it is central, it will profoundly affect vision.

Keratomalacia (X3b): in severe deficiency, the cornea may suddenly melt (keratomalacia). Most common in children aged 1–3 yrs; may be bilateral. At this stage, mortality increases because of generalized susceptibility to other infections.

Corneal scarring (XS): the result of healing (after vitamin A supplementation) of stages X2 and X3. The extent of scarring determines the degree of permanent visual impairment.

Management of vitamin A deficiency

- Give 3 doses of oral vitamin A at day 1, day 2, and in week 3.
- With the 1st dose, give topical antibiotic eye ointment (e.g. tetracycline 1% or chloramphenicol 1%) for 10 days.
- If the cornea is involved, close the eye and gently cover with an eye pad. Refer the patient to a specialist.

Pregnancy: high doses of vitamin A are contraindicated during pregnancy. A pregnant woman with signs of xerophthalmia should be given vitamin A 5,000–10,000 IU PO od for at least 4 weeks. At delivery, give the mother 200,000 IU, which will ensure an adequate supply for both mother and breastfed baby.

Prevention: eat spinach, carrots, sweet potatoes, mangos, papaya, milk, eggs, red palm oil, liver, fish liver oils. A supplementation campaign with vitamin A capsules can be organized every 6 months for children up to 10 yrs and pregnant and lactating women (doses to be given at each supplimentation are given in the box opposite). Any child with measles should be given vitamin A 200,000 IU PO od for 2 days.

Preventive and curative doses of vitamin A

0–6 mths	50,000 IU
6–12 mths	100,000 IU
>1 yr (including adults)	200,000 IU
Vitamin A deficient pregnant women	10,000 IU

200,000 IU of vitamin A is equal to 66 mg of retinyl acetate, or 110 mg of retinyl palmitate equivalent

Iodine deficiency: goitre

Endemic goitre is found in areas where dietary iodine is deficient — usually in mountainous regions with poor soil and high rainfall. It also occurs where goitrogen-containing foods such as cassava (manioc) and cabbage are staples. These vegetables contain compounds that impose an abnormally high demand upon the thyroid or interfere with iodine metabolism within the gland. About 1 billion people are at risk of iodine deficiency.

Clinical features

- Goitre, hypothyroidism, loss of energy
- Miscarriages, stillbirths
- In children: mental retardation (cretinism), deaf mutism, spastic diplegia, strabismus, myxoedema

Classification of goitre due to iodine deficiency

Grade 0: thyroid not palpable or visible
Grade 1: thyroid palpable but not visible when the neck is in normal position
Grade 2: thyroid palpable and visible when the neck is in normal position
Thyroid follicular enlargement occurs due to thyroid-stimulating hormone (TSH) release from the pituitary. Eventually nodules form, with occasional calcification and haemorrhage. Compression can cause dysphagia and hoarseness (recurrent laryngeal nerve involvement). The patient is usually euthyroid. Chronic goitres do not lead to malignancy.

Management: give 1 dose of iodized oil (see box). Repeat after 1 yr (oral) or 2 yrs (IM).
Home-made recipe: make a 0.15% solution of potassium iodide (30 mg of potassium iodide in 20 ml of boiled water) and give 4–6 drops daily.
Lugol's iodine (often kept for sterilization) may also be given as 1 drop every 30 days, or 1 daily teaspoon of a solution containing 1 drop of Lugol's iodine in 30 ml of water.
Massive goitres may need surgery.

Prevention: marketing iodized salt is a sustainable measure. Where >10% of people have a visible goitre, severe iodine deficiency is a problem and mass prevention should be undertaken with IM injections of iodized oil or oral iodine.
Iodine should be given to women in endemic regions before pregnancy to prevent cretinism.

Therapeutic and preventive dosage of iodized oil

	Oral dose in mg of iodine* (Oral therapy will last 12 mths)	IM dose in mg of iodine** (IM therapy will last 1–3 yrs)
Birth–1 yr	100 mg	240 mg
Children 1–5 yrs	200 mg	480 mg
Children 6–15 yrs	400 mg	480 mg
Pregnant women	300–400 mg	480 mg
Non-pregnant women and men <45 yrs	400–1000 mg	480 mg

* Lipodiol capsule (0.4 ml): 1 capsule = 200 mg iodine (oral treatment)
** Lipiodol injectable (ultra-fluid): 1 ml = 480 mg of iodine

Vitamin B₁ (thiamine) deficiency: beriberi

Vitamin B₁ is vital for carbohydrate metabolism and nervous system function. It is present in most food but absent from white rice that has been polished. Pregnant or lactating women and children are vulnerable to beriberi; it may also complicate alcoholism and treatment of trypanosomiasis with nitrofurazone.

Defective carbohydrate metabolism primarily affects CNS and peripheral nerves (dry or paraplegic beriberi) and cardiac muscle (wet or cardiac beriberi) — a mixture of the two forms is common.

Clinical features

Dry beriberi: is a mixed sensory and motor peripheral neuropathy. Gradual onset of weakness and wasting, commencing in legs, often with foot drop and wasted calves. Weakness spreads proximally, eventually involving the arms. The tendon reflexes are lost; affected muscles show oedema and painful contraction when hit. Anaesthesia spreads in a 'stocking and glove' fashion and there is a loss of joint position sense. Ataxia develops requiring the use of a stick. Incontinence occurs in the terminal stages. Death is from generalized and diaphragmatic paralysis.

Wet beriberi: is high-output right heart failure (RHF) with generalized oedema and oliguria. The extremities are initially well perfused; the JVP raised, with marked pulsation due to tricuspid incompetence, and BP low, with a high pulse pressure. The heart sounds become evenly spaced, giving a 'tick-tack' rhythm and dilated valve rings give regurgitant murmurs. Tender pulsatile hepatomegaly, pleural effusions, and ascites may occur. Congestive heart failure causes death.

Infantile beriberi: occurs in infants breastfed from a vitamin B₁-deficient mother. Onset is typically at age 2–3 mths, with irritability and slight oedema that may initially be confused with kwashiorkor, but heart failure occurs rapidly and death may follow in as little as 36 hrs. Older children may have a chronic form similar to adults.

Diagnosis:
ECG and CXR show signs of RHF in cardiac beriberi. There is increased plasma pyruvate (up to 2 mg/dl) and lactate; red cell transketolase levels are low.

Management

Severe acute beriberi: give 50–100 mg thiamine IV tds, followed, when improving, by 10 mg/day PO. Bed rest, fluid restriction, and a high-protein/low-salt diet, supplemented with regular thiamine IM injections or tablets. In moribund patients, venesection of 300 ml blood (in an adult) may relieve the heart failure.

Non-urgent beriberi: give thiamine 10 mg/day PO for 6 weeks. Pain in limbs is relieved rapidly; peripheral neuropathy resolves in months–years.

Infantile beriberi: give 25 mg thiamine IV followed by thiamine 25 mg IM 1–2× daily until symptoms have subsided. Then give thiamine 10 mg/day PO od for 3–4 weeks. Treat the lactating mother with thiamine 10 mg PO for 6 weeks.

Prevention: avoid white rice in favour of parboiled rice (pre-steamed) and whole grain rice. Yeast is an excellent source of vitamin B₁.

Vitamin B₂ (riboflavin) deficiency

Ariboflavinosis is due to vitamin B_2 (riboflavin) deficiency and is found worldwide, often in the presence of other vitamin B deficiencies. Riboflavin is essential for normal oxidative metabolism.

Clinical features: angular stomatitis, sore red lips, increased vertical fissuring of the lips (perleche), purplish raw tongue with enlarged papillae. There may be plugging of sebaceous glands with sebum, giving a roughened appearance to the skin, and scrotal dermatitis.

Management: is with 2–5 mg of riboflavin daily and advice regarding diet. The condition is rapidly cured.

Prevention: the main sources of vitamin B_2 are meat, vegetables, milk, and wholemeal flour.

Nicotinic acid (niacin) deficiency: pellagra

Pellagra is due to deficiency of nicotinic acid (niacin) and its precursors (the amino acid tryptophan). It is common in African communities where maize and sorghum are staples. Nicotinic acid in maize is not bioavailable, and sorghum is rich in leucine which adversely affects nicotinic acid and tryptophan metabolism. Pellagra also occurs in intestinal malabsorption, prolonged high-dose isoniazid treatment, alcoholism, and metastatic carcinoid syndrome. Nicotinic acid deficiency leads to metabolic disturbances, especially in the nervous system. It is often complicated by riboflavine deficiency.

Clinical features: pellagra is characterized by diarrhoea, dermatitis, and dementia. Symptoms may regress and remit according to seasonal and dietary changes, but usually progress over years.

  The patient may initially have vague abdominal symptoms, giddiness, and joint pain (the pre-pellagrous state). The sclerae appear bluish and the patient's character may change, becoming irritable and morose. With time, other signs develop.

Gastrointestinal: gingival swelling and/or bleeding; tongue becomes scarlet, raw, and fissured, and may atrophy; dysphagia due to a burning sensation in the oesophagus. Abdominal discomfort, diarrhoea (often steatorrheic), nausea, and excessive salivation can occur, as well as constipation (occasionally).

Skin: lesions appear at sites exposed to sunlight or subject to pressure. A reddish rash appears on the back of the hands and feet, spreading to the rest of the body in irregular patches. Classically there is a symmetrical lesion at the back of the neck, or a collar-like ring around the neck with a 'v' shape if a shirt is worn (Casal's necklace). Lesions are swollen, itch or burn, commonly have petechiae, and are worse on exposure to sunlight. After 10–14 days, the rash becomes hyperkeratotic and desquamates. Atrophic patches of skin remain between the fingers; the nails become brittle and atrophic.

CNS: signs include insomnia, anxiety, depression, photophobia; acute mania or psychosis (which may be permanent); cogwheel rigidity of the extremities and frontal reflexes. Often there is profound melancholia and suicidal tendencies. Confusion can precede death.

Peripheral nerves: neuropathy and/or paraplegia (spastic or ataxic), tremors, rigidity, paraesthesiae, exaggerated reflexes, upgoing plantar reflex. Cranial nerves are sometimes involved.

Eye: conjunctival oedema, corneal dystrophy, and lens opacities extending from the periphery to the centre.

Diagnosis: plasma nicotinic acid is <0.31 mg/dl in acute disease.

Management: give nicotinamide 150–250 mg PO bd to children and adults until complete recovery (at least 3–4 weeks). Some doctors double the dose in severe disease. Provide a high-energy, balanced diet that is rich in the various B vitamins (e.g. 25–30 g yeast daily).

Prevention: in the case of confirmed outbreaks, weekly vitamin B complex supplementation for the entire population can be undertaken as a short-term measure: give nicotinamide 15 mg/person/day by a weekly distribution of 7 × 15 mg tablets/person.

Vitamin B₁₂ (cobalamin) deficiency

Vitamin B_{12} deficiency is seen in infants/neonates born to, and breastfed by, women deficient in vitamin B_{12}. Vitamin B_{12} and folate are essential for the synthesis of DNA; deficiency produces megaloblastic anaemia. Deficiency may also result from: inadequate intake over years; pernicious anaemia; malabsorption due to ileal disease (e.g. tropical sprue); and disturbed metabolism following nitrous oxide or cyanide poisoning.

Clinical features: the infant/child may show developmental delay, involuntary movements, hypotonia, peripheral neuropathy, optic atrophy, psychiatric disturbances, and subacute combined degeneration of the cord. There may be hyperpigmentation of the palmar and plantar skin and mucous membranes.

Diagnosis: low plasma B_{12}; megaloblastic anaemia with hypersegmented neutrophils and macro-ovalocytes on blood film. The Schilling test diagnoses malabsorption and pernicious anaemia.

Management: give 6 doses of hydroxycobalamin 1 mg IM 3 × per week 2 weeks (6 doses) for to replenish body stores. For patients with malabsorption, continue to give 1 mg IM every 3 months (if necessary, for life). Neonates may be given 0.1 mg per day PO, whilst also treating the deficient mother.

Vitamin C (ascorbic acid) deficiency: scurvy

Scurvy occurs in arid areas where fruit and vegetables are scarce. Vitamin C is essential for the formation of collagen, is an important antioxidant, and helps absorption of iron; it is essential for wound healing and growth.

Clinical features

Adults: gradual weight loss, weakness, swollen painful large joints, muscular stiffness, bruising. The gums swell and become spongy, eventually bleeding and causing loss of teeth. Skin petechiae and purpura occur; wounds fail to heal. There may be microcytic, hypochromic anaemia. Women and the elderly are commonly affected.

Infants: commonly starts at 6–12 months in premature and artificially fed babies. Erupting teeth cause bleeding of the gums; subperiosteal haemorrhage causes limb pain and may be palpable at distal femur and proximal tibia. Costochondral beading may be palpable (scorbutic rosary). Occasionally there is bloody diarrhoea. Anaemia is microcytic and hypochromic, but may be megaloblastic if accompanied by folate deficiency. Bone X-rays show epiphyseal changes and ground glass appearance of the shafts.

Diagnosis: use Hess test — petechiae appear upon occlusion of venous return in the arm with a sphygmomanometer. Measure urinary vitamin C excretion following saturating dose of ascorbic acid; if it is decreased, the patient has scurvy.

Management: ascorbic acid divided in 3 doses for 2 weeks: infants 50 mg/day; children 150 mg/day; adults 500 mg/day. Followed by preventive treatment: children and adults: 50–100 mg/day.

Prevention

- **Vitamin B_{12} deficiency** — eat foods rich in vitamin B_{12}: liver, kidney, clams, eggs, and milk products. Fruit and vegetables are low in vitamin B12.
- **Vitamin C deficiency** — avoid overcooking vegetables (vitamin C is destroyed by prolonged heat), consume fresh fruit (especially oranges, guava, limes); if necessary (e.g. in refugee camps) give tablet supplementation (children and adults: 50–100 mg/day).

Vitamin D deficiency: rickets and osteomalacia

Vitamin D is produced in human skin by the action of sunlight (15 mins/day is enough). The disease therefore tends to affect children and/or women deprived of sunlight due to social or religious reasons. Rickets and osteomalacia are infantile and adult diseases, respectively, of abnormal bone calcification resulting from vitamin D deficiency. They may also result from renal failure, epilepsy treatment, and cirrhosis — all of which alter vitamin D metabolism.

Clinical features

Rickets: onset is within the first 2 yrs of life. The child is pale, irritable, and mentally and physically retarded. There may be delayed closure of the fontanelles and deformities of the spine, chest (pigeon chest, rickety 'rosary' of swollen costochondral junctions), pelvis, and limbs (bow legs, knocked-knees), and softening of the skull (bossing, craniotabes). Hypocalcaemia may cause tetany and laryngeal stridor.

Osteomalacia: usually occurs in women, often during the first pregnancy, and presents with softened, painful bones (pelvis, ribs, femora) and fractures. Hypocalcaemia produces tetany and there may be spontaneous fractures and anaemia.

Diagnosis

Rickets: the line of osteochondral calcification is broadened and rarefied on X-rays, producing cupped, ragged metaphyseal surfaces.

Osteomalacia: uncalcified osteoid tissue at the growing ends of bone results in enlargement. Looser's zones are partial fractures without bony displacement (often of lateral scapular border, inferior femoral neck, or medial femoral shaft). Hypocalcaemia occurs eventually.

Management: give vitamin D weekly for 1 month and then monthly for 3 months. Dose: child 100,000 IU/week PO (or 4000 to 8000 IU/day); adults 300,000 IU/week. 500 mg of calcium should be given daily for the first 15 days of treatment.

Vitamin E deficiency

Vitamin E is an antioxidant, required for cellular protection against oxidative stresses. The best dietary sources are fats and oils but it is destroyed by prolonged storage, heat, or exposure to oxidants. Deficiency affects neonates fed with artificial milk. In adults deficiency may cause myopathy and sensory neuropathy. **Treatment** is with vitamin E 300 mg (400 IU) up to twice daily.

Vitamin K deficiency

Vitamin K is essential for the formation of clotting factors II, VII, IX, and X, and coagulation inhibitors (proteins C and S). Deficiency results in a bleeding tendency. The vitamin is found in leafy green vegetables and is also produced by intestinal bacteria. Deficiency affects poorly fed neonates and adults with malabsorption. The prothrombin time is prolonged. **Treatment** is with vitamin K (up to 10 mg IV as a single dose) in cases of haemorrhage. Dietary advice suffices in most non-bleeding cases.

Obesity

The terms overweight and obese are interchangeable: a person is too heavy for their height compared with standard references. People become obese because they take in more calories in food and drink than they consume in metabolism and work. The extra calories are stored as fat. There is a high calorific intake when people eat large amounts of food at each meal, when they eat snacks between meals, or drink a lot of beer. Obesity tends to be a disease of the better-off, those who live in cities, and those who have sedentary jobs. Obesity increases the risk of coronary heart disease, stroke, hypertension, type II diabetes, gallstones and other digestive disorders, back problems, arthritis of the knees and hips, accidents, fractures, and fatigue.

Diagnosis: obesity can be assessed using the BMI in adults (excluding pregnant women). A BMI >25 indicates probable obesity; >30 definite obesity. Children are obese if they are greater than the 97th centile on either the weight for height curve or the weight for age curve (growth chart) (see p. 599).

Management: weight loss is notoriously difficult.

- Eat foods containing more fibre and less fat or sugar. For snacks, eat fruit or maize cobs; avoid sweets, chips, crisps, and cakes. Cut down on alcohol, especially beer.
- Exercise for >20 mins per day at a level sufficient to raise the pulse and respiratory rates. It is pointless setting your patient an exercise regime more suited to athletes in training — be realistic and always offer encouragement, not scorn.
- Advise stopping smoking as a means of reducing additional risks of vascular disease.

References/further information

Guidelines

MSF (2004) *Nutrition guidelines*

Rajabiun S et al. (2000) *HIV/AIDS: a guide for nutrition, care and support. FANTA project.* Academy for Educational Development, Washington.

UNHCR/WFP (1999) *Guidelines for selective feeding programmes in emergency situation.*

WHO (1999) *Management of severe malnutrition: a manual for physicians and other senior health workers.* WHO, Geneva.

WHO, WFP, UNHCR, IFRC (2000) *The management of nutrition in major emergencies.* WHO, Geneva.

Young H and Jaspars J (1995) *Nutrition matters.* Part I. Intermediate Technology Publication, London, pp. 3–24.

Websites

Commodities: http://www.usaid.gov/hum_response/crg/

Food composition: http://www.fao.org/infoods/software/worldfood.html

Subjects: http://www.fantaproject.org/publications/anthropom.shtml

Subjects medical: http://www.who.int/emc-documents/

Journal: http://www.ennonline.net

Platform: http://www.nutritionnet.net

Injuries, poisoning, and envenoming

Major burns

1. Ask about the nature of the burn; whether there was a blast or whether fumes (? noxious) were inhaled. Was there pre-existing cardiopulmonary disease? Is the patient tetanus immune?
2. Check for signs of a respiratory burn (burnt nasal hairs or soot in the mouth, hoarseness/stridor) and for headache or confusion suggesting carbon monoxide poisoning.
3. Check for associated injuries and circulatory collapse. Get necessary X-rays and ECG (especially for electrical burns).
4. Determine the extent of the burn using **Wallace's 'rule of nines'** (adults):

    Head (whole) = 9%
    Torso (front) = 18%
    Torso (back) = 18%
    Each arm (whole) = 9%
    Each leg (whole) = 18%
    Genital area = 1%
    Thus express any burn as an estimate (%) of total body area (in children head and legs = 14%).
5. Assess the depth of the burn. **Full thickness** burns are brown-white, painless, do not blanch to pressure, and require skin grafting. **Partial thickness** burns are red, blistered, and very painful. They heal in 10–14 days.

Management

- Resuscitate ('A, B, and C'); consider early intubation if the airway is compromised; give 100% oxygen; give 20 ml 1.5% dicobalt edetate IV for cyanide poisoning from burning plastics.
- Stop any major bleeding and replace fluids (for burns >15% in adults or >10% in children): [% area burn × weight (kg)] ÷ 2 = ml of colloid to give over each unit of time since the burn (**not** since time of presentation). Time units; 4 hrs, 4 hrs, 4 hrs, 6 hrs, 12 hrs. Thus, if there has been a delay in reaching hospital, rapid replacement may be necessary. In addition, give 1.5–2.0 ml/kg/hr of 5% dextrose. **NB: adjust all volumes and rates of infusion according to clinical response**.
- Give morphine analgesia; ensure tetanus immunity; dress the burn with vaseline gauze/silver sulfadiazine/saline-soaked gauze and cover. Do not burst blisters.
- Refer all burns >15% area (10% in children) or burns affecting face, hands, or genitals to a burns unit or plastic surgeon if possible.

Trauma and penetrating injuries

Most penetrating wounds will need exploration under GA to repair and exclude damage to deep structures. Even small superficial injuries may hide much internal damage. Cardiorespiratory depression often signifies severe damage, as patients are often young and have large reserves. Do not remove weapons or large foreign bodies from the wound until in the operating theatre as it will increase the risk of bleeding.

Management

Consists of 'A, B, and C' for assessment of **A**irway, **B**reathing, and **C**irculation, with a further 'D' for **D**isability and 'E' for **E**xposure/ **E**nvironmental control. This is best co-ordinated by adopting a standardized routine for assessment as used in the ATLS protocol. This involves:

1. Resuscitation of vital functions along the A, B, and C pathway, not progressing to further stages until each problem is identified and corrected. At all stages the C-spine is protected until injury is ruled out.
2. 2° survey with more detailed head to toe examination, proceeding to X-rays (C-spine, CXR — erect if possible — and pelvic XR as a minimum) and other diagnostic tests such as bloods, peritoneal lavage, etc. Do a rectal examination to check sensation/tone and, if the pelvis is not involved, insert a urinary catheter.
3. Assess disability by careful neurological survey, checking for facial injury.
4. Expose the patient fully and check for evidence of penetrating or blunt trauma. Cover any exposed viscera with saline-soaked gauze.
5. Definitive care is the management of all injuries identified in order of priority, including surgery, fracture stabilization, hospital admission, or transfer if necessary.

Expect serious injuries in the following high-risk patients:

- High-speed impact; ejection or death of another vehicle occupant
- Entrapment within wreckage
- Fall greater than 5 m
- Motorcyclist or pedestrian
- Abnormal vital signs (e.g. systolic BP <90, GCS <12, RR <10 or >30 breaths/min)

Chest wounds: may damage pleura, lung, great vessels, heart, mediastinum, diaphragm, or abdominal viscera. Haemopneumothorax requires a chest drain — if drainage is initially >1500 ml (or 300 ml/hr) thoracotomy may be needed. Close sucking wounds with an air-tight dressing. Be highly suspicious of developing pneumothorax or cardiac tamponade.

Abdominal injuries: all but the most superficial need admission for exploration and observation.

Limb injuries: damage may be to nerves, tendons, vessels, muscle, and bone. Check pulses and sensation distal to the wound; watch for developing ischaemia and compartment syndrome. Never use a tourniquet.

Acute poisoning

Most deaths from poisoning are due to deliberate self-poisoning. Although drug poisoning is common in urban areas of the developing world, the majority of deaths occur in rural areas after ingestion of pesticides. Although outcome seems to be determined purely by the amount ingested for some pesticides, good management for poisoning by others can reduce the death rate.

General management

1. Resuscitate and stabilize using A, B, C. In particular, take care of the airway, intubating any patient unable to support their own airway.
2. Give high-flow oxygen — except for paraquat poisoned patients.
3. Place the patient on their left side. This is important to reduce the risk of aspiration of vomited poison; it will also keep the airway open.
4. If the patient has taken a pesticide, determine whether he/she needs atropine (see p. 648).
5. Suck out secretions as necessary (however, in organophosphate poisoning, atropine will control secretions effectively).
6. Get a history. What has been taken? How much and when? Have a handbook available that lists pesticides by both their chemical class and trade name since many people will only know the latter.
7. Calm the patient. An agitated poisoning patient makes management difficult and increases risk of aspiration — consider giving diazepam.
8. Watch out for and control convulsions. First-line therapy is diazepam; second-line is phenobarbital.
9. Give antidotes according to the poison ingested — poison identity can come from history or recognition of a 'toxidrome' (see box).
10. **Finally, consider** the value of performing gastric emptying or decontamination once everything else is done.

Gastric lavage and induced emesis: are no longer recommended in the routine management of a poisoned patient. Studies have shown little return of poison even when performed in ideal circumstances. Gastric lavage is associated with increased rate of ICU admission and aspiration pneumonia. It should only be considered early, soon after the poisoning, or not at all, and only if it can be done safely in a consenting or intubated patient.

Gastric lavage performed in a non-consenting struggling patient has a high risk of aspiration and death.

Activated charcoal: administered orally, is now the recommended form of GI decontamination (although there are still no trials indicating benefit). Activated charcoal offers a large surface area for the poison to bind to, decreasing the absorption into the body. Give 50–100 mg (15–30 mg for children) dissolved in 200–300 ml of water.

Multiple doses of activated charcoal: some poisons are excreted in the bile and then reabsorbed from the terminal ileum — the enterohepatic circulation. This can be blocked by regular administration of activated charcoal q4h, continued as long as clinically required.

Osmotic cathartics: are no longer recommended. They increase the risk of electrolyte abnormalities with no evidence of benefit.

Toxidromes

Patients are often unable or sometimes unwilling to state the exact poison ingested. This complicates selection of antidotes if a toxicological screen is not available quickly. Toxidromes are collections of signs which narrow the likely poison.

Classification of common pesticides

1. *Insecticides*
   - *Organophosphates (OPs)*: poisoning is often serious, requiring treatment with atropine, pralidoxime, +/− diazepam.
   - *Carbamates*: similar to OPs but AChE inhibition is briefer; however, poisoning may still last a few days and patients require ventilation.
   - *Organochlorines*: being restricted globally due to environmental persistence. Major problem with significant overdose is status epilepticus.
   - *Pyrethroids*: low toxicity but may cause anaphylaxis.

2. *Herbicides*
   - *Chlorphenoxy compounds*: in large overdoses, cause decreased consciousness and rhabdomyolysis resulting in renal failure.
   - *Paraquat*: no treatment is available. Management appears not to alter clinical course.
   - *Propanil*: causes methaemoglobinaemia, few other signs.
   - *Glyphosate*: low toxicity unless pesticide and solvent is aspirated.

3. *Rodenticides*
   - *Aluminium phosphide*: very toxic. Consider giving severely poisoned patients magnesium 1g IV stat, then 1g q1h for three hours, then 1g q6h.
   - *Zinc phosphide*: less toxic. Treat conservatively.
   - *Coumarin derivatives*: long-acting warfarin-like compounds that can be treated conservatively in most cases. Active bleeding requires vitamin K.
   - *Thallium*: highly toxic. Banned in many countries.

There are many other, often newer, pesticides. None have specific antidotes; conservative management with airway support and diazepam for seizures is probably best.

Pesticide poisoning

Careful resuscitation and supportive care of pesticide-poisoned patients, with correct use of antidotes, will save many lives if instituted early. The value of gastric lavage and forced emesis is likely to be low, with a high risk of complications. Most pesticides are dissolved in organic solvents which can cause fatal pneumonia if aspirated. The value of activated charcoal is unknown.

Organophosphates/carbamates — see p. 648.

Organochlorine poisoning: pesticides such as endosulfan, endrin, and the less toxic lindane can cause status epilepticus after large ingestions. *Manage:* with diazepam; give phenobarbital and then GA if no response. Many are now being banned worldwide.

Pyrethroids: synthetic derivatives of the plant-derived pyrethrin. Low toxicity but may cause anaphylaxis. *Manage:* conservatively.

Chlorphenoxy compounds: include MCPA; 2,4-D; 2,4,5-T (latter two are more toxic). In large overdose cause coma and rhabdomyolysis. Observe for black urine of myoglobinuria and muscle pain. *Manage:* keep high urine output with IV fluids. Give sodium bicarbonate if urine is black. Normally have a good outcome if renal failure can be averted.

Paraquat: uniformly fatal if taken in large amount due to multi-organ failure. Lesser doses may result in fatal lung fibrosis. Patients often have marked ulceration of the mouth; while oesophageal damage is a poor prognostic marker (implying that the paraquat was swallowed), mouth ulceration is not, since some patients just take it into their mouth and then spit it out. Intensive haemofiltration may offer some slight benefit; high-dose immunosuppression (cyclophosphamide 15 mg/kg IV od for 2 d; methyl-prednisolone 1 g IV od for 3 d, followed by dexamethasone) has been claimed to prevent lung fibrosis but definite evidence is not available. *Manage:* conservatively. Lavage Fuller's earth, or activated charcoal may be beneficial if given very early (< 30 mins). However, none have been proven to give any clinical benefit. Lavage performed later risks oesophageal perforation.

Propanil: causes methaemoglobinaemia. The patient looks cyanosed but is asymptomatic with metHb levels <20%; headaches and reduced GCS occur as metHb level rises. Death occurs with metHb >70%. *Manage:* give methylthioninium chloride (methylene blue) 1–2 mg/kg IV over 5 mins, repeated after 30–60 mins as necessary, and/or exchange transfusion.

Glyphosate: causes some ulcerative damage to the oesophagus but little else. Do not perform lavage since the main problems with this pesticide occur after aspiration.

Gastric lavage for pesticide poisoning

1. Lavage **must not** be performed in non-consenting conscious patients or in patients with reduced GCS who have not been intubated.
2. It should only be **considered** when patients present less than 1 hr after ingestion of a potentially life-threatening amount of pesticide. Most pesticide poisonings are not life-threatening and do not require gastric lavage — some pesticides are practically harmless to humans, and even highly toxic pesticides are often taken in very small amounts.
3. A 18-gauge NG tube is sufficient for pesticides. Use of a larger bore orogastric tube has a higher rate of complications.

Poisoning with corrosives

Acids cause an immediate mucosal burn that scabs over, limiting damage. In contrast, alkalis produce a liquifactive necrosis that produces much deeper tissue damage.

Clinical features: pain in mouth, throat, and abdomen; dysphagia; drooling. Complications include perforation, haemorrhage, and systemic complications of particular corrosives. Patients with significant poisoning are at high risk of strictures in oesophagus or stomach.

Management: give oxygen and obtain IV access for fluid resuscitation as required. Watch for signs of airway obstruction or GI perforation. Steroids are not recommended since there is no evidence of benefit and they may mask signs of perforation. It is unclear whether there is any role for GI decontamination. Careful endoscopy is recommended to assess damage to GI tract and manage strictures.

Poisoning with hydrocarbons

- Hydrocarbon toxicity occurs after pulmonary aspiration or after systemic absorption; they can be grouped by both volatility/viscosity and systemic toxicity. Poisoning with non-volatile, non-systemically absorbed hydrocarbons such as motor oil does not require any treatment. The risk of aspiration is low.
- Poisoning with more volatile hydrocarbons, with no systemic toxicity, such as kerosene, are very common. Aspiration pneumonia is the main complication with these compounds and so conservative therapy without induction of vomiting or lavage is recommended.
- The management of volatile and systemically toxic hydrocarbons such as phenol is more difficult. Lavage may be indicated in hope of preventing systemic toxicity if the patients have taken a significant dose and been admitted within 1 hr of ingestion. But it is very important not to cause aspiration.

There is no general antidote; steroids are not indicated.
Beware aspiration pneumonia.

Organophosphates/carbamates

These pesticides inhibit acetylcholinesterase (AChE) at autonomic, neuro-muscular, and central synapses, causing acetylcholine (Ach) to accumulate and overstimulate receptors. AChE reactivates quickly in carbamate poisoning; the process is much slower in OP poisoning. Atropine competes with and antagonizes ACh at muscarinic receptors; oximes such as pralidoxime reactivate inhibited AChE. Delay in oxime treatment may allow the inhibited AChE to 'age' and become resistant to reactivation.

Clinical features: result from accumulation of ACh at muscarinic synapses (salivation, bronchorrhoea, urination, diarrhoea, bradycardia, small pupils); nicotinic synapses (muscle fasciculation and weakness, tachycardia, large pupils); and CNS synapses (agitation, confusion, drowsiness → coma). Inhibition of AChE over several days may result in failure of the neuro-muscular junction: the intermediate syndrome (initially neck flexion weakness — ask patient to lift head from the pillow; sometimes cranial nerve palsies; → respiratory muscle weakness and sudden respiratory arrest). Some OPs cause a peripheral motor neuropathy after several weeks.

Diagnosis: is normally clinical, based on the typical features. Blood butyryl-cholinesterase levels may support the diagnosis.

Management

- Resuscitation and supportive care are essential and save lives. They are far more important than gastric emptying.
- Give oxygen. Intubate early — as soon as the patient's GCS drops below 12–13. Give diazepam 10 mg IV slowly over 2–3 mins as required.
- Simultaneously, give atropine 1.2–2.4 mg rapidly as a bolus.
- Watch for a response in the markers of atropinization (see box).
- If no response at 5 mins, double the dose of atropine.
- Continue giving doubling doses of atropine until at least 4 of 5 parameters have been attained and the chest is clear (beware sounds of aspiration). Hundreds of mg may be required.
- Once the patient is atropinized, set up an infusion giving 20–40% of the total bolus dose of atropine required per hour.
- For OPs and where the agent is unknown, give pralidoxime 2 g IV slowly over several minutes (fast injection → emesis and tachycardia), followed by an infusion of 500 mg/hr.
- Treat fits with diazepam 10 mg IV slowly over 2–3 mins; repeated as necessary. Intubate and ventilate if required.

Observe carefully to ensure that (i) the required amount of atropine is being given — increase or decrease as required, and (ii) neck weakness (= early intermediate syndrome) is picked up early so that a patient can be intubated and ventilated before a respiratory arrest.

Markers of atropinization

Sufficient atropine has been given when all of the following are attained:
- Chest clear (no wheeze or creps)
- Pulse >80 bpm
- Pupils no longer pinpoint
- Axilla (or oral mucosa) are dry
- Systolic BP >80 mmHg

Notes
- Aspiration may complicate the chest criteria. Try to differentiate between local creps of aspiration and generalized creps/wheeze of the OP poisoning.
- The pupils may also dilate late — after 30 mins or so. If the other four criteria are attained, there is no need to keep giving atropine until the pupils dilate. Keep under regular observation and they should dilate in time (unless OP has been spilt directly into the eye).
- There is no need to give atropine until the heart rate is 120–140 or the pupils widely dilated. The aim is to reverse the poisoning, not induce atropine toxicity.

Markers of over-atropinization

Too much atropine is being given if:
- Bowel sounds are absent
- Patient is in urinary retention
- Patient is confused (not alcohol-related)
- Patient is febrile

Atropine-induced fevers, particularly in patients agitated by alcohol withdrawal and in hot environments, risk cardiac arrest.

Confusion can be settled with oral or IV benzodiazepines. Reduce temperature by covering the patient with a wet cloth and using a fan.

Poisoning with pharmaceuticals/chemicals

Relatively few pharmaceuticals have specific antidotes — the main aim of management for most patients will be supportive care. There is no evidence for any benefit from lavage, forced emesis, or activated charcoal.

Benzodiazepines: present with drowsiness, slurred speech, ataxia, rarely coma (small pupils/hyporeflexia), or respiratory arrest, due to the drugs' inhibitory effect on the CNS. Most patients can simply be observed. In case of respiratory arrest (often with newer, short-acting drugs), give ventilation. (Severe poisoning can be reversed with flumazenil 0.2 mg IV over 15 secs repeated with doses of 0.1 mg at 60 sec intervals if required, up to a maximum of 1 mg. This drug must not be used if there are signs of tricyclic antidepressant toxicity.)

Cardiac glycosides: can be due to overdose of digoxin medication or ingestion of a source of natural glycoside (e.g. oleander seeds). Main effects are on the heart — arrhythmias and conduction block. Give atropine 0.5 mg IV for bradycardia; repeat if necessary. Temporary cardiac pacing can tide the patient through 3rd degree heart block, but only antidigoxin antibodies can reverse DC-shock resistant VF or cardiogenic shock which occurs with severe poisoning.

Isoniazid: may cause decreased consciousness, convulsions, coma, respiratory arrest, metabolic acidosis. If severe, give pyridoxine IV (quantity equal to the quantity of isoniazid taken; if quantity is not known, give 5 g by slow IV injection) and repeat at 5–20 min intervals if there is no response.

Lithium carbonate: has effects on CNS, heart, and kidney. Haemodialysis is the best method to remove lithium in patients with poor renal function and severe poisoning. Patients with normal renal function do not need haemodialysis. Check serum electrolytes often; if hypernatraemia is present, give 5% dextrose until plasma Na^+ returns to normal. Since most patients on chronic lithium therapy have nephrogenic diabetes insipidus, they will require high fluid maintenance rates.

Opiates: are found in analgesics and recreational drugs. Features include pinpoint pupils, decreased consciousness, and respiratory depression. Give naloxone 0.2–2 mg IV. An infusion may be needed after improvement to sustain it — give 0.4–0.8 mg/hr. The major predictor for naloxone response is respiratory depression. The diagnosis should be reviewed if more than 2mg are required. Observational studies show that the response time is ~9 +/− 4mins for a response as measured by RR >10. Infusions are only needed for long-acting opioids or opioids with prolonged release (e.g. CR preparations and body packers).

Paracetamol: give N-acetylcysteine IV unless paracetamol blood levels can be measured and shown to be safe. Dose = 150 mg/kg in 200 ml of 5% dextrose over 15 mins, followed by 50 mg/kg in 500 ml of 5% dextrose over 4 hrs, and 100 mg/kg in 1 litre over 16 hrs. Continue even if liver failure develops since it may decrease morbidity/mortality. If unavailable, give methionine 2.5 g PO repeated 3×q4h. Check liver and kidney function. Closely monitor blood glucose levels, watching for hypoglycaemia.

Salicylates: severe poisoning may present with CNS depression, haematemesis, hyperthermia. However, lethal doses may not affect consciousness. Lesser poisoning produces GI pain, N&V, tinnitus. Metabolic acidosis occurs in young children; respiratory alkalosis more commonly in older patients. Give charcoal and correct electrolyte imbalances. If there are neurological signs, give 50 mls of 50% dextrose IV; repeat if necessary. Any metabolic acidoisis should be corrected (even if there is respiratory compensation) with sodium bicarbonate.

Tricyclic antidepressants: may present with signs of CNS toxicity (convulsions, ophthalmoplegia, muscle twitching, delirium, coma, respiratory depression), anticholinergic effects (dry mouth, blurred vision, dilated pupils), cardiotoxicity, hypothermia, pyrexia. Control convulsions; monitor heart and correct arrhythmias; control acidosis. Give sodium bicarbonate for any major CVS toxicity or for seizures. The target pH is 7.5 using boluses of 3 meq/kg.

Cyanide: late presentations include dyspnoea, cyanosis, or unconsciousness. Altered mental status, tachypnoea (in absence of cyanosis), unexplained anion gap metabolic acidosis, and bright red blood are earlier signs. Adminster O_2; correct acidosis; give amyl nitrite by inhalation over 30 secs each minute until other drugs are prepared. Then give: dicobalt edetate 300 mg IV over 1 min followed by 50 mls of 50% dextrose. Repeat ×2 if required. (Alternative: sodium nitrite 300 mg by IV injection over 5–20 mins followed by sodium thiosulfate 12.5 g IV over 10 mins.)

Metal ions (e.g. gold, mercury, zinc, lead, copper): acute poisoning can cause coma, convulsions, and death, or affect multiple organ systems. Anticipate and treat shock, renal or hepatic failure. Give penicillamine 1–2 g PO od in 4 divided doses (2 hrs before meals, if possible) for 2–4 weeks. Get a senior opinion. An alternative option (preferred in mercury poisoning) is dimercaprol (BAL) 2.5–3 mg/kg q4h for 2 days; then q6h on the 3 rd day; and bd for days 4–10 or until recovery.

Snake bite

Untreated, less than 10% of people bitten by venomous snakes will die. With treatment, the outcome is even more favourable. Therefore, the first thing to do with a bitten patient is to calm and reassure them. Then attempt to find out the identity of the snake since this may affect which antivenom should be given.

Signs of envenoming: will vary according to the species of snake. However, the effects of most seriously venomous snakes fall into two categories — neurotoxic and haemorrhagic. In the former, the patient may die from respiratory arrest; in the latter, the patient may die from haemorrhagic shock. Some venoms will affect both systems. Other systems affected include muscles and kidneys.

Examine the patient regularly for signs of systemic envenoming. Local symptoms support the idea that the person has been envenomed but are frequently not in themselves an indication for specific antivenom.
- *Local:* pain; swelling; blistering; regional lymphadenopathy.
- *Bleeding:* in gingival sulci; from venepuncture sites, skin wounds, or fang marks; haematuria; if severe, haematemesis or haemochezia may occur. Beware the patient going into shock — raise the foot of the bed and give normal saline. Subclinical bleeding that requires antivenom can be detected with a 20-min whole-blood clotting assay.
- *Neurological:* initial symptoms — blurred vision; heaviness of eyelids; drowsiness; signs: contraction of frontalis muscle; ptosis; ophthalmoplegia; limb weakness. **Check** for signs of respiratory muscle paralysis — dyspnoea, exaggerated abdominal respiration and intercostal muscle contraction, cyanosis.
- *Other systems:* trismus or generalized muscle tenderness indicates rhabdomyolysis; decreased urine output may indicate hypovolaemia or acute renal failure (due to haemolysis and/or direct renal effect of venom); dark urine may indicate either haemolysis or rhabdomyolysis.

If there are no signs of systemic envenoming, keep patient under observation for at least 24 hrs.

Management: give antivenom if there are systemic signs; local swelling involving >half a limb; or other signs recommended locally as an indication for antivenom.
- **There is no point giving a test dose** of antivenom since it poorly predicts the individuals who will have an anaphylactoid response to the antivenom. Instead have adrenalin already drawn up for use if anaphylaxis does occur.
- Give the recommended dose of antivenom by slow IV push over 10–20 mins. (IV infusion in normal saline is another method but the equipment is more expensive and takes longer to set up.)
- Give tetanus toxoid; consider prophylactic penicillin to prevent infection. If the wound has been tampered with give gentamicin. Necrotic tissue must be rapidly excised.

Locally recommended indications for antivenom therapy

-
-
-
-
-

Rehabilitation

Following bites to hands or feet it is essential to think about rehabilitation early. Careful positioning and physiotherapy will reduce complications of the bite and improve the chance of normal function returning.

20-minute whole-blood clotting test

This is a simple test that accurately indicates the need for antivenom in patients with haemorrhagic complications of snake bite.

1. Put 1–2 mls of blood into a new, clean, glass test tube. Do not use a tube that has been washed since left-over detergent may prevent clotting of normal blood.
2. **Leave alone** for 20 mins — do not agitate or keep picking up to inspect since this will alter rate of clotting.
3. At 20 mins, invert once.
4. If the blood flows freely, and there is no clot, then the test is positive and antivenom is indicated. The presence of even a small clot indicates that the clotting system is at least partially functioning and that there is low risk of serious haemorrhage. Antivenom is therefore not indicated.

Positive tests: repeat 6 hrs after giving antivenom. There is little point repeating before this time since it takes 6 hrs for the liver to reconstitute the clotting system after neutralization of the venom components.

Negative tests: observe the patient carefully for signs of bleeding (at fang or cannula site, between teeth). Repeat after 3–6 hrs to check for slow onset of envenoming.

Immunization

Section editor **David Goldblatt**

Introduction

Although the number of children fully vaccinated by the age of 1 yr has increased from 5% in 1974, when the Expanded Programme on Immunization (EPI) was set up, to ~80% in the 1990s, 12 million children under the age of 5 yrs are still dying each year. Many are due to diseases that could be prevented by vaccination in principle, but for which vaccines have not yet been developed. However, 2 million deaths are due to diseases that can be prevented by the vaccines already on offer through the EPI. In 2000 approximately 875,000 children died from measles, almost 500,000 from neonatal tetanus, and 400,000 from whooping cough.

These deaths occur for two reasons — because not all existing vaccines are 100% effective and because each year ~20% of the world's children are not fully immunized in their first year of life with the EPI vaccines. Research work around the world is working to improve the effectiveness of vaccines to work on the first problem. In response to the second problem, the WHO is also working on ways of increasing coverage globally for all EPI vaccines. They have noted that many opportunities to give vaccines are not taken — the so-called 'missed opportunities'. Reduction in these missed opportunities would likely markedly improve global coverage.

Increasing immunization coverage — the importance of missed opportunities

Various studies have identified the following as the most important reasons for a child or woman of childbearing age coming to a health facility and not receiving the vaccines for which he/she is eligible:
- The failure to administer simultaneously all the vaccines for which a child is eligible.
- False contraindications for vaccination — see p. 663.
- Health worker practices, including not opening a multi-dose vial for a small number of persons to avoid vaccine wastage.
- Logistical problems such as vaccine shortage, poor clinic organization, and inefficient clinic scheduling.

Missed opportunities can be reduced by health centres that see women and children by:
- Offering immunizations as often as possible.
- Routinely screening the immunization status of all women and children that the centre serves.
- Teaching health workers which are true and which are false contraindications.
- Ensuring that good practice procedures are followed.

The following section follows the guidelines of the Expanded Programme on Immunization (EPI) for childhood vaccination. However, the epidemiology of the diseases which the EPI aims to combat will differ in each and every country. As a result, the vaccinations that are suitable for a particular country will likely differ between countries. For example, since yellow fever is endemic only in Africa and S. America, vaccination against this disease will be of little benefit in Asian countries. In addition, earlier immunization campaigns have greatly altered the epidemiology of a number of diseases, such as polio, thereby altering the importance of vaccination against these diseases.

To reflect this variation in circumstances, policy needs to be made at national level to decide which vaccines should be included in the country's infant and childhood immunization schedules. These national policies will take precedence over the EPI guidelines presented here. Space has been left on p. 659 for national guidelines to be written into this handbook.

Abbreviations for particular vaccines

BCG	Bacille Calmette Guerin
DT	Double vaccine consisting of diphtheria toxoid and tetanus toxoid for use in children less than 10 yrs old
DTP	Triple vaccine consisting of diphtheria toxoid, pertussis, and tetanus toxoid
MMR	Triple vaccine consisting of vaccines for measles, mumps, and rubella
MR	Double vaccine consisting of measles and rubella vaccines
IPV	Injected polio vaccine (Salk vaccine)
OPV	Oral polio vaccine (Sabin vaccine)
Td	Double vaccine consisting of tetanus toxoid and low-dose diphtheria toxoid for use in children older than 10 yrs old and adults
TT	Tetanus toxoid vaccine

Basic immunization strategies and schedules

The decision to immunize at a particular age is, for the most part, a compromise between:

- The desire to immunize as early as possible, thereby protecting the child before he/she becomes exposed to the infectious agent, and
- The requirement to wait both for the infant's immune response to mature and for the maternally-derived antibodies that crossed the placenta pre-natally to disappear, so that the immunization will be effective.

In general, vaccines are recommended for the youngest age group at risk for developing the disease whose members are known to develop an adequate response to immunization without adverse effects from the vaccine.

The basic schedule calls for all children to receive 1 dose of BCG vaccine, 3 doses of DTP vaccine, 4 doses of OPV, and 1 dose of measles vaccine before their first birthday — see box. In countries where HBsAg carriage rates are >2%, universal infant vaccination with Hep B vaccine is recommended. Where HBsAg carriage rates are lower, adolescent immunization can be considered as an alternative or addition.

Some vaccines require the administration of >1 dose for development of an adequate immune response. The doses should not be given less than 4 wks apart since it may lessen the antibody response. Although increasing the interval will increase the antibody response, the child is then susceptible to infection for a longer time.

It is important to complete the primary series quickly and therefore offer protective immunity to the infant as soon as possible.

Other points:

- As many vaccines as possible should be given in one visit to reduce the number of contacts required.
- If a child has missed the EPI schedule, he/she can receive the first dose of all the vaccines that a child of his/her age should have already received, simultaneously.
- All the EPI vaccines can be safely given at the same time but they should be injected into different sites.
- Different vaccines should not be mixed and administered in one syringe.
- If vaccines cannot be given on the same day, then live vaccines should be spaced at least 4 weeks apart. A shorter interval may result in interference between the vaccines and a reduction in the immune response.

WHO-recommended infant immunization schedule

Age[1]	Vaccines	Hepatitis B[2]	
		Scheme A	Scheme B
Birth	BCG, OPV 0	HB-1	
6 weeks	DTP-1, OPV-1	HB-2	HB-1
10 weeks	DTP-2, OPV-2		HB-2
14 weeks	DTP-3, OPV-3	HB-3	HB-3
9 months	Measles[3] and/or yellow fever		

1. Babies born prematurely should be vaccinated at exactly the same times after birth as babies born at term.
2. Scheme A is recommended where perinatal transmission of Hep B is common (e.g. S.E. Asia). Scheme B may be used in countries where perinatal transmission is less common (e.g. sub-Saharan Africa).
3. Where there is a high risk of mortality from measles among children under 9 months (such as hospitalized or HIV-infected infants, or refugee camps), measles vaccination should be carried out at both 6 and 9 months.

National recommendations

Age	Vaccines
Birth	
6 weeks	
10 weeks	
14 weeks	
6 months	
9 months	

Tetanus immunization of women of childbearing age

The immunization of pregnant women with tetanus toxoid (TT) vaccine is a highly effective means of protecting the newborn child from tetanus. The optimal schedule for this vaccination depends on the immunization history of the woman.

- **Schedule A:** regions in which women were not vaccinated during infancy and childhood, or where there is insufficient documentation for previously vaccinated women to be identified, should administer a full TT 5-dose schedule for all women of childbearing age. The details of these schedules are presented in the box. The regions concerned need to determine the age group to be included in the schedule (e.g. 15–35 yrs or 15–44 yrs).
- **Schedule B:** regions in which women have documentation of previous vaccination with TT-containing vaccines during infancy or childhood can apply more selective schedules for tetanus vaccination — see box. (It is likely that more and more countries will start to fall into this group with the worldwide increase in tetanus vaccination during infancy. The EPI recommends that countries start to use schedule B when DTP vaccination during infancy has reached 80%.)

Adverse reactions

Although modern vaccines are extremely safe, some vaccines may lead to adverse reactions. It is difficult to prove that a vaccination causes a specific event. Instead, population studies must be carried out to look for an association between the vaccination and the adverse event (e.g. clustering of cases in vaccines or a higher incidence in vaccinated compared to unvaccinated groups).

Adverse reactions tend to be caused by:
- *Faults of administration* (programmatic errors): e.g. abscesses after poor mixing of vaccines or use of non-sterile needles or syringes; disseminated disease in immunosuppressed patients after administration of BCG or measles vaccines.
- *Properties of the vaccines:* the reactions may be caused by the immunizing antigen itself or by other components such as antibiotics (used in growth of the virus), preservatives, or adjuvant.

Mild adverse events are common (e.g. 20–50% of DTP recipients experience mild local reactions while some measles vaccine recipients get a rash and fever). Booster doses of toxoids may induce hypersensitivity reactions in some people.

Severe reactions such as encephalitis after mumps or measles vaccines are extremely rare. DTP vaccination has been reported to be associated with many adverse affects but comprehensive studies have failed to link it to many of these adverse effects. Vaccine-associated severe events are much less common than the severe complications caused by the disease itself.

 It is essential to detect serious adverse events and to identify the underlying cause since such reactions will influence community acceptance of the vaccinations and immunization rates.

Schedule A: TT immunization schedule for women of childbearing age

Dose	When to give	Expected duration of protection
TT-1	At first contact or as early as possible in pregnancy	None
TT-2	At least 4 weeks after TT-1	1–3 yrs
TT-3	At least 6 months after TT-2	5 yrs
TT-4	At least 1 year after TT-3 or during subsequent pregnancy	10 yrs
TT-5	At least 1 year after TT-4 or during subsequent pregnancy	All childbearing years

Schedule B: guidelines for TT immunization of women who were immunized in the past

		Recommended immunizations	
Age at last TT immunization	Previous TT immunizations	At present contact	Later (at interval of >1 yr)
Infancy	3 DTP	2 TT	1 TT
Childhood	4 DTP	1 TT	1 TT
School age	3 DTP + 1 DT/Td	1 TT	1 TT
School age	4 DTP + 1 DT/Td	1 TT	None
Adolescence	4 DTP + 1 DT at 4–6 yrs and 1 TT (or Td) at 14–16 yrs	None	None

Contraindications

There are relatively few absolute contraindications to vaccination. Every opportunity to vaccinate a child or woman of childbearing age should be taken, particularly in outpatient clinics (see 'missed opportunities' on p. 656). There is a high risk that delaying vaccination until the child is better will result in that child not getting his/her full complement of vaccinations because he/she did not return again and was lost to follow-up. Many programmes have contraindications which are inappropriate. Such false contraindications are listed in the box.

True contraindications to vaccination include:

- Illnesses severe enough for the child to be hospitalized — if the child is vaccinated but then dies from the pre-existing illness, the vaccine may be thought to have killed the child. However, immunize as soon as the child's general condition improves. Give measles vaccine on hospital admission if possible because of the risk of nosocomial transmission.
- For **live** vaccines, immunodeficiency diseases or immunosuppression due to malignant disease, therapy with immunosuppressive drugs, or irradiation. HIV/AIDS is a special case — see below.
- A severe adverse event (anaphylaxis, collapse or shock, encephalitis, encephalopathy, or non-febrile convulsion) after a previous dose of vaccine. If the adverse reaction occurs with a dose of DTP vaccine, omit the pertussis component and complete the vaccination with the DT vaccine.
- For vaccines prepared in egg (yellow fever, influenza) a history of anaphylaxis following egg ingestion. Vaccines prepared in chicken fibroblast cells (measles or MMR) can usually be given to such people.

Live vaccines should not be routinely administered to pregnant women except where there is a high risk of exposure and the need for vaccination outweighs any possible risk to the fetus. In adult women, pregnancy should be avoided for >1 month after vaccination with a live vaccine. Live vaccines include:

- BCG
- measles
- mumps
- oral polio vaccine (OPV).
- yellow fever
- typhoid
- rubella

Immunization of HIV-infected persons

There has been concern that HIV-induced immune system impairment might make HIV-infected people more susceptible to severe vaccine-associated diseases. There has so far been no evidence to support this concern. Instead, since both measles and TB are associated with higher mortality in HIV +ve patients, there is clearly a great need for these persons to be vaccinated. Most HIV +ve infants and adults are able to mount a good immune response to vaccination and should receive all EPI vaccines as early as possible.

The WHO/UNICEF guidelines for immunization of HIV-infected individuals are presented in the box opposite.

Conditions which are **NOT** contraindications to immunization and which **MUST NOT** prevent a child from being vaccinated

- Minor illnesses such as URTI or diarrhoea, with fever <38.5°C
- Allergy, asthma, other atopic manifestations, hay fever, or snuffles
- Prematurity, small for date infants
- Malnutrition
- Child being breastfed
- Family history of convulsions. (However, if there is a Hx of febrile convulsions, offer advice on the treatment of fever before giving vaccine — for a 2–3 month infant, give 60 mg paracetamol followed by a 2nd dose 4–6 hrs later if required. Advise parents to see a doctor if the fever persists after a 2nd dose of paracetamol.)
- Treatment with antibiotics, low-dose corticosteroids, or locally acting (e.g. topical or inhaled) steroids
- Dermatoses, eczema, or localized skin infection
- Chronic diseases of the heart, lung, kidney, and liver
- Stable neurological conditions, such as cerebral palsy and Down's syndrome
- History of jaundice after birth

WHO/UNICEF recommendations for the immunization of HIV-infected children and women of childbearing age

Vaccine	Asymptomatic HIV infection	Symptomatic HIV infection	Optimal timing of immunization
BCG	Yes[1]	No	Birth
DTP	Yes	Yes	6, 10, 14 weeks
OPV[2]	Yes	Yes	0, 6, 10, 14 weeks
Measles	Yes	Yes	6, 9 months[3]
Hepatitis B	Yes	Yes	As for uninfected children
Yellow fever	Yes	No[4]	
TT	Yes	Yes	5 doses — see above

1. If the local risk of TB infection is low, then BCG should be withheld from individuals known or suspected to be HIV infected.
2. IPV can be used as an alternative in symptomatic HIV +ve children.
3. Because of the risk of severe early measles infection, HIV +ve infants should receive measles vaccine at 6 months and as soon after 9 months as possible.
4. Pending further studies.

EPI vaccines

- Always consult the manufacturer's data sheet before using a vaccine.
- See previous page for general contraindications.
- Some vaccines produce very few reactions while others such as measles and rubella may produce a mild form of disease, with a very small risk of serious complications — see adverse reactions on p. 660. Some vaccines produce discomfort at the site of injection, mild fever, and malaise.
- Anaphylactic reactions are extremely rare but may be fatal.

BCG: is a freeze-dried preparation of a live attenuated strain of *Mycobacterium bovis* that is given in a single ID injection. The vaccine appears to be most effective in preventing TB meningitis and miliary TB in infants, hence its early administration. Its long-term protective effects are unclear as are the stability of the protective immunity induced and the value of booster doses. There is also good evidence that BCG vaccination protects against leprosy. *Cautions:* apart from neonates, any person being considered for BCG vaccination should be given a skin test for hypersensitivity to tuberculoprotein. Except in infants, >3 weeks should be left between administration of any live vaccine and BCG. *Contraindications:* BCG should not be given to subjects with generalized septic skin conditions. *Side-effects:* a small swelling forms 2–6 weeks post-vaccination that may progress to a benign ulcer. Healing occurs in 6–12 weeks.

Diphtheria toxoid vaccine: is a formaldehyde-inactivated preparation of diphtheria toxin, absorbed onto aluminium salts to increase immunogenicity. It is normally given in the form of a triple vaccine with tetanus and pertussis vaccines (DTP), but can be given with tetanus alone when pertussis vaccine is contraindicated. The vaccine does not prevent infection but rather inhibits the toxin's effects, preventing systemic illness. A low-dose vaccine (combined with tetanus: Td) should be used in children >10 yrs old and adults requiring immunization to decrease the risk of serious reactions to the vaccine.

Hepatitis B vaccine: is a suspension of inactivated hepatitis B surface antigen (HBsAg) absorbed onto aluminium salts. It is given by IM injection in 3 doses — the 2nd and 3rd doses are given at 1 month and 6 months (the deltoid muscle is the preferred site in adults, the anterolateral thigh in infants/children; the buttock should not be used as it may decrease vaccine efficacy). It is available as a recombinant vaccine and as a plasma-derived vaccine; both are safe and highly efficacious. If available, one dose of Hep B immunoglobulin should be given immediately to infants newly born to mothers who become infected during the pregnancy or who are Hep e-antigen positive.

Measles vaccine: is a freeze-dried preparation of live attenutated virus that is given by single SC injection. It is normally given at around 9 months but an additional dose can be given at 6 months in those at high risk — see schedules on p. 659. In industrialized countries, it has now been replaced by a triple vaccine that combines measles, mumps, and rubella vaccines (MMR). This vaccine is given after 12–15 months and then again at age 3–5 before school entry. The vaccine can be used to control outbreaks of measles. It should be offered to susceptible children within 3 days of exposure to infection. The vaccine normally contains >1000 units of infectious virus. *Side-effects:* may be associated with a mild measles-like illness with rash and fever 1 week after vaccination. Convulsions and encephalitis are rare complications.

Pertussis vaccine: is available in two forms — whole-cell vaccine (pertussis bacteria killed by chemicals or heat) or the recently introduced, expensive, acellular vaccine. They are normally given by IM injection in a triple vaccine with diphtheria and tetanus vaccines (DTP). The whole-cell vaccine is effective at preventing serious disease but not infection. The induced immunity decreases with time. However, the importance of this vaccine has been shown by a resurgence in disease in the UK and Sweden after vaccine uptake rates fell. Since the vaccine requires 3 doses to elicit a strong immune response, it cannot be used to control an epidemic. The acellular vaccine contains purified immunogenic components of the bacteria — normally the toxoid and 2–4 other components. Side-effects appear to be much less common. **Side-effects:** convulsions and encephalopathy have been reported as very rare complications but it is not certain that they are caused by the vaccine.

Poliomyelitis vaccine: is available in two forms — a live attenuated virus vaccine given by mouth (OPV, Sabin vaccine) and an injectable killed virus vaccine given by IM injection (IPV, Salk vaccine). Each vaccine contains strains of three different types of poliovirus (types 1, 2, and 3), offering wide protection.

The EPI recommends the OPV because of its low cost, ease of administration, superiority in conferring intestinal immunity, and potential for infecting household and community contacts, thereby boosting 2° immunity. OPV has been shown to be the vaccine of choice for eradication due to its ease of administration in campaigns and the dramatic impact gained by breaking chains of transmission. **Cautions:** patients with D&V require a further dose after recovery. **Contraindications:** living with an immuno-deficient person — the IPV should be used for these cases. **Side-effects:** vaccine-associated poliomyelitis in vaccine recipients and contacts is rare — about 1 case per 2 million vaccinations each year in the UK. However, very strict personal hygiene needs to be emphasized, particularly for the contacts of a recently vaccinated baby.

Tetanus toxoid vaccine: is a formaldehyde-inactivated preparation of tetanus toxin absorbed onto aluminium salts that is given by IM or deep SC injection. It is normally given to infants in the form of a triple vaccine with diphtheria and pertussis vaccines (DTP), but can be given with diphtheria alone (DT) when pertussis vaccine is contraindicated. The administration of tetanus toxoid (TT) to a pregnant woman induces antitoxin antibodies which pass across the placenta and prevent neonatal tetanus. Some countries recommend booster doses of TT for all persons at school entry, at school leaving, and then at 10-yr intervals. A full 1° course of immunization can be given to adults who did not receive a childhood course. For serious, potentially contaminated wounds, anti-tetanus immunoglobulin is valuable in addition to wound toilet, vaccination (at a different site), and antibiotic cover. **Cautions:** TT should not be given at <10-yr intervals because of the risk of hypersensitivity reactions.

Yellow fever vaccine: consists of freeze-dried preparation of live attenuated virus (17D strain) that is grown in egg embryos and given by SC injection. It is highly immunogenic and offers at least 10 yrs of immunity. **Contraindications:** do not give to infants under the age of 6 months, unless infection with yellow fever is unavoidable, since there is a small likelihood of encephalitis in this age group.

Other vaccines

Always consult the manufacturer's data sheet before using a vaccine.

Cholera vaccine: is currently a preparation of heat-killed Inaba and Ogawa subtypes of *V. cholera*. Unfortunately this vaccine provides only partial protection of limited duration. Its use is no longer recommended. Oral 1-dose candidate vaccines against the El T or biotype and 01 and 0139 serotypes are currently under development and field trials.

Haemophilus influenzae type b (Hib) vaccines: consist of Hib polysaccharides conjugated to either diphtheria or tetanus toxoids or the meningococcus outer-membrane protein complex. The vaccine is given by IM injection in a schedule of 3 doses during infancy (normally with DTP and OPV), in some countries followed by a booster dose at age 12–18 months. Since the risk of serious Hib infection falls sharply after the age of 4, it is only recommended for individuals at high risk of infection in this age group (sickle-cell disease, during treatment of malignant disease, following splenectomy). *Contraindications:* see p. 663 for general contraindications. *Side-effects:* include fever, headache, malaise, N&V, prolonged crying, anorexia, diarrhoea, rash. Rarer side-effects include convulsions, erythema multiforme, transient lower limb cyanosis.

Hepatitis A vaccine: is a formaldehyde-inactivated preparation of hepatitis A virus grown in human diploid cells that has been absorbed onto aluminium salts. It is given by IM injection, preferably into the deltoid muscle. A booster is recommended at 12 months. *Contraindications:* see p. 663 for general contraindications. *Side-effects:* include transient soreness, erythema, and induration at the injection site. A mild flu-like illness and generalized rashes have been reported.

Influenza vaccine: consists of inactivated influenza virus that has been grown in eggs. Since the virus is continually altering its haemagglutinin (H) and neuraminidase (N) surface proteins, different strains that express the H and N proteins of the prevalent strain must be used each year. The WHO annually recommends which strains should be incorporated into the vaccine after surveying the virus across the world. The vaccine can be given by deep SC or IM injection annually to at-risk people, particularly the elderly, with the following conditions: chronic respiratory (including asthma), renal, and CVS disease, diabetes mellitus, other endocrine disorders, immunosuppression. It may also be of benefit to those living in nursing homes or other long-stay facilities.

Japanese encephalitis vaccine: a formalin-inactivated preparation of virus grown in either mouse brain or cultured hamster cells. The mouse brain preparation has had brain proteins removed and is not associated with CNS damage. This vaccine has been widely used in Asia and shown to be both effective and safe. Two doses are given by SC injection 1–2 wks apart. An additional dose is given at 4 wks and boosters recommended every 1–4 yrs. The hamster cell vaccine has been developed and used extensively in China since 1967. Because of the severity of the disease, the EPI recommend that every country where JE is epidemic consider incorporating this vaccine into their immunization schedules. Research is required to ascertain the earliest age at which this vaccine can be given, the necessity of booster doses, and whether it can be given simultaneously with other EPI vaccines.

Meningococcal vaccines: two forms now exist. One type of vaccine contains capsular polysaccharides purified from various serogroups of *N. meningitidis*. At present, monovalent vaccines exist for groups A and C, bivalent vaccines for both A and C, and a quadrivalent vaccine for serogroups A, C, W-135, and Y. A single dose of the monovalent A group vaccine given by deep SC or IM injection elicits protective immunity for 1–3 yrs in persons >2 yrs. The response is poorer in children <2 yrs — 2 doses are required 3 months apart to achieve protective immunity. Group C vaccines are effective in adults but not children. The current vaccines are not recommended for infant vaccination programmes but may be used together with antibiotics to protect household contacts. They also play an important role in controlling meningococcal A/C epidemics.

A new generation of serogroup C conjugate vaccines are now licensed. They comprise group C polysaccharide conjugated to a mutant diphtheria or tetanus protein. These vaccines are based on the proven technology of Hib conjugate vaccines and have proved highly effective in preventing meningococcal C disease in infants, toddlers, young children, and adolescents in the UK — the first country to introduce them. Three doses are administered in those under 1 yr (although two doses may suffice) and no booster dose is currently given in the UK. Over the age of 1 yr only a single dose is given and is thought to provide lifelong immunity — although this is the subject of ongoing post-licensure surveillance. Bivalent (A/C) and quadrivalent (ACWY) conjugate vaccines are in development and will be of relevance to countries such as those in the African meningitis belt, where serogroup A disease is a major problem.

Mumps vaccine: consists of a live attenuated strain of virus grown in chick embryo cells in tissue culture. It is normally given by IM injection with measles and rubella vaccines in the MMR triple vaccine at age 12–15 months and again at 3–5 yrs. See measles vaccine for side-effects and contraindications (p. 664).

Pigbel vaccine: is an inactivated preparation of toxin from *Clostridium perfringens* type C that is given by IM injection. It is effective in infants and children and has been given routinely to children in Papua New Guinea at ages 2, 4, and 6 months, simultaneously with their DTP vaccination, since 1980. Protection lasts for 2–4 yrs.

Pneumococcal vaccines: two forms of these vaccines now exist. One type of vaccine contains *capsular polysaccharide antigens* from 23 different serotypes of *S. pneumoniae*. Unfortunately these antigens do not induce a protective immune response in children <2 yrs (one of the age groups with the highest attack rate) and protective immunity in older high-risk individuals may be limited or short-lived. The vaccine is recommended for persons >2 yrs who are at high risk for severe infection: sickle-cell disease, CRF, immunosuppression, CSF leaks, HIV infection, asplenia, chronic liver, heart or lung disease, DM. If possible, give the vaccine at least 2 wks before either splenectomy or chemotherapy. *Contraindications:* pregnancy, breastfeeding, during infection. *Side-effects:* hypersensitivity reactions may occur. They are more frequent with re-vaccination, therefore routine re-vaccination is not recommended. However, re-vaccination should be offered where the risk of fatal infection is judged to be high (>4 yrs after 14 serotype vaccine and >6 yrs after 23 serotype vaccine). Children at high risk can be re-vaccinated after 3–5 yrs if they are still <10 yrs old.

A new *pneumococcal conjugate vaccine* was licensed in 2000. The licensed formulation is a seven valent vaccine (serotypes 4, 6B, 9V, 14, 18C, 19F, 23F) conjugated to a mutant diphtheria protein. The vaccine is immunogenic, induces memory, and has been shown to be highly effective in preventing invasive pneumococcal infection as well as providing some protection against pneumonia and otitis media. A 4-dose 1° immunization regime is recommended in infancy with the 4th dose delivered as a booster in the 2nd year of life. A single dose may suffice in older children.

Rabies vaccine: is available as a freeze-dried inactivated preparation of virus grown in either sheep brain or cultured human diploid cells. The former vaccine is still used in some parts of the world but it is associated with an unacceptably high rate of post-vaccination severe neurological complications (~1:1000). This is due to immune responses to sheep brain antigens that contaminate the vaccine. The cultured vaccine is far safer but more expensive. Its use around the world is increasing, however, particularly as novel cheaper ways of administering the vaccine are developed. See p. 412 for prophylactic and post-exposure vaccination schedules.

Rubella vaccine: is a preparation of the live Wistar strain of the virus. It is given by deep SC or IM injection in industrialized countries either to infants as part of the triple measles, mumps, and rubella (MMR) vaccine or as a monovalent vaccine to prepubertal girls between their 10th and 14th birthdays. The purpose is to reduce the incidence of 1° infection in pregnant women and therefore reduce the incidence of congenital rubella syndrome in their offspring. Universal immunization is not recommended at present by the EPI because incomplete coverage would just increase the age at which most infections occur, increasing the likelihood of infection in childbearing women. *Contraindications:* avoid immunizing women during early pregnancy. Advise women not to become pregnant for >1 month after immunization. However, there is no evidence at present that the vaccination is teratogenic.

Typhoid vaccine: occurs in three forms:
- A killed whole-cell suspension
- A purified form of the capsular polysaccharide Vi (both given by deep SC or IM injection)
- An oral live attenuated preparation of the bacteria

None are substitutes for good personal hygiene. All elicit protective immunity in adults and children >2 yrs but not in children <2 yrs. They are therefore not recommended for immunization during infancy.
- The whole-cell vaccine is given in 2 doses 4–6 wks apart but requires boosters every 3 yrs. It is associated with a high incidence of adverse reactions — see below.
- The capsular antigen vaccine is given as a single dose with boosters every 3 yrs.
- The oral vaccine is given in 3 doses on alternate days. Residents of endemic regions who are frequently exposed to *S. typhi* require boosters every 3 yrs; visitors to these regions who will be less exposed require boosters every year.

Cautions: the 2nd dose of the whole-cell vaccine and subsequent boosters should be given by ID injection to reduce adverse reactions. The oral vaccine is inactivated by concomitant administration of antibiotics or sulfonamides. Mefloquine must not be taken for 12 hrs either side of giving the oral vaccine, and preferably should only be started >3 days after vaccine administration. **Side-effects:** local reactions including pain, swelling, and erythema may appear 2–3 hrs after administration of the whole-cell vaccine and 48–72 hrs after administration of the capsular antigen vaccine. Systemic reactions such as fever, malaise, and headache may also occur after administration of the whole-cell vaccine.

New vaccines – under development and required

New and better vaccines are continually required. Important vaccines currently under development include vaccines for:

- Enterotoxigenic *E. coli*
- Malaria
- Dengue
- Para-influenza viruses
- Respiratory syncytial virus
- Human papillomavirus
- HIV
- Meningococcus B
- Rotaviruses
- Shigellae
- Schistosomiasis

Appendix: websites

CDC Health Topics A to Z
http://www.cdc.gov/health/default.htm
A superb site giving information suitable for doctors or the public on most infectious diseases, parasitic diseases, and non-infectious conditions.

CDC Parasitic diseases
http://www.dpd.cdc.gov/dpdx/
Another superb site giving details on parasites, life cycles, diagnostic methods, and an image bank.

Atlas of medical parasitology
http://www.cdfound.to.it/HTML/atlas.htm
Useful images of parasites, life cycles, and some clinical pictures.

CDC Division of Tuberculosis elimination
http://www.cdc.gov/nchstp/tb/default.htm
The starting point for many links to TB information.

University of Iowa – Introduction to Travel Medicine
http://www.vh.org/adult/provider/internalmedicine/TravelMedicine/TravelMedHP.html
A simple on-line textbook of travel medicine.

Malaria Resource (University of Western Australia)
http://www.rph.wa.gov.au/labs/haem/malaria/index.html
Teaches and tests microscopy skills for malaria diagnosis.

Immunisation against infectious diseases (1996 ed.) "The Green Book"
http://www.doh.gov.uk/greenbook/index.htm
The UK guidelines on immunisation.

UK Malaria guidelines (updated Nov 2002)
http://www.hpa.org.uk/infections/topics_az/malaria/pdf/update_guidelines.pdf
Detailed guidance on malaria prophylaxis and stand-by treatment.

AIDS images
http://members.xoom.virgilio.it/Aidsimaging/contents.htm
Clinical pictures, microscope pictures, and X rays of opportunistic infections in HIV.

Index